Pain Management

For Elsevier:

Commissioning Editor: *Timothy Horne*
Development Editor: *Helen Leng*
Project Manager: *Christine Johnston*
Design: *Stewart Larking*
Illustration Manager: *Gillian Richards*
Illustrator: *Barking Dog Art*

SECOND EDITION

Pain Management

Practical applications of the biopsychosocial perspective in clinical and occupational settings

Chris J Main PhD FBPsS
Professor of Clinical Psychology (Pain Management), Keele University, UK

Michael J L Sullivan PhD
Professor of Psychology, McGill University, Montreal, Québec, Canada

Paul J Watson FCSP MSc PhD
Senior Lecturer, Department of Health Sciences, University of Leicester
Visiting Professor, Department of Health Sciences, Leeds Metropolitan University, UK

Contributing authors

Kay Greasley PhD
Senior Research Fellow
Warwick Medical School
University of Warwick, UK

Bengt H Sjölund MD DMSc
Director General, Rehabilitation and Research
Centre for Torture Victims
Copenhagen, Denmark
Professor of Rehabilitation,
University of Southern Denmark

Forewords by

Professor Sir Michael Bond
Vice Principal, Faculty of Medicine,
University of Glasgow, UK

Chris C Spanswick MB ChB FRCA
Pain Physician, Medical Leader of Calgary
Health Region Regional Pain Program
Clinical Assistant Professor in the Department
of Anaesthesia, Faculty of Medicine,
University of Calgary, Canada

CHURCHILL
LIVINGSTONE

ELSEVIER

EDINBURGH LONDON NEW YORK OXFORD PHILADELPHIA ST LOUIS SYDNEY TORONTO 2008

CHURCHILL
LIVINGSTONE
ELSEVIER

An imprint of Elsevier Limited

First Edition 2000
Second Edition 2008

ISBN-13: 978 0 443 10069 7

British Library Cataloguing in Publication Data
A catalogue record for this book is available from the British Library

Library of Congress Cataloging in Publication Data
A catalog record for this book is available from the Library of Congress

Note
Neither the publisher nor the authors assume any responsibility for
any loss or injury and/or damage to persons or property arising out of
or related to any use of the material contained in this book. It is the
responsibility of the treating practitioner, relying on independent
expertise and knowledge of the patient, to determine the best treatment
and method of application for the patient.

The Publisher

Printed in China

Contents

Foreword

Michael Bond

The first edition of this book was published in 2000 and since that time knowledge of pain and its management has broadened and deepened. The advances apply across the biopsychosocial spectrum and yet problems from the past remain. In particular, a widespread tendency to consider the analysis and treatment of pain using only its physical elements and a simple assessment of its severity is a common practice. This, we now know, is an inadequate approach especially in the case of chronic pain with its often complex mixture of physical, psychological and social components. To meet the need for greater understanding of those factors, research has been and is being conducted into them with an associated further development of techniques that permit greater in-depth analysis of psychological and social mechanisms. For example, further evaluation of key psychological mechanisms influencing pain experience and individuals' own ability to cope with it has led to the emergence of the importance of the process of catastrophising because it is a phenomenon closely linked to the development of chronic pain. As a result of such discoveries it has become possible to refine methods of pain management based on the multimodal approach. Another area of progress has been the search for ways in which chronic pain and disability arising out of an episode of acute pain, a classic example being low back pain, might be prevented. Attention has been focused on the risk of such changes occurring and devising ways in which knowledge of the level of risk, and how those factors which give rise to it may be controlled, is of major importance. In line with the drive to reduce the risk of the development of chronic pain and the need to improve the often devastating physical and social consequences of painful injuries in the workplace, research into the processes involved in rehabilitation has led to the development of evidence-based practices which have resulted in significant reductions in morbidity.

The advances mentioned do not remove the necessity of conducting a full clinical examination for pain sufferers, because by paying attention to them the information gained increases the possibility of reaching a balanced opinion about the contribution of physical, psychological, social and occupational factors related to the pain sufferers' current condition and, therefore, the best approach to management.

At the time the previous edition of this book was written, facilities for pain management programmes were developing rapidly and primarily within the setting of tertiary care where, usually, the team was lead by an anaesthetist aided by nurses, physiotherapists and at times, by psychologists. More recently, the recognition of pain as a speciality and a need to make adequate provision for pain management has led to an improvement in the availability of management programmes based on the full biopsychosocial model for pain. In addition, pain management has spread to the important areas of community care and the workplace where the opportunities for the prevention of the development of chronic pain and disability are greatest. Therefore, it is a matter of importance that pain education is available for a wide range of clinicians and others who may be involved with those who suffer from acute pain, which has the potential for becoming chronic, and requires the full range of physical, psychological, social and occupational techniques available for its management.

Several distinguished authors led by Professor Chris Main are responsible for this exceptionally well-written and informative book. It provides up-to-date information about the nature of pain and the many factors which contribute to its variations within and between individuals, together with methods for assessing them. It deals with the important issue of the risk of pain becoming chronic and describes techniques which can be applied to those variations in order to reduce the level of pain and disability and to increase the range of social activities and occupational possibilities for individual pain sufferers. When I wrote a foreword to the first edition of this book I said that it should be on the shelves for clinicians involved in pain management. The wealth of information, the clarity of the writing and the high level of practicality in the second edition, make it even more necessary for all professionals dealing with people in pain to possess a copy of it.

Foreword
Chris C Spanswick

This is not simply an updated version of the first edition of this book, *Pain Management: an Interdisciplinary Approach* (Main & Spanswick, 2000). The focus of that edition was primarily to act as a 'bench book' for those wishing to set up and run 'Pain Management Programmes' in tertiary care. The reader should be aware that in the UK the term 'Pain Management Programme' refers to the group-based therapy rather than the whole department, which is its usual meaning in North America and other places.

In the conclusion of the first edition, the editors hinted that the principles behind pain management applied in other clinical and occupational areas, and not just in tertiary pain treatment centres. It is no surprise that this book focuses on the application of pain management principles in those areas. It includes much of the detail of assessment and delivery of a cognitive/behaviourally-based pain management programme and it draws on the text of the previous book to do this.

This book is structured in a different way, and the content that is shared with the first edition has been brought up to date. The style is still both very readable and understandable, and is backed by a very evident review of the current literature and up-to-date references. The appraisal of the evidence is honest, even to the point of noting the current lack of published evidence that early CBT-based interventions in primary care is effective in preventing the development of chronicity. The authors point out that despite a lot of progress there is still much to do in terms of knowing what to deliver, how to deliver it, and in training health professionals in primary care to a sufficient level of competence to deliver it.

The book looks in depth at how pain management principles can be applied in the office in primary care. The first section gives a very readable account of the scientific background and current knowledge of models of pain and factors influencing the development of disability. The subsequent sections build on this body of knowledge and describe screening, assessment and treatment options in detail.

Whilst retaining its scientific basis, this is still a very practical book, and is illustrated with case examples as well as guidance on 'how' to do things as well as 'what' to do. There is a particularly good section, for example, on 'therapeutic groups' in Chapter 11. Many of us end up working with groups of patients without any training, which can be a daunting and sometimes bruising experience, and Chapter 11 provides many useful practical ideas on how to do it.

This book is both suitable and essential reading for all professionals. For example, the chapter on psychological mechanisms is written in language that the non-psychologist can understand, but also in sufficient depth that a general psychologist would find it helpful in their clinical work should they have to treat a patient with chronic pain.

Perhaps most importantly this book looks carefully at occupational perspectives. Many of our patients have difficulty in functioning at work and are often not able to work. Returning to work is often not regarded as a prime outcome for some pain management programmes, but it is a vitally important issue that cannot be ignored, both for the individual and for society. The costs of chronic pain and associated disability to individuals are of course not insignificant, but the costs to society are huge. The authors review the literature on the socio-economic aspects of chronic pain and disability in depth. They discuss the importance of both individual and organizational issues. This section is fascinating as the authors have attempted to 'grasp the nettle' and address issues such as litigation, malingering and dealing with departments of human resources. These are the practical everyday issues that patients and their therapists deal with regularly.

Finally, the authors look to the future in their concluding chapter. There are still many challenges ahead, in research, service delivery in different settings, training of professionals, dealing with workmen's compensation boards and insurers, influencing politics and policies, serving the ageing population and minority populations. The authors advocate for appropriate use of language in dealing with patients with chronic pain, a re-look at professional roles in the delivery of care and encouragement of active participation of the pain patient in their own treatment and management. Pain Management is evolving and is the responsibility of every healthcare professional. This book is vital reading for all, whether they work single-handedly in an office or within a team.

Preface

It is often said that that the process of writing and attempting to formulate ideas change the very nature of those ideas. At the time of gestation of the original edition of this book (1998), the intention was to attempt to systematise what was known at that time about the nature and practice of pain management. The impetus behind such a tricky endeavour was apparent increase in interest, although frequent misunderstandings, about the nature of pain management, and interdisciplinary pain management in particular.

The origins of the previous edition were in a self-help manual prepared for patients attending the Salford Pain Management Programme and associated teaching materials presented for pain clinicians of different disciplines who attended our teaching and training workshops (and courses). The term 'pain management' was applied originally to interdisciplinary pain management as developed from the original North American programme at the University of Washington in Seattle. At that time the term could be contrasted with 'pain relief', the expressed purpose of most of the UK pain clinics, usually focused primarily on the biomedical aspects of pain and often run single-handed by an anaesthetist with a specific interest in pain. With the passage of time, associated partly with the uncomfortable realisation that much pain could not be cured, the term 'pain management' was adopted by traditional pain clinics and the original distinction between the two types of approaches became blurred. In retrospect the development of a wider approach to the treatment and management of pain was of course to be welcomed, but we felt there was a danger that the distinctive features of interdisciplinary pain management were in danger of becoming subsumed under and constrained by the narrower conceptualisation of pain. Some might argue that over the ensuing years, promulgation of a biopsychosocial approach has led to a neglect of the 'bio' part of the term, and certainly some professionals are still fairly Cartesian in their understanding of pain and practice of pain management. Nonetheless we set out in 1998 to try to articulate what we believed about pain, what we had found helpful in working with patients, and attempted to offer a framework linking our understanding of fundamental pain mechanisms with the patient's own understanding and experience of pain.

It is interesting to reflect that our primary focus at that time was tertiary pain management, not only because of our particular professional backgrounds, but because pain management was viewed very much as a form of rehabilitation for the chronic patient. In the concluding chapters of the book we recognised the potential for a more 'upstream' approach to prevention of prolonged pain and unnecessary disability and offered an introduction to the challenges of tackling occupational rehabilitation, but these chapters represented approaches to pain management which had not as yet been incorporated within the perceived remit of traditional pain management.

It turned out, however, that we had anticipated a change in the 'Zeitgeist'. Those original speculations are rapidly becoming core to the performance of pain management. Furthermore, the principles of pain management are more widely accepted in both primary care and in occupational medicine. Everyone seems to be 'sold' on the pain management approach. But we believe we cannot simply transfer the lessons from secondary and tertiary pain management straight into these arenas. When the publishers suggested a new edition of the book, we originally conceptualised an update of the original, with, as might be expected, incorporation of recent research studies, but with major alteration to no more than 25–30% of the book at most. As we began to undertake the revision, however, it became clear that there had been such a major change in understanding of, and opportunities for, pain management, that a much more radical approach was needed. Although there will be much material that is familiar to the reader we hope that we have extended the remit of the book to include the new and exciting material that has come from the extension of pain management.

Coincidently, changes in authors' commitments (and indeed location) necessitated a fairly fundamental reconsideration of the whole enterprise. A new team was put together and the book developed much more into a multi-author volume than an edited textbook. This has led to a new title, and new authors, but despite the major changes in the book, we still feel that it should be understood as having evolved from the previous edition, and owes much to the contributors to the previous edition, whose efforts we gratefully acknowledge.

We have attempted therefore to retain the link between theory, assessment and intervention, but we have tried to develop a much sharper focus on newer applications, while hopefully retaining much of the clinical guidance from the first edition. Ultimately the success, or not, of our endeavours can be gauged only by the extent to which we have been able to assist our colleagues in the settings in which they have the opportunity to assist people who are troubled by pain.

Chris J Main
Michael J L Sullivan
Paul J Watson

Acknowledgements

The gestation of this book has been an unduly long process. We could offer all the usual reasons and excuses, but in recognising this fact, we have to warmly acknowledge the encouragement, support, assistance and forbearance of Mary Law and Helen Leng of Churchill Livingstone (now Elsevier), and Sara Keepence, with whom it has been a real pleasure to work.

As stated in the preface, we owe a considerable debt to the contributors to the first edition, since although this new volume is significantly different, we hope we have managed to retain the general perspective and wisdom of our former colleagues, in particular Chris Spanswick, who has done more than almost anyone in the UK to promulgate and indeed demonstrate patient-centred pain management.

It has been hard to strike a balance between acknowledgement of the continually evolving evidence base for pain management in all its guises and provision of practical advice about the management of people with pain, but the inspiration in particular of our research-oriented clinical colleagues has underpinned the whole book. We have attempted to acknowledge and reference where appropriate the work of many of our colleagues, and have attempted to paraphrase much of their work, often explicitly, but also unwittingly since of course good ideas evolve and sometimes travel so far that their origins become obscure. We can only apologise unreservedly for unintentional misrepresentations, and ignorant or ill-considered omissions.

We should, however, like to make special mention in this edition of Gordon Waddell and Kim Burton, whose influence can be seen throughout the book. We would also like to acknowledge the artist Stephen A. Read who was commissioned to draw the original artwork that was used for Figure 2.2.

Finally we acknowledge the support of, and give our warmest thanks to, our nearest and dearest, our families, who have suffered significant neglect as a consequence of the many hours we have stolen from them in producing this book.

Section **One**

Models and mechanisms

Chapter 1 begins with a historical review of important theories of pain which underpin modern pain management. Investigation of the link between pain and disability leads to the development of biopsychosocial models of illness and introduces the new biopsychomotor model of pain.

In Chapter 2, consideration of behavioural, cognitive and emotional influences on pain leads to a wider discussion on the influences of cognitive processes on the experience of pain. The chapter continues with discussion of the nature of communication, pain coping styles and strategies, and concludes with consideration of the role of psychological factors in interventions and obstacles to recovery.

In Chapter 3 the psychological impact of pain and disability is reviewed. Depiction of the relationship between chronic pain and psychopathology precedes consideration of the nature of clinical decision making. Description of presenting psychological characteristics in patients with pain is offered as an introduction to the identification of psychiatric illness, with consideration of implications for pain management and risk identification.

In Chapter 4, the focus is on cultural and social influences on pain and disability. Reflections on the influence of culture lead to discussion of the socio-communications model, the nature of social learning and widespread influence of social factors on the interpretation and meaning of pain. In the next part of the chapter, consideration is given to the important influences of demographic factors, particularly age and gender. After appraisal of the specific influences of the family context, the chapter concludes with reflections on the important topic of professional–patient communication.

In Chapter 5, after an overview of the nature and purposes of risk identification and screening, risk factors for the persistence of pain and persisting pain-associated limitations are reviewed. In considering the utility of classification, clustering and screening the need for an overarching conceptual framework is stressed.

Chapter One

Models of pain and disability

CHAPTER CONTENTS

Introduction

The nature of pain has puzzled humanity for centuries. As a personal experience, pain has an immediacy and impact. This experience seems difficult to capture in words, yet such is the power of its impact that it could be considered that pain can be described adequately only in picture or metaphor (Fig. 1.1).

For centuries there has been a sustained attempt to develop a philosophical and scientific understanding of pain. Many different models of pain have been offered and it is sometimes difficult to appreciate the extent to which our thinking is constrained by the prevailing conceptual models, or Zeitgeist. This chapter begins with consideration of pain from a historical perspective through the eyes of influential thinkers from a variety of disciplines. Interestingly, although theoretical models are a product of their time, they can cast a long shadow. Contemporary conceptualisations about the nature of pain echo thinking from the past. An overview of earlier theories about pain is offered to identify their influences on contemporary thinking and illustrate how our assumptions about the nature of pain and its relationship with impairment and function have changed over the centuries, and how this broader understanding has informed a progressively wider range of options for treatment and intervention.

We are indebted to Bonica (1990) for much of the historical source material.

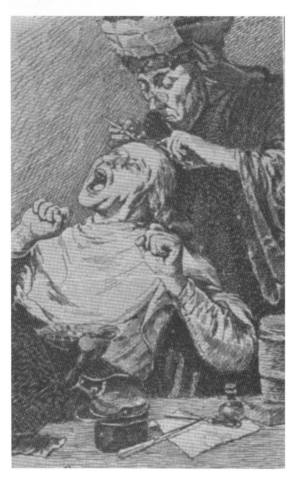

Figure 1.1 • Surgery prior to the development of anaesthesia (Fulop-Miller 1938).

Early theories of pain

Pre-Cartesian

Although any contemporary model of pain will include both physiological and psychological factors, early theories of pain were very different (Table 1.1). Early civilisations offered a variety of explanations for pain and attributed it to such factors as religious influences of gods, the intrusion of magical fluids, the frustration of desires and deficiency or excess in the circulation of Qi.

The early Greeks gave more specific consideration to the nature of pain. Plato believed that the heart and liver were the centres for appreciation of all sensation, and that pain arose not only from peripheral sensation but as an emotional response in the soul, which resided in the heart. Aristotle believed that the brain had no direct function in sensory processes. There was even less understanding of pain from internal or visceral causes. It was frequently attributed to the influence of evil spirits or the gods.

Hippocrates considered that pain was a consequence of deficiencies or excesses in the flow of one of the four fluids, or humours (blood, phlegm, yellow bile or black bile). Galen, in contrast, clearly established the anatomy of the cranial and spinal nerves. He distinguished three types of nerve: 'soft' nerves, 'hard' nerves and pain nerves. He also considered that the centre of sensibility was the brain.

Nonetheless, Aristotle's theories had considerable influence. For a long time pain was still considered to be an emotion or sensation experienced in the heart or an effect possibly of the entry of evil spirits. The brain

Table 1.1 Models of pain and their origins I: pre-Cartesian

Epoch	Key figures	Pain sources and mechanisms
Primitive		Magical fluids; exorcism; sorcery; women healers; medicine men
Ancient Egyptian		Influences of gods; spirits of dead; network of 'metu'; object intrusion
Ancient India		Frustration of desires; all joy/pain in heart
Ancient China		Yin–Yang balance; vital energy (Qi); network of 14 meridians; acupuncture
Ancient Greece (6th–4th BC)	Alcmaeon	Brain centre of sensation
	Anaxagoras	All sensations associated with pain

(continued)

Table 1.1 (continued)

Epoch	Key figures	Pain sources and mechanisms
	Hippocrates	Four humours; pain as deficit/excess
	Plato	Pain from both peripheral sensation and heart; pain/pleasure affect whole body; pain as a 'passion of the soul'
	Aristotle	Five senses; brain no direct function in sensation; pain as increased sensitivity of every sensation; caused by vital heat
Ancient Rome (3rd BC)	Galen	Central and peripheral nervous system; brain as centre of sensibility Three classes: soft nerves with 'psychic pneuma' (sensory), hard nerves (motor) and pain nerves
Middle Ages (10th AD)	Avicenna	Five 'external' and five 'internal' senses (in brain); 15 different types of pain (due to humoral changes)
	Magnus	Sensation in anterior cerebral ventricle
	Mondino	Brain seat of sensation with power to cool heart
	da Vinci	Brain centre of sensation; nerves tubular; spinal cord as a conductor

Abstracted from Bonica (1990, pp. 2–17), with permission.

was thought to play no part in the experience of pain. Indeed, the controversy over whether pain should be regarded as a sensation or as an emotion has continued to the present day and has led to an overstated dichotomy between sensory and emotional factors. Descartes' new theory was, therefore, a massive leap in the understanding of the mechanism of pain, and drew significant criticism from his contemporaries at the time.

Cartesian model

Descartes' explanation of pain (Descartes 1664) needs to be understood against the background of his philosophy. Descartes (Fig. 1.2) attempted to show that humans consisted of an earthly machine (*machine de terre*) inhabited by and governed by a rational soul (*ame raissonnable*). He tried to explain how blood, itself derived from food, gave rise to animal spirits by means of which the special earthly machine, the brain with its nerves, carried out the behests of the rational soul. The spirits dilated the brain, thus enabling it to receive the impressions of external objects, and flowed from the brain along the nerves into the muscles, thus enabling the nerves to serve as 'the organs of the external senses'. Animal spirits constituted a very subtle fluid amenable to the physical laws governing fluids, and the nerves were hollow tubes along which the spirits flowed in a wholly mechanical manner (Foster 1901). The nerves were not merely hollow tubes, but contained also delicate threads which spread all over the body from their origins at the internal surface of the brain and served as organs of sense. These threads were easily set in motion by the objects of the senses and at the same instant pulled upon the parts of the brain from which they originated.

Descartes offered the example of a foot coming into contact with fire (Fig. 1.3):

If for example the fire comes near the foot, the minute particles of this fire, which as you know have a great velocity, have the power to set in motion the spot of skin of the foot which they

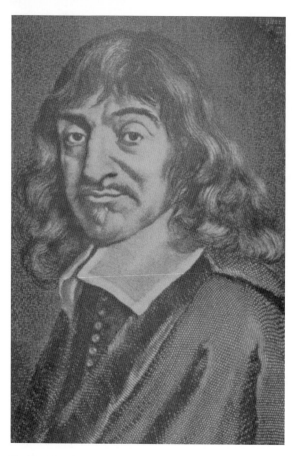

Figure 1.2 • Rene Descartes.

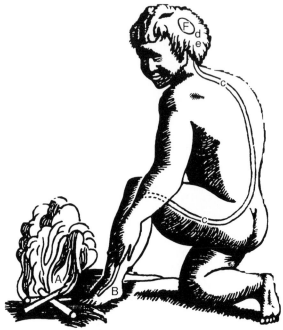

Figure 1.3 • Descartes' model of pain. From Waddell (1998).

touch, and by this means pulling upon the delicate thread which is attached to the spot of the skin, they open up at the same instant the pore against which the delicate thread ends, just as pulling at one end of a rope one makes to strike at the same instant a bell which hangs on the other end.

(Descartes 1664, translated by
Foster 1901, p. 265.)

As Foster points out, Descartes' theory required these nerves to have physical properties for which he had no evidence.

Descartes offered a dualistic view of mind and body. The body essentially was a machine whose workings could be explained by the laws of nature. The 'rational soul' was the 'conductor of the orchestra'. Descartes never really satisfactorily resolved the relationship between the two. There certainly does not seem to be any central 'processing' of the information, although it is consistent with the notion of summation.

The Cartesian legacy

In understanding pain mechanisms, there have been two major assumptions that have been inherited from Descartes: first that of a one-to-one relationship between the amount of damage (or nociception) and the pain experienced, and, secondly, the separation of mind and body.

The model of a one-to-one relationship between the amount of tissue damage and the amount of pain experienced has attractiveness, in that it seems to be consistent with the everyday experience of acute pain. It has to be remembered of course, that pain is first and foremost a biological warning signal. Pain is necessary to protect us from damage. There are well-recorded instances of children with an insensibility to pain who unknowingly injure themselves. They are unable, for example, to experience pain from internal disease and need to have their temperature monitored regularly in order to alert their carers to the possibility of internal pathology. They do not have a normal life expectancy. Thus, the function of pain in alerting us to actual or potential tissue damage is extremely important. We are programmed to react rapidly to pain. Sudden pain produces an instinctive withdrawal response. We attend immediately to it. We attempt to escape from the source of pain and we try

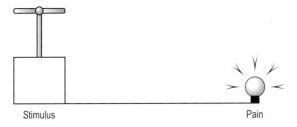

Stimulus   Pain

Figure 1.4 • The patient's model of pain. This model of pain demonstrates a direct relationship between stimulus (the pressure on the T bar) and the amount of pain (the brightness of the electric bulb). It implies information travelling in one direction only, and does not allow for any modulation of the stimulus. This model implies that a small stimulus may not cause pain, a large stimulus will always cause pain and when pain in sensed there is always damage causing it. Stopping the stimulus is the way of stopping the pain. Cutting the wire is the only other alternative.

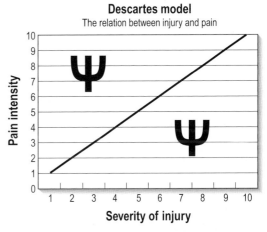

Figure 1.5 • Injury, pain and the imputation of psychological factors.

to protect the injured tissue from further damage. The pain is giving us important information about its source, nature and intensity. On occasions, such information may be of life-threatening importance. Avoidance of further painful experiences will necessarily avoid damage, aid healing and enable a return to the 'normal' state. The assumption that a higher level of pain is indicative of more serious physical damage is therefore useful, but an *accurate* appraisal of the pain is not necessary. This is illustrated in Figure 1.4.

This model of pain demonstrates a direct relationship between stimulus (the pressure on the T bar) and the amount of pain (the brightness of the electric bulb). It implies information travelling in one direction only, and does not allow for any modulation of the stimulus. This model implies that a small stimulus may not cause pain, a large stimulus will always cause pain and when pain is sensed there is always damage causing it. Stopping the stimulus is the *way* of stopping the pain. Cutting the wire is the only other alternative.

Four hundred years later, clinicians and patients alike continue to think of pain according to a Cartesian model. Pain is viewed as part of the 'mechanical' processes of the body, arising directly from injury or illness. Pain is viewed as a signal of damage or the threat of damage, and pain is expected to be relieved once injury or illness has healed.

Most patients have little understanding of the complexity of the neurophysiology and anatomy of nociceptive pathways and pain experience and indeed do not require such knowledge. They are unlikely to have experienced pain in the past without some injury or cause. The concept of pain experience as *not* directly

associated with the amount of tissue damage is alien and illogical to them. Perhaps we should not be surprised, for unless the pain persists there is usually no need for a patient to understand pain mechanisms. Furthermore, the medical profession and allied disciplines will, to a large extent, have reinforced this model of pain and damage. Rest is usually prescribed for any painful injury, along with pain killers and other treatments. Certainly, patients are advised not to move something if it hurts. The message 'let the pain be your guide' is commonly given to patients recovering from an acute injury, reinforcing the notion of pain being a direct measure of tissue damage.

A legacy of the 'mind–body split' has been the conceptualisation of pain as being *either* physical *or* psychological. Patients' general defensiveness about considering anything from a psychological viewpoint has made contemporary pain management, which accepts an interaction between physical and psychological factors, difficult for patients to accept. (Some patients view discussions about 'non-physical' influences on pain with disbelief, suspicion and sometimes downright hostility.) Attribution to a psychological influence on the perception of pain by a professional may be taken by the patient as synonymous with an implication of some sort of mental illness, a suggestion that the pain is imaginary or even that the patient is malingering.

As shown in Figure 1.5, a Cartesian model predicts a one-to-one relation between the severity of injury and pain intensity. We expect that minor injuries will be associated with minor pain and that severe injury will be associated with severe pain. Even though years of research have questioned the tenability of this model, we continue to believe in it. When situations arise that do not conform to our Cartesian view of the world, it is then that we are likely to invoke psychological explanations. When we observe someone who has experienced a minor injury express very intense pain, we become suspicious that the patient might be exaggerating his or her experience. We entertain this psychological explanation because the patient's situation is at odds with

Table 1.2 Models of pain and their origins II: 17th–mid-20th century

Epoch	Key figures	Pain sources and mechanisms
17th and 18th centuries		
1628	Harvey	Heart as site of pain
1664	Descartes	Body as a machine; nerves as tubes containing threads; pineal gland and ventricles as reservoirs of animal spirits; spirits flow along tubes; bell-rope mechanism
1794	Darwin (E.)	Pain as 'phase of unpleasantness'; intensity
19th century		
1827	Bell	Dorsal and ventral roots
1839	Muller	Special nerve energies
1859	Schiff	Specificity (sensory) theory
1894	von Frey	Pain as fourth cutaneous modality
1895	Erb	Intensity (summation) theory
1895	Goldscheider	Skin sensory input summated at dorsal horn; spinal 'summation path'
1895	Marshall	Pain as an affect
1895	Strong	Pain includes original sensation plus psychic reaction
20th century		
1900	Sherrington	Pain having both sensory and affective dimensions
1920	Head	Pain centre in the thalamus
1932	Nafe	Spatial and temporal patterning of impulses
1943	Livingston	Central summation theory; T cells critical
1951	Gerard	Nerve lesions and 'synchronously firing pools'
1952	Hardy	4th theory–primary perception and secondary reaction
1955	Sinclair	Peripheral pattern theory
1959	Nordenboos	Sensory interaction theory

Abstracted from Bonica (1990, pp. 2–17), with permission.

our implicit model of pain. Similarly, when we observe someone who has sustained severe injury express little or no distress, we wonder whether the individual is doing something psychologically to control his or her pain. Our tendency to invoke psychological explanation for situations that do not conform to our Cartesian world view is a factor that has undoubtedly contributed to defensive reactions in many of our patients.

In conclusion, the Cartesian theory represented a significant advance on its predecessors, in postulating a mechanism of pain transmission from the periphery of the body to higher centres in the brain, but every theory has its limitations. It was unable to explain clinical phenomena such as phantom pain (where pain is felt in a part of the body that has been amputated), the absence of pain in the presence of injury (such as battle wounds that are noticed only when the threat to life has passed), or the persistence of pain beyond tissue-healing time (as in chronic pain conditions). Finally it could be argued that its assumptions of a one-to-one relationship between nociception and pain experience, and its dualistic separation of mind and body, have been particular hindrances to the development of an adequate theory of pain.

Post-Cartesian developments

Two major physiological theories of pain became the object of research in the 19th century (Table 1.2). Descartes had developed the concept of a pain pathway linking the periphery of the body with higher centres in the brain. It led to the specificity theory, in which pain was considered to be a *specific sensation* independent of other sensations. According to the intensive (summation) theory, however, touch was experienced as a painful sensation only when it reached a certain threshold (following intense stimulation). Both these theories and their later derivatives were essentially physiological in nature and the *perception* of pain was not specifically addressed. They offered a relatively simple relationship between tissue damage and pain perception. The sensory system responsible for mediating pain was regarded as relatively rigid and straightforward in that any tissue damage initiated a sequence of neural events that inevitably produced pain. An unfortunate inference from this simplistic view was that pain was fixed solely by characteristics of the noxious stimulus and that the nociceptive system functioned primarily as a passive relay mechanism. Neither of the theories could explain either pain in the absence of tissue damage or variation in pain between individuals with (apparently) the same amount of tissue damage. The latter tended to be attributed to long-term personality characteristics rather than be seen as a feature of the psychological impact of the pain itself.

We now know that pain perception depends on complex neural interactions where impulses generated by tissue damage are modified both by ascending systems activated by innocuous stimuli and by descending pain-suppressing systems activated by various environmental and psychological factors.

With the addition of the later sensory interaction theory (postulating a fast and a slow system of pain transmission), the foundation of the gate control theory (GCT) (Melzack & Wall 1965) was laid.

The gate control theory

Melzack & Wall (1965) (Fig. 1.6) proposed the original gate theory of pain, or GCT-I (Fig. 1.7). This theory marked a turning point in our understanding of pain. It was of landmark importance in two respects: first in terms of the mechanisms of the transmission and modulation of nociceptive signals, and secondly in terms of its recognition of pain as a psychophysiological phenomenon resulting from the interaction between physiological and psychological events.

The GCT incorporated physiological specialisation, central summation patterning and modulation of input by psychological and other factors into a new model that has formed much of the contemporary psychology of pain.

The GCT postulated spinal 'gates', in the dorsal horn at each segmental level in the spinal cord, determining which of the competing impulses (pain, heat or touch) was transmitted at any particular moment. Successful transmission through the gate was affected not only by the intensity of the stimulation, and competing local

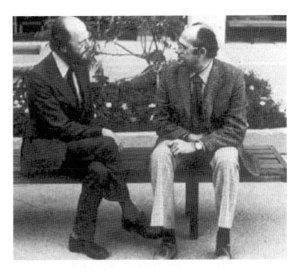

Figure 1.6 • Melzack and Wall.

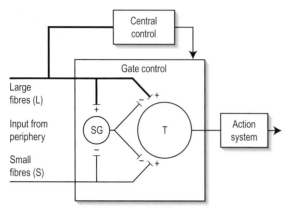

Figure 1.7 • Gate control theory I (GCT-I). L, the large diameter fibres. S, the small diameter fibres. The fibres project to the substantia gelatinosa (SG) and first central transmission (T) cells. The inhibitory effect exerted by the SG on the afferent fibre terminals is increased by activity in L fibres and decreased by activity in S fibres. The central control trigger is represented by a line running from the large fibre system to the central control mechanisms; these mechanisms, in turn, project back to the gate control system. The T cells project to the action system (+, excitation, −, inhibition). From Melzack & Wall (1965, p. 971), reproduced with permission.

stimuli, but also by descending impulses from the higher central nervous system. In contrast to the model of Descartes, the transmission of information about events in the periphery is not a simple one-way system. There is continual modulation of information from the periphery – in the gate theory's case, nociception.

Figure 1.8 is a schematic representation of the sensory input at each segmental level in the dorsal horn of the spinal cord. The large fibres (L) and the small fibres (S) project into the substantia gelatinosa (SG) and the first transmission cells (T). It can be seen that input from large fibres will *reduce* the amount of nociceptive traffic, whereas input from the smaller fibres will *increase* nociceptive traffic going further up to the action system.

The diagram also shows the influence of 'central control' (at the dorsal horn). This central control is initiated by input from the large fibres and feeds back into the 'gate control system'. These large fibres carry specific information about the nature and location of the stimulus. They conduct rapidly, not only potentially setting the sensitivity of the cortical neurons but also influencing the sensory input in the gate itself. This may occur not only at the level of the original input but also at other levels.

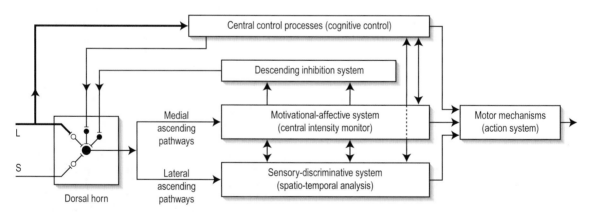

Figure 1.8 • Gate control theory II (GCT-Ib). The output of the T cell in the dorsal horn projects to the sensory-discriminative system via the lateral ascending system and to the motivational-affective system via the medial ascending system. The central control 'trigger', composed of the dorsal column and the dorsolateral projection systems, is represented by a heavy line running from the large fibre system to the central control processes, which take place in the brain. These in turn project back to the dorsal horn as well as to the sensory-discriminative and motivational-affective systems. Added to the scheme of Melzack & Casey is the brainstem inhibitory control system activated by impulses in the medial descending system, and which provides descending control on the dorsal horn. Moreover, there is much interaction between the motivational-affective and the sensory-discriminative systems as indicated by the arrows. The net effect of all of these interacting systems is activation of the motor (action) system. Modified from Melzack & Casey (1968). Courtesy of Charles C. Thomas, Publisher Ltd, Springfield, Illinois, USA.

This rapid transmission allows the brain to identify, evaluate and modulate input before the action system is activated by the T cells. The final common pathway is provided through the T cell, which, when the output from this exceeds a critical level, sends information further on to the action system. This system describes those areas of the brain responsible for the behavioural responses to pain and the 'experience' of pain itself.

Soon after the first publication, the theory was expanded (Melzack & Casey 1968) to describe the neural system beyond the gate (Fig. 1.9). The expanded theory suggested different systems for the motivational, affective and cognitive aspects of pain experience. The neospinothalamic projection serves to process *sensory discriminative* information (location, intensity and duration). The information passing through the paleospinothalamic system activates the reticular and limbic areas, giving rise to the unpleasant affect and aversive (*motivational*) drive, which ultimately produces action. The higher centres in the brain (neocortical) influence the sensory-discriminative and the motivational-affective systems having evaluated the input in the light of past experience.

Melzack & Wall (1983) modified the GCT model in the light of new information. The model retained the excitatory and inhibitory links from the substantia gelatinosa and added the expanded version of the central controls as described by Melzack & Casey (1968) (Fig. 1.9). Melzack & Wall's (1965) gate control theory of pain was an effort to provide an integrative model of pain that could account for the wide range of pain phenomena that their theoretical predecessors could not. The gate control theory of pain also included psychological factors as defining features of the pain experience.

Melzack's (1996, 1999) work on phantom-limb phenomena led him to postulate that the brain areas (and processes) that typically gave rise to pain sensation could generate a pain sensation even in the absence of sensory input. In other words, the mechanisms that underlie the experience of pain arise from patterns of brain activation that can operate completely independently of sensory input. Melzack used the term 'neuromatrix' to describe the spatial distribution of the network of neurons implicated in pain experience. The specific architecture of brain activation during pain has been termed the neurosignature of pain.

A modern understanding of pain mechanisms

Further developments from the GCT

Much work has been done over the last 30 years to tease out the details of Melzack & Wall's theory and much more is now known about the complexity of the neurophysiology and neuroanatomy of the pain pathways, in particular the mechanisms of ongoing transmission of nociception that take place in the dorsal horn of the spinal cord. Anatomical pathways, neurotransmitters and gene expression have all been described.

Some of the major strands in further development are shown in Table 1.3. The traditional view of two parallel circuits for sensory and affective components, mapping onto two discrete pain centres in the brain has had to be revised, because it is now known that the brain circuits are much more complex than was first believed. Central neural mechanisms associated with such phenomena as placebo/nocibo, hypnotic attention, distraction and ongoing emotions are now thought to modulate pain by decreasing or increasing neural activity within many brain structures (Price & Bushnell 2004).

In addition to the 'cross-talk' between systems, the process is dynamic and recursive. We know little about change in the individual across time but recent research suggests that the brain is 'active' rather than a passive processor of information. This is seen in neuroplastic

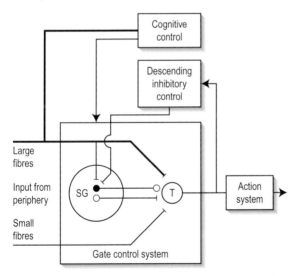

Figure 1.9 • Gate control theory II (GCT-II). The new model includes excitatory (white circle) and inhibitory (black circle) links from the substantia gelatinosa (SG) to the transmission (T) cells as well as descending inhibitory control from brainstem systems. The round knob at the end of the inhibitory link implies that its actions may be presynaptic, postsynaptic, or both. All connections are excitatory, except the inhibitory link from SG to T cell. Modified from Melzack & Wall (1983), reproduced with permission of Penguin Books Ltd.

Table 1.3 Models of pain and their origins III: since the gate control theory

Epoch	Key figures	Pain sources and mechanisms
1962, 1965	Melzack & Wall	GCT-I: competition at dorsal horn for transmission
1966	Mendell	Wind-up
1968	Melzack & Casey	Ascending and descending influences; motivational, cognitive and behavioural aspects of pain experience
1983	Travell	Myogenic pain theory
1991	Jones	Limbic system mapping (PET)
1991	Dubner	Neuroplasticity
1994	Flor	Psychophysiological mechanisms
1996	Orbach	Stress–hyperactivity theory
1996	Melzack	Neuromatrix theory

changes in peripheral nociceptive mechanisms in complex regional pain syndromes in which, after injury, the body fails to repair itself properly, and as a consequence of new connections established through neuronal sprouting, plastic changes at the spinal cord level lead to chronic pain of increasing severity out of proportion to the original injury.

Research into phantom sensation following amputation (Flor et al 1998) has demonstrated that central processing of peripheral nociceptive information can also become distorted, in that the somatosensory map may no longer correspond to the changed pattern of nociceptive signals, leading to phantom pain perceived in a body part which is no longer there.

A third strand of challenging evidence comes from the studies on memory where it appears that memory of pain, without any new peripheral input, can be sufficient to trigger the experience of pain. Research suggests that aversive pain memories may have a powerful influence on the perception of new pain stimuli (Bryant 1993). The phenomenon is not fully understood but may be associated both with central neuroplasticity and with secondary conditioned responses, possibly mediated by the limbic system.

Psychobiology

Psychobiology is a vastly expanding field with a plethora of theoretical perspectives, and legions of research studies into specific mechanisms of potential relevance to an understanding of pain mechanisms.

Pain and consciousness

The recently emerging field of consciousness research offers an interesting path from biology to psychology based on evolutionary principles. According to Chapman et al (1999), consciousness is 'an emergent property of the brain: a dynamic self-organising process operating in a distributed neural network' leading to a set of hierarchical processes. The constructivist framework assumes that the brain deals not with reality itself but with an internal representation of reality that constructs from moment to moment, using sensory information, a network of association and memory stores. Pain is viewed as a threat to the biological integrity of the self. Although this type of reductionist model is not to everyone's taste, in offering a bridge between biology and phenomenology it would appear to merit consideration as one way of understanding the psychological impact of pain. Thus some of the core features of human consciousness such as coherence, sense of self, purposiveness and the personal nature (and affect) become a link between pain, dysfunction and distress. The development of *schemata* as types of conceptual templates which emerge as a network of associations in response to the challenge of pain may offer a basis for the development of psychological strategies directed at the perception of pain and pain-associated incapacity (Ch. 10).

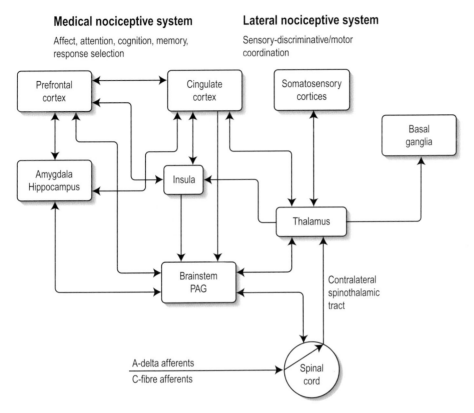

Medical nociceptive system

Affect, attention, cognition, memory, response selection

Lateral nociceptive system

Sensory-discriminative/motor coordination

Figure 1.10 • Main anatomical components of the 'pain matrix' and their possible functional significance. PAG = periaqueductal grey matter. From Jones (2005), reproduced with permission of IASP Press, Seattle.

The interface between psychological processes and events in the brain

It has been shown in non-human primates that manipulation of attention influences descending pathways from the brain to the first synapse of the spinal cord (Bushnell et al 1985) thus confirming a core postulate of the GCT. Developments in new technology have allowed investigation of attention and distraction on pain-evoked activity in the brain in humans. According to Jones (2005):

The most important features of brain imaging techniques is that they are able to measure many aspects of nociceptive processing such as anticipation of pain and neurochemical changes associated with pain, which cannot be measured by any other means (p. 61).

A recent depiction of pain mechanisms is shown in Figure 1.10. According to Jones (2005) the main division of function between the medial and lateral systems is likely to be that of affective and sensory-discriminative

processing, respectively, with intensity probably being processed through the matrix. The perigenual cingulate and associated structures are most likely to be concerned with processing the affective responses to pain, whereas the mid-anterior cingulate is more likely to be concerned with affective processing (response selection and monitoring) and control of attention. However, he cautions against attempts as yet to move towards a physiological reclassification of pain and concludes 'when such a classification does become possible, it is likely to be simpler, with less emphasis on localisation and duration, and with greater emphasis on the psychological context of the pain and the pathophysiological mechanisms resulting in its maintenance' (p. 66).

The influence of psychological factors on muscle and movement

The culmination of Melzack & Wall's original GCT can be seen in Melzack's recent neuromatrix theory, but this seems far removed from the earlier myogenic pain model

Box 1.1

Psychophysiological models of pain

- Spasm–pain–spasm
- Muscle hyper-reactivity model
- Diathesis–stress model.

After Watson (2002)

Box 1.2

Pain and muscle activity in workers

Westgaard (1999) recorded the muscle activity during a typical working day in a group of office workers and another group working on a production line, and subjects were asked to rate their neck and shoulder pain and the perception of muscle tension.

- The best predictor of the development of pain in the *production line* workers was indeed the actual level of muscle activity
- However, in the *office workers*, who demonstrated much less muscle activity, the best predictor of the development of pain was the *perception* of muscle tension even though there was no relationship between self-report of muscle tension and measured EMG
- This further appears to have been closely related to the *psychological status* of the worker at the time, calling into question the presumed linearity of the relationship between pain and muscle activity in the office workers.

(Travell & Simons 1993) which focused primarily on the relationship between pain, muscle function and movement and gave little recognition to the influence of central processing on pain perception.

There are several parallel and related lines of research which illuminate the emergence of this new theory: firstly psychophysiological research examining the influence of psychological factors on muscle and movement; and secondly diathesis-stress models (based primarily on the influence of pre-existing psychological vulnerabilities on pain and function).

Watson (2002) distinguished the three major types of psychophysiological pain models (Box 1.1).

The spasm–pain–spasm model

Initial models of myogenic pain tried to explain the perseverance of pain following injury according to a model which suggested that, following injury, muscle activity increases around the affected area to protect it. This triggers neuronal activity precipitating hyper-reactivity, spasm and local ischaemia, thus reducing the sensitivity of wide dynamic range neurones causing previously non-nociceptive stimuli (e.g. pressure) to become painful (Coderre et al 1993; Mense 1997; Gifford 1998a, 1998b).

This model might serve in the acute state or in short-term acute flare-up in recurrent or chronic pain states where increased muscle activity can be demonstrated in some muscle groups, in particular over injured joints. However, inhibition of other muscle groups also occurs and the relationship between the muscle activity and the report of pain is unclear (Simons & Mense 1998). Research into identifying elevated muscle activity in chronic pain states without obvious spasm has not substantiated a role for consistently elevated levels of muscle tension (Ahern et al 1988; Arena et al 1991; Letchuman & Deusinger 1993; Watson et al 1997a, 1997b) and when chronic pain patients are compared to pain-free controls using electromyography most research has failed to demonstrate any difference in muscle activity at rest.

Muscle hyper-reactivity model

In order to overcome the apparent limitations of the above model, researchers have suggested that the increase in muscle activity may not be permanent but occur with sufficient frequency to perpetuate the painful condition. In this model, both physiological and psychological stress can increase muscle activity.

An example of an experimental investigation into pain, muscle activity and work is shown in Box 1.2. The fact that the postures the subjects maintained during their work did not lead to high levels of muscle tension and that their beliefs and perception of muscle tension appeared to be most influential in reporting pain offer important support for the interaction between physical and psychological factors in understanding the impact of pain.

The data further demonstrated that muscle tension *increased* proportionately with the *complexity* of the task to a point where pain was reported. In another study of healthy controls Waersted & Westgaard (1996) found that the biomechanical demands of the task (sitting at a VDU) alone were insufficient to cause increases in muscle tension sufficient to cause pain, but increasing the complexity of the task and the attention required to perform it, were of greater importance in the development of myogenic neck/shoulder pain. (This experimental work maps onto the later discussion of the relationship between *perceptions* of work and *objective* work characteristics in Chs 14 and 15.)

The diathesis–stress model

The integration of pain research and psychophysiological research, however, led to more complex formulations of the nature of pain mechanisms such as the stress–hyperactivity–pain theory, offered as a further development of the myogenic pain theory (Orbach & McCall 1996).

Flor et al (1991) proposed a *diathesis–stress model* to explain pain-increased muscle activity among chronic pain patients in response to stressful experiences. In experimental studies, as predicted by the model, the chronic low-back pain (LBP) group responded to the personally relevant stressors in the lumbar muscles, and temporomandibular joint (TMJ) subjects responded in the jaw muscles (Flor & Birbaumer 1994). The concept of pre-existing vulnerability or 'diathesis' of some sort is, however, a clear contender as a possible explanatory factor for the otherwise unexplained individual differences both in the development and severity of chronic pain syndromes. The construct has been useful in clarifying the relationship between pain and depression (Ch. 3).

More recently, following a recent review of the experimental literature, Watson arrived at a number of conclusions (summarised in Box 1.3).

The neuromatrix theory

As aforementioned, much of the strands of research can be seen as culminating in the neuromatrix theory (Melzack 1999), the key features of which are summarised in Box 1.4. The theory would seem to offer an explanation in terms of homeostasis for the development of chronic pain and disability. The emotional impact of chronic pain can be understood in terms of the stress of pain and other stressors (including specific pain-associated incapacities). The development of chronic disability can be understood within a homeostatic framework in terms of attempts to restore 'equilibrium' by engaging in attempts to minimise pain, if not escape from it, or attempts to avoid pain altogether.

The development of the 'disuse syndrome', fear-mediated responses and guarded movements (frequently observed characteristics of patients attending pain management programmes) can also be understood within this general psychobiological framework as an example of a way of coping with persistent pain and are echoed in the potential clinical implications of the experimental studies described above.

Box 1.3

Summary of experimental findings

- Beliefs (fears) about injury and ability to cope with pain change muscle action in chronic LBP patients, these are unconscious but objectively observable
- In chronic LBP the resolution of abnormal dynamic muscle activity is mediated by changes in fear of movement and confidence in the patient's ability to manage their pain
- Chronic pain patients demonstrate abnormal muscle responses to stressful situations including pain
- Responses to palpation are highly influenced by fear of reinjury in chronic pain patients
- Perceptions about increases in muscle tension may be more important in the development of pain than objectively measured increases in some situations
- Stereotypical responses to pain can be conditioned in normal subjects. Once conditioned an associated stimulus is sufficient to elicit the muscular response independently from pain
- The combined effect of psychological stress and physical stressors on the development and maintenance of chronic pain is under-researched.

From Watson (2002)

Box 1.4

Key elements of Melzack's neuromatrix theory

- Pain is a multidimensional experience, produced by characteristic 'neurosignatures' or patterns of nerve impulses generated by a widely distributed neural network: the 'body-self-neuromatrix'
- Neurosignature patterns may be triggered by sensory inputs but also independently
- The neuromatrix is genetically determined and modified by sensory experience
- Injury disrupts the body's homeostatic regulation systems, thereby producing stress and initiating complex programmes to restore homeostasis
- Stressors activate programmes of neural, hormonal and behavioural activity aimed at restoring homeostasis
- If stress responses continue, they lead to immune system suppression and activation of

(Continued)

the limbic system (which has a role in emotion, motivation and cognitive processes)
- Stress and pain perception possess overlapping mechanisms
- Neuromatrix output determines whether pain will be experienced or suppressed
- Pain suppression must be determined not only by the release of endorphins and other opioids, but also by sensory, discriminative and evaluative processes
- Prolonged activation of the stress-regulation systems will lead to tissue breakdown and 'set the stage' for the development of fibromyalgia, osteoporosis and other chronic pain conditions
- The limbic system, being the neural substrate of the affective–motivational dimension of pain, is so interdependent that it should be considered to be part of a single system
- A number of chronic pain syndromes, as well as depression, may be linked to the stress-regulation system
- All psychological stressors may contribute to the neuro-endocrine processes that give rise to pain syndromes
- Individual variation in the enhancement of a given stress is a function of: other concurrent stresses; cumulative effect of prior stresses; kinds of concurrent or prior stresses; and the severity and duration of stresses
- Even when pain is experienced, it may be a stressor if it implies danger and threat to the survival of the self, physically or psychologically.

Adapted from Melzack (1999)

Pain perception

The role of attentional mechanisms

There are now a large number of human studies showing variation in brain activity in response to pain, under varying conditions of attention and distraction (Bushnell et al 2004). Some of the methodology has its origins in the field of experimental psychology in which there has been considerable interest in the psychophysiological impact of manipulation of attention, often requiring perceptual discrimination under conditions of distraction. Thus identical stimuli may be presented to different receptive fields (such as different body regions for somatosensory stimuli) or the subject may be required to discriminate among different dimensions of the same stimulus, and attend to a particular feature of the

stimulus such its colour or shape. Thus we are able to study attentional processes such as accuracy and vigilance, but also their emotional and psychophysiological correlates such as anxiety, mood and arousal. These paradigms have also been used to investigate both experimental and clinical pain and confirmed the influence of attention on nociceptive processing (Bantick et al 2002; Legrain et al 2002) and vigilance on the perception of pain (discussed more fully in Ch. 2).

It might be expected that anticipation of pain, coloured by previous experience, might contribute to increased vigilance and attentional focus, and indeed the physiological and neuro-anatomical correlates of anticipation have provided further evidence of the impact of psychological processes on the neural substrate. According to Bushnell et al (2004), 'Anticipation-related changes in cerebral activity . . . may underlie numerous behavioural responses associated with changes in emotional state, preparation for dealing with the impending stimulus, and even activation of endogenous analgesic processes,' although they note 'there is no firm evidence that anticipation of pain, without the actual noxious stimulus, results in the perception of pain itself' (p. 111).

Pain perception: the emotional component

Negative emotion has long been recognised as a concomitant of pain and certainly merits some consideration in its own right. However, it is sometimes difficult to differentiate attention and emotion and this difficulty is reflected in the influence of emotion on pain intensity rating. There is, however, now widespread recognition that ratings of pain intensity and pain unpleasantness need to be distinguished and it appears that the desire to avoid or escape pain appears to be associated with pain unpleasantness, independent of pain intensity (Rainville 2004).

Animal studies have produced both behavioural and physiological evidence of an influence of acute threat, threat anticipation and aversive stimulation (including pain) on endogenous pain modulation (Manning 2004) but mapping onto the human is problematic.

It has been suggested that pain sensations may be considered as specific inducers of a primitive emotional response in the context of biological adaptation (Rainville 2004), consistent with the first two stages of the four-stage model (Price 1999), discussed below, in which immediate pain appraisal is followed by an immediate affective response. This view is consistent with the evolutionary view (Williams 2002) and the significance given to facial expression in neonates with painful conditions (Craig 2003).

According to Rainville (2004) pain-related emotions may affect pain perception in several ways, as shown in Figure 1.11. According to this formulation, goal-directed desires appear to influence mainly pain unpleasantness, whereas goal-directed expectations influence both pain sensation intensity and pain unpleasantness. Emotion-related physiological arousal may contribute to the felt arousal and to pain unpleasantness.

Rainville makes a distinction between pain-related negative emotions and negative emotions unrelated to pain. He considers that such experiential factors may in part explain individual differences in response to pain but that we are some way yet from fully identifying the precise relationship between the brain areas and mechanisms underlying the multiple dimensions of pain and emotion.

Many normal and adaptive psychological processes can become maladaptive, but the stage at which this occurs is difficult to delineate. Thus apprehension can turn into significant fear/avoidance and appraisal can turn

into hypervigilance. The nature of *fear* and of *hypervigilance* in the context of painful conditions is discussed in more detail in the chapter on psychological mechanisms (Ch. 2) and also in the context of therapeutic interventions (Chs 9, 10 and 11).

The four-stage model: a dynamic view of pain mechanisms

The distinctions between the sensory and affective components of pain, set in an evaluative framework linked with behavioural responses as anticipated by the GCT, offer a radically new view of pain and pain mechanisms. Little is known as yet about the 'cross-talk' between systems, how the response to pain is shaped across time or about individual differences in these processes. A helpful integrated conceptual framework has been offered in the four-stage model (Price 1999), shown in Figure 1.12.

According to Riley & Wade (2004) this model consists of an initial sensory discriminative stage of which the major ingredient is the perceived intensity of the pain sensation. This stage is related to immediate appraisals associated with the sensory features of pain, automatic and somatomotor activation and perception of the immediate context surrounding the pain. The second stage of pain processing, termed *immediate unpleasantness* reflects an individual's immediate affective response and involves limited cognitive processing, including reflection about the immediate implications of having pain including emotional response and the accompanying arousal. The third phase of pain processing involves longer-term cognitive processes relating to the meaning and longer-term implications accompanied by *extended pain affect* reflecting the experiential side of suffering.

Recent research has identified specific areas of the brain most closely affected with each of the stages. According to Price & Bushnell (2004) pain sensation and pain unpleasantness represent two distinct dimensions of pain differentially relating to nociceptive stimulus intensity and separately influenced by various psychological factors. Indeed according to Bushnell et al (2004) 'There is now overwhelming evidence that psychological

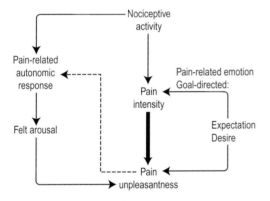

Figure 1.11 • Rainville's model of pain-related emotion and perception. Pain-related emotions are suggested to affect pain perception in several ways. Goal-directed desires appear to affect mainly pain unpleasantness, whereas goal-directed expectations influence both pain sensation intensity and pain unpleasantness. Emotion-related physiological activity may contribute to the felt arousal and to pain unpleasantness. From Price & Bushnell (2004), reproduced with permission of IASP Press, Seattle.

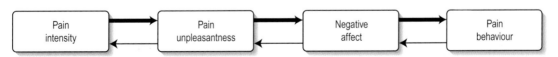

Figure 1.12 • Four-stage model of pain processing. The recursive arrows acknowledge that, although the earlier stages give rise to later stages over time, there is a reciprocal effect in that past and current levels of later stages can influence future levels of earlier stages. From Price & Bushnell (2004), reproduced with permission of IASP Press, Seattle.

modulation of pain has genuine physiological underpinnings' (p. 112).

Thus the four stages of pain processing are consistent with neurophysiology. Underlying neural mechanisms of sensory as well as primary and secondary affective dimensions of pain include multiple ascending spinal pathways to the brain with both serial and parallel processing in the brain (Price & Bushnell 2004). Serial interactions between pain sensation, immediate pain unpleasantness and extended pain-related affect are respectively associated with serial interactions between somatosensory cortices, insular and cingulate cortices, and prefrontal and temporal areas.

Influences of moderators and mediators within the four-stage model

Riley & Wade (2004) also offer interesting observations on an illuminating conceptualisation of influences of additional factors, such as ethnicity, age, gender and personality on stages of pain processing. However, many of the studies are correlational or cross-sectional in nature, the mechanisms are unclear and the size of the putative effects relatively modest. Indeed Riley & Wade concede that 'the manner in which the four stages of pain are processed is similar across various demographics (diagnosis, ethnicity and gender) with perhaps the exception being age', though they caution against over-reliance on interpretation of group differences.

From an intuitive point of view, given the clearly multifactorial nature of chronic pain, the pain-processing stages must be influenced by external factors, but a clearer picture would require large data sets, serial measurement, complex research design and sophisticated statistical analysis. The influence of demographic, psychological and social factors on chronic pain and disability is considered in much more detail in later chapters of this book.

Pain mechanisms: summary of key points

The GCT has offered a testable model of how psychological factors could activate descending pain-inhibitory systems, influence nociceptive processing and thereby modulate pain. It offered a way of integrating concepts of pain behaviour, both as a response to pain and as behaviour that could come under environmental control. The theory has stimulated interest into beliefs, appraisal and fears about pain and pain-related coping strategies. It has encouraged the investigation of the nature of pain-associated disability and led to the development of biopsychosocial models, which have attempted a wide

Box 1.5

Legacy of the GCT

- Offered a testable model of how psychological factors could activate descending pain-inhibitory systems, influence nociceptive processing and thereby modulate pain
- Offered a way of integrating concepts of pain behaviour, both as a response to pain and as behaviour that could come under environmental control
- Has stimulated interest into beliefs, appraisal and fears about pain and pain-related coping strategies
- Has encouraged the investigation of the nature of pain-associated disability and led to the development of biopsychosocial models, which have attempted a wide integration of physical, psychological and social perspectives.

integration of physical, psychological and social perspectives. The importance of psychological influences on the perception of pain has been increasingly recognised. Experimental studies into pain threshold and tolerance have highlighted the importance of fatigue, depression and fear. Several research groups are currently investigating the role of attentional mechanisms and memory. Studies in phantom pain have led to the formulation of the neuromatrix theory (Melzack 1999), which has stimulated much debate into cognitive representation of sensation. Finally, the link between psychology and physiotherapy has led research away from the myogenic pain theory of Travell & Simons (1993) to the investigation of psychophysiological responses to pain and the influence of central mechanisms. The key features of the legacy of the GCT are summarised in Box 1.5.

From pain mechanisms to models of illness

The new understanding of pain mechanisms has paved the way for a number of new therapeutic approaches focused directly on the manipulation and modification of attention and distraction as therapeutic tools, in fields such as placebo-induced analgesia, hypnosis and cognitive–behavioural therapy (Price & Bushnell 2004). Specific psychological influences on the experience of pain will be considered in the next chapter. There has, however, been a much wider effect on clinical practice resulting from the conceptualisation of new clinical models of pain and illness.

The traditional disease model

There are similarities between the Cartesian model of pain and the traditional disease model of illness in their assumption of a direct one-to-one relationship between physical signs of disease and accompanying symptoms. Virchow (1858) in his model of cellular pathology established the basis of the medical model of illness and disease that has influenced medical treatment for the last century. In arriving at a diagnosis and treatment, the physician proceeded through a number of stages. On the basis of the patient's presenting symptoms (complaints), the doctor investigated the presence of associated physical signs. Having identified treatable pathology and arrived at a diagnosis, treatment was then prescribed with the expectations that the disease would be cured, the physical signs would disappear and the patient would no longer be troubled by the presenting symptoms. Consider, for example, patients who present with ear pain. Doctors will inquire further about the nature of the ear pain and consider a range of possible causes for the pain. They will then examine the patient to confirm their provisional diagnosis. Doctors will see an inflamed ear drum and infer that the patient has an infection that is causing the pain. They will prescribe antibiotics to cure the infection and both doctors and patients expect the symptoms (the pain) and the signs (the redness of the ear drum) to improve. In other words, an explanation for the symptoms and signs has been found. By treating the cause of the symptoms and signs it is expected that they will be cured.

This model is dependent, however, on there being a close relationship between symptoms, signs and disease. It does not take into account the variability of the patient's response to illness and in the self-report of symptoms. Despite these shortcomings, the model works well for most acute medical and surgical conditions.

Limitations of the traditional medical model for the treatment of pain

Syndromes and diagnoses

Medicine has categorised disease and illness in order to aid diagnosis and subsequent treatment. Textbooks abound with 'clinical syndromes'. These indicate a number of different symptoms and physical signs, which when present should lead the doctor to reach a specific diagnosis. The 'diagnosis' may then be further confirmed or refuted by performing specific tests. The results of these tests may be included in the description of the clinical syndrome.

It is not necessary, usually, to have all the recognised symptoms, signs or test results to make a diagnosis of the clinical syndrome. The observations may be given different emphasis so that some features of the syndrome may be more heavily weighted than others with the result that sometimes patients may be given a diagnosis on very little evidence. Furthermore, many of the symptoms, signs and even test results may be found also in other clinical syndromes (the diagnosis of complex regional pain syndrome (CRPS) is a good example of this), thus making a specific diagnosis more difficult and highly subjective. In some cases it may not be considered possible to confirm the diagnosis until the response to treatment is known. In such situations it is difficult to have full confidence in the accuracy of the initial diagnostic process.

The variations detected in the types, number and severity of symptoms, signs, tests and even responses to treatment are usually attributed to variations in the disease process rather than in the patient. If the level of 'complaints' made by the patient is high, this is usually attributed to long-term personality characteristics and is often ignored. Failure to respond to treatment following diagnosis usually leads to re-evaluation to assess the diagnosis. This will usually entail at least further investigations in the hope of 'turning up something'. It may also lead to repeated attempts at treatment that unfortunately have a high chance of failure. This in turn may lead to different diagnoses from doctor to doctor, which is very confusing for patients.

If patients cannot be classified into a known syndrome or diagnosis and fail to improve following several trials of treatment, they may end up with the label of 'hysteria', 'hypochondriasis' or 'functional overlay'. The difficulty may be to do more with limitations of the classification system than with the nature of the patient's response to illness. Nonetheless, some patients are left with no clear diagnosis and, having failed to respond to treatment, are discharged without the prospect for any further treatment and told to 'learn to live with it'. It can be seen how strict adherence to the disease model of illness can leave patients without an adequate explanation for their pain, may offer no prospect of helpful treatment and may lead to the suggestion that their fundamental problem is one of mental attitude or psychiatric disorder.

Implications of failure to recognise the importance of variability in response to pain

There is a large variation of self-report of symptoms with (apparently) the same pathology and recent research has demonstrated large variation in complaints of pain with specific pathology. In one study (McAlindon et al 1992) only 50% of patients with demonstrable major arthritis of the hip joint as identified by X-ray complained of pain. An early magnetic resonance imaging (MRI) study of the lumbar spine found that 76% of asymptomatic volunteers demonstrated a disc herniation at one or more levels (Boos et al 1995). There is clearly no direct relationship between disc abnormalities and pain. The reasons for this are not fully understood, but the data suggest that the disc bulge is often not the pain source. Without doubt, psychological factors are important influences on the perception of pain, decision to consult and response to treatment, but it is clear that the physical basis of pain is still inadequately understood. Recent research suggests that ascription of all patient variability to the 'mental realm', in the sense of discrediting it, would appear to be extremely unwise; yet this has been an inevitable consequence of overstrict adherence to the narrow medical model.

From theoretical models to clinical practice

Patients demonstrate a wide range of responses to acute pain (ranging from the understated or stoical to the highly florid and dramatic). In most cases of acute pain, the cause of pain will be clear, the diagnosis is unambiguous and the only issue of concern will be matching up the analgesic strategy with the patient's particular response. Marked pain behaviour may or may not accompany the pain experience. Usually, particularly with episodes of acute pain, treating the cause of the pain successfully will also have a significant effect on the 'pain behaviour' and the latter becomes of little concern. Analgesia may be effective even when behaviour is quite bizarre. This may be taken to confirm the view that all pain behaviour, however bizarre, is secondary to nociception and consequently that targeting treatment solely at the nociceptive source is all that is required to manage both the pain and the consequent behaviour. If the treatment of the pain does not change the pain behaviour then the pain is often regarded as psychological or imagined. Although this may not be made explicit to the patient, the patient often picks up such implications from the behaviour and manner of the treating staff.

Understanding pain behaviour

In order to emphasise the importance of the interpretation of pain behaviour, we have posed two theoretical questions about pain behaviour and offered some

Q Why do some patients exhibit more pain behaviour than others?

A 1. They may be frightened of the pain, and emphasise their discomfort lest it is underappreciated (and undertreated)
2. They may have suffered poorly controlled pain in the past
3. It may be part of their style
4. They may have learned to behave like this.

Q How do clinicians respond to pain behaviour and why?

A 1. They may disregard the behaviour as 'random noise', simply ignore it and continue to treat with analgesia
2. They may seek to alleviate the distress and ignore the requests for analgesia
3. They may seek to alleviate the distress as part of their overall management
4. They may give the patient inadequate treatment and reject them.

alternative answers, which are further illustrated by case examples. Each strategy represents a way of understanding the patient's needs and reflects the model of pain adopted by the clinician.

Consider Case Studies 1.1–1.3. Which answer do you consider to be appropriate in each case? Consider each option in terms of its recognition of pain and distress and whether a narrow medical or a cognitive–behavioural approach is being adopted.

Influence of symptom presentation on the treating doctor

Without a definitive diagnosis it is difficult for doctors to form a clear treatment plan. Doctors often do not know what to do with the patient and this may lead them to adopt a number of strategies as shown in Box 1.6.

The very fact that the patients' symptoms and signs do not match with the traditional model of the illness can have a subtle effect on the way that doctors communicate with and manage them. Firstly it colours doctors' beliefs about the veracity of the complaints. Doctors will tend to be dismissive of 'non-organic' findings. They will tend to ignore them at best or regard them as signs of malingering, faking, secondary gain or psychiatric problems at worst. Such 'behavioural findings' are often described as 'bizarre'.

Doctors, having made certain judgements about patients and their illnesses, begin (unwittingly) to

Case study 1.1

Straightforward case of uncontrollable pain behaviour that stops as soon as an epidural is working

Mrs G. was 32 years old and having her first baby. She had been admitted during the night having started in labour. Her contraction pains had increased steadily over the early morning, but she was still early on in labour. She became increasingly distressed by her pain and by mid-morning was literally screaming with pain. She became very restless and difficult for the midwives to manage. Clinical examinations were virtually impossible and she began to become progressively agitated. She became abusive, shouting and swearing. She would not let anyone near her to perform a vaginal examination to assess progress. She started throwing the Entonox around saying it was useless but would not listen to any instructions that would enable her to use it more successfully.

With much difficulty an epidural was successfully given. Mrs G.'s behaviour changed rapidly as the epidural became effective. Assessment was completed and there appeared to be no obstetric problems or cause for alarm. She apologised for her outburst and her labour continued uneventfully.

Case study 1.2

Marked pain behaviour that is not helped by an epidural

Mrs H. was 28 years old and was making very slow progress in labour. Her previous labour had also been difficult. She complained of a lot of pain, but this had not responded well to the usual pethidine. The pain had reached unbearable levels and she pleaded for something to be done. An epidural was given. The siting of the epidural, however, was difficult and painful and Mrs H. asked for a consultant to be brought to complete it. Not only was a consultant not available but unfortunately the epidural did not work perfectly. She continued to complain, demanded to know why it hadn't worked and requested that something further be done.

Mrs H. became even more agitated and started to complain about the soreness of the drip site, the epidural catheter in her back and a number of other things. The staff gradually became disaffected with her and began to ignore her complaints, giving them progressively less credence.

Unfortunately, when Mrs H. later became extremely distressed, the staff dismissed her pain complaints as being 'rather exaggerated'. It transpired that she was in obstructed labour and in fact needed an emergency caesarean section.

Case study 1.3

A patient with profound pain behaviour and little to find in the way of objective signs of nociception

Mr A. presented with chronic low back pain and a high level of disability. There were no positive neurological findings to suggest a prolapsed intervertebral disc or any major structural pathology. Apart from guarded movements and some behavioural responses to examination there was little else to find. Thorough physical examination and a review of health did not reveal any other problems. X-rays of lumbar spine were reviewed and a diagnosis of degenerative spinal disease was made. The degeneration was considered to be the principal cause of his pain.

Mr A. was very angry as he had been told in the past that there was nothing wrong with him. He was convinced that he had a serious problem with his back. He could walk only short distances with the aid of two walking sticks and spent most of his day resting because any activity caused intense pain. He had undergone a number of treatments without any relief. His doctors had given up on him.

Box 1.6

Interview strategies frequently adopted by doctors

- Further or repeated investigation on the assumption that something 'has been missed'
- Referral to another/different pain specialist
- A trial of treatment on the 'assumed' best bet diagnosis
- Communication in body language, if not explicitly, that the problem is psychiatric and possibly even referral to psychiatry
- No further offering of assistance.

communicate this to the patient. This is done in the way they talk to the patient, their (the doctor's) non-verbal behaviour and sometimes what they explicitly say to the patient. Often doctors are not aware that they communicate anything to the patient, but our experience has shown that most patients whom we have seen for assessment for pain management feel that it has been implied by their previous doctors that 'it is all in the mind'. This, of course, colours how patients interact with their doctors.

Effect on the patient of the doctor's 'difficulties'

The fact that the doctor appears not to make any sense of the physical findings is quickly perceived by the patient, who is then likely to lose confidence in the doctor. From the patient's point of view the doctor does not understand their problem or does not know enough about it. This in turn colours the way the patient communicates with the doctor. If patients suspect that their doctor does not believe them they may be reluctant to disclose more worrying symptoms. Furthermore, the patient will be less likely to accept the doctor's formulation or recommendations.

Unfortunately, patients may have no one else to turn to. If doctors order some more physical tests in the unremitting search for a purely physical explanation of patients' problems, then they will tend to go along with it, hoping that something will be found. Usually such hopes are dashed, the patient becomes even more distressed and the doctor–patient relationship is significantly damaged. This experience may be repeated with other doctors until patients then begin to lose faith in all doctors. They have become damaged and distressed by the process of seeking treatment. Their pain persists and they may believe they have to try even harder to persuade specialists that their pain is not 'all in the mind'. Unfortunately, the attempt to convince them often enhances their pain behaviour and therefore makes it even more likely for other doctors to be dismissive, especially if the patient has been previously described in their case notes as showing 'functional overlay'.

It can be seen how an attempt to understand chronic pain in terms of the narrow medical model not only fails to do justice to the complexity of the problem, but can be harmful to the patient and, in many cases, is probably responsible for a considerable proportion of the distress associated with chronic pain problems.

Models of disability

Discussion of clinical models is presented in this chapter. Discussion of a number of models with a particular occupational focus is deferred until Chapters 13–15.

Development of the biopsychosocial perspective

Many theoreticians and several different research groups have developed models of disability. Although some of the models are labelled as 'pain models', they are perhaps more appropriately understood as 'disability' or 'illness models'.

Engel (1977) is credited with the first use of the term 'biopsychosocial', but although his advocation of a better integration of mind and body, with inclusion of the social context of illness, was a significant advance on the

somewhat simplistic 'physical–mental dichotomy', his formulation focused heavily on psychodynamic constructs. Although not empirically based, his writings have had a huge influence, particularly on the development of liaison psychiatry (White 2005) and can be said to have inspired more recent statistically constructed biopsychosocial models such as the Glasgow Illness Model (see below).

Loeser model of pain and suffering

Loeser (1980) produced a hugely influential depiction of the relationship between pain and suffering illustrating an alternative to the mental–physical dichotomy (Fig. 1.13). Essentially it located nociception within a set of concentric 'shells' incorporating suffering, pain behaviour and the social context (or environment). The implication that one could not understand the impact of pain without incorporating these other elements represented a major conceptual shift in the understanding of pain and inspired the diagrammatic representation of the Glasgow Illness Model.

Glasgow Illness Model (GIM)

The GIM (Waddell et al 1984) was an early empirical attempt to disentangle physical and psychological factors in an attempt to explain why some patients, with (apparently) the same amount of physical impairment were more disabled than others. New measures of pain and disability (Waddell & Main 1984) were constructed, and using multiple regression models, the relationship between the two were examined. The additional influence of a large number of other variables, particularly psychological variables, and also pain measures were then

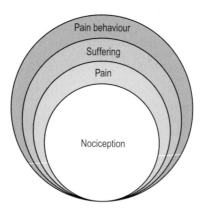

Figure 1.13 • Loeser's conceptual model of the dimensions of chronic pain. From Waddell (1998), reproduced with permission of Elsevier Ltd.

examined. The major findings of the set of research studies are shown in Box 1.7 and illustrated as in Figure 1.14.

These studies were important principally for three reasons. They demonstrated firstly that in patients with chronic non-specific low-back pain, their level of disability was only partly explicable by physical examination findings. Secondly the studies showed that the ways patients reacted to their pain were probably more important than had previously been understood. Finally, they suggested that explanation for high level of disability was more likely to be to do with the persistence of the pain and its effects, rather than some sort of pre-existing abnormality of personality.

There were three major limitations of the studies:

1 They were primarily cross-sectional cohort studies and so it was not possible to do more than suggest possible causal pathways.
2 Little more than a rudimentary attempt was made to examine social and occupational variables.
3 The psychological measures available at that time did not include specific measures of beliefs about pain, fear or coping strategies.

The studies nonetheless have been influential.

The model has been progressively refined and further developed, most recently in Waddell (2004) where the basic elements of the biopsychosocial model have been mapped onto the WHO-ICF model, as shown in Figure 1.14.

From models to classification

The complex issues of assessment and classification in relation to screening and targeting are considered in detail in later chapters, but it is important to appreciate at this juncture that models of pain and disability influence the design and development of descriptive systems attempting to incorporate biopsychosocial aspects of pain and disability. One such assessment system designed for chronic pain patients, based on the empirical integration of biomedical, psychosocial and behavioural data,

Box 1.7

Findings of the Glasgow illness studies

- The physical impairment variables explained about 40% of the variance in patients' disability scores
- There were slight gender differences
- Psychological factors explained about an additional 30% of variance in the disability scores
- Long-standing personality traits such as introversion or neuroticism, and hysteria or hypochondriasis were relatively unimportant
- Current distress, in the form of heightened somatic awareness and depressive symptoms, and pain behaviour, in the form of behavioural signs and symptoms were much more powerful influences on disability
- Even with statistical control for gender, and for differences in physical examination findings, distress and pain behaviour were significantly predictive of disability
- Development of pain behaviour was associated with the amount of previous failed treatment.

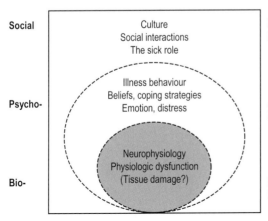

Figure 1.14 • A biopsychosocial model of low back pain and disability. ICF, International Classification of Functioning, Disability and Health: WHO, World Health Organization. From Waddell (2004), reproduced with permission of Elsevier Ltd.

Box 1.8

Turk and Rudy's MAP Classification

- *Dysfunctional*, characterised by patients who perceive the severity of their pain to be high, who report a high level of interference of pain in activities; indicate a high level of emotional distress and report a low level of activity
- *Interpersonally distressed*, who view others as not very understanding or supportive of their problems
- *Adaptive copers*, characterised by high levels of social support, relatively low levels of pain, low perceived interference, low distress, higher activity and a higher level of perceived control.

was the *Multi-axial Assessment of Pain (MAP)* (Turk & Rudy 1988). The system was developed originally from a 64-item questionnaire called the West Haven–Yale Multidimensional Pain Inventory, or WHYMPI (Kerns et al 1985). The first two sections of the questionnaire relate to patients' appraisal of pain and its effects on various aspects of life. The second part addresses patients' views of the reaction of others to their pain and its effects. The third part of the questionnaire assesses the frequency with which patients perform a range of activities. The authors claim wide empirical support for the validity of the questionnaire (Turk & Rudy 1990). The authors used cluster-analytic and multivariate classification methods to identify three different types of patient, which they have replicated across a wide range of pain patients with different pain diagnoses. The distinct patient profiles are shown in Box 1.8.

The MAP classification has been important in demonstrating that similar types of patients present with different sorts of pain disorders, and it has recently been recommended for the matching of patients to treatment (Turk 2005).

A similar attempt was offered by the P-A-I-N clustering of MMPI profiles by Robinson et al (1989). The MAP classification, however, seems to have better statistical and clinical validation. It would appear to have merit as a general screening system, but it is insufficiently accurate in the assessment of some of its elements to be used as a basis for individual clinical decision making in pain management.

Chronic disability and its development

During the last 25 years there has been a considerable amount of research into the identification, measurement and interpretation of the psychological components of the biopsychosocial model at various stages of chronicity. Once a chronic pain syndrome is clearly established, intensive therapeutic effort in the form of an interdisciplinary pain management programme (Ch. 11) may be required, but an overview of pain models and mechanisms would be incomplete without recognition of the complexity of the clinical syndrome which can develop and there have also been a number of attempts to depict interrelationships diagrammatically. Main & Spanswick (2000) offered a way of conceptualising chronic disability in a model comprising a number of stages. It is discussed in more detail in Chapter 11.

Linking pain experience and pain behaviour: the biopsychomotor conceptualisation of pain

According to Sullivan (2006) the current focus on the sensory dimensions of the pain system, and in a related fashion, the neglect of behaviour as an integral component of the pain system has limited theoretical advance and has also impeded the development of effective treatment approaches for individuals with pain conditions. A case can be made for viewing pain as a multidimensional system that includes behaviour as a *central and defining feature*. The biopsychomotor reconceptualisation is important both from a theoretical and from a clinical perspective.

Can pain be adaptive without behaviour?

From an evolutionary perspective, pain signals have been discussed as an internal mechanism that increases the probability of survival (Wall 1999). Central to the survival value of the pain system is the mobilisation of behaviour that will act on the source of the pain, or tend to the consequences of pain. Indeed, it could be argued that without a pain behaviour system, there would be no adaptive value to the pain signal itself.

A pain system without behaviour is as adaptive as a fire station without firemen.

The behaviour of pain involves more than the reflexive withdrawal of a limb from a pain stimulus. Individuals experiencing pain will often display a range of verbal and non-verbal pain behaviours. There is also a social response to pain behaviour where others might engage in protective or caring behaviour toward the injured individual.

The biopsychomotor model of pain retains two elements of Descartes' model; the lesion and the experience of pain but suggests that in addition to the sensory component of the pain system, it is important to consider two main intra-individual behavioural systems; the communicative behaviour system and the protective behaviour system (Sullivan et al 2006). The content of the model and its potential for identifying and implementing interventions is discussed further in the next chapter. It is to be hoped that research aiming to elucidate the meaning or significance of different pain behaviours might lead to the development of assessment or intervention tools that will improve the treatment experiences and treatment outcomes of individuals suffering from persistent pain conditions.

The biopsychosocial conceptualisation of pain and disability has been important in changing the way we think about pain and its treatment.

Concluding reflections

In so far as we can tell, pain has always been an aspect of the human condition, but its precise characterisation has been elusive. It has been regarded both as a sense and as an emotion, but prior to the time of Descartes there does not seem to have been any clear recognition that there was central processing of pain signals in the brain. The role of sensory transmission and central registration in the brain of pain signals was recognised by Descartes, but the 'divorce' of the mind from the body, which was explicit in his Cartesian dualism, posed considerable difficulties in explaining the relationship between the experience of pain and underlying physiology. The advent of Melzack & Wall's gate control theory of pain in 1965, however, has led to developments in both the physiology and the psychology of pain such that modern pain management requires consideration not only of the perception of pain, but of the reaction to it (whether behaviourally, cognitively or emotionally). The move from unidimensional explanations to multidimensional perspectives offers not only a formidable intellectual challenge but also a wonderful opportunity to improve our understanding of chronic pain and its management.

Key points

- **Chronic pain differs from acute pain and has to be understood in terms of a complex interplay between physical and psychological features**
- **The narrow disease model needs to be replaced with a broader illness model recognising the influence of both the social context of pain and suffering and the adaptive function of pain behaviour**
- **Decision making and management are coloured by the doctor's own implicit model of pain**
- **Inconsistencies in diagnosis and prescription of ineffective or ineffectual treatments may profoundly distress patients, thereby confounding their management**
- **Adequate formulation of the patient's problem requires a multidimensional perspective**
- **Chronic pain patients require illness management not just disease management**
- **Proper management of chronic pain requires recognition of the interplay between physical and psychological factors and the socioeconomic context in which the consultation occurs.**

References

Ahern D K, Follick M J, Council J R et al 1988 Comparison of lumber paravertebral EMG patterns in chronic low back pain patients and non-pain controls. Pain 34: 153–160

Arena J G, Sherman R A, Bruno G et al 1991 Electromyographic recordings of low back pain subjects and non-pain controls in six different positions: Effect of pain levels. Pain 45:23–28

Bantick S J, Wise R G, Ploghaus A et al 2002 Imaging how attention modulates pain in humans using functional MRI. Brain 125:310–319

Bonica J J 1990 History of pain concepts and therapies. In: Bonica J J (ed) The management of pain, 2nd edn. Lea & Febiger, New York, ch 1

Boos N, Rieder R, Schade V et al 1995 The diagnostic accuracy of magnetic resonance imaging, work perception and psychosocial factors in identifying symptomatic disc herniations. Spine 20:2613–2625

Bryant R A 1993 Memory for pain and affect in chronic pain patients. Pain 54:347–351

Bushnell M C, Duncan G H, Dubner R et al 1985 Attentional influences on noxious and innocuous cutaneous heat detection in humans and monkeys. Journal of Neuroscience 5:1103–1110

Bushnell M C, Villemure C, Duncan G H 2004 Psychophysical and neurophysiological studies of pain modulation by attention. In: Psychological methods of pain control: basic science and research perspectives. Progress in pain research and management, vol 29, Price D D, Bushnell M C (eds). IASP Press, Seattle, ch 5, pp 99–116

Chapman C R, Nakamura Y, Flores L Y 1999 Chronic pain and consciousness: a constructivist perspective. In: Gatchel R J, Turk D C (ed) Psychosocial perspectives in pain. The Guilford Press, New York, ch 3, pp 35–55

Coderre T J, Katz J, Vaccarino A L et al 1993 Contribution of central neuroplasticity to pathological pain: Review of clinical and experimental evidence. Pain 52:259–285

Craig K D 2003 A new view of pain as a homeostatic emotion. Trends in Neuroscience 26:303–307

Descartes R 1664 L'homme. E Angot, Paris

Engel G 1977 The need for a new medical model: a challenge for biomedicine. Science 196:129–136

Flor H, Birbaumer N 1994 Focus article: acquisition of chronic pain. Psychophysiological mechanisms. APS Journal (Pain Forum) 3(2):119–127

Flor H, Birbaumer N, Turk D C 1991 The psychobiology of chronic pain. Advances in Behavioural Research and Therapy 12:47–84

Flor H, Elbert T, Muhlnickel W 1998 Cortical reorganisation and phantom phenomena in congenital and traumatic upper-extremity amputees. Experimental Brain Research 119:205–212

Foster M 1901 Lectures on the history of physiology during the 16th, 17th and 18th centuries. Cambridge University Press, Cambridge

Fulop-Miller R 1938 Triumph over pain. Literary Guild of America. Republished 2005 by Kessinger Publishing, Kila, MT

Gifford L S 1998a Tissue and input related mechanisms. In: Gifford L S (ed) Topical issues in pain 1. Whiplash – science and management. Fear-avoidance beliefs and behaviour. CNS Press, Falmouth, pp 57–65

Gifford L S 1998b The 'central' mechanisms. In: Gifford L S (ed) Topical issues in pain 1. Whiplash – science and management. Fear-avoidance beliefs and behaviour. CNS Press, Falmouth, pp 67–80

Jones A K 2005 The role of the cerebral cortex in pain perception. In: Justins D M (ed) Pain 2005 – An updated review: refresher course syllabus. IASP Press, Seattle, ch 7, pp 59–68

Kerns R D, Turk D C, Rudy T E 1985 The West Haven-Yale Multidimensional Pain Inventory (WHYMPI). Pain 23:345–356

Legrain V, Guerit J M, Bruyer R et al 2002 Attentional modulation of the nociceptive processing into the human brain: selective spatial attention, probability of stimulus occurrence, and target detection on laser evoked potentials. Pain 99:21–39

Letchuman R, Deusinger R H 1993 Comparison of sacrospinalis myoelectric activity and pain levels in patients undergoing static and intermittent lumbar traction. Spine 18:1361–1365

Loeser J D 1980 Perspectives on pain. In: Turther P (ed) Clinical pharmacy and therapeutics. Macmillan, London, pp 313–316

McAlindon T, Snow S, Cooper C et al 1992 Radiographic patterns of osteoarthritis of the knee joint in the community: the importance of the patellofemoral joint. Annals of the Rheumatic Diseases 51:844–849

Main C J, Spanswick C C 2000 Pain management: An interdisciplinary approach. Churchill Livingstone, Edinburgh

Manning B H 2004 Preclinical studies of pain modulation. In: Psychological methods of pain control: basic science and research perspectives. Progress in pain research and management, vol 29, Price D D, Bushnell, M C (eds), IASP Press, Seattle, ch 3, pp 43–71

Melzack R 1996 Focus article: Gate control theory: on the evolution of pain concepts. Pain Forum 5:128–138

Melzack R 1999 Pain and stress: A new perspective. In: Gatchel R J, Turk D C (eds) Psychosocial perspectives in pain, The Guilford Press, New York, ch 6, pp 89–106

Melzack R, Casey K L 1968 Sensory, motivational and central control determinants of pain. In: Kenshalo D R (ed) The skin senses. Charles C Thomas, Springfield IL, pp 423–439

Melzack R, Wall P D 1965 Pain mechanisms: a new theory. Science 150:971–979

Melzack R, Wall P D 1983 The challenge of pain. Basic Books, New York

Mense S 1997 Pathophysiologic basis of muscle pain syndromes. An update. Physical Medicine and Rehabilitation Clinics of North America 8:23–53

Orbach R, McCall W D 1996 The stress-hyperactivity-pain theory of myogenic pain: proposal for a revised theory. Pain Forum 5:51–66

Price D D 1999 Psychological mechanisms of pain and analgesia. Progress in pain and analgesia, vol 1. Seattle, IASP Press

Price D D, Bushnell M C (eds) 2004 Psychological methods of pain control: basic science and research perspectives. Progress in pain research and management, vol 29. IASP Press, Seattle

Rainville P 2004 Pain and emotions. In: Psychological methods of pain control: basic science and research perspectives. Progress in pain research and management, vol 29, Price D D, Bushnell, M C (eds), IASP Press, Seattle, ch 6, pp 117–141

Riley J L III, Wade J B 2004 Psychological and demographic factors that modulate the different stages and dimensions of pain. In: Psychological methods of pain control: basic science and research perspectives. Progress in pain research and management, vol 29, Price D D, Bushnell M C (eds), IASP Press, Seattle, ch 2, pp 19–41

Robinson M E, Swimmer G I, Rallof D 1989 The P-A-I-N MMPI classification system: a critical review. Pain 37:211–214

Simons D G, Mense S 1998 Understanding and measurement of muscle tone as related to clinical muscle pain. Pain 75:1–17

Sullivan, M J L 2006 Toward a biopsychomotor conceptualisation of pain. Clinical Journal of Pain (in press)

Sullivan, M J L, Stanish, W D, Thibault et al 2006 The influence of communication goals and physical demands on different dimensions of pain behavior. Pain (in press)

Travell J G, Simons D G 1993 Myofascial pain and dysfunction: the trigger point manual. Williams & Wilkins, Baltimore, MD

Turk D C 2005 The potential of treatment matching for subgroups of patients with chronic pain: lumping versus splitting. Clinical Journal of Pain 21:44–55

Turk D C, Rudy T E 1988 Towards an empirically derived taxonomy of chronic pain patients: integration of psychological assessment data. Journal of Consulting and Clinical Psychology 56:233–238

Turk D C, Rudy T E 1990 The robustness of an empirically derived taxonomy of chronic pain patients. Pain 42:27–35

Virchow R 1858 Cellular pathologie in ihrer Begrundurg auf physiologische und pathologische. A Hirschwald, Berlin

Waddell G 1998 The back pain revolution. Churchill Livingstone, Edinburgh

Waddell G 2004 The back pain revolution, 2nd edn. Churchill Livingstone, Edinburgh

Waddell G, Main C 1984 Assessment of severity in low back disorders. Spine 9:204–208

Waddell G, Bircher M, Finlayson D et al 1984 Symptoms and signs: physical disease or illness behaviour? British Medical Journal 289:739–741

Waersted, M, Westgaard R H 1996 Attention-related muscle activity in different body regions during VDU work with minimal physical activity. Ergonomics 39(4):661–676

Wall P D 1999 Pain: the science of suffering. Weidenfeld and Nicholson, London

Watson P J 2002 Psychophysiological models of pain. In Gifford L (ed) Topical issues in pain, vol 3. CNS Press, Falmouth, pp 181–198

Watson P J, Booker C K, Main C J et al 1997a Surface electromyography in the identification of chronic low back pain patients: the development of a flexion relaxation ratio. Clinical Biomechanics 12(3):165–171

Watson P J, Booker C K, Main C J 1997b Evidence for the role of psychological factors in abnormal paraspinal activity in patients with chronic low back pain. Journal of Musculoskeletal Pain 5(4):41–56

Westgaard, R H 1999 Effects of physical and mental stressors on muscle pain. Scandinavian Journal of Work, Environment and Health 25(Suppl 4):19–24

White P (ed) 2005 Biopsychosocial medicine: an integrated approach to understanding illness. Oxford University Press, Oxford

Williams A C de C 2002 Facial expression of pain: an evolutionary account. Behavioral and Brain Sciences 25:439–455

Chapter Two

2

Psychological mechanisms

CHAPTER CONTENTS

A diverse array of cognitive, behavioural, emotional and environmental factors have been identified as key components of a complex pain modulation system. As has been stated in the previous chapter, the critical role of psychological factors in the perception of pain has now been demonstrated.

Lessons from the history of medicine

Perhaps one of the earliest persuasive demonstrations of the role of psychosocial factors in pain perception came from the work of Anton Mesmer in the mid-1700s. Mesmer, a student of divinity, law and medicine first experimented with the healing power of magnets (Fulop-Miller 1938). He found repeatedly that magnets applied to the body of an ailing person appeared to alleviate pain and suffering. Later, Mesmer believed that the 'vital magnetism' emanated not from within the magnets, but from within his own body. Soon he claimed he was able to alleviate pain and suffering simply by passing his hands over ailing persons.

Mesmer's treatment became so popular that he was unable to treat all who sought his help. The demand for his treatment led him to develop ways of treating many individuals at once. Mesmer realised that he could magnetise objects which then could hold the healing vital magnetism for a period of time. In Paris, Mesmer magnetised trees and water fountains where people could gather and be cured of their condition.

In his clinic (Fig. 2.1), Mesmer built *baquets* to facilitate the treatment of several individuals at once.

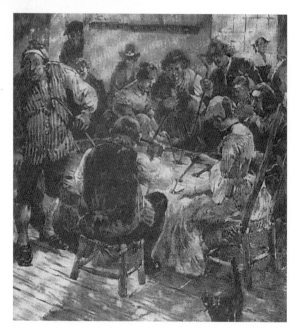

Figure 2.1 • Patients attending Anton Mesmer's clinic. From Coleman J (1950). Individuals suffering from pain conditions crowded Anton Mesmer's clinic to receive the healing powers of 'vital magnetism'.

The *baquets* were large tubs built of wood and filled with water. On the bottom of the baquet, Mesmer carefully arranged pieces of glass and metal. Once the *baquets* were infiltrated with his healing magnetism, patients would gather around the *baquet*. They would place large metal rods into the *baquet* and touch one end of the rod to the part of their body that was in pain. The healing forces of vital magnetism flowed up the metal rod and into the body of the ailing person, thus curing them of their affliction.

A disciple of Mesmer, Puységur discovered that through magnetism, patients could be made to experience an artificial sleep, or trance state. For decades to follow, surgeons in France, Scotland and England would claim that surgeries could be performed painlessly once patients had been 'mesmerised' into artificial sleep.

In a world that had yet to develop effective analgesics for the control of pain, magnetism was deemed a divine gift. The Scottish surgeon John Elliotson declared that 'God, in His infinite mercy, had implanted in the human body the healing power of animal magnetism' (Fulop-Miller 1938). However, Mesmer's magnetism soon fell into disfavour as a means of controlling pain and suffering. In 1785, the Academy of Sciences rejected the claims of Mesmer and his followers, and concluded that magnetism was devoid on any medical or scientific value.

In 1803, Friedrich Serturner discovered morphine (Rey 1993). Although the analgesic properties of opium had been recognised long before as in the laudanum preparations described by Paracelsus and later Sydenham, these preparations were crude and were considered unsafe by the medical community. But the purification of the active substance in the poppy seed was to forever change the relationship between humans and pain. The powerful analgesic properties of morphine drew increased attention to the physical basis of pain and interest in the psychosocial basis of pain perception waned.

It was not until the 1950s that questions about psychosocial factors in pain perception began once again to draw the attention of clinicians and researchers. Beecher's (1956) naturalistic observations of war casualties sparked renewed debate on the psychosocial aspects of pain. Working as a military physician, Beecher was struck by the wide range of soldiers' responses to injury and pain. Beecher (1956) provided vivid descriptions of soldiers who had sustained severe wounds in combat yet did not request narcotics to alleviate their pain. He suggested that for many soldiers, the wounds may have represented their 'ticket to safety' and that their pain experience may have been lessened by this positive reinterpretation.

By the mid-1960s, mounting clinical and scientific evidence was calling for a model of pain that would consider both the physiological and psychological mechanisms involved in pain perception. The call was most compellingly answered by Melzack and Wall's Gate Control Theory of Pain (Melzack & Wall 1965).

Historical foundations of the modern psychology of pain

The study of individual differences in the clinical field, however, was dominated by four separate paradigms which led to a number of integrative models, as shown in Box 2.1.

The psychodynamic model was heavily influenced by psychosomatic theories and purported to explain disease in terms of emotional mediation. According to classical psychoanalytical tradition, the psychological component was to be understood in terms of unconscious conflicts, established during childhood, 'reactivated' during situations of stress during adulthood and 'expressed' in a range of somatic symptoms that, if sufficiently severe, could lead to illness. Initially physicians believed that pain was caused by organic *or* psychological factors. Persistent pain that eluded diagnosis or

Box 2.1

Major paradigms in the psychology of pain

- Psychodynamic (derived from psychosomatic theory)
- Personality theory (derived from classical psychopathological theory)
- Behavioural model (derived from the experimental analysis of behaviour)
- Cognitive model
- Integrated models:
  - cognitive–behavioural models
  - psychophysiological and psychobiological models
  - biopsychomotor model.

treatment was labelled as hysterical or psychogenic and relegated to the psychiatric domain. Pain was explained as a defence against psychic conflict and psychoanalytic approaches were used in treatment. According to this model, ideas or conflicts that were too anxiety provoking to be experienced consciously were suppressed and 'converted' into pain symptoms. In essence, pain symptoms were seen as an expression of underlying 'psychic pain' (Blumer & Heilbronn 1982). Typically, the patient continued to suffer pain while the psyche was examined and 'treated'.

Personality was also invoked as a factor that might explain pain conditions. Engel (1959) suggested that individuals with certain personality features might be predisposed to develop chronic pain conditions. Although the early work in this area was anecdotal, ostensibly 'objective', approaches were later employed where personality profiles of pain patients were investigated using tests such as the Minnesota Multiphasic Personality Inventory (MMPI) and the later MMPI-2 (Hathaway & McKinley 1967, Butcher et al 1989).

The personality model with its understanding of individual differences in terms of personality profiles seemed to offer an advance on the previously largely unsubstantiated clinical observations, or on the 'pseudo-objectivity' of projective tests such as the Rorschach ink-blot test. Research in this area was not very rigorous and led to inconsistent findings. Although there is no consensus about the role of personality in pain experience, the bulk of research has not supported the view that there exists a 'pain-prone' personality.

Fordyce (1976) offered the most radical departure from the disease model of illness and applied principles of learning theory to account for the behavioural displays observed in pain patients. According to the principles of operant conditioning, behaviours are influenced by their consequences. A particular behaviour (e.g. moaning) that is followed by a positive consequence (e.g. empathic attention) will have a higher probability of being emitted in the future, regardless of the level of pain. In this case, 'moaning' becomes instrumental in achieving empathic attention. Fordyce (ibid) argued that while pain behaviours might be reactive to pain experience in the short term, in the long term these behaviours increasingly come under the control of environmental reinforcement contingencies. Pain *behaviour* became the focus of therapeutic investigation and intervention, and led to the development of behaviourally based rehabilitation programmes, the forerunners of modern interdisciplinary pain management programmes.

Cognitive-behavioural approaches have dominated recent intervention research on psychosocial factors associated with pain and disability. Cognitive-behavioural perspectives proceed from the view that an individual's interpretation, evaluation and beliefs about their health condition, and their coping repertoire with respect to pain and disability will impact on the degree of emotional and physical disability that they will experience (Turk & Gatchel 1999, Gatchel & Turk 2002, Vlaeyen & Linton 2000). It is important to note that the term cognitive–behavioural does not refer to a specific intervention but, rather, to a class of intervention strategies. The strategies included under the heading of cognitive–behavioural interventions vary widely and may include self-instruction (e.g. motivational self-talk), relaxation or biofeedback, developing coping strategies (e.g. distraction, imagery), increasing assertiveness, minimising negative or self-defeating thoughts, changing maladaptive beliefs about pain, and goal setting (Turk et al 1983, Linton & Andersson 2000). A client referred for cognitive–behavioural intervention may be exposed to varying selections of these strategies.

Psychophysiological and psychobiological models have attempted to integrate the psychological aspects of pain with physiology and offer a bridge between the experience or pain, and its physiological and biochemical substrates, whether in terms of peripheral or central mechanisms. The inherent attractiveness in terms of explanatory power and level of integration, however, is tempered somewhat by the inherent difficulties in measurement and in replication of full-blown clinical pain in experimental environments. (They are discussed in more detail in Ch. 1.)

In terms of psychological models, perhaps the most helpful model, from both the theoretical and the clinical point of view, is the recently developed biopsychomotor model (Sullivan 2006). It is discussed later in this chapter.

Psychological influences on pain and incapacity: a clinical overview

Psychological factors have a wide-ranging effect on the perception of pain and its effects. These are summarised in Box 2.2.

As observed in the previous chapter, there is now convincing evidence that central mechanisms can influence the perception of nociceptive signals from the periphery of the body. It is commonly observed clinically that pain 'feels worse' when patients are feeling tired or depressed. Pain often seems to feel worse during the night when the brain has 'less to do'. Attentional factors are also important (Eccleston 1995); some patients can be taught to distract themselves quite successfully from pain. Research has also shown that individuals differ not only in pain threshold but also in their ability to discriminate pain of different qualities and intensities. The reasons for this are not fully understood. Research into memory for pain, however, suggests that aversive pain memories may have a powerful influence on the perception of new pain stimuli (Bryant 1993). Finally, psychobiological investigations have demonstrated a wide range of conditioned peripheral and central responses to pain involving both physiological and biochemical events (Flor & Turk 1989).

In conclusion, it would appear that the significance of fundamental psychological mechanisms in the perception of clinical pain may be of much more importance than has been recognised hitherto.

Psychological influences on health-care seeking are well recognised. Decisions to seek health care are dependent on perception of physiological functioning and interpretation of symptoms. These in turn have to be understood in terms of the individual's 'model of illness'. Simply put, unless an individual perceives a symptomatic abnormality that is defined in health terms, the issue of consultation does not arise. The individual has to believe further, however, that it is appropriate to consult with the symptom: that the doctor or therapist is likely to be able to help and some good will result from the consultation. Of course these beliefs are themselves multiply determined and will have been influenced by the individual's sociocultural background, tolerance of symptoms and the impact of symptoms on quality of life and work (Skevington 1995).

Some of the more important psychological factors influencing response to treatment are shown in Box 2.3.

Patients attending pain clinics or pain management programmes have often seen several other professionals. Failed treatment can have a profoundly demoralising effect. The patient may have lost confidence in the likely benefit of *any* further treatment. They may be concerned that 'something has been missed' (e.g. cancer). They may be significantly disaffected with healthcare professionals, particularly if they feel they have been misled in terms of likely benefit from treatment, if they feel that they have not been believed or it has been implied that the problem is 'all in their mind'. Such iatrogenic factors can have a significant influence both on a patient's decision to accept treatment or to comply with it.

At times it is helpful to consider the psychological influence on pain from a familial rather than an individual perspective. Individuals' reactions to pain are heavily influenced by the limitations imposed by it. Inability to sustain the previous role in the family, whether as a breadwinner or as a care provider, can have a profound effect on morale. Changes in role necessitated by pain-associated incapacity may not only have practical and financial implications, but they may also have a significant effect on relationships within a family.

Box 2.2

Influence of psychological factors on pain and incapacity

- Fundamental mechanisms
- Health-care seeking
- Response to treatment
- The family context
- Recovery from injury and development of chronic incapacity.

Box 2.3

Influence of psychological factors on response to treatment

- Patient's expectation
- Non-specific (placebo) responses to treatment
- Compliance with treatment (including adherence to treatment protocols)
- Acceptance of appropriate responsibility for the management of their symptomatology.

Pain affects families, not just patients. Sleep disturbance, depressed mood, increased irritability and disturbed sexual functioning can be difficult to tolerate by those living with the pain patient. This change in affairs may lead in turn to distress, disaffection and hostility directed towards the patient. Alternatively it may lead to oversolicitous behaviour and the reinforcement of maladaptive behaviours and (eventually) to chronic invalidism.

Several recent studies in back pain have demonstrated not only that psychological factors are predictive of a wide range of treatments but also that they are more powerful predictors than demographic factors, clinical history or clinical examination findings. Their influence is seen in the treatment response not only of patients with chronic pain, but also of those with acute pain (Burton et al 1995). The implications of these findings are important and have led to a shift of emphasis from tertiary care to secondary prevention both in health care and in occupational settings.

Psychological impact of different types of pain

Features of pain experience such as its intensity, duration, probable cause, predictability and controllability can impact in important ways on an individual's emotional state. Different sorts of pain may also have widely differing psychological impacts, and different types of pain are perceived differently by doctors as well as by patients. Of general concern to patients is the cause of their pain, its likelihood of responding to treatment and what they can expect in the future. Pain associated with disease (such as rheumatoid arthritis) may have a predictable relationship with recurrence of inflammation. Such pain is not necessarily easier to tolerate, but it is more easily comprehended and consistently managed. Several of the special problems are shown in Box 2.4.

Box 2.4

Special problems in the psychological impact of pain

- Difficulties in diagnosis
- Degree of successful pain control
- Impact on everyday life
- Likely future course.

With acute pain, clear diagnosis often can be made with little disagreement amongst diagnosticians. With chronic pain problems, however, patients may have been offered a variety of diagnoses. Lack of consistency and clarity in diagnosis can be extremely distressing for patients because they may worry that the 'real' cause of their pain has not been established. Such diagnostic confusion in turn undermines their confidence in their treating doctors or therapists and can lead to the sort of iatrogenic distress described above.

Different pains are controllable to different extents. Neurogenic pain is particularly unresponsive to analgesics and can therefore be particularly distressing. Alternatively some types of pain may be responsive to analgesics or non-steroidal drugs but only in doses that produce significant side-effects that are difficult to tolerate. Radicular pain may be eased by resting and exacerbated by walking. Headache may be predominantly stress related, postural or cardiovascular in origin, and therefore manageable to different extents.

Pain differs not only in quality and severity but also in its impact on activities of daily living, quality of life and work. There is evidence that whether or not people become depressed with pain is dependent primarily, perhaps surprisingly, not on the severity of the pain but on the extent to which it interferes with their life. Emotional distress states such as depression and anxiety are common consequences of pain and may in turn reduce pain tolerance. (The impact of pain on mental health is discussed in more detail in the next chapter.) The likely *effects* of the pain therefore have to be considered in evaluating the likely psychological impact of a particular pain condition.

The probable future course also varies amongst pain conditions. This is also unrelated to the severity of the pain. Patients are often able to muster resources to cope reasonably successfully with pain of short duration. Pain that is likely to become chronic requires a much wider range of coping skills and may require a range of alternative coping strategies.

In summary, although there are many similarities in the nature and management of chronic pain problems, it is important to allow for variations in the likely psychological impact of different sorts of pain.

Pain and emotion

The experience of pain

It has long been recognised that there is no one-to-one relation between injury and pain experience. At times, severe injuries may be associated with little or no pain. At other times, seemingly insignificant injuries can be associated with excruciating pain. There will also be instances, such as is the case in many chronic pain conditions, of significant pain in the absence of any discernible organic pathology or at least physical findings considered insufficient to explain the severity of the pain (Waddell 2004). It is becoming increasingly apparent, however, that there is a direct influence of psychological factors on the experience of pain. Emotional distress states such as depression or anxiety can increase the amount of pain a person will experience in a painful situation. It has been repeatedly shown that increased attention to pain sensations will lead to increased perception of pain. Indeed some investigators have suggested that attention might be the final common pathway through which psychological factors influence pain experience (Sullivan et al 2002). Any psychological factor that draws attention to pain will increase pain perception. Conversely, any psychological factor that draws attention away from pain will decrease pain perception.

The direct emotional impact of pain

The link between pain and emotion in terms of physical mechanisms was addressed in the previous chapter but the topic also commands considerations from the clinical perspective. Thus the level of distress is not simply explained by the pain intensity, but appears to be mediated by a number of cognitive factors (concerning beliefs about the nature of pain and the significance attached to it), discussed below, but also influenced by the nature and extent of the impact of the pain on function and quality of life. Arguably the almost exclusive focus on sickness and disability, as opposed to factors which may protect us from, or minimise the emotional impact, has led us to underestimate the importance of self-reliance in the battle against pain.

The emotional impact of pain can range from the mildly distressing to the overwhelming, with the level of emotional distress characterising patients presenting to clinics as lying usually between these two extremes. It should be appreciated that a certain degree of distress is *appropriate* when confronted with persisting pain or pain-associated limitations. Level of emotional impact is a predictor of chronicity and thus should be viewed as a 'yellow flag' (Ch. 5), although if of sufficient intensity it should be viewed as an 'orange flag' (Ch. 3) and specialist help should be sought.

A brief introduction to the concept of flags is presented at the end of this chapter and the impact of pain from a mental health perspective is considered further in the next chapter.

The emotional impact of pain-associated limitations

Clinically it is well recognised that in addition to altered mood, chronic pain is frequently associated also with disturbed sleep, strain on relationships, and diminished quality of life. The demoralising effects of pain can be enhanced still further if it has a significant financial impact. Economic hardship resulting from unemployment is well recognised, but an individual's economic situation can also directly influence treatment seeking and response to treatment.

The major spheres of influence are summarised in Box 2.5.

Increase in family hardship

The economic impact may be felt not only by the individual, but also by their family. This can further enhance feelings of despair, frustration and sometimes guilt. As aforementioned, the family may or may not have the arrangements or opportunities to mitigate the economic impact.

Strain on relationships

Families of chronic pain patients sometimes seem to have made remarkable adjustments to mitigate financial loss without apparent strain on relationships, but even the strongest of relationships can be strained by economic adversity. Even if it is possible to mitigate the hardship, this may be only at the cost of placing a significant strain on relationships. Frequently, the partner of the major breadwinner will feel obliged to increase

Box 2.5

Possible adverse effects of economic factors

- Increase in personal stress
- Increase in family hardship
- Strain on relationships
- Treatment seeking and legitimisation of symptoms
- Acceptance of treatment by the patient
- Acceptance or rejection for treatment by the health-care professional.

their hours of work or find a new or better paid job to compensate for the shortfall. This may result in increasing tiredness, impaired quality of life and resentment at having to make major changes to the pattern of family life. There may be effects also on relationships with the extended family, if help with childcare becomes necessary in order to obtain further paid work.

Treatment seeking and legitimisation of symptoms

First and foremost, consultation with doctors is motivated by a search for a diagnosis and cure. There are, however, other factors affecting treatment seeking. Sick certification by a medical practitioner may be necessary for entitlement to benefits of various sorts. In the UK, self-certification is permitted for up to 5 days, after which medical ratification is required for entitlement to benefit. Employers vary in the amount of self-certification they will tolerate in an individual period before formal appraisal of health status is initiated, but it is certainly the case that legitimisation of the complaint is a major factor in consultation with doctors. In families under strain, particularly with prolonged sickness absences, doubts may have been raised about the 'legitimacy' of the pain, and whether the patient is genuinely as incapacitated as they claim. (As discussed below, such doubts may have been raised within medicolegal reports.)

Cognitive influences on the experience of pain

The term 'cognitive' has come to refer to a wide range of factors influencing the perception of pain and response to treatment, but it is perhaps helpful to think of these in terms of three distinct fields of enquiry, shown in Box 2.6.

It should be remembered, however, that even though it is possible to distinguish separate aspects of cognition, each patient is characterised by an individual combination of cognitive features, which underpins the appraisal of pain and the response to treatment. The complexity of these interrelationships is indicated in the following quotation:

> *Patients who believe they can control their pain, who avoid catastrophising about their condition; and who believe they are not severely disabled appear to function better than those who do not. Such beliefs may mediate some of the relationships between pain severity and adjustment.*

(Jensen et al 1991, p. 249)

Health beliefs models (HBMs)

Within the field of health psychology there have been a large number of theoretical models attempting to link thoughts, emotion and behaviour in health-care contexts. Indeed many of the theoretical constructs underpinning measurement instruments used in the pain field have their origins in other aspects of health care. Some of the earlier research into the influence of fear on health threats suggested that there was a parallel processing of health information and that beliefs or appraisals (cognitive representations) of events could be distinguished from the emotional representation in terms of fear or arousal. Furthermore, these cognitive representations of threats could be distinguished from resulting actions or action plans.

According to Petrie & Weinman (1998) these attributes

> *provided the basis for the coping responses or procedures for dealing with the health threat. Thus, in being faced with a situation such as the experience of an unusual symptom, or the provision of a diagnosis from a doctor, individuals will construct their own representation which, in turn, will determine the behaviour and other responses, including help-seeking and medicine-taking. In addition to their representations of the threat, the individual will also draw upon their expectations and beliefs about the different behavioural choices (pp. 2–3).*

Although pain has certain distinct features that make it more puzzling and potentially problematic than other symptoms, the representational perspective is helpful in offering a possible framework for understanding the response to pain. Recent interest in self-help approaches to health is based on the recognition that individuals can influence their own health and well-being in a wide variety of situations. Indeed the notion of self-help is fundamental to the philosophy of pain management.

Social cognition models (SCM) are now widely employed in health psychology. According to Conner &

Box 2.6

Aspects of cognition

- The nature of cognitive processes
- Specific beliefs about pain and treatment
- Pain coping styles/strategies.

Norman (1998) they can be divided into 'attribution models', focusing primarily on individuals' beliefs about cause (causal attributions) and a second more diverse set of models (of which the best known are probably the theory of planned behaviour, or TPB, and the theory of reasoned action, or TRA) invoked to try to predict future health-related behaviours and outcomes. There are three major concerns about the usefulness of these theoretical models. First, although conceptually illuminating, there is as yet little research on the predictive value of these models (Quine et al 1998). Secondly, there is controversy about the relative utility of beliefs 'supplied' by the models and individually generated beliefs (Agnew 1998). Finally, different cognitions may be important at different stages of the initiation and maintenance of health behaviour.

There has been little research specifically into the utility of HBMs to either the treatment of rehabilitation in general or pain in particular. Kerns et al (1997) have tried to apply the transtheoretical model of change (Prochaska & DiClemente 1982) to pain patients, but in a recent review Dijkstra (2005) considered that the theory needed further development and refinement.

In conclusion, the utility of HBMs to the understanding of pain or its treatment needs to be systematically investigated. Most of the development and discussion of such models seems to have been in the 1980s and 90s. There would appear to be a number of promising avenues for exploration, but the specific value of these models in the pain field has not as yet been demonstrated empirically.

The self-regulation model or SRM (Leventhal et al 1998) as a conceptual framework does, however, have some intuitive appeal, perhaps because it offers a way of linking a patient's understanding of illness with their response to it. Horne (2006) identifies seven major components of the theory. They are summarised in Box 2.7.

Health threats. Internal threats (such as experience of symptoms) or external threats (such as medical warnings) lead us to build up an illness representation (or 'mental map') of our condition.

Illness representations ('mental maps'). There are five major components of these maps: the nature of the problem (identity); how long we expect it to last (timeline); what caused it (cause); its likely effects (consequences); and its prognosis (control/cure). Our answers to these questions, including our emotional reaction, make up our mental map.

Symptom experiences and labels. Our experience of these symptoms and the way they are labelled and managed as part of our interactions with the health-care systems is progressively shaped, and in the case of chronic illness may become characterised by iatrogenic confusion and distress. According to Horne (2006), 'Perpetual experiences are generally more persuasive than abstract ideas' (p. 122).

Search for coherence. We try to understand the illness in common-sense terms (find coherence).

Representations influencing action. Our mental maps strongly influence our decision about how to respond to the illness (and whether or not to follow medical advice).

Dynamic interaction of beliefs and behaviour. Our beliefs and behaviour mutually interact and influence each other. In the course of a chronic illness there may be a whole plethora of such interactions, changing across time.

Role of emotion. Cognitive and emotional processing occur in parallel, and some reactions thus may appear to be irrational and lead to unhelpful, and sometimes medically inadvisable responses to the perceived threat.

The themes are explored further with reference to the understanding and management of medically unexplained symptoms by Salmon (2006) who considers persistent medically unexplained medical symptoms to be not so much a 'property of the patient' but a 'consequence of the doctor's inability to explain symptoms' and depicts patients as 'casualties of the dualistic structure of medical care and beliefs' (p. 153).

Cognitive processes and the experience of pain

Within this complex set of inter-relating mechanisms, there appear to be a number of key elements which

---

Box 2.7

Main tenets of the Self-Regulation Model (SRM)

- Health threats
- Illness representations ('mental maps')
- Symptom experiences and labels
- Search for coherence
- Representations influencing action
- Dynamic interaction of beliefs and behaviour
- Role of emotion.

individually, and in combination, influence the experience of pain. They are shown in Box 2.8.

Attention

The role of attention is central in pain perception. We know from experience that distraction is a valuable clinical technique in the management of pain, as for example in the management of children undergoing invasive medical procedures (Kuttner 1989). We know from the neuroimaging research referenced in the previous chapter that attentional processes modulate pain perception at multiple brain areas, and that experimentally induced pain can be altered by the manipulation of patients' expectations and that these 'top-down mechanisms' related to expectation may contribute to the modulation of pain (Chapman & Okifuji 2004).

Anticipation

The important role of anticipation of pain has not always been recognised. Anticipation, based on prior (or imagined) experience, in the context of specific beliefs about illness, in conjunction with emotional responses can establish unhelpful patterns of escape and avoidance resulting in some control of pain, but at a cost of unnecessary pain-associated limitations. According to Flor & Hermann (2004) there are three important ways in which anticipation may influence the experience of pain: explicit expectation of uncontrollable painful stimulation may make subsequent nociceptive input more noxious; higher perceived levels of pain lead to avoidance; and the presence of pain may affect the way in which pain-related and other information is processed.

Differences in the way information is processed

Experimental studies of various sensory modalities have shown differences in how different people process

Box 2.8

Important mechanisms in the cognitive processing of pain

- Attention
- Anticipation
- Differences in the way information is processed
- Cognitive distortion
- Memory
- Worry
- Vigilance and hypervigilance.

information in terms of accuracy and consistency of judgement. The 'demand characteristics' of the experimental setting can exert a profound influence on the responses elicited from a subject.

Studies of subjects faced with experimental pain stimuli have also shown consistent individual differences in how subjects respond to the same stimulus. Researchers have wondered whether such differences are consistent across other different pain stimuli (such as cold, heat and pressure) and whether it is possible to identify differences in the manner or style of response. Unfortunately, with clinical pain it is not possible to examine the phenomenon with the same degree of precision since the 'pain stimulus' cannot be controlled with the same level of accuracy. Researchers, however, offered a number of ways of considering differences in how patients respond to pain.

Cognitive distortion

Psychosomatic theorists interpreted coping with pain in terms of defences against physical threat. Subjects (or patients) thought to be underestimating the severity of pain (or perceived threat) were considered to be using 'denial' or 'repression'. This defensive style of coping was thought to be an automatic response to threat. Typically 'repressors' have low scores on self-report measures of anxiety, and high scores on measures of defensive avoidance or social disapproval. Such psychological mechanisms are considered to have their physiological and biochemical correlates. Simply put, the extent to which 'denial' or 'repression' is successful in reducing perceived threat or anxiety determines its success as a coping strategy.

Memory

According to Flor & Hermann (2004), memory of pain may lead to selective focus on stimuli which predict pain and increase avoidance. Furthermore such memories may themselves become triggers for pain. Thus Rimm & Litvak (1969), in an early study demonstrated that subjects showed physiological arousal merely by thinking about painful experiences. More recently Flor & Hermann (2004) have investigated the importance of somatosensory pain memories in the process of cortical reorganisation after phantom limb injury. They conclude:

> *We assume that the operant conditioning processes may lead to the establishment of both explicit (conscious) and implicit (subconscious and automatic) memories for pain leading to the*

formation of cortical and sub-cortical cell assemblies with a large associative network . . . thus such memories increase the likelihood that a chronic pain sufferer will maintain a host of learned pain responses on the subjective-verbal, the physiological and the motor-behavioural level and on all levels of the nervous system (p. 65).

Worry

According to Eccleston & Crombez (1999), 'The cognitive reality of chronic pain patients is one of repetitive preoccupation with threatening thoughts about pain and its effects on oneself.' Worry is thought to be useful in problem solving. Aldrich et al (2000), in conceptualising the nature of worry in the context of pain have argued that the two important features of chronic pain are that:

- The pain represents a persistent aversive signal of threat
- The pain constitutes a problem without an acceptable solution.

Eccleston et al (2001) compared pain-related and non-pain-related worry in patients with chronic pain. They concluded:

The pattern of results suggests that the characteristics of worrying in chronic pain patients do not arise from a general disposition to worry . . . or from a general disposition to anxiety . . . worrying about pain is a normal process which is triggered in many cases by an increase in pain and is specifically related to current distress and awareness of somatic sensations . . . In the presence of a threat of pain, a normal vigilance to pain and other somatic sensations is established . . . in the absence of an immediate escape from pain, worrying about pain and its consequences emerges. This worry about pain is intrusive, attentionally demanding and difficult to disengage from (p. 316).

Vigilance and hypervigilance (HV)

According to Crombez et al (2005), early researchers understood vigilance to be characterised by dependence on a currently activated goal (i.e. goal-dependent) and to involve conscious and intentional alertness to task-relevant targets. However, many chronic pain patients present with persistent, distressing and preoccupying pain, showing evidence of a dysfunction attentional process which has been described as *hypervigilance.*

Hypervigilance to pain emerges when a person's goal is related to avoidance and escape from pain. However, recent research has shown that hypervigilance is primarily automatic or non-intentional rather than intentional. According to Crombez et al (ibid, p. 6):

Hypervigilance is an unintentional and efficient process that emerges when the threat value of pain is high, the fear system is activated, and the individual's current concern is to escape and control pain. It can be controlled but not without costs.

The mechanisms thought to underpin vigilance are shown in Box 2.9, as are some clinical implications for treatment.

In fact HV has been investigated not only in the context of experimentally induced pain in the laboratory, but also in conditions such as fibromyalgia. In one recent study (Crombez et al 2004) although fibromyalgia patients reported significantly greater vigilance to pain, the difference between the groups was explained by pain intensity and catastrophic thinking.

Beliefs about pain and treatment

Conceptual overview

Beliefs and attitudes are important concomitants of the experience of pain. According to DeGood & Tait (2001):

Beliefs about the nature of pain and about coping with pain should not be viewed as artifacts of the chronic pain experience that will disappear once a correct diagnosis is made and corresponding treatment initiated. Rather, maladaptive cognitions can lie at the heart of the chronic pain problem (p. 321).

In considering the cognitive component of pain, it is sometimes difficult to differentiate clearly amongst beliefs, expectancies, appraisals and cognitive processes. However, *beliefs* are best understood as pre-existing views, shaped by our social and cultural history, about the nature of pain. *Expectancies* are beliefs about the future course of pain. They include *self-efficacy* beliefs which reflect personal expectations about being able personally to influence the future course (and thus include elements of beliefs about control), and *outcome expectancies* which concern beliefs about specific outcomes, irrespective of the person's role in effecting them. *Appraisals* incorporate an element of judgement.

Box 2.9

Hypervigilance (HV): theoretical and clinical implications

- HV is primarily a *goal-dependent attentional process:*
  - should not be confused with other central pain mechanisms
  - cannot easily be studied in paradigms which instruct participants to *attend* to pain
  - standard assessment of pain threshold/ tolerance inadequate as operationalisation of HV
  - may be best studied in situations of *competing* attentional demands, i.e. when attention directed away from pain, or when pain irrelevant to task at hand.
- Because HV is unintentional and efficient, it may *undermine* distraction strategies
- HV facilitates the detection of pain and pain-related information
- HV is strongly related to action tendencies to escape or avoid
  - thus pain expectancies in clinical samples do not amplify pain intensity per se but intensify escape or avoidance tendencies
  - so-called 'amplification of pain' is instead the consequence of repeated failure to successfully distract oneself from pain
  - possible also that pain evokes a more intensive defensive and fear response in those hypervigilant to pain.
- Since HV emerges when threat value is high, it is not unique to a particular pain syndrome
- Since HV is dependent on the goal to escape and avoid, a valuable treatment option is to target the fear system and threat value of pain:
  - this may be accomplished by challenging erroneous beliefs about pain
  - or by learning to accept that a meaningful life is possible despite pain.

Adapted from Crombez, van Damme & Eccleston (2005, p. 6)

Individuals differ not only in specific matters of appraisal, but also more generally in terms of their tendency to view events in a certain way.

Investigation of cognitive factors in pain patients was stimulated initially by research into depression and anxiety. Clinical investigation of distressed individuals commonly reveals patterns of predominantly negative thinking. This observation led Beck (1976) to identify patterns of thoughts in depressed and anxious individuals that he termed 'negative cognitive triads'.

The triad for depression is believed to consist of a negative view of the *self* (perceived as deficient, inadequate or unworthy), a negative view of the *world* (any and all interactions are perceived as frustrating, unrewarding and unsuccessful) and a negative view of the *future* (current difficulties or suffering will continue indefinitely). These thoughts exacerbate feelings of sadness, indecisiveness, apathy, avoidance, helplessness and hopelessness.

The negative triad of anxious patients relates to themes of personal danger. They view themselves as *vulnerable* people living in a world that is personally *threatening* (but not universally so), facing an *unpredictable future*. In addition to depressive symptomatology, anxiety is characterised by cognitive hypervigilance and heightened autonomic arousal.

A comparison can be made with pain patients who also demonstrate features of anxiety and depression. Similar pessimistic or negative beliefs are found regarding pain and outcome of treatment. Thus they believe that *hurt is synonymous with harm*, that *pain uniquely determines physical functioning* and that they face *inevitable structural and/or physiological decline* over the next few years. Such beliefs lead not only to demoralisation but also to debilitation. Patients avoid interactions or activities that are expected to elevate pain and/or suffering, and they become more socially isolated and physically deconditioned.

Research has tended to focus on a number of different types of belief or appraisal about the nature of pain, and the development of new tests assessing different aspects of beliefs has become something of a 'growth industry'. DeGood & Tait (2001) identify four principal dimensions of belief (regarding aetiology, diagnostics, treatment expectations and outcome goals). Some illustrations of these different types of beliefs are shown in Box 2.10.

Although these are listed as individual specific beliefs, patients of course consult with a profile of such beliefs. Failure to identify cogent beliefs at the time of initial assessment may lead to poor clinical decision making and recommendation of ineffective or inappropriate treatment. The perception of pain thus is complex and varies from individual to individual. Research studies, however, have highlighted a number of key themes that are commonly found amongst pain patients.

Beliefs assessed by one of the most widely used instruments, the Survey of Pain Attitudes, or SOPA (Jensen et al 1994) are shown in Box 2.11.

In practice three of the most important clinical constructs are beliefs about the nature of pain, self-efficacy

Box 2.10

Sample dimensions of beliefs about chronic pain and pain treatment

- Aetiology of pain
- Somatic only vs interaction of multiple factors
- External vs internal (e.g. accident vs ageing)
- Consequence of a negligent act vs natural or chance act
- Pain as a symptom of disease vs pain as a benign condition
- Diagnostic expectations regarding
- History taking
- Clinical medical examination
- Laboratory tests
- Psychosocial evaluation
- Treatment expectations
- Active vs passive treatments
- Invasive vs noninvasive procedures
- Cure vs rehabilitation mindset
- Medical vs multidisciplinary perspective
- Somatic/medical vs psychological/behavioural
- Outcome goals
- Complete cure vs partial relief
- Rapid vs gradual improvement
- Sensory comfort vs improved quality of life
- Full or partial return to prior functioning.

Adapted from DeGood & Tait
(2001, Table 17.1, p. 323)

Box 2.11

Beliefs assessed by the SOPA

- Perceived control over one's pain (control)
- Belief that one is unable to function because of pain (disability)
- Belief that pain is a signal of damage and that exercise and activity should be limited (harm)
- Belief that one's pain is influenced by one's emotional state (emotions)
- Belief that taking medication is appropriate (medication)
- Belief that aid should be received from family members (solicitude)
- Belief that a medical cure exists (cure).

beliefs and fears of hurting/harming. Most of the important theoretical constructs can be subsumed under one of these headings.

The nature of pain

Patients often express puzzlement about the nature of their pain. The fact that their pain has persisted may seem to be a mystery. Questions about the nature of pain may need to be addressed as part of the initial clinical evaluation, and of course the nature of pain and disability is an integral part of the educational component of all pain management programmes.

Beliefs about control

Beliefs about the extent to which pain can be controlled would appear to be one of the most powerful determinants of adjustment to pain and the development of incapacity. In the psychological literature there has long been interest in the extent to which individuals believe they can control, or gain control over, aspects of their lives. The role of perceived self-control as a factor that mediates pain and depression was explored by Rudy et al (1988) using structural modelling techniques. Although the *direct* association between pain and depression was minimal, depression developed principally when pain significantly interfered with family, work and social interactions, and/or existed in conjunction with pessimism about being able to control pain. The issue of 'controllability' may be even more important in relationship to adjustment to pain and incapacity. In one interesting study (Affleck et al 1987), judgements of illness predictability were associated with perceptions of greater personal control over daily symptoms and disease course. Perception of a high degree of influence over medical care and intervention was associated with positive mood and psychosocial adjustment. Conversely, the belief that providers had greater control over *daily symptoms* was related to negative mood. Those who had a more severe disease and who believed they had no personal control over *disease course* experienced mood disturbance and exhibited less positive psychosocial adjustment. Optimal adaptation to a chronic condition thus seems to depend upon patients' ability to come to terms with what they can and cannot control. During the 1980s and 90s, there was some interest specifically in pain locus of control beliefs (Main & Waddell 1991, Toomey et al 1991) but more recently the focus has shifted to self-efficacy.

Self-efficacy beliefs

Closely linked with the concept of controllability is that of self-efficacy. Described initially by Bandura (1977), self-efficacy refers to individuals' belief that they have about their capability to execute a behaviour required to produce a particular outcome. This general idea has been investigated in terms of the relationship between such beliefs and resultant behaviour in relation to treatment outcome. The theoretical perspective offered by Bandura can be paraphrased as follows: once a situation has been perceived as involving harm, loss, threat or challenge and individuals have considered a range of coping strategies open to them, what they do will be dependent on what they believe they can achieve. The action taken is a consequence of:

1 their conviction that they have the skill/ability to execute the behaviour required in order to produce the desired outcome (self-efficacy expectation)

2 their estimation that a chosen behaviour will lead to the desired outcome (outcome expectancy).

Turk (1996) describes four sources of information from which individuals make efficacy judgements: past performance on the task ('I've done it once, I can do it again'), or a similar task, performance of others judged to be similar to oneself ('If they can do it, so can I'), verbal encouragement from others that one can complete a task, and finally perception of state of physiological arousal.

Self-efficacy beliefs therefore both predict present behaviour yet can be used as mechanisms of change. Efforts, however, are not always successful. Clinical and experimental investigations suggest that perceived coping *inefficacy* may lead to preoccupation with distressing thoughts and concomitant physiological arousal, thereby increasing pain, decreasing pain tolerance and leading to increased use of medication, lower levels of functioning, poorer exercise tolerance and increased invalidism.

Such beliefs in combination with negative emotional responses frequently can lead to the following state of affairs (DeGood & Shutty 1992, p. 221):

Pain patients who perceive themselves lacking the capacity to acquire self-management skills might be less persistent, more prone to frustration, and more apt to be non-compliant with treatment recommendations. Hence, some patients might demonstrate adequate understanding of particular treatment rationale, yet be non-compliant due to their perceived inability to produce the behaviour necessary to follow treatment recommendations.

Most research into self-efficacy has ignored the outcome expectancy component of Bandura's theory, but a notable exception is a study conducted by Lackner et al (1996). They explored the relative contribution of predictors of disability, such as pain and reinjury expectancy, and self-efficacy beliefs in a sample of patients with chronic low-back pain (LBP). Their results demonstrated that self-efficacy accounted for the greatest proportion of variance in physical performance even after anticipated pain and reinjury had been excluded. Pain intensity was also a significant (albeit limited) predictor of performance on four of the five tasks. The researchers challenge the view that harm expectancies and pain catastrophising are primary causal determinants of function, and argue that they are components of one's confidence of successful task performance. (Treatment recommendations derived from this interpretation emphasise the importance of goal and quota setting, and monitoring of pain and task performance as components of pain management.) According to Asghari & Nicholas (2001) pain self-efficacy beliefs are an important determinant of pain behaviours and disability associated with pain, over and above the effects of pain, distress and personality variables.

Specific fears of hurting, harming and further injury

Behavioural theorists such as Fordyce (1976) explained the development of 'avoidance learning' where successful avoidance of pain established a behavioural pattern that was successful in reducing pain but with the cost of maintaining the 'disability'. During the last decade, particularly since the landmark study of Vlaeyen et al (1995) who found that fear of movement and reinjury were more related to depressive symptoms and catastrophising than to pain itself, there has been a burgeoning of research into the role of fear and anxiety on the development of chronic pain-associated disability. It is crucial to recognise the role of fear and avoidance as obstacles to rehabilitation following injury.

A number of recent studies have tried to disentangle the specific mechanisms involved. According to Geisser et al (2004) pain-related fear is directly associated with musculoskeletal abnormalities and is also associated with limitation in movement and thus implicated in the development and maintenance of chronic low-back pain. In an experimental study, De Jong et al (2005) demonstrated that graded exposure in vivo activated cortical networks and opined that the meaning people attached to noxious stimuli influenced its experienced painfulness. In another study pain-related fear and pain catastrophising were stronger predictors of overall disability even than pain intensity, and in a lifting task, pain-related fear was the strongest predictor of performance (van den Hout 2001). It would appear thus that *perceptions* may be more strongly associated with the development of disability than actual performance and that explanation of disability needs to incorporate consideration both of the cognitive and emotional components as well as the behavioural one. Thus Keefe et al (2004) have recommended the targeting of pain-related anxiety and fear in order to reduce pain-associated disability.

Many of the early studies investigated patients with established pain problems, particularly chronic low-back pain; there has been a shift of emphasis towards secondary prevention (Ch. 9). In an early study of 300 patients with acute back pain attending their family doctor, fear-avoidance beliefs predicted outcome at 2 and 12 months (Klenerman et al 1995). But in a recent study of acute low-back pain (with median duration of episode of 5 days) Sieben et al (2005) found only modest correlations among pain intensity, pain-related fear, avoidance behaviour and disability, and suggested that the chronic LBP model may not be entirely appropriate for acute back pain patients. They recommended a focus on the *transition* from acute to chronic back pain, although the challenges in terms of research design are daunting. It seems probable that there are a large number of potential 'pathways to chronicity' and as a precursor to the design of further interventions, we will require a clearer understanding of the nature of change and the underlying processes involved (Morley 2004), with inclusion of both study of the individual patient and also his/her social environment, including the percepts and behaviours of care-givers (Keefe et al 2004).

Nonetheless the importance of addressing such beliefs and associated psychological mechanisms within a reactivation framework would seem to be compelling and the correction of mistaken beliefs has become an integral part of new approaches to the prevention of chronic incapacity both in health-care settings (Ch. 9) and in occupational settings (Chs 14 and 15). The relationship between fear and pain is shown in Box 2.12.

The assessment of pain-related fears is discussed in detail in Chapter 8.

Pain behaviour

Over a quarter of a century has passed since Fordyce (1976) advocated the application of behavioural principles to the formal analysis and modification of dysfunctional behaviour in patients suffering with pain. In his focus on pain *behaviour* he advocated an approach to the management of pain that was radically different from the traditional medical model. Pain behaviours may be verbal (e.g. complaints of pain and suffering, groans

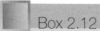

Box 2.12

Fear and pain: key points

• Fear is a biological response to an aversive stimulus
• We are programmed to escape such stimuli and restore 'normality' (homeostasis)
• Pain produces such imbalance
• Fear therefore is a natural response to pain
• It can be understood in terms of its emotional, cognitive and behavioural components
• In the context of severe, traumatic or prolonged pain it can produce a phobic response characterised by marked avoidance
• Fear of pain thus can become more disabling than pain itself
• Recent research into the components of pain-related fear and avoidance are leading to the development of sharply targeted interventions with the potential for reducing the impact of pain and preventing unnecessary disability.

or sighs), postural and gestural (e.g. bracing, guarding, rubbing or grimacing) and are evident in patterns of behaviour that differ from the normal (e.g. excessive resting or reclining). The early behaviourally oriented pain management programmes applied experimental principles specifically to the analysis and modification of such behaviour and behaviour patterns.

Strictly controlled behavioural change programmes are difficult to deliver, but even in less strictly controlled programmes an understanding of the basic principles of learning theory can be of enormous help in recognising the patient's response to change and to professional guidance.

The key aspects of pain behaviour are shown in Box 2.13.

Respondent and operant conditioning

Respondent conditioning (or learning) refers to the learned association between a *neutral* stimulus and a *reflexive* response as a result of frequent co-occurrences. For example, when patients with temporomandibular joint (TMJ) pain experience a surge in nociceptive input they may wince. Chewing does not normally produce pain behaviour, but if, upon chewing, individuals expect *intense* pain they may emit learned responses in the form of pain behaviours such as grimacing, raising shoulders, or other signs of agitation. Thus pain behaviour that was previously produced by TMJ pain comes to be produced

Box 2.13

Key aspects of pain behaviour

- Observable
- May contain verbal, subverbal and non-verbal components
- May contain both respondent and operant features
- Often highly context dependent
- Patients not always aware of their own pain behaviour
- Can be influenced by cultural and social factors
- In treatment and familial contexts, best understood as a form of communication
- May be highly influential in clinical decision making.

by chewing. This is an example of *classic conditioning* (like Pavlov's experiments on his dogs).

Pain behaviours can also come under the influence of environmental factors. If a pain patient receives sympathetic attention when they show signs of pain, a pattern of pain behaviour may become established (because of the sympathetic attention). In this example, the mechanism is one of *operant conditioning*. The pain behaviour can be understood not simply as a response to nociceptive input but also as a behaviour that is being operantly maintained. It is important to stress that couples are often completely unaware of the interrelationships amongst these behaviour patterns. With the passage of time, pain behaviours that were originally *responses* to nociception come to be *stimuli* for the behaviour for others, which thereby reinforce the behaviour.

Yet pain continues to be defined primarily in terms of its sensory or experiential dimensions, as illustrated by the IASP definition of pain: *An unpleasant sensory and emotional experience associated with actual or potential tissue damage, or described in terms of such damage* (Merskey & Bogduk 1994). Although pain is frequently discussed in terms of its adaptive value, models of pain have restricted their focus to the processes involved in the experience of pain, almost to the complete neglect of the processes involved in the expression of pain. For a pain system to have any adaptive value, it must not only signal tissue damage but it must also mobilise the necessary behavioural programmes required to act on the situation causing pain. A pain system without behaviour is as adaptive as a fire station without firemen.

The importance of behavioural systems as integral components of pain phenomena is being increasing

recognised. Damasio (1994) discussed pain as a lever for decision and action, although he did not specify the processes by which this would occur. In his later years, Wall (1999) suggested that pain symptoms were probably linked to motor systems for escape and minimisation of injury. Williams (2002) has been most explicit in bringing behaviour into the world of pain by suggesting that communicative behaviours such as facial displays might have played an important role in the evolution of the human species.

The behavioural programmes associated with pain might include actions designed to escape a situation that could cause an injury, to protect or care for an injury, to communicate a need for assistance, or to alert others to potential danger. The consistency with which these categories of behaviour are associated with pain suggests that they are not simply shaped through learning, but are integral components of the pain system (Williams 2002).

Pain behaviour and communication

The subjective experience of pain has been shown to play a significant role in the expression of pain behaviour (Labus et al 2003). However, the relation between the experience of pain and pain behaviour is modest, with self-reports of pain intensity rarely accounting for more than 10–15% of the variance in indices of pain behaviour (Fuchs-Lacelle et al 2003, Labus et al 2003, Sullivan et al 2004). It appears, therefore, that pain experience and pain behaviour are only partially overlapping constructs (Hadjistavropoulos & Craig 2002). Pain experience and pain behaviour serve different functions, they may be influenced by different internal and external contingencies, they likely have different correlates, and may well respond differentially to treatment interventions (Fordyce et al 1986, Sullivan et al 2004).

Non-verbal communication

A considerable amount of research has been conducted on the facial displays that accompany the experience of pain (Craig 1999, Williams 2002). The configuration of that face rapidly communicates to observers information about the internal state of the person experiencing pain. There are indications that observers weight facial information heavily when inferring the pain of others (Prkachin & Craig 1995, Sullivan et al 2006a). Whether a mother is responding to her injured child, or a physician is attending to a patient, information displayed in the face will alert the care giver to the care needs of the individual expressing pain.

There is likely an innate component to facial displays of pain (Craig 1999, Williams 2002). Newborn facial response to tissue damage is very similar to that of older children and adults. Albeit innate, facial displays of pain, like any other form of human behaviour are likely to be influenced by a variety of factors such as individual differences in expressivity, communication goals and environmental contingencies.

Individual differences in the expression of pain

There are marked individual differences in the manner in which people will express pain. Numerous investigations have reported that women display more pronounced facial expressions of pain than men (Craig et al 1992). One explanation of sex differences in pain expression is that women's more pronounced displays reflect their more intense experience of pain (Unruh 1996). Another explanation is that men might be actively suppressing facial expression of pain as a form of self-presentation strategy (Unruh 1996). It is likely that both factors play a role. Gender differences are discussed in more detail in Chapter 4.

There is recent evidence suggesting that individuals who are high in pain catastrophising are particularly likely to display marked facial expressions in response to painful stimulation (Sullivan et al 2000, 2004, 2006b) In one study, high pain catastrophisers displayed more intense facial responses to painful stimulation when they were in the company of a research assistant than when they were alone (Sullivan et al 2004). It has also been shown that individuals who are depressed are also very likely to display intense facial responses to painful stimulation (Keefe et al 1986).

Protective behaviour and escape behaviour

One of the functions of pain behaviour is to minimise pain and reduce the probability of injury exacerbation (Craig 1999, Fridlund 1994). For example, the use of limping to minimise weight bearing on an injured limb reduces the probability of injury exacerbation. Holding or guarding an injured arm might also be used in order to protect the compromised arm from further injury.

Escape behaviour (e.g. discontinuation of behaviour causing pain) is another component of protective behaviour. Escape behaviour is considered to be one of the defining criteria of pain-related disability (Vlaeyen & Linton 2000). In other words, disability due to pain emerges when individuals either discontinue or avoid activities that are associated with pain. These activities may be activities of daily living, social and recreational activities, or occupational activities.

Following injury, individuals may need to engage in protective behaviour in order to promote recovery. There are indications, however, that psychological factors associated with fear play a significant role in the degree of protective behaviour in which individuals will engage when experiencing pain.

Clinical and experimental research continues to accumulate, showing that individuals who score high on measures of fear of pain are less active (Bussman et al 1998), they have reduced range of motion (McCracken et al 1992), they are prone to discontinuing activities that are associated with pain (McCracken & Gross 1993; Vlaeyen et al 1995), and they avoid activities that they expect will be associated with pain. Fear of pain has been shown to be a better predictor of disability than medical status variables or pain itself (Waddell et al 1993).

Coping styles and strategies

Since the publication of the textbook by Turk et al (1983), there has been considerable interest in the styles and strategies demonstrated by patients in coping with pain. Jensen et al (1991) and Lazarus (1993) provide excellent early overviews of the coping literature. Geisser et al (2004) and DeGood & Tait (2001) provide more recent reviews. According to DeGood & Tait (2001):

> Coping is a fluid process, subject to change across situations and over time . . . a process composed of appraisal, responses and reappraisals. Appraisals and responses are both coloured by individual differences, including differences in beliefs, expectancies, personality and biological characteristics and social roles (p. 327).

Given the multiple influences on coping it is perhaps unsurprising therefore that there appears to be such a wide variation in patients in response to pain. This was recognised in the development of the influential *Ways of Coping Checklist* (Folkman & Lazarus 1980) which is not only useful as a clinical screener, as discussed below, but has also stimulated a range of more focused measurement instruments (Ch. 8). As a consequence, a number of different constructs have entered general parlance. The principal conceptual 'landmarks' are illustrated in Box 2.14.

Box 2.14

Coping styles and strategies

- Styles:
  - avoiders and copers (confronters)
  - assimilative and accommodative.
- Strategies:
  - active versus passive
  - adaptive versus non-adaptive
  - emotion-focused versus problem-focused
  - avoidant and attentional
  - efficacy of coping strategies.

It is perhaps helpful to begin with an operational definition of 'coping'. It has been defined as 'ongoing cognitive and behavioural efforts to manage specific external and/or internal demands that are appraised as taxing or exceeding the resources of the person' (Lazarus 1993, p. 237). This appears to be a useful starting point, but in practice, of course, patients employ a range of coping *styles* and types of *strategy* in order to limit the effects of pain.

Coping styles

Letham et al (1983) described patients as *confronters* or *avoiders*; it has been observed (Waddell et al 1993) that fear and avoidance of pain can become more disabling than pain itself as, although avoidance at early stages may reduce nociception, the avoidance behaviours may persist in anticipation of pain rather than simply as a response to it. Whether this stable disposition leads to psychological and physiological consequences for pain patients may be extrapolated from research using global measures of flexible-accommodative versus rigid, less adaptive coping style. (According to Weinberger 1990, 'true' low-anxiety individuals are flexible copers, whereas repressors have compulsive tendencies.)

Brandstadter (1992) distinguished two fundamentally different styles of coping with chronic pain: *assimilative coping* (tenacious goal pursuit), involving active attempts to alter circumstances in line with personal preferences, and *accommodative coping* (flexible goal adjustment), or 'downgrading' of goals or expectations when goals are seen to be unattainable through active coping efforts. Two scales, tenacious goal pursuit and flexible goal adjustment, have been developed to measure these aspects of coping (Brandstadter & Renner 1990). In a recent study of coping style and pain-associated distress, it was concluded (Schmitz et al 1996, p. 41):

> *accommodative coping functions as a protective resource by preventing global losses in the psychological functioning of chronic pain patients and maintaining a positive life perspective. Most important, the ability to flexibly adjust personal goals attenuated the negative impact of the pain experience (pain intensity, pain-related disability) on psychological well-being (depression). Furthermore, pain-related coping strategies led to a reduction of disability only when accompanied by a high degree of flexible goal adjustment.*

Coping strategies

The overall efficacy of coping techniques appears to be moderated by levels of pain intensity and appraisals of perceived pain control abilities (Jensen & Karoly 1991). Their role in pain management needs to be understood in the context of the specific beliefs and expectations already discussed. Individuals' choice of strategies will depend on their beliefs about pain, their confidence in being able to influence events (i.e. self-efficacy) and of course on their repertoire of coping behaviours. Over the last 20 years a wide range of psychological instruments have attempted to identify different ways of coping with pain and incapacity. A number of the more commonly used instruments are described in Chapter 8. The best known is the Coping Strategies Questionnaire (CSQ) (Rosenstiel & Keefe 1983) of which there have been a number of variants. The original questionnaire of 48 items yielded scores on six cognitive coping strategies (Diverting Attention; Reinterpreting Pain; Coping Self-Statements; Ignoring Pain; Praying/Hoping; and Catastrophising) one behavioural coping strategy (Increasing Activity) and two specific self-efficacy items. The original structural validity of the CSQ as published was weak, but because of its strong clinical content it has continued to be used. There have been attempts, however, to strengthen the instrument. According to DeGood & Tait (2001), two lines of research have emerged from it: firstly factor analytic studies aimed at identifying superordinate constructs relevant to coping; and secondly studies of the utility of individual scales for the identification of coping strategies associated with good or poor outcome of treatment. A number of the derived constructs are shown in Box 2.15.

> ### Box 2.15
>
> **CSQ-derived composite coping measures**
>
> - Coping Attempts (including all of the cognitive scales except Catastrophising)
> - Pain Control and Rational Thinking (including the Catastrophising scale and the two self-efficacy items)
> - Active and Passive Coping (constructed from sets of specific items)
> - Coping Flexibility (defined simply as the number of coping strategies (excluding Catastrophising).

An insufficient number of studies have been done as yet on different clinical populations and stages of illness to distinguish real clinical variance from inaccuracy of measurement and no new composites have as yet emerged as 'brand leaders'). Indeed as Boothby et al (1999) have pointed out, because most of the constructs were empirically derived, their composition typically varies somewhat across samples. Of all the CSQ scales and composites, catastrophising has proved the strongest predictor of outcome (usually measured in terms of function or self-reported disability) and it has stimulated the development of the Pain Catastrophising Scale, or PCS (Sullivan et al 1995). There has been some disagreement about whether catastrophising should be viewed as a coping strategy or as a type of appraisal (belief).

It should be recognised that there is a considerable degree of overlap amongst a number of these dimensions and constructs and that the categories are not mutually exclusive in that individuals may use combinations of coping strategies and further research is needed into their distinctiveness and utility.

For practical purposes, therefore, an attempt will be made to reflect upon the more important clinically relevant dimensions.

Adaptive vs maladaptive coping strategies

As described above, CSQ (Rosenstiel & Keefe 1983) provides measures of both cognitive and behavioural coping strategies but it makes a major distinction between adaptive (or positive) and maladaptive (or negative) coping strategies. As Turner (1991) has pointed out, however, specific coping strategies are not inherently adaptive or maladaptive. A strategy useful at one point in time may be of little value at another, and some strategies may be of benefit if used in moderation but not if used to the exclusion of others. Indeed, as Keefe et al (1992) have observed, the assessment of behavioural coping strategies can be problematic in that the distinction between behavioural coping efforts and outcomes of coping can become difficult to distinguish. While these caveats seem fairly persuasive, the concept appears to have inherent clinical utility. The questionnaire is discussed further in Chapter 8.

Active and passive coping strategies

The 19-item Vanderbilt Pain Management Inventory, or VPMI (Brown & Nicassio 1987) distinguished between active (adaptive) and passive (non-adaptive) coping strategies, the distinction depending on the relationship that a strategy has to variables such as psychological adjustment. This distinction still appears to have some clinical utility. Active strategies (e.g. taking exercise) require the individual to take a degree of responsibility for pain management by attempting either to control pain or to function despite pain. Passive strategies (e.g. resting) involve either withdrawal or the passing on of responsibility for the control of pain to someone else. Brown et al (1989) found that depression was more severe when patients used high levels of passive coping strategies at high levels of pain intensity. No relationship between active coping and depression was found and it would appear that the use of active coping strategies does not act to mitigate the relationship between pain and depression.

Keefe et al (1992) have criticised the concept of active and passive coping strategies arguing that no strategy is truly passive in nature. As they point out, strategies such as taking medication may actually require the patient to comply actively with a treatment regimen.

Emotion-focused and problem-focused coping strategies

Lazarus & Folkman's (1984) theory of stress and coping makes a clear distinction between problem-focused and emotionally focused coping. Emotion-focused coping strategies aim to control stress, in contrast to problem-focused coping strategies, which are aimed at attempting to relieve or solve a problem. This distinction seems to have inherent appeal and is certainly fundamental to psychologically oriented pain management programmes. These features can be assessed by the Ways of Coping Checklist (Folkman & Lazarus 1980). This instrument, which is widely used in the general stress and coping literature, measures the use of two major categories of coping efforts: problem-focused coping and emotion-focused coping.

Attentional vs avoidant coping strategies

Coping strategies have also been described as being attentional (e.g. seeking information) and avoidant (e.g. distraction). There is evidence to suggest that the different types of strategy are differentially effective at different stages in pain, thus in acute pain the use of avoidant strategies is associated with decreased distress, whereas in chronic pain the converse is the case. This perspective has not as yet been fully researched.

Coping strategy effectiveness

The relationship between the use of these strategies and psychological adjustment is complex (Jensen et al 1991) and it has been suggested by Jensen & Karoly (1991) that pain duration has a moderating influence in that, for those with longer duration of pain, there is no relationship between the use of such strategies and psychological adjustment. The overall efficacy of pain-specific coping strategies in enhancing pain tolerance was evaluated by Fernandez & Turk (1989) using meta-analytic techniques. Six major classes of cognitive coping strategies were conceptualised: external focus of attention, neutral imaginings, pleasant imaginings, dramatised coping, rhythmic cognitive activity and pain acknowledgement. They concluded that each class of coping strategy significantly attenuated reports of pain, imagery being the most effective and strategies involving repetitive cognitions or sensory focus being the least effective.

At present little is known about changes in use of coping strategy over time, about individual differences in use of coping strategy or about how the effectiveness of the same coping strategy varies from person to person. For example, some individuals may use a variety of techniques, others only one. One of the few studies to examine the relationship between the day-to-day use of coping strategies, their perceived efficacy, and the effects on pain intensity and affect was conducted by Keefe et al (1997) in a sample of rheumatoid arthritis patients over a period of 30 consecutive days. Between-subject analysis demonstrated that individual differences in daily judgements of coping efficacy failed to correspond to either pain intensity or type of strategy used; greater pain intensity was associated with the use of a wider variety of coping strategies than low pain states. Using the day instead of the person as the unit of analysis, the authors demonstrated that perceived coping efficacy for that day was associated with greater

use of relaxation, redefining of pain, spiritual support seeking and a consequent reduction in pain and negative affect and enhancement of positive mood. Furthermore, individual judgement of coping effectiveness resulted in lower pain levels on the following day, and improvements in next-day mood were also attributed to use of relaxation strategies.

DeGood & Tait (2001) stress the importance to address further the assessment of coping in outcome research, coping across the lifespan and the role of moderating variables, particularly those which may moderate or mediate coping efficacy such as readiness for change, flexibility in goal-setting and self-efficacy. We are still some way from the development of effective care pathways for the individual patient but research over the last decade into coping strategies holds promise for the development of more effective care pathways.

Catastrophising: an interpersonal perspective

Researchers have consistently identified 'catastrophising' as a major clinical feature both in the chronic patient's symptom complex and also as a predictor of chronicity. Initially catastrophising was conceptualised fairly specifically as a type of cognitive distortion (similar to the sorts of cognitive distortion found in depressed patients). According to Beck (1976), negative bias in information processing is maintained by general and systematic errors in logical appraisal. Catastrophising, as originally defined, was characterised by profoundly negative ruminations about one's present and future ability to cope, though often included in measures of coping strategies, is probably best understood as a set of dysfunctional beliefs or appraisals (Jensen et al 1991). The tendency towards negative appraisal (or undue pessimism) has consistently been shown to be a better predictor of low pain tolerance, disability and depression than measures of disease activity or impairment, both at the time of testing and at long-term follow-up (e.g. Keefe et al 1989). It may be based on mistaken beliefs about pain and outcome of treatment, but is most clearly associated with depression. The cognitive distortion is not, however, simply a facet of depression, for it has been shown to be a significant predictor of self-reported disability and work loss even when the influence of pain severity and depression has been taken into account (Burton et al 1995, Main & Waddell 1991).

More recently, it has been suggested that the expressive features of pain catastrophising might reflect a communal approach to coping with pain (Sullivan et al 2000, 2001). Within this framework, it is assumed that individuals differ in the degree to which they adopt interpersonal goals in their efforts to cope with stress (Coyne & Fiske 1992, Lyons et al 1995, Sullivan et al 2000). Sullivan et al (2001) suggested that pain catastrophisers might engage in exaggerated pain expression in order to maximise proximity, or to solicit assistance or empathic responses from others in their social environment. The Communal Coping Model (Lyons et al 1995, Sullivan et al 2001, Thorn et al 2003) represents a marked departure from traditional cognitive frameworks in positing that the coping efforts of individuals experiencing pain are not necessarily directed toward the management of pain. Rather, it is suggested that for pain catastrophisers, the experience of pain might provide the stage for the pursuit of interpersonal goals.

Pain as a multidimensional bio-behavioural system

In response to tissue damage, a cascade of neurochemical events are likely to be triggered, ultimately giving rise to the subjective experience of pain. This is the domain of pain systems that has been addressed in current models of pain transmission (Ch. 1). What has received little or no attention, at least within formal models of pain, is what happens after pain has been experienced.

There are significant interpersonal and clinical implications to the behavioural dimensions of pain.

Social influences on the perception and report of pain

The report of pain can be influenced by the social context not only through behavioural mechanisms (see above) but also by social desirability (or the desire to present oneself in a favourable light). Both Deshields et al (1995) and Haythornthwaite et al (1991) found that patients with high scores on the Social Desirability Scale reported less depression, anxiety and disability than patients characterised as less susceptible to self-denial or impression management. The latter researchers accept this result as evidence that repressors (not described as such in either study) were a 'subgroup of chronic pain patients whose experience is less severe' than their counterparts.

Pain behaviour as a social response

Expressions of pain behaviour typically occur in a social context. Overt expressions of pain are very likely to draw the attention of others in the vicinity of the individual experiencing pain. Increasingly, research is pointing to the social responses of others as key determinants of the degree of pain behaviour that will be exhibited by an individual experiencing pain. Supportive encouragement and solicitousness can have a significant influence on the display of pain behaviour and on communication about pain (Romano et al 1991, 1995). This is illustrated in the adaptation to Descartes's model shown in Figure 2.2.

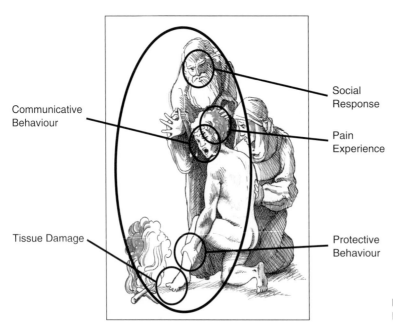

Communicative Behaviour

Tissue Damage

Social Response

Pain Experience

Protective Behaviour

Figure 2.2 • Sullivan's adaptation of Descartes' model (Sullivan 2006).

Pain behaviour has to be understood in terms of its *social context*. Indeed pain has been described as an interesting social communication, the meaning of which has still to be determined (Fordyce 1976). Chronic pain patients can display widespread changes in behaviour following injury. Pain may affect a wide range of activities, and displays of pain behaviour can produce marked and unpredictable reactions in others. This is particularly true in social situations, when the reaction of others to any display of incapacity can be unpredictable. The responses of others may range from displays of concern to downright unpleasantness. There may be no apparent reaction at all. In patients who lack confidence and self-assurance such unpredictabilities can be daunting.

The biopsychomotor model: the integration of the psychological components

The recently developed biopsychomotor model (Sullivan 2006) has been offered as a way of reintegrating the distinctive psychological facets of pain. Its essential features are shown in Box 2.16.

The biopsychomotor model of pain has clear implications for the breadth of processes that will be considered as integral dimensions of the pain system. The model has important clinical implications as well. Traditional medical approaches to pain have given

Box 2.16

Key features of the biopsychomotor model

- Pain cannot be understood as a purely sensory phenomenon
- The experience of pain is intimately related to pain behaviour
- Pain behaviour is adaptive and has to be understood from within an evolutionary and functional perspective
- Pain behaviour is both respondent to the sensory component and shaped by the social environment
- Communication about pain needs to be understood as a bidirectional process between the pain patient and those in his/her environment
- The model offers new understandings of pain, both in terms of understanding fundamental mechanisms and also in the development of new therapeutic interventions.

some recognition to the behavioural dimensions of pain, but these have been regarded as secondary or reactive to pain. The implicit assumption has been that effective treatment of pain (sensation) will lead to the disappearance of pain behaviour. Research, however, suggests that the behavioural dimensions of pain (e.g. disability) may persist in spite of reductions in pain, and that disability can be reduced in the absence of reduction in pain.

It has been suggested further that new avenues for intervention might become apparent if we consider the different behavioural dimensions of the pain system to be at least partially independent. Some patients may present with an over-representation of the communicative dimension of the pain system, others may present with an over-representation of the protective behaviour dimension. Since these components are determined by different cognitive and affective factors, intervention techniques specifically designed to target the determinants of different behavioural components might yield better outcomes than interventions aimed simply at reducing pain intensity.

Targets for intervention and obstacles to recovery

Risks, flags and obstacles to recovery

Over the last decade the use of the term 'flag' as marker for, or predictor of, the future course of pain-associated incapacity has become fairly widespread in publications and clinical practice. Since psychological factors constitute a major part of the flag system, they will be described briefly at this juncture. They are an important illustration of a shift in psychological focus from older constructs of psychopathology to the burgeoning of interest in normal psychological processes which has been stimulated by the Gate Control Theory (Ch. 1).

The major flags, and their sources, are shown in Box 2.17.

Red flags. In the field of back pain the signs and symptoms considered indicative of possible spinal pathology or of the need for an urgent surgical evaluation became known as 'red flags'. These 'risk factors' for serious pathology or disease became incorporated into screening tools recommended for use in primary care by clinicians to identify those patients in whom an urgent specialist opinion was indicated (CSAG 1994, AHCPR 1994).

Yellow flags. In New Zealand, increasing costs of chronic non-specific low-back pain stimulated the development of a psychosocial assessment

Table 2.1 Flag model with implications for action

Type of flag	Recommendation for action
Red	Triage for specialist medical opinion
	Reassess if appropriate
Orange	Triage to mental health specialist
	Reassess after specialist treatment
Yellow	Biopsychosocial management
	Develop integrated approach to reactivation with removal of perceived obstacles to recovery
Blue	Identify modifiable work perceptions
	Develop integrated approach to reactivation with removal of perceived obstacles to recovery
	Consider liaison with employer in context of RTW or work retention plan
Black	Appraise significance as potential rehabilitation 'showstoppers'
	Check black flags with employer and investigate possibility of accommodation
	Reset patient expectations and develop integrated approach to reactivation *or* do not accept for treatment

system designed systematically to address the psychosocial risk factors which had been shown in the scientific literature to be predictive of chronicity (Kendall et al 1997). These 'yellow flags' were developed not only from a clinical perspective but also from an occupational perspective and consisted of both psychological and socio-occupational risk factors.

Orange flags. Yellow flags should be thought of as aspects of normal psychological processes, but they have sometimes been confused with psychiatric disorder, such as major mental illness or major personality disorder, including illicit drug use and ongoing forensic involvement. Orange flags can be thought of as the psychiatric equivalent of red flags in that they require specialist assessment/referral and render the individual unsuitable (at that time) for a straightforward biopsychosocial approach (Main et al 2005).

Blue flags. It became clear, however, that implicit within the yellow flag initiative was the possibility of a range of different solutions, involving both health-care providers and occupational personnel. It was decided that insufficient attention had been given to specific occupational factors and it was decided therefore to subdivide the yellow flags into clinical yellow flags and occupationally focused blue flags (Main & Burton 2000). The blue flags have their origins in the work reported stress literature. They are those perceived features of work, generally associated with higher rates of symptoms, ill-health and work loss, which in the context of injury may delay recovery, or constitute a major obstacle to it, and for those at work may be major contributory factors to suboptimal performance or

'presenteeism'. It should be emphasised that blue flags incorporate not only issues related to the perception of job characteristics such as job demand, but also to the perception of social interactions (whether with management or fellow-workers).

Black flags. Finally, from a work retention or work rehabilitation perspective, a further distinction has been made between two types of occupational risk factors: those concerning the perception of work (blue flags), and organisational obstacles to recovery, comprising objective work characteristics and conditions of employment (black flags) (Main & Burton 2000).

The flag model essentially has both strengths and weaknesses (Linton et al 2005). It has the advantage that it distinguishes clinical from occupational factors, it attempts to distinguish 'internal' or Type I factors from 'external' or Type II factors (Sullivan et al 2005), its focus is primarily on *modifiable* risk factors, and in adopting a 'system's perspective' recognises the importance a range of contextual factors both in the development/ maintenance of the pain-associated limitations, and also, more importantly, as offering a number of differing therapeutic options. However, the model is a conceptually rather than empirically derived statistical model, and therefore is offered simply as one of a number of possible ways of thinking about pain in context.

A brief overview of the flags and general recommendations for action are shown in Table 2.1. Their utility in the context of screening, assessment and management in a variety of settings are discussed further in Chapters 3, 5, 9, 14 and 15.

Conclusion

Psychological issues are at the heart of interdisciplinary pain management. The shift from the narrow biomedical model to the biopsychosocial model now permeates clinical service delivery and social policy. It is important to recognise, however, that the investigation of such factors has to be every bit as rigorous and systematic as investigation of fundamental physiology, anatomy and biochemistry. In historical terms, the psychology of pain is still a relatively young field of enquiry.

In this chapter the nature of psychological influences on pain has been considered from a number of distinct perspectives. The ground-breaking work of the behavioural perspective offered by Fordyce (1976), and the cognitive framework stimulated by Turk et al (1983), has established the foundations for the psychology of pain in the context of interdisciplinary pain management. The multidimensional framework offered by the biopsychosocial model has required the integration of psychological concepts with both biomedical and socioeconomic perspectives.

Recent research within the psychological domain has offered new insights into the influences on the perception of pain and adjustment to residual pain-associated limitations. However, the influence of Cartesian dualism has been hard to shake off. Reintegration of core psychological features within a 'style of life' is illustrated in the recent biopsychomotor model, which appears to have some potential as one of the newer integrative models. The broadening of perspective from targets for intervention to include obstacles to recovery illustrated in the flag model illustrates the advantage of a move from

a major focus on psychopathology to an investigation of normal psychological processes influencing the perception of pain and adjustment to it. These more recent insights into the nature of psychological processes would seem to offer new opportunities for reshaping the nature of interventions to enhance outcome, whether in the context of rehabilitation or in terms of secondary prevention. It seems that psychological factors are needed not only in understanding the nature of pain and adjustment to it, but need to be considered also in the context of screening, assessment, design of interventions and the prevention of unnecessary chronicity, whether in clinical or occupational settings. Each of these issues will be considered in depth in other chapters.

In conclusion, it seems that since the GCT there have been significant advances in the clarification of the nature of psychological factors, but in terms of a clear understanding of the specific influence of psychological factors and their interaction, however, much remains to be done.

Key points

- **Psychological factors have a considerable influence on pain and disability**
- **They have a stronger influence on outcome than do biomedical factors**
- **The shift from medical to biopsychosocial models of illness highlights the major importance of psychological factors**
- **The most important factors are distress, beliefs or attitudes, pain behaviour and pain coping strategies**
- **Further research is needed into the interaction amongst these factors at various stages of illness**
- **Psychological factors in response to acute pain are predictive of chronic incapacity**
- **There needs to be a redirection from investigations into the nature of pain towards obstacles to recovery**
- **Distress at and confusion about previous treatment have a powerful influence on patients' reactions to pain and disability**
- **Better management of psychological reactions at early stages of treatment has the potential for reducing iatrogenic distress and preventing unnecessary chronicity, and this suggests a need to develop the integration of psychological perspectives into the clinical practice of other professions.**

References

Affleck G, Tennen H, Pfeiffer C et al 1987 Appraisals of control and predictability in adapting to a chronic disease. Journal of Personal and Social Psychology 53:273–279

Agnew C 1998 Modal versus individually derived behavioral normative beliefs about condom use: comparing measurement alternatives of the cognitive underpinnings of the theories of reasoned action and planned behaviour. Psychology and Health 13:271–287

AHCPR 1994 Management guidelines for acute low back pain. Agency for Health Care Policy and Research, US Department of Health and Human Services, Rockville MD

Aldrich S, Eccleston C, Crombez G 2000 Worrying about chronic pain: vigilance to threat and misdirected problem solving. Behavior Research and Therapy 38:457–470

Asghari A, Nicholas M K 2001 Pain self-efficacy beliefs and pain behaviour. A prospective study. Pain 94:85–100

Bandura A 1977 Self-efficacy: towards a unifying theory of behaviour change. Psychological Review 84:191–215

Beck A 1976 Cognitive therapy and the emotional disorders. International University Press, New York

Beecher H K 1956 Relationship of significance of wound to pain experienced. Journal of the American Medical Association 161:1609–1613

Blumer D, Heilbronn M 1982 Chronic pain as a variant of depressive disorder: the pain-prone disorder. Journal of Nervous and Mental Disorders 170:381–406

Boothby J L, Thorn B E, Stroud M W et al 1999 Coping with pain. In: Gatchel R J, Turk D C (eds) Psychosocial factors in pain: critical perspectives. Guilford Press, New York, pp 343–359

Brandstadter J 1992 Personal control over development: some developmental implications of self-efficacy. In: Schwarzer R (ed) Self-efficacy: thought control of action. Hemisphere, Washington DC, pp 127–145

Brandstadter J, Renner G 1990 Tenacious goal pursuit and flexible goal adjustment: explication and age-related analysis of assimilative and accommodative strategies of coping. Psychology and Ageing 5:58–67

Brown G K, Nicassio P M 1987 The development of a questionnaire for the assessment of active and passive coping strategies. Pain 31:53–65

Brown G K, Nicassio P M, Wallston K A 1989 Pain coping strategies and depression in rheumatoid arthritis. Journal of Consulting and Clinical Psychology 57:652–657

Bryant R A 1993 Memory for pain and affect in chronic pain patients. Pain 54:347–351

Burton A K, Tillotson K M, Main C J et al 1995 Psychosocial predictors of outcome in acute and subchronic low back trouble. Spine 20:722–728

Bussman J B J, van de Laar Y M, Neleman M P et al 1998 Ambulatory accelerometry to quantify motor behavior in patients after failed back surgery. Pain 74:153–161

Butcher J N, Dahlstrom W G, Graham J R et al 1989 Manual for the administration and scoring of the Minnesota Multiphasic Personality Inventory-2: MMPI-2. University of Minnesota Press, Minneapolis

Chapman C R, Okifuji A 2004 Pain: basic mechanisms and conscious experience. In: Psychosocial aspects of pain: a handbook for healthcare providers. IASP Press, Seattle, ch 1, pp 3–27

Coleman J C 1950 Abnormal psychology and modern life. New York: Scott, Foresman and Company

Conner M, Norman P 1998 Editorial: social cognition models in health psychology. Psychology and Health 13:179–185

Coyne J, Fiske V 1992 Couples coping with chronic illness. In: Akamatsu T, Crowther J, Hobfoll S et al (eds) Family health psychology. Hemisphere, Washington, DC, pp 129–149

Craig K D 1999 Emotions and psychobiology. In: Wall P, Melzack R (eds) Textbook of pain, 4th edn. Churchill Livingstone, Edinburgh

Craig K D, Prkachin K M, Grunau R V E 1992 The facial expression of pain. In: Turk D C, Melzack R (eds) Handbook of pain assessment. Guilford Press, New York, ch 15, pp 257–276

Crombez G, Eccleston C, van den Broeck A et al 2004 Hypervigilance in pain and fibromyalgia. The mediating role of pain intensity and catastrophic thinking about pain. Clinical Journal of Pain 20:98–102

Crombez G, van Damme S, Eccleston C 2005 Hypervigilance to pain: an experimental and clinical analysis. Clinical Journal of Pain 116:4–7

CSAG (Clinical Standards Advisory Group) 1994 Report on back pain. HMSO, London

Damasio A 1994 Descartes' error: emotion, reason and the human brain. Macmillan, New York

DeGood D E, Shutty M S Jr 1992 Assessment of pain beliefs, coping and self-efficacy. In: Turk D C, Melzack R (eds) Handbook of pain assessment. Guilford Press, New York, ch 13, pp 214–234

DeGood D E, Tait R C 2001 Assessment of pain beliefs and coping. In: Turk D C, Melzack R (eds) Handbook of pain assessment, 2nd edn. Guilford Press, New York, ch 17, pp 320–345

De Jong J R, Vlaeyen J W S, Onghena P et al 2005 Reduction of pain-related fear in complex regional pain syndrome type I: the application of graded exposure in vivo. Pain 116:264–275

Deshields T L, Tait R C, Gfeller J D et al 1995 Relationship between social desirability and self-report in chronic pain patients. Clinical Journal of Pain 11:189–193

Dijkstra A 2005 The validity of the stages of change model in the adoption of the self-management approach in chronic pain. Clinical Journal of Pain 21:27–37

Eccleston C 1995 The attentional control of pain: methodological and theoretical concerns. Pain 63:3–10

Eccleston C, Crombez G 1999 Pain demands attention: a cognitive-affective model of the interruptive function of pain. Psychological Bulletin 125:355–366

Eccleston C, Crombez G, Aldrich S et al 2001 Worry and chronic pain patients: a description and analysis of individual differences. European Journal of Pain 5:309–318

Engel G L 1959 Psychogenic pain and the pain-prone patient. American Journal of Medicine 26:899

Fernandez E, Turk D C 1989 The utility of cognitive coping strategies for altering perception of pain: a meta-analysis. Pain 38:123–135

Flor H, Hermann C 2004 Biopsychosocial models of pain. In: Psychosocial aspects of pain: a handbook for healthcare providers. IASP Press, Seattle, ch 3, pp 47–75

Flor H, Turk D C 1989 Psychophysiology of chronic pain. Do chronic pain patients exhibit symptom-specific psychophysiological responses? Psychological Bulletin 105:215–259

Folkman S, Lazarus R 1980 An analysis of coping in a middle-aged community sample. Journal of Health and Social Behaviour 21:219–240

Fordyce W E 1976 Behavioral methods for chronic pain and illness. C V Mosby, St Louis, MS

Fordyce W E, Brockway J A, Bergmann J A et al 1986 Acute back pain: a control-group comparison of behavioral vs traditional management methods. Journal of Behavioral Medicine 9:127–140

Fridlund A 1994 Human facial expression: an evolutionary view. Academic Press, San Diego, CA

Fuchs-Lacelle S, Hadjistavropoulos T, Sharpe D et al 2003 Comparing two observational systems in the assessment of knee pain. Pain Research and Management 8:205–211

Fulop-Miller R 1938 Triumph over pain. Literary Guild of America. Republished by Kessinger Publishing 2005, Kila, MT

Gatchel R J, Turk D C 2002 Psychological approaches to pain management, 2nd edn. Guilford Press, New York

Geisser M E, Haig A J, Wallbom A S et al 2004 Pain-related fear, lumbar flexion, and dynamic EMG among persons with chronic musculoskeletal low back pain. Clinical Journal of Pain 20:61–69

Hadjistavropoulos T, Craig K 2002 A theoretical framework for understanding self-report and observational measures of pain: a communication model. Behaviour Research and Therapy 40:551–570

Hathaway S R, McKinley J C 1967 Minnesota multiphasic personality inventory manual, rev edn. Psychological Corporation, New York

Haythornthwaite J A, Sieber W J, Kerns R D 1991 Depression and the chronic pain experience. Pain 46:177–184

Horne R 2006 Beliefs and adherence to treatment: the challenge for research and clinical practice. In: Halligan P, Aylward M (eds) The power of belief. Oxford University Press, Oxford, ch 8, pp 115–136

Jensen M P, Karoly P 1991 Control beliefs, coping efforts and adjustment to chronic pain. Journal of Consulting and Clinical Psychology 59:431–438

Jensen M P, Turner J A, Romano J M et al 1991 Coping with chronic pain: a critical review of the literature. Pain 47:249–283

Jensen M P, Turner J A, Romano J M et al 1994 Relationship of pain specific beliefs to chronic pain adjustment. Pain 57:301–309

Keefe F, Wilkins R, Cook W, Crisson J et al 1986 Depression, pain and pain behavior. Journal of Consulting and Clinical Psychology 54:665–669

Keefe F J, Brown G K, Wallston K A et al 1989 Coping with rheumatoid arthritis pain: catastrophising as a maladaptive strategy. Pain 37:51–56

Keefe F J, Salley A N Jr, LeFebvre J C 1992 Coping with pain: conceptual concerns and future references. Pain 51:131–134

Keefe F J, Affleck G, Lefebvre J et al 1997 Pain coping strategies and pain efficacy in rheumatoid arthritis: a daily process analysis. Pain 69:35–42

Keefe F J, Rumble M E, Scipio C D et al 2004 Psychological aspects of persistent pain: current state of the science. Journal of Pain 5:195–211

Kendall N A S, Linton S J, Main C J 1997 Guide to assessing psychosocial yellow flags in acute low back pain: risk factors for long term disability and work loss. Accident Rehabilitation and Compensation Insurance Corporation of New Zealand and the National Health Committee, Wellington NZ

Kerns R D, Rosenberg R, Jamison R N et al 1997 Readiness to adopt a self-management approach to chronic pain: the Pain Stages of Change Questionnaire (PSOCQ). Pain 72:227–234

Klenerman L, Slade P D, Stanley I M et al 1995 The prediction of chronicity in patients with an acute attack of low back pain in a general practice setting. Spine 20:478–484

Kuttner L 1989 Management of young children's acute pain and anxiety during invasive medical procedures. Paediatrician 16:39–44

Labus J S, Keefe F J, Jensen M P 2003 Self-reports of pain intensity and direct observations of pain behavior: when are they correlated? Pain 102(1–2):109–124

Lackner J M, Carosella A M, Feuerstein M 1996 Pain expectancies, pain and functional self-efficacy expectancies as determinants of disability in patients with chronic low back disorders. Journal of Consulting Clinical Psychology 64:212–220

Lazarus R S 1993 Coping theory and research: past, present and future. Psychosomatic Medicine 55:234–247

Lazarus R, Folkman S 1984 Stress appraisal and coping. Springer-Verlag, New York

Letham J, Slade P D, Troop J D G et al 1983 Outline of a fear-avoidance model of exaggerated pain perception. Behaviour Research and Therapy 21:401–408

Leventhal H, Leventhal E A, Contrada R J 1998 Self-regulation, health and behavior: a perceptual-cognitive approach. Psychology and Health 13:717–733

Linton S J, Andersson T 2000 Can chronic disability be prevented? A randomised trial of a cognitive-behavior intervention and two forms of information for patients with spinal pain. Spine 25:2825–2831

Linton S J, Gross D, Schultz I Z et al 2005 Prognosis and the identification of workers risking disability: research issues and directions for future research. Journal of Occupational Rehabilitation 15:459–474

Lyons, R, Sullivan, M J L, Ritvo P et al 1995 Relationships in chronic illness and disability. Sage, Thousand Oaks, CA

McCracken L, Gross R 1993 Does anxiety affect coping with pain? Clinical Journal of Pain 9:253–259

McCracken L M, Zayfert C, Gross R T 1992 The Pain Anxiety Symptoms Scale: development and validation of a scale to measure fear of pain. Pain 50(1):67–73

Main C J, Burton A K 2000 Economic and occupational influences on pain and disability. In: Main C J, Spanswick C C (eds) Pain management: an interdisciplinary approach. Churchill Livingstone, Edinburgh, ch 4, pp 63–87

Main C J, Waddell G 1991 A comparison of cognitive measures in low back pain: statistical structure and clinical validity at initial assessment. Pain 46:287–298

Main C J, Phillips C J, Watson P J 2005 Secondary prevention in health-care and occupational settings in musculoskeletal conditions (focusing in particular in low back pain). In: Schultz I Z, Gatchel R J (eds) Handbook of complex occupational disability claims: early risk identification, intervention and prevention. Kluwer Academic/Plenum, New York, sect IV: ch 1, pp 387–404

Melzack R, Wall P D 1965 Pain mechanisms: a new theory. Science 150:971–979

Merskey H, Bogduk N 1994 Classification of chronic pain. IASP Press, Seattle

Morley S 2004 Editorial: Process and change in cognitive behaviour therapy for chronic pain. Pain 109:205–206

Petrie K J, Weinman J A (eds) 1998 Perceptions of health and illness: current research and applications. Harwood Academic, Amsterdam, pp 2–3

Prkachin K, Craig K 1995 Expressing pain: the communication and interpretation of pain signals. Journal of Nonverbal Behavior 19:191–205

Prochaska J O, DiClemente C C 1982 Transtheoretical therapy: toward a more integrative model of change. Psychotherapy: Theory Research and Practice 19:276–288

Quine L, Rutter D R, Arnold L 1998 Predicting safety-helmet use among schoolboy cyclists: a comparison of the theory of planned behaviour and the health belief model. Psychology and Health 13:251–269

Rey R 1993 History of pain. Edition La Decouverte, Paris

Rimm O L, Litvak S B 1969 Self-verbalisation and emotional arousal. Journal of Abnormal Psychology 74:181–187

Romano J, Turner J, Friedman L et al 1991 Observational assessment of chronic pain patient-spouse behavioral interactions. Behavior Therapy 22:549–567

Romano J, Turner J, Jensen M et al 1995 Chronic pain patient-spouse interactions predict patient disability. Pain 65:353–360

Rosenstiel A K, Keefe F J 1983 The use of coping strategies in chronic low back pain patients: relationship to patient characteristics and current adjustment. Pain 17:33–44

Rudy T E, Kerns R D, Turk D C 1988 Chronic pain and depression: a cognitive mediation model. Pain 35:129–140

Salmon P 2006 Explaining unexplained symptoms: the role of beliefs in clinical management. In: Halligan P, Aylward M (eds) The power of belief. Oxford University Press, Oxford, ch 9, pp 137–159

Schmitz U, Saile H, Nilges P 1996 Coping with chronic pain: flexible goal adjustment as an interactive buffer against pain-related distress. Pain 67:41–51

Sieben J M, Portegijs P J M, Vlaeyen J W S et al 2005 Pain-related fear at the start of a new back pain episode. European Journal of Pain 9:635–641

Skevington S 1995 Psychology of pain. John Wiley, Chichester

Sullivan, M J L 2006 Toward a biopsychomotor conceptualisation of pain. Clinical Journal of Pain (in press)

Sullivan M, Bishop S, Pivik J 1995 The Pain Catastrophizing Scale: development and validation. Psychological Assessment 7:524–532

Sullivan M, Tripp D, Santor D 2000 Gender differences in pain and pain behavior: the role of catastrophizing. Cognitive Therapy and Research 24:121–134

Sullivan M J L, Thorn B, Haythornthwaite J A et al 2001 Theoretical perspectives on the relation between catastrophizing and pain. Clinical Journal of Pain 17:52–64

Sullivan M J, Rodgers W M, Wilson P M et al 2002 An experimental investigation of the relation between catastrophizing and activity intolerance. Pain 100(1–2):47–53

Sullivan M J, Adams H, Sullivan M E 2004 Communicative dimensions of pain catastrophizing: social cueing effects on pain behaviour and coping. Pain 107:220–226

Sullivan M J, Feuerstein M, Gatchel R et al 2005 Integrating psychosocial and behavioral interventions to achieve optimal rehabilitation outcomes. Journal of Occupational Rehabilitation 15:475–489

Sullivan, M J L, Martel, M O, Savard, A et al 2006a The relation between catastrophizing and the communication of pain experience. Pain 122:282–288

Sullivan M J L, Thibault, P, Savard A et al 2006b The influence of communication goals and physical demands on different dimensions of pain behavior. Pain 125:202–203

Thorn B E, Ward L C, Sullivan M J et al 2003 Communal coping model of catastrophizing: conceptual model building. Pain 106(1–2):1–2

Toomey T C, Mann J D, Abashian S et al 1991 Relationship between perceived self-control of pain, pain description and functioning. Pain 45:129–133

Turk D C 1996 Biopsychosocial perspective on chronic pain. In: Gatchel R J, Turk D C (eds) Psychological approaches to pain management: a practitioner's handbook. Guilford Press, New York, ch 1, pp 3–32

Turk D C, Gatchel R J (eds) 1999 Psychosocial factors in pain. The Guilford Press, New York

Turk D C, Meichenbaum D H, Genest M 1983 Pain and behavioral medicine: a cognitive-behavioral perspective. Guilford Press, New York

Turner J A 1991 Coping and chronic pain. In: Bond M R, Charlton J E, Woolf C (eds) Proceedings of the VIth World Congress on Pain. Elsevier, New York, pp 219–227

Unruh A 1996 Review article: Gender variations in clinical pain experience. Pain 65:123–167

van den Hout J H, Vlaeyen J W, Houben R M et al 2001 The effects of failure feedback and pain-related fear on pain report, pain tolerance and pain avoidance in chronic low back pain patients. Pain 92:247–257

Vlaeyen J, Kole-Snijders A M J, Boeren R G B et al 1995 Fear of movement/(re)injury in chronic low back pain and its relation to behavioral performance. Pain 62:363–372

Vlaeyen J W, Linton S J 2000 Fear-avoidance and its consequences in chronic musculoskeletal pain: a state of the art. Pain 85:317–332

Waddell G 1998 The back pain revolution, 1st edn. Churchill Livingstone, Edinburgh

Waddell G 2004 The back pain revolution, 2nd edn. Churchill Livingstone, Edinburgh

Waddell G, Somerville D, Henderson I et al 1993 A fear avoidance beliefs questionnaire (FABQ) and the role of fear avoidance beliefs in chronic low back pain and disability. Pain 52:157–168

Wall P D 1999 Pain: the science of suffering. Weidenfield and Nicholson, London

Weinberger D A 1990 The construct validity of the repressive coping style. In: Singer J L (eds) Repression and dissociation. University of Chicago Press, Chicago, pp 337–386

Williams A C de C 2002 Facial expression of pain: an evolutionary account. Behavioral and Brain Sciences 25: 439–455

Chapter Three

3

The psychological impact of pain and disability

Historical perspective

The relationship between pain and mental health has a long history. Paradoxically, the mental health practice of antiquity was more concerned with the infliction of pain than its alleviation. Demonology dominated early views of mental illness. Archaeological records suggest that shamans of the Stone Age bored holes in the skulls of 'affected' individuals in order to provide an escape route for the evil spirits which were thought to be possessing them (Selling 1943). Similarly, priests of the middle ages engaged in practices such as exorcism in order to rid the body of evil spirits (White 1896). When unsuccessful, rituals of exorcism were supplemented by flogging, starving, immersion in cold water and other torturous methods. These methods were devised to create such an unpleasant environment within the body that no evil spirit would wish to remain. Torturous techniques were later adopted by medical practitioners of mental asylums as useful techniques to calm agitated patients (Fig. 3.1).

It is only within the last century that mental health practice has turned its attention toward the treatment of individuals with chronic pain conditions. However, in current conceptualisations of chronic pain there remain vestiges of the conceptual models of antiquity. Even certain aspects of demonology have remained central to current explanatory models and methods of intervention for chronic pain. For example, Freudian theory suggests that certain psychological conflicts suppressed from consciousness can find expression as physical symptoms such as pain and disability. Within this framework, analytical and abreactive techniques are used to 'free' sufferers from the subconscious

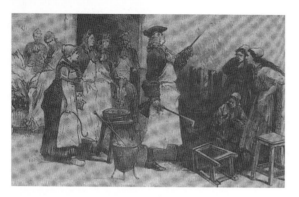

Figure 3.1 • Boerhaave's treatment of hysteria. 'In the insane asylum at Leyden, hot irons were applied to the head to bring patients to their senses. Here, Boerhaave, a medical authority of the time, is threatening hysteric women patients with cauterisation' (White 1896).

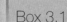

Box 3.1

Reasons for the identification of psychopathology

- Unrecognised and untreated psychopathology can compromise successful rehabilitation
- Psychopathology may increase pain intensity and disability thus perpetuating pain-related dysfunction
- Anxiety decreases pain threshold and tolerance
- Anxiety and depression are associated with symptom magnification
- Emotional distress may be associated with autonomic arousal, hypervigilance, misinterpretation of symptoms or somatic amplification.

Adapted from Dersh et al (2002, p. 773)

conflicts that are at the root of their pain problems (Breuer & Freud 1893). The notion that some form of noxious agent is locked within the individual with chronic pain and that this agent must be released in order to bring about a cure continues to find expression in many domains of mental health practice associated with chronic pain (Weintraub 1988).

Despite a century of clinical and theoretical discussions of the relation between pain and mental health, there is a sense that no significant advance has occurred. Progress in our understanding of the links between pain and mental health, and in our ability to effectively treat mental health conditions associated with pain has been modest. The billions of dollars spent each year on the disability-related costs of chronic pain, and the extensive waiting lists of hundreds of pain clinics speak of the magnitude of the pain problem in our society. The all-too-frequent negligible impact of treatments offered at pain clinics highlights the limits of the tools available to bring about meaningful change in the suffering and disability associated with chronic pain.

Chronic pain and psychopathology

Chronic pain is associated with a high rate of diagnosable psychopathology. According to Dersh et al (2002), there are a number of reasons to identify psychopathology in chronic pain patients (shown in Box 3.1). There is certainly statistical evidence for such associations,

but the interpretation of such relationships is far from straightforward.

Clearly the treatment of major mental health problems is primarily the responsibility of mental health professionals, but many chronic-pain patients show evidence of significant distress, and it has been reported that approximately 50% of psychiatric inpatients will report having some pain. At a practical level, therefore, the pain professional of any discipline must have some understanding of the nature of psychopathology, particularly with respect to when patients should be referred to other services and when their distress should be managed within the context of a multidimensional pain management approach.

To treat or not to treat? The nature of clinical decision making

Having identified the issue of mental health problems, which shall be considered in more detail later in this chapter, with further discussions on assessment in Chapter 8 and on management in Chapter 10, there are a number of key questions that need to be answered in order to determine the patient's likelihood of deriving benefit from a pain management programme (PMP). These questions are listed in Box 3.2.

Thus, one must judge whether the mental health problems constitute an absolute or temporary barrier to full participation in the PMP. Then, assuming

Box 3.2

Key clinical questions

- Is the patient likely to benefit from pain management?
- Are there any psychiatric obstacles to participation in a PMP at this time?
- Is the patient in need of a specialist mental health review?
- If the patient is currently receiving psychiatric treatment should this be completed before undergoing a PMP?
- Would the patient benefit from in-house psychological intervention as a precursor to full participation in the PMP?

Box 3.3

Major types of orange flag

Flags indicative of unsuitability for pain management

Major personality disorder:

- evidence of aggressive or disruptive behaviour
- clear evidence of unwillingness to take any personal responsibility
- marked irritation at having to 'share treatment' (i.e. be part of a group).

Substance abuse disorder:

- concentration, cooperation or participation likely to be compromised by major recent or ongoing illicit drug use or markedly excessive alcohol use.

Current forensic involvement:

- scheduling of treatment or negotiation of reasonable rehabilitation goals not possible until resolution of ongoing forensic involvement.

Flags indicative of need for specialist referral

Active psychiatric disorder:

- showing evidence of psychotic symptoms such as disordered thinking, marked agitation
- under psychiatric management for ongoing psychiatric illness
- experiencing significant cognitive side-effects from medication.

Difficulties in comprehension (apart from medication side-effects):

- post-traumatic cognitive impairment
- other neuropsychological difficulties of a severity likely to compromise participation in programme.

Very high level of distress:

- unable to fully participate in assessment because of distress
- not able to participate in the establishment of treatment goals because of distress.

Major communication problems:

- illiteracy
- unable to communicate in the language of the programme.

---

the patient is considered potentially suitable for pain management at all, the need for primary psychological treatment in addition to pain management needs to be considered.

Appraisal of significant mental health problems: identification of orange flags

The nature of the conceptual system of flags was described at the end of the previous chapter. To recap, yellow flags should be thought of as aspects of *normal* psychological processes, but they have sometimes been confused with psychiatric disorders, such as major mental illnesses or major personality disorders, including illicit drug use and ongoing forensic involvement. Such factors have been termed *orange flags*. Orange flags can be thought of as the psychiatric equivalent of red flags in that they require specialist assessment/referral, marking the individual as unsuitable (at the time) for a straightforward biopsychosocial approach. More specifically, they should be thought of as psychological symptoms or behavioural patterns that render the individual unsuitable (at the time) for routine pain management, indicating instead that the individual should be referred to a mental health specialist.

Note: Flag identification should not be confused with detailed psychological or psychiatric assessment; it should be thought of more in terms of signposting and triage.

The major orange flags are shown in Box 3.3.

Flags indicative of unsuitability for pain management

Evidence of any of these flags at the time of initial assessment should raise serious questions about whether the patient is suitable for the sort of PMP that is essentially based on self-help, requires application and focus, and uses therapeutic groups as part of its approach.

(Problematic use of appropriate medication, whether analgesics, NSAIDs, antidepressants or hypnotics, is not an orange flag, and should be managed by the pain team, as discussed in Part 3 of Chapter 11.)

Flags indicative of the need for specialist referral

Evidence of any of these flags may also eventually turn out to be 'showstoppers', and will require, at the very least, assessment by a mental health professional (from within or without the pain service) and the development of a shared treatment protocol or (preferably) the reappraisal of the patient's suitability for pain management at the conclusion of his/her psychiatric treatment.

Identification of orange flags as a management process

Screening for orange flags should be thought of as a management process rather than a psychiatric or psychological assessment. The categories are rudimentary and should be considered as no more than signposts towards specialist assessment/management. As such, they should be conceptualised as part of an early-warning system, identifying patients who require specialist evaluation before consideration for 'routine' biopsychosocial management. Whether such flags are absolute or only temporary obstacles to full engagement in self-directed management will need to be evaluated on a case-by-case basis, following a detailed clinical assessment.

Caveats

Exclusion or deferment on the basis of orange flags should be extremely rare, except in health-care systems permitting direct self-referral without any sort of screening.

It is particularly important that, in general, the management of pain-associated distress should be considered to fall within the remit of the pain management team, and that it should be viewed, essentially, as a yellow flag, rather than as a contra-indication to pain management. It is not unusual, for example, for a patient to

be involved in a number of initial sessions of individualised psychological therapy as a means of enabling full participation in the PMP.

Presenting psychological characteristics

Assuming that psychological factors of orange flag significance have led to appropriate patient referral or triage, it is now appropriate to consider the nature of the psychological components characterising the patient with chronic pain. These psychological components are usually a consequence of the persistence of pain, and of the extent of the concomitant impact of pain on function, participation and well-being. In this chapter, the nature of the main psychological characteristics will be described. Assessment and management will be discussed in later chapters.

The principal psychological characteristics of patients presenting with pain are shown in Box 3.4.

Anxiety, depression and anger are the three emotions that best characterise the distress of chronic pain sufferers, and much of this distress is evidenced in the display or expression of pain behaviour. It is possible to consider these psychological phenomena in terms of their specific cognitive and behavioural features or in terms of their psychobiological or psychophysiological substrates, but the focus of this chapter is on the psychological *impact* of pain and disability. In practice, patients often present with a mixed bag of symptoms of varying severity and significance. In primary care, among patients presenting with less entrenched and less severe pain-associated problems, it is not appropriate to focus heavy-duty psychological management on any but the most dramatic of symptoms (e.g. declared suicidal intent or self-harm). With the passage of time, however, the impact of pain increases so that there is a much higher level of identifiable psychological symptoms of

Box 3.4

Principal presenting psychological disorders accompanying pain

- Depression
- Anxiety
- Post-traumatic stress disorder
- Phobias and generalised anxiety disorder (GAS)
- Somatisation
- Anger and hostility.

greater severity. This trend is reflected in the increasing rate of identifiable psychological disorders with the passage of time, and with the number of failed treatments. Such clusters of symptoms may merit management in their own right and if sufficiently developed may constitute an identifiable mental illness requiring treatment.

The rest of this chapter will focus on the description of the major psychological symptom clusters, all of which map onto DSM-IV (1994) criteria for mental disorders and which may be indicative of minor psychiatric illnesses requiring treatment in their own right or treatment as part of a comprehensive pain management package.

Identification of psychiatric illness

An excellent review of the relationship between emotion and pain is offered by Robinson & Riley (1999). Chronic pain patients are frequently distressed, but the level of distress or the manner of symptom presentation occasionally raises the question of a primary or coexistent psychiatric disorder requiring treatment in its own right. Some clinics include formal psychiatric assessment as part of their initial evaluation. This chapter will appraise the validity and utility of some of the older psychiatric constructs, such as hysteria and hypochondriasis, as well as the more frequent of the psychological syndromes accompanying chronic pain. A full debate of the content and nature of systems of psychiatric classification is beyond the scope of this textbook. The formal DSM-IV diagnostic criteria for some of the most frequently ascribed diagnoses in chronic pain patients are presented in the Appendix to Chapter 8.

Depression

Of all mental health outcomes associated with chronic pain, depression is by far the most prevalent. Depression is a clinical syndrome characterised by emotional distress, negative thinking, motivational deficits and vegetative symptoms. Depression not only negatively impacts on the quality of life of the individual suffering from persistent pain, but there are indications that depression adds to the burden of impairment associated with persistent pain. It has been suggested that the pessimistic thinking or motivational deficits associated with depression may compromise an individual's progress in rehabilitation and recovery. As such, the assessment and treatment of depression are considered integral components of the management of patients with persistent pain. For decades, the pain–depression interface has been the focus of research and vigorous debate. For convenience, depression will be considered under a number of headings.

The spectrum of depression

The term 'depression' can be misleading. In common parlance, it is used to refer to a wide spectrum of emotions ranging from the slightly demoralised or fed-up to the suicidal. On the one hand, it can be considered to be a normal human emotion of variable intensity, but if sufficiently severe, it may be better understood as a major mental illness (in which individuals may no longer be capable of taking charge of their own affairs).

Similarities between chronic pain and depression

Undoubtedly, pain patients frequently seem to be demoralised or depressed. The similarities between chronic pain patients and depressed patients have led to a vigorous debate about the nature of depression in pain patients. Widely varying reported estimates in rates of depression among pain patients illustrate differences in the methods used to assess depression as well as differences across diagnostic groups and stages of chronicity. It is important, therefore, to distinguish dysphoric mood from depressive *illness*, for which there are clear diagnostic criteria (shown in Ch. 8). Even using these criteria, diagnosis is not always straightforward. It is important to note that the somatic symptoms of depression (weight change, sleep disturbance and fatigue) may also be a function of the chronic pain state, and that cognitive intrusion is a common experience in both acute and chronic pain. Substance abuse and anxiety are also concomitants of depression.

Prevalence of depression

Community surveys indicate that approximately 20% of individuals with chronic pain symptoms suffer from a diagnosable depressive condition (McWilliams et al 2003). Much higher rates are seen in specialty pain treatment centres (France et al 1986). For the clinician working in a specialty pain treatment centre, statistics suggest that at least every second patient seen will likely meet diagnostic criteria for a depressive disorder.

Numerous reviews have commented on the high rate of depressive disorders in samples of chronic pain patients (Banks & Kerns 1996, Romano & Turner 1985, Sullivan et al 1992). The high levels of comorbidity of pain and depression have prompted considerable

Box 3.5

Key issues in pain-associated depression

- Depressive symptoms are to be expected in patients presenting with chronic pain and indeed there are similarities in the clinical presentation of chronic pain patients and depressed patients
- There is a wide spectrum in severity of depressive symptoms but if sufficiently severe the symptoms may constitute a depressive illness
- Depression and pain are mutual risk factors, although research gives stronger support to chronic pain as a precursor of depression rather than vice versa
- Pain-associated depression can have a significant impact not only on psychological well-being but on work
- With significant depressive symptoms it may be worth considering a multimodal approach combining pharmacological interventions with pain management
- There recently has been an increasing research focus on vulnerability and resilience factors as influences on the development of pain-associated depression and its amelioration
- Strong contenders as potentially important psychological mechanisms in ameliorating pain-associated depressive symptoms appear to be cognitive factors, such as perceived control over pain and catastrophising, but further research into the determinants of outcome of treatment is needed and explanatory models will undoubtedly need to be multifactorial rather than unidimensional
- At this time it seems likely that the depressed patient with persistent pain may benefit most from multidisciplinary approaches that combine pharmacotherapy, depression management strategies and activity mobilisation strategies.

debate over the putative mechanisms that might underlie both pain and depression (Blumer & Heilbronn 1982, Dworkin & Gitlin 1991, Turk & Salovey 1984). A number of the key issues are shown in Box 3.5.

Severity of symptoms

Like all mental health problems, depressive symptoms vary in terms of their number and severity. A depressed mood is considered to be a normal reaction to events that are characterised by prolonged stress or loss. When examined in relation to stress or loss, it is not surprising that individuals with persistent pain show elevated

symptoms of depression. The stresses that can be associated with chronic pain include persistent physical distress, loss of employment, loss of financial security, loss of independence, adversarial relations with third-party payers, disrupted family relationships, etc. For example, it has been reported that depressive symptoms associated with chronic pain may arise in the context of negative spouse responses to pain (Cano et al 2000), low social support (Trief et al 1995), marital dissatisfaction (Cano et al 2000) and low family cohesion (Nicassio et al 1995).

Impact on work

Recent studies suggest that depressive symptoms associated with musculoskeletal disorders may increase the risk for prolonged work disability (Sullivan et al 2005, Vowles et al 2004). Individuals with pain-related musculoskeletal conditions with elevated depressive symptoms are away from work on sick leave for twice as long as individuals with musculoskeletal conditions who do not have depressive symptoms (Currie & Wang 2004). Depressive symptoms in individuals with musculoskeletal conditions have also been associated with a longer duration of wage replacement benefits following work injury or surgical intervention (Dozois et al 1995, Schade et al 1999).

Is there a predisposition to the development of depressive symptoms?

A considerable amount of research has aimed at identifying potential vulnerability factors that might predispose the development of depressive symptoms. Initial pain intensity and pain frequency have been shown to be concurrently and prospectively associated with elevated depressive symptomatology (Haythornthwaite et al 1991, Magni et al 1994). Investigations have suggested that pain intensity might be indirectly related to depression through mediating factors such as perceived life control, perceived life interference, and attributions (Maxwell et al 1998, Turk et al 1995). Given that there is significant stability to depressive symptoms, numerous investigations have noted that a substantive proportion of variance in outcome or follow-up depression is accounted for by initial levels of depression (Banks & Kerns 1996).

Several investigations also highlighted the potential contribution of negative cognitions to the development or maintenance of depression. Appraisal-related variables such as perceived disability (Geisser et al 2000), perceived interference due to pain (Maxwell et al 1998), perceived inadequacy of problem-solving skills (Kerns et al 2002), cognitive distortions (Smith et al 1994) and pain catastrophising (Sullivan et al 2006b) have been associated with elevations of depressive symptomatology. Factors such as self-efficacy for pain management (Arnstein et al 1999), self-control (Maxwell et al 1998) and greater acceptance of pain (McCracken 1998) have been discussed as protective or resilience factors that might decrease susceptibility to depression in individuals with persistent pain.

Surprisingly, there has been limited research on the treatment of depression associated with persistent pain. There is accumulating evidence that interventions that lead to reductions in pain catastrophising are associated with improvement in depressive symptoms (Burns et al 2003, Sullivan et al 2006b). Reductions in the helplessness dimension of pain catastrophising appear to contribute most strongly to reductions in depression (Burns et al 2003). Intervention programmes that specifically target catastrophic thinking may be those associated with the best outcomes (Sullivan et al 2006a). Given that persistent pain and depression are both associated with activity withdrawal, the depressed patient with persistent pain may benefit most from multidisciplinary approaches that combine pharmacotherapy, depression management strategies and activity mobilisation strategies.

Conclusions: key issues in depression

The conclusions of this overview are summarised in Box 3.5.

Anxiety

A number of the major considerations in the evaluation of anxiety in pain management patients is shown in Box 3.6.

Anxiety: the importance of the clinical history

Anxiety can vary in its severity from little more than a mild irritation to an emotionally crippling psychiatric disorder. A certain degree of anxiety is normal in many aspects of everyday life. In small amounts it acts as a 'motivator', and is a component of enhanced performance in different sorts of tasks. In contrast, excessive anxiety leads to demoralisation, disturbed concentration and impaired performance.

A degree of anxiety is a common feature of pain patients, particularly when they have not been given a clear explanation for their pain and its likelihood of responding to treatment. From the diagnostic point

Box 3.6

Key considerations in the assessment of anxiety

- Clarification of the nature and severity of symptoms
- Eliciting the patient's interpretation of symptoms
- Clarifying the specific focus of anxiety and somatic concern
- Evaluating the influence of anxiety on pain perception and response to treatment
- Implications for clinical management.

of view, it is important to take a careful clinical history of the development of an individual's anxiety. Widespread, long-standing anxiety may require treatment in its own right.

Importance of determining the focus of anxiety

Furthermore, patients differ in their *interpretation* of symptoms. In an exposition of the 'cognitive-perceptual model of somatic interpretation', Cioffi (1991) reviewed evidence supporting the view that the meaning patients assign to physical symptoms is profoundly influenced by their beliefs, assumptions and 'common-sense explanations' (causal attributions) and those of other influential individuals. These psychosocial processes and cognitive styles of thinking in turn guide behaviour. The primary task of the clinician is to determine the specific focus of the anxiety and whether patients' fears are based on misunderstandings about the nature of the pain or its future course. (Specific assessment of fear and anxiety will be discussed in Ch. 8.)

If an individual's anxiety is primarily focused on pain and its likely future course, however, the anxiety may be better understood as an incapacitating fear based on mistaken beliefs. Diagnostically, the anxiety may be better viewed as a pain-associated psychological dysfunction rather than as a primary psychiatric disorder. To the non-specialist, such distinctions may seem a little contrived (and indeed require careful assessment), but they are highly significant with regard to the appraisal of an individual's suitability for pain management.

Anxiety as an orange flag

If an individual's anxiety is sufficiently severe or widespread, it may preclude the patient's active engagement in a PMP. If it antedates the development of a pain condition, it may confuse and complicate assessment and make the identification of achievable goals of treatment difficult to attain. Stress reduction is a fundamental part of PMPs (Ch. 11), but if the level of anxiety is such as to compromise active participation in the PMP, some preparatory individualised anxiety management may be considered. Otherwise, it should be viewed as an orange flag and the individual referred to mental health services.

The diagnostic features of clinical anxiety are shown in Chapter 8.

Clinical management as an important facet of pain management

The role of stress reduction in management is discussed in detail in Chapters 10 and 11, but a brief overview may be helpful at this juncture. In terms of clinical management, the therapeutic goal is to attempt to modify the way in which anxiety, heightened somatic concern, or fear may have led to the misinterpretation of a patients' symptoms and the subsequent *labelling* of relatively normal sensations as abnormal, if not pathological. Often, apparently unfocused anxiety is based on specific fears of hurting/harming or of pain becoming uncontrollable or progressively increasing pain-associated incapacity. Individuals with high levels of somatic anxiety have a strong propensity for catastrophic thinking and, whereas a post-treatment report of catastrophic thinking is significantly diminished, levels of somatic anxiety are little changed. It may be that in individuals who are somatically focused it is the degree of catastrophising that governs emotional and physiological arousal. Failure to 'correct' these distortions during the pain management process will prevent successful rehabilitation and perhaps reinforce further mistaken beliefs about symptoms and convictions regarding pathology or disease.

Recommendations for the management of anxiety in pain patients are shown in Box 3.7.

Post-traumatic stress disorder

The nature of PTSD

Characteristics of events associated with the onset of a pain disorder have a bearing on the nature of mental health outcomes that might be experienced. Road accidents or occupationally related traumatic events can expose individuals to stresses that are so severe as to overwhelm their coping resources and leave them struggling to keep their emotional world intact (Asmundson

Box 3.7

Recommendations for the management of anxiety in chronic pain patients

- There is a spectrum of anxiety ranging from mild to significantly disabling
- Elicitation of a careful clinical history is extremely important
- Most anxiety should be manageable as part of the stress reduction component of the PMP
- Some patients may be helped by individualised anxiety management prior to the PMP
- If the nature or severity of the anxiety is such as to be likely to compromise optimal benefit from a PMP, it should be managed as an orange flag (rather than a yellow flag) and referral to the mental health services should be instigated

et al 1998). Incidents characterised by high levels of threat or exposure to horrific or disturbing circumstances can lead to symptoms of post-traumatic stress disorder (PTSD). The diagnostic criteria of PTSD are discussed more fully in Chapter 8.

PTSD and chronic pain

Diagnoses of PTSD are being made with increasing frequency in individuals with pain conditions associated with traumatic onset (Asmundson et al 1998, Mayou et al 2002). The comorbid experience of chronic pain and PTSD appears to be associated with more severe presenting symptomatology than in cases of either condition alone (Geisser et al 1996). Diagnoses of PTSD are also being discussed as a significant obstacle to rehabilitation progress in individuals with persistent pain (Sharp & Harvey 2001).

The lifetime prevalence of PTSD in the general population is estimated between 1% and 14% (DSV-IV 1994). Prevalence estimates of PTSD among chronic pain patients vary widely across studies. Polatin et al (1993) recruited 200 chronic low-back pain patients to assess the current and lifetime incidence of psychiatric disorders. Among their subjects, only 1% met lifetime prevalence of PTSD and 1% met current PTSD criteria. These results are similar to the lifetime prevalence of PTSD in the general population. On the other hand, in a large population survey, McWilliams et al (2003) reported a point prevalence rate of 10% for individuals with chronic pain compared to 3% in individuals without chronic pain.

Other studies have reported higher prevalence rates, particularly in individuals who were involved in motor vehicle accidents. Chibnall & Duckro (1994) examined 42 patients with chronic post-traumatic headache subsequent to a motor vehicle accident. A diagnosis of PTSD was made for 29.3% of subjects, and 19.5% met the criteria for partial PTSD. Other studies have shown that the prevalence of PTSD among motor vehicle automobile victims with chronic pain may range between 37% and 75% (Sullivan et al 2006a).

Risk factors for the development of PTSD

Although there are no studies directly addressing the prevalence of PTSD as a function of type of onset, it appears that PTSD symptoms might be more likely in pain conditions associated with traumatic onset than insidious onset (Geisser et al 1996). Pain alone is probably not sufficient to give rise to symptoms of PTSD; however, the incident that gave rise to the pain may have characteristics that can lead to PTSD symptoms (Asmundson et al 1998). A history of early trauma might heighten the risk of PTSD in individuals who develop pain conditions such as fibromyalgia (Cohen et al 2002). It has been suggested that pain might contribute to the persistence of PTSD symptoms by acting as a 'trigger' for memories of the traumatic incident (Mayou et al 2002, Sharp & Harvey 2001).

Treatment of PTSD symptoms in patients with chronic pain

There have been few discussions of approaches to the treatment of PTSD specific to chronic pain samples. Interventions will typically proceed by implementing a number of symptom reduction techniques that will vary as a function of the symptom profile of specific patients (Rothbaum et al 2000). There has been research to suggest that selective serotonin reuptake inhibitors (SSRIs) such as fluoxetine, sertraline and paroxetine can yield clinically meaningful reductions in the debilitating symptoms of emotional distress and social impairment associated with PTSD (Davidson et al 2001). Cognitive-behavioural interventions have also been shown to be effective in reducing PTSD symptoms and appear particularly useful in minimising anxiety and avoidance-related symptomatology (Hembree & Foa 2000). The use of anxiolytics in the management of PTSD symptoms has met with limited success (Braun et al 1990). In spite of available treatments, for approximately 50% of individuals who receive a diagnosis of PTSD, symptoms are likely to follow a chronic trajectory (Kessler et al 1995).

Box 3.8

PTSD: conclusions and recommendations

- In chronic pain patients with a traumatic onset of symptoms, routine screening for PTSD should be undertaken as a matter of routine
- If PTSD symptoms are of little more than nuisance value, they are likely to be helped by the stress reduction and sleep hygiene parts of the PMP
- If the symptoms are non-trivial they should be treated as a orange flag and specific treatment directed at the amelioration of the PTSD symptoms *prior* to acceptance on to the PMP
- Usually this will require referral to external mental health services, but if only a brief course of treatment is indicated, and if there is appropriate expertise within the pain team, this can sometimes be undertaken on an individual basis as part of preparation for the full PMP.

Conclusions and recommendations regarding treatment are summarised in Box 3.8.

Phobias and generalised anxiety disorder

In addition to PTSD, anxiety disorders that have been discussed in relation the chronic pain include simple or social phobias, and generalised anxiety disorder (McWilliams et al 2003). Fears are common experiences that are adaptive in many circumstances, but can lead to significant life interference when they become extreme or out of keeping with the actual danger associated with a particular event or circumstance. In some cases, PTSD symptoms partly resolve to the extent that they no longer require treatment for the widespread symptoms of emotional arousal, but the individual is left with specific fears (as a consequence of conditioning) that may have a phobic component and thus be amenable to treatment as such.

Prevalence of specific phobias and general anxiety disorder in chronic pain patients

In a community sample of chronic pain patients, McWilliams et al (2003) reported prevalence rates of

7% for generalised anxiety disorder, 6% for panic disorder, 15% for social phobia and 11% for simple phobia. In each case, the prevalence rates were found to be significantly greater than those observed in individuals without chronic pain. Although point prevalence rates of anxiety disorders in individuals with chronic pain might be higher than those of the general population, some investigators have suggested that lifetime prevalence might not differ significantly between chronic pain samples and the general population (Polatin et al 1993).

Anxiety disorders as the 'poor cousin' in terms of focused research

As a class of mental disorder, anxiety-related conditions associated with chronic pain may be as prevalent as depression (McWilliams et al 2003). However, relative to depression, anxiety disorders associated with chronic pain have received surprisingly little research attention. The reasons for the lack of systematic investigation of anxiety disorders in chronic pain patients are not entirely clear. It is possible that anxiety disorders might not be considered as debilitating as depressive disorders or PTSD. Along a similar vein, anxiety might be viewed as a normal reaction to chronic pain. For example, Gatchel (1991) suggested that anxiety might be a normal reaction to the onset of persistent pain, but its expression and associated disability might become dysfunctional or pathological as the pain condition transitions from an acute to a chronic phase. It has also been suggested that symptoms of generalised anxiety disorder observed in chronic pain patients might reflect pre-existing emotional dysfunction as opposed to a reaction to chronic pain (Polatin et al 1993).

Recommendations for management

If during the initial clinical appraisal of chronic pain patients, evidence of specific phobias or anxiety disorders emerge, then a clinical judgement needs to determine whether they are of sufficient importance to compromise the patient's probable benefit from the PMP. In such a case, these symptoms should be viewed as an orange flag and the individual should be referred to the appropriate mental health service, with the option of pain management reappraisal at a later date. However, if the problem is sufficiently circumscribed and does not compromise the establishment of appropriate goals for the PMP, it may be that it could be reassessed in terms of specific therapeutic attention following the PMP. An alternative within the PMP

might be to use the fear as a focus for the mastery of a problem-solving self-help approach and perhaps, therefore, as a means of tackling an obstacle to recovery (or optimal participation), as a first stage in the PMP itself.

Somatic awareness and concern ('somatisation')

The nature of somatisation and somatic concern

The term 'somatisation' is both controversial and ambiguous and the clinical literature is full of studies using similar or related terms ranging from a simple awareness, focus on, or concern about somatic symptoms to a full-blown psychiatric disorder in which psychological conflicts are assumed to have been transformed into physical symptoms. (Further discussion is offered in Ch. 8. Key features are shown in Box 3.9.)

Box 3.9

Key features of somatic awareness and concern ('somatisation')

- Somatic awareness and concern are part of the process of psychological appraisal of the presenting symptom (pain)
- It is perhaps best viewed as a biological response interpreted according to the patient's understanding of and familiarity with pain, shaped by social learning encounters with health-care professionals
- Iatrogenic distress and confusion (in the context of failed treatment and disappointment with outcome) may heighten somatic concern
- For the majority of chronic pain patients such concerns will be alleviated with the contextual view of pain offered in PMPs and it is likely that concern about symptoms, although not necessarily awareness of them, can be alleviated with the yellow flag approach within a PMP
- In a minority of patients there is evidence of longstanding and significant concerns about symptoms, and their current pain concern may be illustrative of a perpetuation of this process

(Continued)

- Such patients, if suffering from a somatoform disorder, are unlikely to benefit from a PMP and should be referred to the mental health services (i.e. orange flag triage) but patients may find it difficult to accept such a course of action, since a direct relationship between their present pain and their pain onset may be a matter of firm conviction. Thus even referral for *assessment* by a mental health specialist may provoke resistance.

Concern about symptoms can be viewed along a continuum from an essentially appropriate and normal response to the symptom of pain (and to be understood and managed, therefore, as a yellow flag) to a disorder requiring specialised mental health treatment (and treated, therefore, as an orange flag).

This distinction is more than just academic, since the two perspectives illustrate widely diverging views as to the genesis and nature of the somatic concern.

Implications of 'diagnosis'

Reframing concern about pain as a primary psychiatric disorder is a serious matter, and should not be undertaken lightly. Such a reframing may not be accepted by the patient and indeed may establish a basis for iatrogenic distress, most marked in cases of personal injury litigation in which a case may be made for a pre-existing or ongoing somatoform disorder to be considered as an alternative explanation for the persistence of pain resulting from a traumatic accident.

'Somatisation' as a normal phenomenon

Heightened awareness of all sorts of symptoms is characteristic of some pain patients (Main 1983). This heightened somatic awareness can be indicative of somatic anxiety. The process of somatisation has been defined in a number of ways, but is perhaps best understood as a *normal* phenomenon rather than as a psychopathological one. According to Sullivan & Katon (1993, p. 141):

A primary care perspective on somatization reveals it to be a ubiquitous and diverse process linking the physiology of distress and the psychology of symptom perception. Nearly all somatization is transient and treatable through modification of

physician behavior and the proper application of psychiatric and psychological therapies.

If such a concern is long standing and the focus has been on a wide range of different types of bodily symptoms, the patient may fulfil the criteria for a somatisation disorder; most pain patients, however, do not. The experience of somatically focused anxiety is, though, a common and apparently stable characteristic of pain sufferers and it is perhaps best understood as a cognitive distortion or misperception. A study of temporomandibular disorder (TMD) pain found that high-somatisation patients were three times more likely than low-somatisation patients to report pain in sites unrelated to the disorder (Wilson et al 1994).

Concluding reflections

Somatic awareness and concern is an essentially normal phenomenon and should be thought of as part of the process of psychological appraisal of the presenting symptom (pain). Patients vary in the extent of their somatic concern but there is little research into the determinants of this variation. Somatic awareness and concern can perhaps be thought of as a biological response interpreted according to the patient's understanding of and familiarity with pain. It is probable that social learning is further shaped by encounters with health-care professionals. Amongst chronic pain patients, there is often evidence of iatrogenic distress and confusion (in the context of failed treatment and disappointment with outcome) and it is likely that this heightens somatic concern.

For the majority of chronic pain patients, such concerns will be alleviated with the contextual view of pain offered in PMPs, and it is likely that concern about symptoms, although not necessarily awareness of them, can be alleviated with the yellow flag approach within a PMP. In a minority of patients, there is evidence of long-standing and significant concerns about symptoms, and their current pain concern may be illustrative of a perpetuation of this process. Such patients, if suffering from a somatoform disorder, are unlikely to benefit from a PMP and should be referred to mental health services.

However, a clear diagnosis of somatoform disorder can only be made by a mental health specialist. This may require an orange flag triage (if there is no appropriate expertise within the pain team), and patients may find it difficult to accept such a course of action since a direct relationship between their present pain and their pain onset may be a matter of firm conviction.

Box 3.10

Anger: most frequent themes

- Persistence of pain
- Failure of treatment
- Lack of clear and specific diagnosis
- Inconsistent diagnoses
- Perpetrator of injury
- Current/previous employer
- Benefit system
- Lawyers.

Thus even referral for *assessment* by a mental health specialist may provoke resistance. To make matters worse, there is little evidence of the efficacy of treatment for somatoform disorders.

Anger and hostility

Anger is commonly observed amongst pain patients and is a common feature of the chronic pain syndrome. According to Fernandez & Milburn (1994), anger, fear and sadness together are significant predictors of the affective component of pain, yet the literature examining the relationship between chronic pain and adjustment has focused primarily on the influence of anxiety and depression. Free-floating anger, like anxiety, is a mood disturbance and is not clearly focused. More commonly, anger has a declared focus. Some of the common themes are shown in Box 3.10.

Patients express anger in a number of ways. Anger is often evident from the manner and content of their communication. Patients may be disaffected with many aspects of their situation. They may be angry about how they have been treated in the past, or they may believe that they were referred to a PMP simply because their doctor could offer no better alternative. Emotional intensity may range from mild annoyance to hostility or even frank aggression.

Psychosomatic theorists have attempted to make a distinction between suppressed anger and expressed anger, but the distinction is of little value except in so far as it affects the decision whether or not to offer the patient assistance, or whether it compromises the patient's response to and compliance with treatment. Provided that the patient has sufficient trust in the staff to enable participation in the programme, most of the issues of concern will be addressed during group treatment.

The themes in Box 3.10 include both aspects of medical care and the socioeconomic consequences of pain-associated incapacity. In groups, individuals can be assisted to come to terms with their anger and disappointment. (The use of therapeutic groups is discussed further in Part 6 of Ch. 11.) Adjustment to pain also seems affected by the responses of others, such as family. Anger may be expressed as hostility to others, although there appear to be gender differences in the interaction between response to pain, style of anger management, level of hostility and response of spouse (Burns et al 1996). In men with the highest ratings of anger expression, the degree of pain severity and activity interference was partly accounted for by the perceived negative responsiveness of their wives. This relationship between anger, hostility and adjustment remained even when the effects of depression had been taken into account.

According to Fernandez & Turk (1995) and Robinson & Riley (1999), the role of anger in chronic pain and the removal of anger as part of the healing process have not so far been investigated sufficiently. Anger has physiological effects and persistent anger clouds judgement. This avenue of research would seem to merit much further investigation.

Conclusion

Chronic pain and pain-associated limitations on function, participation, quality of life and well-being are recognised. The impact of such factors on patients is variable. Population studies have indicated subgroups of patients with apparently high levels of reported pain who appear to have adjusted psychologically to the reality of ongoing pain as part of their life. They no longer consult health-care professionals and do not show evidence of high levels of distress. The research focus has primarily been on health-care consulters as viewed from a sickness or disability perspective, and appraised with a view to probable benefit from treatment. We know little about positive or adaptive coping strategies that may buffer the psychological impact of pain, but we can certainly state that the psychological impact of pain cannot entirely be explained simply by pain severity.

We know that in health-care consulters, with the passage of time, the nature and severity of the psychological impact appears to increase. Further, amongst chronic-pain consulters, there is clear evidence of an adverse psychological impact, at times of a severity indicative of a specific identifiable psychological disorder. In a sense, however, an adverse psychological response in the face of chronic pain and its unpleasant/disruptive effects is to be expected, and is, therefore, part and parcel of the lot of the chronic pain patient.

The challenge for the pain clinician is to determine whether the negative psychological impact can be limited by the approach offered by the pain service and the interdisciplinary PMP. Many chronic pain patients are characterised by marked emotional responsiveness, distorted cognitions and maladaptive pain behaviours, and, as such, they could reasonably be characterised as presenting with a psychologically mediated chronic pain syndrome (Main 1999). The treatment of choice for such patients is a cognitive–behavioural approach, or CBA (Morley et al 1999).

In a minority of patients, psychological difficulties are so severe as to compromise response to a PMP and to require primary psychological/psychiatric treatment in their own right. In this chapter, a range of such conditions has been identified. In such cases, orange flag triage should be undertaken.

However, this may be difficult for patients to accept, and may undermine the patients' confidence in the pain management team. Therefore, triage needs to be approached sensitively, and only when appropriate.

Finally, a general distinction has been made between flags indicative of unsuitability for pain management and flags indicative of need for specialist referral. In the latter case, the possibility of reappraisal of suitability for a PMP at a later date should be kept open for those patients considered likely to benefit clinically from initial orange flag management.

Key points

- **Chronic pain has an adverse psychological impact on patients**
- **There are a number of core psychological symptoms (and clusters) by which patients can be characterised**
- **The most important of these are depression, PTSD, anxiety, PTSD, phobias and general anxiety disorder, somatisation and anger (hostility)**
- **Patients vary in type and extent of psychological impact**
- **If sufficiently severe these psychological features may require assessment in their own right by mental health specialists**
- **The task for the pain management clinician is to determine whether any of these features, if unaddressed, are likely to compromise benefit from pain management**
- **There are two functions of orange flag appraisal:**
  - **firstly to identify those patients who are unlikely to benefit on psychological or behavioural grounds from pain management at all**
  - **secondly to identify those in which specialist mental health assessment should be undertaken to assess whether primary psychological treatment should be undertaken instead of, or as a precursor to, pain management.**

References

Arnstein P, Caudill M, Mandle C L et al 1999 Self-efficacy as a mediator of the relationship between pain intensity, disability and depression in chronic pain patients. Pain 80:483–491

Asmundson G, Norton G, Allerdings M et al 1998 Post-traumatic stress disorder and work-related injury. Journal of Anxiety Disorder 12:57–69

Banks S M, Kerns R D 1996 Explaining high rates of depression in chronic pain: a diathesis-stress framework. Psychological Bulletin 119:95–110

Blumer D, Heilbronn M 1982 Chronic pain as a variant of depressive disease: the pain-prone disorder. Journal of Nervous and Mental Disease 170:381–394

Braun P, Greenberg D, Dasberg H et al 1990 Core symptoms of post traumatic stress disorder unimproved by alprazolam treatment. Journal of Clinical Psychiatry 51:236–238

Breuer J, Freud S 1893 Studies on hysteria. Republished 1957, Basic Books, New York

Burns J W, Johnson B J, Mahoney N et al 1996 Anger management style, hostility and spouse responses: gender differences in predictors of adjustment among chronic pain patients. Pain 64:445–453

Burns J W, Kubilus A, Bruehl S et al 2003 Do changes in cognitive factors influence outcome following multidisciplinary treatment for chronic pain? A cross-lagged panel analysis. Journal of Consulting and Clinical Psychology 71:81–91

Cano A, Weisberg J N, Gallagher R M 2000 Marital satisfaction and pain severity mediate the association between negative spouse responses to pain and depressive symptoms in a chronic pain patient sample. Pain Medicine 1:35–43

Chibnall J T, Duckro P N 1994 Post-traumatic stress disorder in chronic post-traumatic headache patients. Headache 34:357–361

Cioffi D 1991 Beyond attentional strategies: a cognitive-perceptual model of somatic interpretation. Psychological Bulletin 109:25–41

Cohen H, Neumann L, Haiman Y et al 2002 Prevalence of post-traumatic stress disorder in fibromyalgia patients: overlapping syndromes or post-traumatic fibromyalgia syndrome? Seminars in Arthritis and Rheumatism 32:38–50

Currie S R, Wang J L 2004 Chronic back pain and major depression in the general Canadian population. Pain 107:54–60

Davidson J R, Rothbaum B O, van der Kolk B A et al 2001 Multicenter, double-blind comparison of sertraline and placebo in the treatment of post traumatic stress disorder. Archives of General Psychiatry 58:485–492

Dersh J, Polatin P B, Gatchel R J 2002 Chronic pain and psychopathology: research findings and theoretical considerations. Psychosomatic Medicine 64:773–786

Dozois D J A, Dobson K S, Wong M et al 1995 Factors associated with rehabilitation outcomes in patients with low back pain (LBP): prediction of employment outcome at 9-month follow-up. Rehabilitation Psychology 40:243–259

DSM-IV 1994 Diagnostic and statistical manual of mental disorders, 4th edn. American Psychiatric Association, Washington DC

Dworkin R, Gitlin M 1991 Clinical aspects of depression in chronic pain patients. Clinical Journal of Pain 7:79–94

Fernandez E, Milburn T W 1994 Sensory and affective predictors of overall pain and emotions associated with affective pain. Clinical Journal of Pain 10:3–9

Fernandez E, Turk D C 1995 The scope and significance of anger in the experience of chronic pain. Pain 61:165–175

France R D, Houpt J L, Skott A et al 1986 Depression as a psychopathological disorder in chronic low back pain patients. Journal of Psychosomatic Research 30:127–133

Gatchel R J 1991 Early development of physical and mental deconditioning in painful spinal disorders. In: Mayer T G, Mooney V, Gatchel R J (eds) Contemporary conservative care for painful spinal disorders. Lea & Febiger, Philadelphia, pp 278–289

Geisser M E, Roth R S, Backman G E et al 1996 The relationship between symptoms of post-traumatic stress disorder and pain, affective disturbance and disability among patients with accident and non-accident related pain. Pain 66:207–214

Geisser M E, Roth R S, Theisen M E et al 2000 Negative affect, self-report of depressive symptoms, and clinical depression: relation to the experience of chronic pain. Clinical Journal of Pain 16(2):110–120

Haythornthwaite J A, Sieber W J, Kerns R D 1991 Depression and the chronic pain experience. Pain 46:177–184

Hembree E A, Foa E B 2000 Posttraumatic stress disorder: psychological factors and psychosocial interventions. Journal of Clinical Psychiatry 61:33–39

Kerns R D, Rosenberg R, Otos J D 2002 Self-appraised problem solving and pain-relevant social support as predictors of the experience of chronic pain. Annals of Behavioral Medicine 24(2):100–105

Kessler R C, Sonnega A, Bromet E et al 1995 Post traumatic stress disorder in the National Comorbidity Survey. Archives of General Psychiatry 52:1048–1060

Magni G, Moreschi C, Rigatti-Luchini S et al 1994 Prospective study on the relationship between depressive symptoms and chronic musculoskeletal pain. Pain 56:289–297

Main C J 1983 The Modified Somatic Perception Questionnaire. Journal of Psychosomatic Research 27:503–514

Main C J 1999 Medicolegal aspects of pain: the nature of psychological opinion in cases of personal injury. In: Gatchel R, Turk D C (eds) Psychosocial aspects of pain. Guilford Press, New York, ch 9, pp 132–147

Maxwell D, Gatchel R J, Mayer T G 1998 Cognitive predictors of depression in chronic low back pain: toward an inclusive model. Journal of Behavioral Medicine 21:131–143

Mayou R A, Ehlers A, Bryant B 2002 Posttraumatic stress disorder after motor vehicle accidents: 3-year follow-up of a prospective longitudinal study. Behavioral Research and Therapy 40:665–675

McCracken L M 1998 Learning to live with the pain: acceptance of pain predicts adjustment in persons with chronic pain. Pain 74:21–27

McWilliams L A, Cox B J, Enns M W 2003 Mood and anxiety disorders associated with chronic pain: an examination in a nationally representative sample. Pain 106:127–133

Morley S, Eccleston C, Williams A 1999 Systematic review and meta-analysis of randomized controlled trials of cognitive behavior therapy and behavior therapy for chronic pain in adults, excluding headache. Pain 80:1–13

Nicassio P M, Radojevic V, Schoenfeld-Smith K et al 1995 The contribution of family cohesion and the pain-coping process to depressive symptoms in fibromyalgia. Annals of Behavioral Medicine 17:349–356

Polatin P B, Kinney R K, Gatchel R J et al 1993 Psychiatric illness and chronic low-back pain: the mind and the spine – which goes first? Spine 18:66–71

Robinson M E, Riley J L III 1999 The role of emotion in pain. In: Gatchel R J, Turk D C (eds) Psychosocial factors in pain. Guilford Press, New York, pp 74–88

Romano J M, Turner J A 1985 Chronic pain and depression: does the evidence support a relationship? Psychology Bulletin 97:18–34

Rothbaum B O, Meadows E A, Resick P et al 2000 Cognitive-behavioral therapy. In: Foa E B, Keane T M, Friedman M J (eds) Effective treatments for PTSD: practice guidelines from the International Society for Traumatic Stress Studies. Guilford, New York, 320–325

Schade B, Semmer N, Main C J et al 1999 The impact of clinical, morphological, psychosocial and work-related factors on the outcome of lumbar discectomy. Pain 80:239–249

Selling L S 1943 Men against madness. Greenberg, New York

Sharp T J, Harvey A G 2001 Chronic pain and post-traumatic stress disorder: mutual maintenance? Clinical Psychology Review 21:857–877

Smith T W, O'Keeffe J L, Christensen A J 1994 Cognitive distortion and depression in chronic pain: association with diagnosed disorders. Journal of Consulting and Clinical Psychology 62:195–198

Sullivan M J L, Katon W 1993 Focus article: somatization: the path between distress and somatic symptoms. APS Journal 2:141–149

Sullivan M J L, Reesor K, Mikail S et al 1992 The treatment of depression in chronic low back pain: review and recommendations. Pain 50:5–13

Sullivan M J L, Feuerstein M, Gatchel R et al 2005 Integrating psychosocial and behavioural interventions to achieve optimal rehabilitation outcomes. Journal of Occupational Rehabilitation 15:475–489

Sullivan M J L, Gauthier N, Tremblay I 2006a Mental health outcomes of chronic pain. In: Wittink H (ed) Evidence, outcomes and quality of life in pain treatment: a handbook for pain treatment professionals. Elsevier, Amsterdam (in press)

Sullivan M J L, Adams H, Thibault P et al 2006b Initial depression severity and the trajectory of recovery following cognitive-behavioural intervention for chronic pain. Journal of Occupational Rehabilitation (in press)

Trief P M, Carnike, Jr, C L M, Druge O 1995 Chronic pain and depression is social support relevant? Psychology Reports 76:227–236

Turk D C, Salovey P 1984 Chronic pain as a variant of depressive disease: a critical reappraisal. Journal of Nervous and Mental Disease 172:398–404

Turk D C, Okifuji A, Scharff L 1995 Chronic pain and depression: role of perceived impact and perceived control in different age cohorts. Pain 61:93–101

Vowles K E, Gross R T, Sorrell J T 2004 Predicting work status following interdisciplinary treatment for chronic pain. European Journal of Pain 8:351–358

Weintraub M I 1988 Regional pain is usually hysterical. Archives of Neurology 44:914–915

White A D 1896 A history of the warfare of science with theology in Christendom. Appleton, New York

Wilson L, Dworkin S, Whitney C et al 1994 Somatization and pain dispersion in chronic temporomandibular disorder pain. Pain 57:55–61

Chapter Four

4

Cultural and social influences on pain and disability

Introduction

In Chapter 2, the influence of beliefs and emotions on the perception of pain was reviewed. The response to pain in terms of pain-associated incapacity (or functional disability) has also been discussed and it is clear that *adjustment* to pain is also subject to a wide variety of influences. How we interpret pain and how we respond, and when or indeed whether we seek treatment, is subject to social learning. We learn which symptoms to take seriously and which require treatment. This may bear little relationship to the seriousness of the pathology. Serious symptoms may be dismissed as trivial, whereas relatively minor problems initiate treatment seeking. Without reference to the social framework of the patient and how they see their symptoms we cannot really understand their behaviour.

The evidence suggests that social factors have an influence on pain ranging from earliest experiences as a neonate to adjustment to chronic pain and incapacity in adulthood and old age. Prior to consideration of their specific spheres of influence it is important to consider briefly some of the underlying cultural, subcultural and social mechanisms which may shape our perceptions.

Cultural influences

Cultural and subcultural factors are not in themselves obstacles to rehabilitation except in so far as they translate into difficulties in comprehension, mistaken beliefs about the nature of pain and disability, resistance to seek treatment, unwillingness to comply with treatment

Box 4.1

Potential influence of cultural and subcultural factors

- Lack of adequate service provision:
  - difficulties in language or comprehension
  - failure in provision of culturally appropriate services.
- Mistaken beliefs about pain and disability
- Resistance to treatment seeking
- Unwillingness to comply with treatment
- Failure to accept responsibility for treatment outcome.

procedures or failure to accept a degree of personal responsibility for the outcome of rehabilitation. Each of these factors should be assessed as an obstacle in its own right (Box 4.1).

It can be seen that, with the exception of the first factor in Box 4.1, these potential obstacles are not culturally or subculturally specific. In appraisal of the influence of clinical history, however, it is important to consider whether such biases may have influenced the manner and content of treatment that has previously been offered to the patient.

Culture can be defined in terms of individuals' sense of ethnicity, religion, historical roots and general value systems. Culture, as reflected in similarities among individuals within a society, forms the basis for the development of stereotypes, which essentially maximise the similarity within groups and focus on the differences between the groups. Cross-cultural differences are evident in many aspects on human behaviour, and certainly in prevalence of illness and in health-care usage.

Cross-cultural differences in response to pain

Historical context

In the 1950s and 60s, Zborowski laid the groundwork for investigations of relationship between ethnicity and the experience of pain (Zborowski 1952, 1969), emphasising that pain is not only a neurological or physiological experience, but it is also shaped by experience, learning and culture. The global population is in a pattern of migration never seen before in history. The health-care practitioner, especially in urban areas, regularly comes into contact with people from other countries and cultures who may not speak the language of the host

nation. There are also subtler issues to deal with which depend on the way in which people of different cultures interpret the meaning of pain, their perceptions about the need for treatment and how pain behaviour varies between cultures and in those who are not able to communicate verbally due to language difficulties.

Difficulties in classification

There are difficulties in precise definition of terms, and this has an impact on research findings (Bhopal & Donaldson 1998). 'Ethnicity' is a cultural term implying a group of people with a shared distinctive culture and common language, and as such represents a shared identity (Njobvu et al 1999) and this may or may not be the national identity. In this context, classification by race alone is insufficient for research into pain (Turk 1996). Some studies use religion to define ethnicity (e.g. Hindu, Sikh, Muslim), whilst others use language (e.g. Hispanic), despite possible geographical separation and difference in racial grouping (e.g. West African and Indonesian Muslims). Furthermore the cultural influences in response to pain and injury may be viewed at a macroscopic (at the level of national identity) or at a microscopic level (such as in a work group or factory).

Accepting the previous caveat, in the UK ethnic minorities represent 7.9% of the total population. The largest group, which accounts for 50% of the ethnic minority population, describe themselves as South Asian or British South Asians of Indian, Pakistani, Bangladeshi or other South Asian origin (National Statistics Office 2001). Many of these groups are located in specific urban areas where previous immigrants have settled. In the city of Leicester in the UK for example, 36% of the population described themselves as Asian or British Asian in the last census and the demographic changes in that city predict that by 2011 the ethnic 'minorities' will constitute more than 50% of the population. In the USA the main ethnic groups are African Americans and Hispanics and like the South Asian people in the UK they are not distributed evenly but are concentrated in particular geographical regions.

Differences in language and pain expression

In Europe there is a stereotypical view of stoical northern Europeans and more emotionally expressive southern Europeans in reaction to pain, but it is not clear whether differences in pain expression are a product of different beliefs about pain and injury or differing acceptability of types of expression regardless of the pain beliefs. Therefore in practice, while it is unwise uncritically to adopt general classifications (Caucasian/ European, African, Asian) without an understanding of the underpinning beliefs about pain and the cultural norms for the expression of pain, it may be helpful to adopt such distinctions prior to the establishment of a better descriptive system.

Confounds of the link between ethnicity and pain

People newly arrived in a country rarely enjoy the standard of living of those who are native to the country or well established there. Newly arrived immigrants tend to be represented better in the lower socio-economic groups and there is strong evidence for a link between low socioeconomic status and poor health, including the report of more pain (Eden et al 1994, Nazroo 2003) and this may explain much of the variance in health between ethnic groups and the host nationals. There is some evidence that acculturation, whereby the immigrant takes on the values, beliefs and behaviours of the host nationals, may ameliorate ethnic differences in pain report and health. Those who are more acculturated report similar levels of pain and illness to the host population, in particular those who are second- and third-generation immigrants are more likely to share these beliefs and behaviours. However, this is still poorly researched. African Americans have lived in the United States for many generations, indeed many descend from people who have lived there for more generations than many white Americans, and still differences in pain beliefs and responses are reported. The fact that the descendants of ethnic groups often continue to live marginalised from the main stream society and continue to experience poorer socioeconomic positions and poorer health care may remain the key factor.

Differences in the experience and perception of pain

Ethnic differences in the reporting of low-back pain have been observed; in Australian Aborigines one-third of men and half of the women experienced back pain. However, they did not perceive it as a health issue and consequently did not report symptoms openly, display behaviour or seek medical treatment (Honeyman & Jacobs 1996). A study in rural Nepal reported that back symptoms were very common, although virtually no-one sought help for symptoms when medical services were made available. It appeared that the symptoms of back trouble were perceived as part of normal ageing processes (Anderson 1984). This demonstrates that the importance of a symptom like back pain and what a

person does as a consequence is subject to social norms. Some countries have tried to harness this social conditioning by trying to effect a cultural change through changing perceptions about back pain in the population to reduce consulting and give people a more benign impression of back pain through an intensive media campaign (general educational approaches are discussed further in Ch. 9).

Interestingly, there may be psychological differences as well as social differences related to ethnicity. Greater psychological disability, increased report of post traumatic distress syndrome and more sleep impairment has been demonstrated in African Americans and Hispanic groups with chronic pain compared with non-Hispanic whites. Black Americans also demonstrate greater affective pain scores in report of their pain and in response to experimental stimuli. To support this observation, increased activity in the limbic system during experimental pain stimuli has been demonstrated in African Americans when compared to white non-Hispanic Americans (McCracken et al 2001).

Health-care inequalities

Recently there has been concern that people who are ethnically different from a host nation are at a disadvantage with respect to treatment for painful conditions (Green et al 2003). Research into the health care for ethnic groups has demonstrated that people from such groups receive less health care than the host groups with respect to the provision of preventative health care, provision of medication and secondary care referrals (Atri et al 1996, Balarajan et al 1991, Green et al 2003, Shaya & Blume 2005, Todd et al 2000, Todd et al 1997).

One obvious explanation for the undertreatment of people from ethnic minority groups is the problem of communication. Newly arrived immigrants and those who live in close-knit communities may not be fluent in the language of their adopted country, and health-care providers may not have easy access to interpretation services. Inability to access information about available treatments or screening because of poor access to language specific literature and problems with literacy in the host language or own language have been identified as barriers to health care.

The differences may be more subtle; some people from ethnic minorities may perceive the doctor as the 'expert' and deferentially accept treatment unquestioningly – externalising their locus of control. The Medical Outcomes Study (Hays et al 1994), demonstrated that ethnic minority people were less likely to become involved in medical decisions about their own treatment than non-minority groups. However, this is ameliorated somewhat if the treating physician is of the same ethnic group as the patient.

Differential consultation rates for painful conditions, increased pain report and disability and lower quality of life have been observed for ethnic groups (Edwards et al 2001, McCracken et al 2001, Riley et al 2002) in comparison to the host nation. Higher primary care consultation rates for musculoskeletal pain have been reported in South Asian people in the UK who also report more back pain and widespread body pain than white British subjects (Allison et al 2002, Gillam et al 1989) and being from a South Asian ethnic group is a significant risk factor for reporting back and neck pain (Webb et al 2003).

Despite this increase in primary care consultations there is no evidence to demonstrate that these primary care consultations are translated into increased secondary or tertiary referrals. Indeed there is evidence that people from South Asian groups are less likely to be referred to specialist services (Balarajan et al 1991, Gillam et al 1989). In the USA where there is no social health-care system, people from ethnic minorities are less likely to consult primary care physicians, this has been attributed to financial reasons and/or the relatively larger number of Hispanic and African Americans who do not have comprehensive health insurance cover.

Acceptability of treatment and manner of health-care delivery

Treatments for pain provided in the West have been developed primarily from a western perspective of the causes and appropriate way to manage it. This applies particularly to the psychological and behavioural management of pain since there has been virtually no research into how this approach fits with the views of chronic pain in people from other cultures. We need to examine not only the philosophical approach of our programmes but also the way in which they are delivered. Such an analysis may lead to fundamental differences in how pain management is delivered, particularly in those with chronic pain.

Furthermore, the manner of health-care delivery often does not take account of cultural differences. Some cultures cannot accept mixed treatment groups delivered by both male and female health-care professionals. In some cultures women may not be able to venture out of the house for long periods unaccompanied. These issues need to be addressed to ensure that those who need treatment are receiving it. Most good health-care providers have advisors from different ethnic groups who can be a fund of information when developing services, and it is necessary now to integrate the insights into the development and evaluation of culturally competent

Box 4.2

Ethnic influences on pain: key features

- Difficulties in classification
- Confounding of links between pain and ethnicity
- Differences in language and pain expression
- Possible differences in the perception and experience of pain
- Health-care inequalities
- Acceptability of treatment and manner of health-care delivery
- Need for ethnic sensitivity and culturally grounded pain management.

pain management approaches for people from ethnic minorities.

Need for ethnic sensitivity and culturally grounded pain management

The advantages of ethnic diversity in multicultural societies are clearly evident in matters of culture such as arts, cuisine and the physical environment. In recent decades, however, problems such as social exclusion, poverty and discrimination have also become features of multiculturalism. There have been attempts through legislation to enable integration into society of immigrants from widely varying ethnic backgrounds. The need to address matters of language, educational and vocational skill development has been recognised and reflected to an extent in specific government-driven initiatives.

In order to address health inequalities, in terms of health-care provision, take-up and improved outcome for ethnic minorities, specific attention must now be directed at the content and manner of health-care provision. More specifically, in management of pain problems we need to develop culturally grounded pain management based on an ethnically sensitive and informed understanding of the ethnic influences on pain and its effects.

The key points regarding ethnic differences are summarised in Box 4.2.

Cultural and subcultural context as a framework for socialisation mechanisms

As aforementioned, little is known in fact about differences in *perception* of pain. The stereotype of the stoical northern European and the more emotionally

Box 4.3

Socialisation mechanisms

- Long-term social influences on pain experience, beliefs, appraisals, pain behaviours and pain coping strategies
- Role of direct instruction, reinforcement and punishment and observational learning
- Influence of emotional stress factors in the family context on pain experience and illness behaviour
- Specific influences of attachment, marital stress, family disturbances and family violence including physical and sexual abuse
- Role of sex differences in the socialisation of individual differences in pain and illness behaviour
- Influence of marital status, ethnicity and other socio-demographic characteristics on styles of socialisation
- Cross-cultural differences in the influence of health systems.

expressive southern European can be seen in the television coverage of reaction to disasters of various sorts. While it may be helpful for some purposes to focus on features in common across cultures, ignoring differences can lead to overgeneralisation and caricature. In understanding how individuals react, subcultural factors may be more illuminating. Cultural factors can be best understood perhaps in terms of socialisation mechanisms, and how these may affect both the *perception* of pain and the *response* to pain (including both treatment seeking and response to treatment).

Socialisation mechanisms

A number of the key aspects of social aspects of pain have been identified (IASP 1997). They are summarised in Box 4.3.

A considerable body of research has been undertaken into many of these mechanisms (reviewed by Skevington 1997). Even although it may be extremely important to understand such factors from a societal perspective, and therefore from the viewpoint of education and social policy, individuals are seldom able to give a clear understanding of such mechanisms in their particular case. They will tend to recall significant events, and may be quite unaware of some of the social forces which have shaped their perception. In clinical decision making, clinicians have to rely primarily on the information immediately available to them in terms of medical documentation, and in terms of the clinical

history and symptoms as presented by the patient. Some events of course may have considerable clinical significance (such as a history of sexual or physical abuse), but patients' clinical recall will tend to be focused on the supposed genesis of the current pain problem and the attempts to treat it. They will tend to be more accurate in their recall of aspects of history which are relatively recent and may be unable to clarify the origins of their beliefs about their pain. Such information frequently emerges during pain management as patients refine objectives for treatment and become aware of obstacles to recovery. It is important therefore to consider some of these social mechanisms.

A socio-communications model of pain

Although anecdotally, pain would seem to be relatively common, relatively little is known precisely about the prevalence of acute, recurrent and chronic pain in children, in part because of variability and imprecision in pain assessment, poor sampling frames and unknown generalisability of findings.

According to Craig (2002) 'understanding pain in infants, children and adolescents requires a broad perspective. Pain is a more plastic phenomenon than traditional sensory formulations acknowledge, with developmental factors and the social contexts in which children live their lives having a substantial impact.' He offers a 'socio-communications model' to illustrate the complex interdependence between the experience of pain, its expression and influence of and on care-givers (Fig. 4.1).

Assessment and interpretation of pain or pain behaviour and decisions about therapeutic interventions represent challenges, not only because of the subjective nature of pain (a problem also in pain assessment in adults) but also because of the influence of the stage of cognitive development on perception and communication within the child's social environment.

Further social learning

Arguably one of the most important influences on the development of modern pain management has been the recognition that chronic illness needs to be understood in a social context. Pain behaviour can also be viewed from a social learning perspective. A key feature in the early behavioural explanations was the recognition that pain behaviour was a consequence not just of nociception but of its social context. As such it needs to be understood not only as a response to nociception but also as a social event which may be subject to a wide variety of influences.

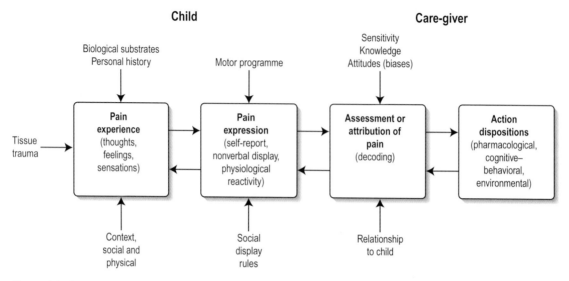

Figure 4.1 • The socio-communications model. From Craig (2002), reproduced with permission of IASP Press, Seattle.

Most developmental psychologists would agree that a major feature of 'learning', as normally understood, is the conscious assimilation of information. The term 'social learning', in the context of the development of chronic pain behaviour, needs to be understood somewhat differently as a process by which pain behaviour, and even the experience of pain, may be shaped by the context in which it occurs.

Furthermore, it is not always appreciated that social learning is an ongoing process and needs to be understood not only from the perspective of the young child, but also as a powerful force in the development of pain behaviour in adulthood. In the context of clinical pain management, the power of social influences can often be identified particularly in the contexts of family interactions, and as an important aspect of the health-care consultation process. Patients may be mostly unaware of the power of such influences, and indeed may resist the suggestion that their incapacity is more than a direct result of nociception.

Spheres of influence of social factors

The major spheres of influence of social factors are shown in Box 4.4.

Understanding the meaning of pain

Although we are biologically programmed to respond immediately to sudden unexpected pain in terms of escape or withdrawal, our response to pain frequently

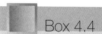

Box 4.4

Major spheres of influence of social factors

- Understanding the meaning of pain
- Communication about pain
- Treatment seeking
- Response to treatment
- Development of pain coping strategies.

also has to be understood in a social context. We arrive in the world with a set of instinctive responses which are then 'shaped' by social processes. The constructivist perspective on pain (Ch. 1) has deep roots in evolution and pain is viewed not as an accident of human development but as a protective factor that fosters adaptation and survival in a primitive world. Pain has to be understood as emerging from a biological substrate anchored in social processes.

According to Hadjistavropoulos & Craig (2002), observational measures of pain, such as non-verbal components, reflect involuntary features of pain under the control of lower levels of brain activity to a greater extent than those associated with language and they describe non-linguistic vocalisations and facial expressions as 'prime survival mechanisms' and not dependent on the conscious regulation of behaviour. Thus, for example, neonatal cries are largely reflexive and command attention, which caring adults are 'programmed' to provide. Craig et al (1992) have developed a sophisticated videotape rating system called the Neonatal Facial Coding System, or NFCS, which has enabled research into the expression of pain in neonates.

During the last decade there have been still further levels of sophistication in computerised analysis of expression.

Later, as we mature from neonates into infants and then young children, we learn about the meaning and significance of sensations, including pain. We observe how others react to situations and in turn develop behaviour repertoires of our own, initially by observation, then by imitation. Our first clumsy attempts are met with a variety of responses, but gradually through social learning processes, we come become more skilled and effective in our interactions with others, such that our needs are met. These learning processes have been specifically investigated in children with pain. They report striking similarities between newborn and adult facial responses to events that are painful to adults. Parents are 'programmed' into responding to expressions of distress in their children. As non-verbal characteristics are integrated with verbal utterances, more sophisticated communication patterns are established between parent and child. Young children learn to attribute significance to various sensations and thus develop a set of responses which become established behaviour patterns. 'Meaning' thus is learned and children learn to react to various levels of pain intensity. The dual process of observation and receiving various sorts of responses from others leads the child to develop not only a set of behavioural responses, but also a set of beliefs about pain and expectations about how others will respond. (A more detailed analysis of socialisation mechanisms is presented below.) As they grow older, children may experience new and different pain problems, and experience a different set of responses from others to their presentation of pain.

Communication about pain

As children mature into adults, they develop a wide range of communication skills. How they communicate about pain will depend on their experience of it. It is commonly observed among very young children who hurt themselves that their immediate response is to look at their parent. The response of the parent not only influences the child's response to that particular incident but begins to establish a set of expectations and behaviour patterns in the child. By the time the child has reached adulthood they may have encountered other people with pain, and their understanding of pain may have been further developed.

Treatment seeking

Pain is a common fact of life, yet not everyone consults a professional about it. Whether individuals seek treatment seems to be determined not only by the severity of the pain but by a further set of considerations such as the significance given to the pain, the treatment options available and access to health care. Treatment seeking can also be understood from a social perspective, and indeed the term 'illness behaviour' was originally a social construct. These ideas have had a powerful influence on more recent terms such as chronic illness behaviour 'invalidism', or the more specific 'pain behaviour' and 'chronic pain syndrome' (as viewed from a behavioural perspective).

Response to treatment

Prediction of an individual's response to treatment for pain is difficult, and their response seems to be determined by many factors. There is no doubt, however, that beliefs exert a powerful influence on response to treatment and may represent significant obstacles to treatment or recovery. Burton et al (1995) have shown that psychosocial factors are more important than medical factors in predicting future levels of disability one year later. The most important feature of the psychological profile was found to be the individual's beliefs about the likely future course of their symptoms.

Beliefs have many origins, ranging from specific information conveyed to them by health-care staff, to the views of family members or acquaintances, to articles in popular magazines and television programmes. A key aspect in assessment of suitability for interdisciplinary pain management is the appraisal of such beliefs.

Social factors may have a powerful influence on the degree of conviction with which a patient adheres to a particular belief. Trust or confidence in influential friends or family may underpin development of a near unshakeable conviction in a belief which has been expressed by them about the nature of pain or treatment. If such an opinion is unhelpful or misguided, it may constitute an obstacle to recovery which is difficult to overcome.

Many patients who develop chronic pain problems express distress about opinions given to them by doctors. Unfortunately, information received by patients can be sketchy, inconsistent and sometimes wrong. Furthermore, information received from health-care professionals can also be contradictory or misleading. (As discussed in Ch. 11, with chronic pain patients such iatrogenically produced misunderstandings can lead to confusion and distress.) Understanding and managing *social* aspects of the communication therefore is essential not only in the delivery of effective pain management, but also in the prevention of unnecessary incapacity. It is discussed in more detail later in this chapter.

Development of pain coping strategies

Individuals present with a wide range of coping strategies which they have learnt, sometimes through trial and error, but frequently from their social and family environment (Ch. 2). These coping strategies may be considered appropriate or inappropriate, depending on the specific context. Many different social influences may have had a bearing on the development of the particular repertoire of coping strategies evident at initial assessment. A detailed clinical history may indicate strong family influences. Locating management advice within an *appropriate* educational framework has been the guiding principle behind evidence-based guidelines for the management of back pain in primary care (CSAG 1994, Cost B13 Working Group 2004, Waddell 1998). These newer initiatives are discussed further in Chapter 9.

Conclusion

A proper understanding therefore of the social context in which the response to pain has been developed will often assist clinical decision making concerning both decisions about whom to accept for treatment, and also in the specific development of a therapeutic strategy.

The influence of demographic factors

The biopsychosocial model allows for wide variation in response to pain and in the first part of this chapter a powerful influence of cultural and social factors on pain has been identified. It is important also, however, to take into account perhaps more 'fundamental' differences in matters of age and gender which may influence service provision, clinical decision making and response to treatment. If in a society it is argued that there should be equal access to fundamental health care for all, then clinical service provision has to take into account the influence of demographic factors. In a cash-constrained health-care system such as the NHS in the UK, with devolution of health-care budgets to self-governing trusts, cash constraints have led to variation in levels of service provision of certain types of treatment (such as certain types of pharmacological treatment for cancer) being described in terms of a 'postcode lottery', so that whether or not treatment is provided is determined not only by clinical need but also by the district in which

---

Box 4.5

General influences of age and gender

- Initial biases and assumptions
- Manner of assessment
- Whether to offer treatment and what treatment to offer
- Expectations of treatment outcome.

---

a patient resides. This situation, properly a matter for ethical debate, illustrates that whether or not someone receives treatment is not dependent solely on their clinical profile. Such considerations might be seen in the first instance as lying within the purview of the politician.

There is, however, an additional obligation on those charged with health-care provision and that is to optimize the match or 'fit' between the treatment options and the patient receiving it. Potential differences between the pain management needs of the infant and those of the elderly patient are clearly evident, but there are also important sex/gender differences in health-care seeking and response to treatment. The 'one size fits all' is clearly inappropriate. While it might be argued that ensuring equality of health-care provision across communities is a matter for the politician rather than the clinician, in delivery of a person-centred approach to treatment, it is necessary to examine the influences of age and gender on perception of pain and response to treatment.

A number of general influences of age and gender on perception of pain and response to it are shown in Box 4.5.

The influence of age

Pain in neonates, children and adolescents

Pain in this age group has already been addressed from a social learning perspective, but there are additional influences on perception of pain. As McGrath & Gillespie (2001) have pointed out, the nociceptive system is plastic, having the capacity to respond differently to the same amount of tissue damage, so that even routine procedures such as injections are to an extent context-dependent and thus experienced differently. Maturation of the nervous system gradually permits the influences of descending pathways from the higher brain and modulates the nociceptive signals. Cognitive development influences not only the experience of pain but also understanding of the pain and appraisal of its emotional significance. Choice of assessment measure therefore has to reflect the developmental stage. In addition to the cognitive developments in infants and young children, the advent of puberty and the psychohormonal changes associated with adolescence can complicate matters still further, particularly in the context of chronic pain, not only in terms of assessment but also in terms of interventions. Chronic and recurrent pain in children has a point prevalence of at least 15% (Goodman & McGrath 1991) and as Eccleston & Malleson (2003) have pointed out, 'a noteworthy number of children and their families are severely affected by pain'. Delay in diagnosis and assignment of unhelpful and inaccurate diagnoses can compromise psychological adjustment, heighten family distress and decrease pain tolerance. Eccleston & Malleson (2003) observe further, 'The path to chronicity of pain is characterised by failed attempts to adjust and cope with an uncontrollable, frightening and adverse experience' (p. 1409).

Studies have shown that the best predictors of adolescent emotional distress are the extent to which adolescents catastrophise and seek social support to cope with the pain (Eccleston et al 2004). Fortunately, multidisciplinary programmes tailored for the needs of adolescents are now being developed and new assessment tools are becoming available (Eccleston et al 2005).

Pain in older people

The vast majority of treatments for chronic pain have been developed in younger people and there have been few investigations of age differences over the life span. As a consequence, clinicians have had to extrapolate from guidelines developed for young people (Farrell & Gibson 2004). Yet ageing is a 'prime candidate as a pain modulating factor' (ibid, p. 495) and although complications such as comorbidity can accentuate differences and complicate management, and the magnitude of age-related changes in pain presentations is not always substantial, it is important to appreciate the influence of age.

Most clinical series of patients suggest that the peak incidence of back pain and sciatica is at about 40 years of age, and epidemiological studies (Consumer's Association 1985, Croft et al 1994) suggest that lifetime prevalence increases from the late teens up to the 45–55 age group. According to Waddell (1998), 'these studies all suggest that the peak prevalence of back pain is somewhere between 40 and 60 years. There is probably a slight fall later in life' (p. 87). However, all forms of disability increase with age, and particularly affect the elderly, and the proportion of individuals reporting *restricted activity* rises linearly until retirement age.

Most epidemiological studies of older people have not been designed specifically to identify pain problems, and studies carried out in hospital populations cannot be considered equivalent to community samples (Helme & Gibson 2001). There is variation according to site of pain (Jones & Macfarlane 2005). However, pain prevalence appears to rise until the seventh decade of life, after which the overall prevalence does not appear to increase, but there is a higher proportion of certain types of painful conditions such as arthritis. In one of the few population studies, Thomas et al (2004) found an overall four-week prevalence of 72.4% (with a slightly higher prevalence among females) with pain causing interference in activities of daily living in 38.1% of the population. Physical changes in the musculoskeletal system are recognised as part of the ageing process. In the evaluation of the effects of accidents in cases of personal injury (such as road traffic accidents), there is frequently dispute among the medical assessors about the extent to which degenerative changes identified on X-rays can be attributed to the effects of injury received in the accident. Concepts such as 'acceleration' of pre-existing degeneration are based upon assumptions about normal changes in physical features with increasing age. To the extent that limitation in function is related to such changes, it is important therefore to evaluate an individual's disability in comparison with a reference group of the same gender and of a comparable age (Waddell & Main 1984).

According to Gibson & Helme (2001), there is some evidence of a modest age-related increase in experimental pain threshold, but it is not clear how or indeed if this translates directly into clinical pain experience since the picture is complicated by increased levels of comorbidity with age in the context of multiple influences on pain reporting. (Thus, for example, increasing levels of depression associated with lack of social support may adversely influence pain tolerance and enhance treatment seeking.) Thus while there are clear implications from such factors for the design and delivery of person-centred pain management, the role of specific age-related changes in pain perception remains unclear.

Of more interest in the context of pain management, however, are the psychological and social changes which accompany increasing age. Unsurprisingly, work interference as such becomes statistically less problematic as older people move to part-time work or cease work, but there is more to life than work. It is known that adjustment to pain is affected by the extent to which it interferes with valued activity (Rudy et al 1988). Increasing age may bring increasing leisure opportunities, but also increasing dependence and the need for practical and social support. As far as pain management is concerned it is important therefore to consider age not necessarily as a barrier to treatment but as a factor which may influence the understanding of the individual's adjustment to pain-associated incapacity. It is important also to identify treatment goals which are appropriate for the individual's age and circumstances. It should be remembered that older patients are sometimes reluctant to disclose the extent of their difficulties to health-care professionals and may even hold the inappropriate view that they are 'troubling the doctor' in consulting for treatment.

Finally, although our understanding of the effects of age on pain has become increasingly sophisticated, the interplay of pain and comorbidity generally, and of pain and dementia specifically are critical issues that remain largely unresolved (Farrell & Gibson 2004).

Some of the key features of the influence of age on pain are presented in Box 4.6.

Sex and gender

According to LeResche (2000) the prevalence of most pain conditions appears to be higher in women than men, although it is not possible to disentangle the extent to which these differences are attributable to female sex or the degree to which they are attributable to different rates of exposure to other risk factors for pain in men and women. In some conditions for example there is a clear interaction between age and gender. Although women are more likely to report multiple pain problems, at most body sites, this is not the case for every pain condition at every stage in the life-cycle. Thus while for back pain differences in prevalence are small, there are more marked differences in joint pain, chronic widespread pain, fibromyalgia, headache and TMJ pain. However, the fact that most common conditions show at least somewhat higher prevalence in women than men suggests that a generic gender factor (or factors) are present.

The reason for these differences is not immediately apparent but according to Unruh (1996), they are not likely to be explained simply by biological factors. In her judgement the key issues to be understood in trying to explain these differences are:

- *the way in which women and men perceive and respond to pain,*
- *the biological, social and developmental factors which may affect gender variations in the pain experience, and*
- *the response of the health-care system to the pain presented by men and women.*

(Unruh 1996, p. 124)

Box 4.6

Key features of the influence of age

- The pre-linguistic pain behaviour of neonates is illustrative of a primitive biological response to pain
- The neuroplasticity of the nervous system allows the modulation of pain by descending influences of the higher brain
- The experience of pain is progressively shaped and powerfully altered by the social context of pain
- The role of language and development of communication is fundamental to this process
- The psychohormonal changes of adolescence further influence the experience of pain, pain expression and psychological adjustment
- Chronic pain management in the adolescent requires a broadly based multidimensional approach within a biopsychosocial framework
- There appears to be a rise in the prevalence of pain until about the seventh decade of life
- There may be age-related differences in pain threshold in older people but on the evidence available these are likely to be of much less significance than the psychosocial and economic changes associated with older people
- Higher levels of comorbidity in the elderly, in terms both of physical illness, dementia and psychiatric disorder are likely to have an increased influence on pain tolerance and treatment seeking
- An increasing burden of pain is more likely to be influenced by psychosocial rather than biological factors and comprehensive pain management will need to be customised to the individual patient needs with recognition of the multiple influences on pain.

Some of the challenges in explaining the differences between the sexes in response to pain are shown in Box 4.7.

Sex differences in the experience of pain

The experience of pain from adolescence through adulthood is different in men and women. Women are more likely to have had experience of recurrent pain as a result of menstruation. Pregnancy and childbirth are further biological events which are sex-specific, and a proportion of women suffer chronic pain as a consequence of gynaecological problems or the physical demands of childbirth. Women need to distinguish between manageable

Box 4.7

Challenges in explaining the differences between men and women with pain

- Differing overall prevalence
- Differences across pain conditions
- Pain associated with sex-specific disease conditions
- Biological and physiological mechanisms
- Central mechanisms
- Responses to experimental pain procedures
- Implications for understanding clinical pain
- The psychosocial context of clinical pain
- Differences in pain perception
- Beliefs; emotional responses and coping strategies
- Social learning and health-care usage
- Clinical and research implications.

and excessive pain due to normal processes. There is a danger that opportunity for appropriate pain treatment may be overlooked because the pain is viewed as a 'normal' phenomenon rather than as a consequence of disease or injury. As Unruh (1996) has observed:

pain for women is a monitor for health as well as a potential symptom of injury, illness or disease . . . men have recurrent pains of lesser intensity, frequency or duration than women; however men are more likely to experience pain from injury, and acute and chronic life-threatening diseases (p. 157).

Pain associated with sex-specific disease conditions and surgery

These cases are important in terms of general medical management but of less relevance specifically to issues of pain management unless they have led to a chronic pain problem. In the latter event, the factors maintaining the chronic pain, and the associated obstacles to recovery may be of more relevance than the genesis of the pain.

Biological mechanisms

There has been little research as yet on specific sex differences in biological mechanisms, although there appear to be some differences in brain chemical metabolism and in the biological mechanisms of pain transmission (Polleri 1992).

In their review of sex differences in pain, Miaskowski & Levine (2004) contrast experimental

pain studies and clinical pain studies. They cite the Riley et al (1998) meta-analysis of the influence of gender in 22 experimental pain studies identifying an effect size of 0.55 for pain threshold and 0.57 for pain tolerance and a more recent study by Chesterton et al (2003) in which a sex difference of 28% was found. Finally, Riley et al (1999) in a further meta-analysis of the influence of sex steroid hormones on pain sensitivity found a clear impact of stage in the menstrual cycle in response to pressure stimulation, thermal heat stimulation and ischaemic muscle pain, although a different pattern was found for electrical stimulation.

Experimental pain research in animals has found differences in analgesic response, raising the possibility of oestrogen-dependent pain mechanisms as a partial explanation for sex differences. There do appear to be gender differences in pain regulatory systems, although it remains to be determined which aspects of the pain response differ according to gender. Miaskowski & Levine (2004) review a number of studies investigating sex differences in response to opioid and non-opioid analgesics but consider there to have been a 'paucity of studies'.

Central mechanisms

Experimental researchers have investigated both central and peripheral mechanisms and have postulated differences in primary afferent input to the CNS (i.e. both long-term developmental and phasic menstrual cycle-dependent changes in primary afferent function and coding), and central differences in the processing of sensory-discriminative and motivational-affective information at several levels of the nervous system.

Peripheral physiological responses to noxious stimuli

Although gender differences in cardiovascular response to non-painful stressors have been documented, there appear to have been fewer studies on gender differences in physiological response to tissue damage. According to Fillingim & Maixner (1995), 'Collectively, these findings suggest aversive stimuli and stressful tasks are less likely to evoke sympathetic nervous system and pituitary-adrenal responses while evoking greater negative psychological responses in females compared with males' (p. 216).

A number of more specific conclusions also emerge from their review.

- Overall, females exhibit greater sensitivity to laboratory pain compared with males
- These gender differences do not appear to be site specific

- Although gender differences are reported for all pain induction procedures, some forms of stimulation have produced more consistent findings than others (e.g. pressure vs thermal)
- Gender-associated differences appear to occur most consistently with pain induction procedures which mimic pain sensations similar to those experienced clinically (e.g. headaches, cramps and muscle soreness).

However, the authors acknowledge that further research is needed into different types of experimental pain, since experimental and biological factors do not appear to explain adequately gender differences, and that 'pain responses are characterised by great inter-individual variability and this variability likely contributes to the discrepancies across studies' (p. 210).

Implications of experimental pain studies for understanding clinical pain

The specific relevance of experimental pain findings for the understanding of clinical pain or its management has always been problematic, and this is particularly true in the investigation of sex differences. As an example, greater use of morphine post-operatively by men has also been found, but it is not clear whether the difference is in nociception or in pain tolerance. In contrast, human laboratory studies have shown that women may have somewhat lower pain thresholds and increased muscle tenderness. Indeed the incidence of fibromyalgia is much higher in women.

Thus while there may be a biological component explaining some of the differences in pain perception between men and women, the size of the effect is neither large nor consistent. Even if it is accepted that there may be differences in how women and men react to pain this difference does not appear to be attributable simply to differences in pain threshold. Even if it were accepted that experimental pain tolerance was an appropriate methodological framework within which to investigate sex differences, there is abundant evidence that *clinical* pain tolerance is influenced significantly by psychosocial factors. Investigation of differences in response to pain by men and women would seem to require a broader biopsychosocial framework including a focus on gender role rather than the narrower biological construct.

Implications of clinical pain studies for understanding clinical pain

According to Miaskowski & Levine (2004), acute and chronic clinical pain studies suggest that in comparison to men, women report greater pain with the same pathology, greater pain with the same degree of tissue injury, report a greater number of painful sites and are more likely to develop chronic pain syndrome after a clinical trauma. However, according to Robinson et al (2004), the size of the differences between men and women in clinical studies is less marked and less consistent, and the large discrepancy between experimental and clinical studies suggests situationally specific effects.

It appears improbable that the well-documented sex differences in use of health care, in consultation rates, and in beliefs about and expectations of health care will be explicable entirely on the basis of basic biological mechanisms. Differences in clinical presentation by men and women is suggestive of differences in social learning and in the experience of pain, possibly mediated or moderated by differences in beliefs about pain, in emotional impact and in pain coping strategies. The magnitude of such influences, however, and their interaction with fundamental biological mechanisms remains to be determined. Prior to attempting to derive some conclusions about the specific impact of sex difference on our understanding of pain and its management, it is necessary to move beyond biologically determined sex differences to differences in gender, and adopt a psychosocial rather than a biological perspective.

The influence of gender

Men and women appear to differ in the significance they attribute to painful events. The reason for this is not entirely clear, but may be related to differences in the interpretation of pain as well as socially determined differences in how they respond to pain. Some of the more important factors are shown in Box 4.8.

The interpretation of pain

It has been observed that gender differences in the prevalence of recurrent pain appear from adolescence

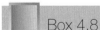

Box 4.8

The influence of gender

- Interpretation of pain
- Need to consult
- Reasons for consulting
- Willingness to consult
- Response to treatment
- Recovery from injury.

onwards. Interpretation is shaped by experience. It is easy to understand how differences in familiarity with different sorts of pain may lead to differences in the attribution of significance (and therefore action as a result of it). A key facet of clinical assessment is an appraisal of the individual's specific understanding of their pain, and the significance they attach to it (see Ch. 3). In the context of pain management it is important first and foremost as a determinant of consultation and may determine whether or not a patient is likely to benefit from pain management (see Ch. 11). There is clear evidence of gender-specific differences in the interpretation of pain as such, but there may be important differences in the reasons for consulting.

Differences in consulting behaviour

A number of different explanations have been offered for differences in consulting rates between men and women. Three possible such explanations are differences in reasons for consulting, differences in the emotional response to pain and differences in the readiness to consult health-care professionals.

Reasons for consulting

As mentioned above, men and women have different needs to consult health-care professionals, not only with reference to their own gynaecological and obstetric needs, but also as a consequence of their role as primary carers within the family. They may attend to pain sooner to prevent disruption of their wider social obligations to their family. Men may be more likely to consult if pain is perceived as a threat to work. The complexity of modern social structures and the marked variation within gender in consultation rates, however, make such generalities not only hazardous, but unhelpful. In the context of pain management, the reasons for consulting would seem to be much more relevant.

Emotional response to pain

Differences in consulting also may be a consequence of gender differences in the emotional response to pain and in types of coping strategies. Thus, while women may be more worried and irritated about pain, men may be more embarrassed about it (Klonoff et al 1993). Men and women may differ in their use of coping strategies, whether 'problem-focused' or 'emotionally focused' (Folkman & Lazarus 1980, Lazarus & Folkman 1984) (see Ch. 2) and in their adoption of shorter-term or longer-term strategies (because of the potentially disruptive effects of the pain). Stress and depression may be more closely associated with pain in women

than men (Magni et al 1990), although not all studies have found this.

Readiness to consult

Finally, there may be differences in the willingness to consult. There may be an element of truth in the ascription of gender differences in consultation to differences in the 'threshold' of self-disclosure or in willingness to discuss emotional issues. Difference in the manner of presentation of symptoms, and in particular the emotional component may have a significant effect on the patient–doctor communication process and the treatment actually received (see below).

Response to treatment

There are no controlled studies specifically on the influence of gender on outcome. Ascription of differences in treatment response specifically to gender would require control for possible biases in assessment, selection for treatment, goals for treatment and extent of engagement in treatment. (Unpublished data on the outcome of the inter-disciplinary PMP at the Manchester and Salford Pain Centre has, however, shown some differences between men and women in the value they place on different aspects of the teaching programme, when reviewed 6 months post-treatment. It seems that women particularly appreciate discussing their difficulties within a group, while men often seem to find the re-activation part of the programme more helpful.)

Recovery from injury

Although there is no clear evidence of differing effects of pain on activities of daily living in men and women, according to Unruh (1996), there is some evidence that there is a difference between men and women in the factors influencing return to work. She reports the study of Crook (1993) who found that men made more efforts to return to work, and returned sooner, while women had significantly more psychological distress and functional handicap than men as the time post-injury increased. It was reported also that the total number of painful sites and the extent of the psychological distress influenced the likelihood of a woman's return to work.

Specific influences of the family context

A number of the specific influences of the family context are shown in Box 4.9.

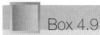

Specific influences of the family context

- Complex role of family and social network in understanding of pain
- Types of interaction between pain sufferers and their care-givers
- Contributions of the family and significant others to the maintenance of disability
- Physical and psychological effects on the principal care-giver
- Economic effects of treatment on the family
- Potential of the family and its members as powerful intervention agents.

Complex role of family and social network in understanding of pain

By the time many patients are considered for pain management, their pain behaviour is usually well established and it is often difficult to obtain a clinical history of sufficient accuracy to determine the precise mechanisms involved. It is important to appreciate that the report of pain intensity may be coloured by the patient's suffering, the pain-associated disability influenced by responses of various family members and ability to work affected by economic consequences of sickness not only on the patient but on their family. Thus a pain problem which began with impact only on the patient may have become a problem of major significance to the entire family.

Types of interaction between pain sufferers and their care-givers

Interpersonal communication comprises a complex set of signals, both verbal and non-verbal. Misunderstandings and miscommunications characterise dysfunctional families. When a pain problem arises among individuals who do not normally communicate adequately, major distress and disruption can arise. Families vary in sensitivity to self-report and non-verbal pain behaviour. It may be essential to identify and rectify such misunderstandings at the time of initial assessment before a pain management programme can be instigated. Indeed specific training in communication skills, such as appropriate assertiveness, forms a key part of the psychological component of many pain management programmes.

Contributions of the family and significant others to the maintenance of disability

The most common interpersonal problems characteristic of chronic pain patients are anger (or hostility) and over-solicitousness.

Anger

Chronic pain and pain-associated incapacity are frequently very stressful (and indeed if there are no indications of distress, then the patient may be insufficiently motivated to make a success of pain management). More specifically, chronic pain can create a profound sense of helplessness, resulting in feelings of frustration manifest as irritability, and sometimes anger, directed at other members of the family. Relationships may deteriorate. The patient may become even more demoralised and stressed. The diminished self-confidence may lead to avoidance of activities anticipated to be painful and they may feel unable to contemplate participation in active rehabilitation.

Over-solicitousness

Over-solicitousness on the part of family members is frequently easy to identify, but more difficult to address. Neither the patient nor the family member may be aware of the powerful influences their behaviour can exert on each other. It is important to consider over-solicitousness from two perspectives: firstly in the context of fear/avoidance and secondly in the context of enhanced well-being. If a patient is confronted with an activity which is anticipated to be painful, since pain is unpleasant at best, they will be somewhat reluctant to undertake the activity. If their partner offers to assist them, they no longer have to face the situation. They feel relieved. Unfortunately, this pattern of interpersonal behaviours can become generalised to more and more situations, until the patient becomes progressively more disabled. Unless the patient is distressed about their level of disability and increasing dependence on their partner, it is perhaps unwise for the therapist to intervene. Many patients, however, become increasingly frustrated by their lack of independence. It can be difficult for both patient and partner to accept that the over-solicitousness has contributed to the problem. The partner may have to be shown a more appropriate way of helping.

If the patient feels much happier with the increased attention, then provided the partner is willing to continue to provide it, it is perhaps necessary to view the over-solicitousness as an interactive pattern which

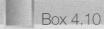

meets the emotional needs of the parties concerned. As such the over-solicitousness may constitute a sufficiently serious obstacle to rehabilitation and to permit acceptance for pain management. It may be of course that although it is possible to agree rehabilitation objectives which are achievable despite the over-solicitousness, they are not likely to be achieved. Certainly, where there is evidence of a clear mismatch between the needs of the patient and their partner, some therapeutic attention may have to be directed at their relationship prior to the pain management programme. Only if the situation is successfully resolved, will it be possible to proceed further with pain management.

Physical and psychological effects on the principal care-giver

It is not always appreciated that members of the family can become significantly disaffected with chronic pain in their relative. They also may become tired, exhausted, demoralised and depressed. It is frequently found amongst chronic pain patients assessed for treatment, that the needs of the partner have never been identified or even considered. As stated above, however, chronic pain can become a family problem. In some cases, the partner is the driving force behind treatment seeking. It is important therefore wherever possible to assess the needs of the partner as well as the patient in considering pain management. Sometimes the partner will be demoralised to the extent of requiring treatment in their own right.

Economic effects of treatment on the family

For families in a difficult situation, the economic implications of continued incapacity may be considerable. Such difficulties are frequently found in the context of litigation.

In considering pain management, it is important to attempt an appraisal in the context of the family unit and decide whether the perceived risk of improved function in terms of possible loss of benefits constitutes an obstacle to acceptance for treatment. (The impact of pain on the family is discussed further in Ch. 2.)

Potential of the family and its members as powerful intervention agents

The previous parts of this chapter have addressed possible mutually adverse influences of pain within

families. Family members, however, can often be powerful influences on the *success* of rehabilitation (Keefe et al 1996, 2001). As aforementioned, it is important to include their contribution to the nature of the patient's difficulties. If they are given an appropriate understanding of the principles of pain management, with its core emphasis on the re-establishment of self-control, partners can help encourage and motivate patients; especially at times when their confidence wavers. They can be facilitators of change in family activity and equal beneficiaries of improvement in quality of life. Furthermore, following the pain management programme, they may be able to provide the encouragement necessary to overcome 'flare-ups' and continue to improve function after completion of the programme, when the patient is likely to miss the support and encouragement of their fellow patients. (The role of the family in the context of therapy is discussed further in Ch. 11.)

Professional–patient communication

In addressing aspects of professional–patient communication from a social perspective, it is important to appreciate the complexity of clinical assessment, and during a typical assessment, there will be many and varied types of interaction. Strategies for maximising the effectiveness of interviewing will be addressed more specifically later, but in this chapter the focus specifically will be on the factors which influence the communication process.

A number of social aspects of the clinical assessment are shown in Box 4.10.

> **Box 4.10**
>
> **Social aspects of clinical assessment**
>
> - Purposes of the clinical assessment
> - Patient objectives for interview
> - Factors affecting communication
> - Potential factors affecting professional judgement
> - Patient factors affecting self-disclosure
> - Special features of different professional encounters
> - Overview of the nature of communication.

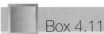

Box 4.11

Purposes of the clinical assessment

- Eliciting information
- Clinical history
- Appraisal of presenting symptoms
- Seeking confirmatory physical signs
- Arriving at a clinical formulation
- Arriving at a clinical decision
- Communicating findings to patient
- Eliciting patient support for plan of action.

Purposes of the clinical assessment

Communication is at the heart of clinical assessment, yet the complexity of the communication process is seldom appreciated. It can only be understood with reference to the specific matter in hand. Simply put, even short interchanges on clearly focused topics contain a complex pattern of individual verbal and non-verbal communications which are then meshed so that responses from one person serve as cues not only as acknowledgements that the message has been received, but also as a cue for further discourse. In addressing the social aspects of clinical assessment, it may be helpful initially to consider the major purposes of clinical assessment. They are shown in Box 4.11.

By the time many pain patients come to see an interdisciplinary team, they may be confused and distressed, and the assessment of suitability for pain management can represent another ordeal, particularly for patients who are apprehensive about doctors or have difficulty in communicating their fears and anxieties. It is most important not to further contribute to their confusion or distress by failing to communicate clearly and unambiguously the clinical formulation and associated decision. If further information is required prior to arriving at a clinical decision, the reasons for this should be clearly explained. If possible, the patient's partner or friend should be invited to attend the feedback session. Some clinics have a patient 'advocate' such as a nurse who will explain the outcome of the assessment in more detail to them after the formal clinical interview. It is also good practice to summarise the clinical formulation and associated treatment decision to all interested parties in the form of a letter.

Patient objectives for interview

As has been already stated almost all patients, if given a choice, would elect for a cure over and above all other

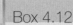

Box 4.12

Patient objectives for interview

- Obtaining cure or symptomatic relief
- Seeking diagnostic clarification
- Seeking reassurance
- Seeking 'legitimisation' of symptoms
- Expressing distress, frustration or anger.

possible outcomes. By the time chronic pain patients are referred to pain clinics, however, they may no longer believe that a cure is possible, and may present with a number of other, or additional, requirements. A summary of the most important patient objectives are shown in Box 4.12.

Obtaining cure or symptomatic relief

Pain is the single most common complaint presenting to hospitals. Direct referral from general practitioners, or referral to a pain clinic from other specialists is often couched specifically in terms of pain relief or sometimes complete cures. This may have been 'promised' to the patient, possibly in an attempt to get them to agree to the referral. In the majority of cases such an outcome is unattainable.

Seeking diagnostic clarification

Seeking diagnostic clarification is almost equally important. Any competent pain clinic should attempt to offer this. In pain management programmes in particular, clarification of the presenting characteristics in terms of the biological, psychological and socio-occupational dimensions is fundamental both in terms of specifying possible treatment targets (Chs 10 and 11) as well as identifying obstacles to recovery (Ch. 5).

Seeking reassurance

Some patients primarily are seeking reassurance. They may have come to terms with the fact that there is no cure for their chronic pain. They may wish simply to confirm that there is no serious pathology (such as cancer) which has been missed, or that there has been no new treatment developed which would be of assistance to them. While it is often easy to reassure such patients, a thorough assessment nonetheless should be provided.

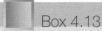

Seeking 'legitimisation' of symptoms

If patients have seen a large number of specialists, and been offered a wide range of different diagnoses, they may develop significant iatrogenic confusion and distress. The intensity of such distress can be magnified by the medicolegal process, in which claimants may read reports expressing doubt about the validity of their symptoms or even describing themselves as malingerers. Alternatively, they may have heard doubts expressed by members of their family about the genuineness of their pain-associated symptoms. They may even have begun to worry themselves that the persistence of their pain may be indicative of psychological disorder. In reassuring patients, it is important to identify the origin of the seeds of doubt. The powerful influence of the family has already been addressed earlier in this chapter. If the family are suspicious, it will be important to communicate also with them. Satisfactory 'legitimisation' of symptoms is a prerequisite for pain management.

Expressing distress, frustration or anger

By the time they are assessed in pain clinics, chronic pain patients may have developed significant distress and disaffection with health-care professionals. Referral to a tertiary centre specialising in interdisciplinary pain management may have necessitated a long wait before being seen. Whatever the reasons for the patient's distress, frustration or anger, it is important to give the patient time to express it. Preliminary questionnaires may have indicated a high level of emotion. Frequently, emotionally charged issues are raised or become apparent only at the time of the initial interview. It is important to be empathic without becoming overtly supportive of an excessively negative view of previous treatment. It is important to remember of course that, in cases of medical negligence, that patients have every right to redress. It should be made clear, however, that the purpose of the clinical assessment is to offer them appropriate advice or treatment, and not to offer an opinion whose prime purpose is to serve as part of a legal claim. If necessary, this should be made explicit.

Factors affecting communication

Communication can be viewed from two distinct perspectives: technical–sociopsychological, focusing primarily on the nature of the communication process, or psychotherapeutic, in which the emotional components of the doctor–patient relationship become the key ingredients of the therapeutic exchange. A number

> **Box 4.13**
>
> **Factors affecting communication**
>
> **Communication characteristics**
> - Verbal:
>   - clarity
>   - complexity.
> - Non-verbal:
>   - general demeanour
>   - eye-contact
>   - signalling continued attention.
> - Meshing of verbal and non-verbal signals
>
> **Aspects of the therapeutic relationship**
> - Practical considerations
> - Familiarity
> - Liking
> - Trust
> - Importance of the 'placebo response'.

of the elements of communication (viewed from both perspectives) are shown in Box 4.13.

Communication characteristics

Analysis of communication has become almost a science in itself. It will be possible to consider only some of the major features in this chapter. Detailed analyses of communication using the Neonatal Facial Coding System (Gruneau & Craig 1990) described above have illuminated understanding particularly of non-verbal communication of pain. As reported above, researchers have found striking similarities between newborn and adult facial responses to events that are painful to adults. An important finding of such research studies has been the importance of context. Development of florid pain behaviours can best be understood in a social context within which chronic pain behaviour patterns are displayed alongside a number which may be more 'context-dependent' and 'triggered' by the consultation process itself. In clinical situations, during the course of a clinical assessment a vast quantity of social signals is emitted. The information is somehow integrated into a clinical opinion.

Verbal characteristics

A common language is a prerequisite for good communication. Special efforts need to be made to ensure adequate communication with patients who have a different first language. Interpreters may be needed. Where standardised questionnaires constitute part of the assessment procedure, care should be taken to validate the questionnaires properly. Cultural differences in the meaning of pain are recognised (see above), but careful elucidation of their precise significance may necessitate a qualitative rather than a quantitative approach.

In addition to consideration of the meaning of the words used, the complexity of the communication must also be addressed. Wherever possible, clear and simple sentences should be used. The time for interview is frequently constrained and patients may recall only the major points. Opinions should be stated clearly and the patient's understanding should be confirmed. It should be noted in passing that patients will tend to recall the points of most emotional significance, and sometimes to the neglect of other important topics. (When one of our patients was told by a previous doctor that 'I am sure everything is all right, but I would like to ask Mr X, the consultant neurosurgeon, to have a look at you,' she completely forgot the first part of the sentence and became convinced that she had been told she probably had a brain tumour.)

Non-verbal aspects of communication

There are many non-verbal aspects of communication and only some of the more important will be highlighted here. It should be recognised, however, that these can have a very powerful influence on the whole interaction. Many patients are apprehensive about consulting health-care professionals.

Patients can be encouraged or discouraged in their presentation of symptoms simply by the professional's general demeanour. The power of 'social signalling' is perhaps most easily recognised amongst young people attempting to develop an intimate relationship. Establishment of eye contact, and signalling interest by expression, orientation and reducing interpersonal distance are only some of the cues or signals learned in the socialisation process. Signals of course can be misunderstood.

In doctor–patient communication, the importance of establishing eye contact, signalling attention and willingness to listen are particularly important. Patients who are apprehensive about the encounter may become particularly aware of apparent 'mismatch' between cues (where for example the professional states interest, but communicates the opposite in terms of body language).

Satisfactory meshing of verbal and non-verbal signals, and keeping the discussion flowing (with appropriate reassurance or encouragement) is important in the facilitation of communication.

The therapeutic relationship

The nature of communication is complex (Gask & Usherwood 2003) and it can also be considered in terms of its emotional characteristics. Many encounters with primary care personnel are straightforward, focused and not particularly emotionally loaded. Chronic pain is frequently accompanied by 'emotional baggage' and chronic disability is often best characterised as a 'psychologically mediated chronic pain syndrome'. The distress which accompanies chronic pain can be viewed from many aspects. Whatever its precise configuration, however, the level of distress can have a markedly inhibiting effect on self-disclosure, and thus compromise a clear assessment.

Practical considerations can have a powerful limiting effect on the quality of the therapeutic relationship. Making adequate time available for consultation and ensuring confidentiality (both in terms of records and privacy) are prerequisites of a good therapeutic context. The typical 8–10-minute general practice interview is ill-suited to a more than rudimentary exchange.

Many people find it difficult to disclose their feelings to others. In the assessment of chronic pain patients it is essential to facilitate this process. While it may not be essential for patients actually to like their health-care professional, it is important that they respect and trust them. Appropriate confirmation or clarification of the particular professional role may facilitate this process.

The 'placebo response' has long been recognised in medicine. It gained prominence in demonstration of so-called 'non-specific effects' in treatment. In a recent review of randomised controlled trials Hrobjartsson & Gotzsche (2006) concluded there was no evidence that placebo treatments in general have important effects, although they may have small effects on patient-reported outcomes such as pain. However, factors such as characteristics of the therapist have long been considered to be potentially important influences on treatment (Richardson 1994), and aspects of the therapeutic relationship in relationship to patient expectancies, treatment satisfaction and outcome in the treatment of pain would seem to merit much more attention.

The same considerations should be borne in mind in establishing a satisfactory context for therapeutic exchange.

Potential influences on professional judgement

Clinical decision making requires the integration of information of bewildering complexity. Studies on the inter-rater reliability of individual clinical signs have demonstrated that even in the assessment of so-called objective physical signs, clinicians can vary considerably in their judgement (Waddell & Main 1984). There are

Box 4.14

Potential factors affecting professional judgement

Technical skill
- Accuracy in identification of physical signs
- Estimation of severity
- Integration of elements.

Prejudicial biases
- Race, culture and gender
- Nature of symptoms
- Patient's clinical history
- Ongoing litigation.

two principal types of influence on clinical judgement: technical accuracy and prejudicial bias. Details are shown in Box 4.14.

Technical accuracy

Differences in the frequency with which certain features are identified by different raters indicate that the raters differ in skill, in the way in which they are applying criteria or in prejudicial bias. There may be differences in the identification of specific clinical features, in estimation of their impact (or severity), or in their integration into a composite clinical grading or judgement. Many clinicians are unaware of their inaccuracies in assessment. Technical problems can be improved with training to criterion. (In clinical research trials for example it is customary to train interviewers or raters until they have reached an acceptable degree of consistency.)

Prejudicial biases

For the purpose of this chapter, inconsistency in judgement will be examined from the standpoint of prejudicial bias which can influence the judgement of the clinician, irrespective of the symptoms the patient presents or of the manner in which they are presented.

Race, culture and gender

Deliberate discrimination on the grounds of race, culture or gender is illegal. Unconscious or unwitting bias is harder to detect. Differences in diagnostic rates, in clinical features, or in selection for different sorts of treatment may indicate such bias. It is important of course to examine referral patterns; such a selected

subgroup may have been referred. Comparisons within the team can, however, be made to determine whether clinicians indicate preferential bias of whatever sort.

Nature of symptoms

Clinicians may differ in the interpretation they place on different sorts of symptoms, or on the manner in which they are presented. Evidence of distress during clinical assessment may lead certain clinicians to pay insufficient attention to other aspects of symptom presentation and clinical history. Florid demonstration of pain behaviour may be viewed inherently with suspicion. This phenomenon is well illustrated in the medicolegal field in the interpretation of behavioural responses to examination (Main & Waddell 1998). Routine audit of decision making should indicate whether different clinicians place different weightings in arriving at an overall clinical judgement.

Patient's clinical history

It may become quickly apparent that a particular consultation is only the latest in a long 'patient career'. Expression of anger about previous health-care encounters may make a clinician disinclined to be sufficiently objective in their assessment. If a treatment has not worked, it is easy to blame the patient. The patient may have been willing to undergo treatment and fully compliant with it. The treatment itself may have been ineffective, inappropriate or frankly contra-indicated.

Ongoing litigation

In an increasingly litigious society, with the length of time until litigation is sometimes concluded, a significant number of pain patients may be still involved in litigation at the time of initial assessment. Determination of whether litigation should be considered a barrier to improvement can be difficult, but should not be taken as an excuse for an inadequate assessment. Economic influences are discussed further in Chapter 12.

Patient factors affecting self-disclosure

Clinical judgement has to be based on the best possible quality of information. The richest source of information is the patient. The patient's perception of their symptomatology and the interpretation they place on it are the cornerstones of modern pain management. Elicitation of the impact of pain on self-confidence, on relationships with others, on physical intimacy and on quality of life requires sensitivity on the part of the assessor. It is important to be aware therefore of a number of factors which can inhibit self-disclosure. These are shown in Box 4.15.

Patient expectations

It is important, first and foremost to clarify the patient's initial expectations from the assessment. If some information has not already been obtained from questionnaires filled by the patient, clarify the issue at the outset of the interview. Do not assume that a third party (such as a referring doctor) has fully determined this.

Misunderstandings

It is equally important to address misunderstandings which may have arisen concerning the purpose, timing or content of the assessment. Dealing competently and promptly with such misunderstandings is important in establishing trust.

Nature of previous consultations

If you have a clear referral letter, and have obtained all relevant previous medical records, you may believe that there is little need to discuss the nature of previous consultations with the patient. It is important, however, to confirm the accuracy of the information which has been made available to you, and identify any discordance between the patient's perception of these encounters and those of the professional involved. A specific appraisal of their clinical history may be important not only regarding matters of fact, but also in terms of the emotional impact.

Distress

Many patients show evidence of distress. The reasons are not always immediately apparent. It is important to encourage the distressed patient to clarify their concerns. This may take tact and patience. All clinical staff

participating in pain management programmes have to be able to facilitate self-disclosure in chronic pain patients. Videotaped training is recommended.

Fear

Patients may appear to be fearful. Patients may worry that they have significant structural damage or pathology which has been missed, that they are becoming mentally unstable or that they will become a permanent invalid. It is essential to establish a relationship with the patient such that they feel able to disclose such fears to you. (Assessment directed specifically at fear of further injury is discussed in Ch. 8.)

Anger

As indicated in Chapter 3, many chronic pain patients present with a mixture of emotions. Establishing a therapeutic climate with angry or hostile patients can be particularly difficult. As with the assessment of distress and fear, it is important to try to find out particularly what the patient is angry about. They will usually tell you. If it is a matter over which you might have been expected to have some control, make an appropriate apology. If the matter lies outwith your control, empathise as appropriate. Usually you will be unable to right the wrongs of the past. Your task, in the context of a clinical assessment, is to try to help the patient to 'move forward'. Some patients can be 'defused' successfully at the time of the initial assessment. Others need the support of a therapeutic group. You will have to decide whether the intensity or focus of anger can be dealt with therapeutically or whether it constitutes a major obstacle to rehabilitation.

Special features of different professional encounters

Finally, it is important to recognise that there are some differences in the social psychology of assessment in different sorts of assessment and therapeutic clinics.

Encounters will differ not only in the specific objectives of the encounter, but also in the patient expectations of it. In general, however, the same principles regarding communication still apply. Whatever the purpose of the assessment, the patient's trust must be established, the purpose of the assessment agreed and a therapeutic style and context designed to maximise self-disclosure must be employed. A number of practical recommendations likely to lead to more successful interviews, particularly for single-handed practitioners, are discussed in Chapter 9.

Overview of the nature of communication

It is hard to overemphasise the importance of focused, sensitive and skilled communication in the assessment of chronic pain patients. In most professions, such skills are not taught to a satisfactory level. New staff joining pain management teams frequently appear bemused about the nature of the interactions in which they find themselves. In the context of psychologically mediated chronic pain syndromes, attention to the communication process itself is as fundamental as is the use of MRI in the determination of structural damage. Individual communication skills are essential in careful assessment. Competent interdisciplinary clinical decision making requires furthermore adequate communication among members of the interdisciplinary pain management team. Finally, feedback to the patient at the conclusion of the clinical assessment often represents a critical moment in the patient career. Turning the patient from passive 'doctor shopping' towards active self-directed pain management sometimes requires finely tuned communication skills.

The special influence of compensation and litigation

Arguably, few issues in clinical medicine generate as much emotion as the nature of pain and pain-associated incapacity in the context of personal injury litigation. The powerful influences of economic factors in general and of compensation and litigation in particular on the presentation of pain complaints, on pain adjustment and on response to treatment are addressed in Chapter 12.

Summary and conclusion

In conclusion, the experience of pain and response to it can only be understood within the individual's social and cultural framework. Beliefs about the nature of pain have a powerful influence on adjustment to pain and the development of incapacity. In addressing the impact of chronic pain within the context of pain management, it is important to consider not only the *content* of communication process but also the *process* of communication. Consideration of the social factors may illuminate clinical history and help understand the patient's response to assessment. Furthermore, establishment of an appropriate 'atmosphere' or social climate is a prerequisite in gaining confidence of the patient and in facilitating self-disclosure. Finally, social factors can also have a powerful influence on response to treatment, not only in the context of group interventions, but also in the influence of staff and significant others, whether in the maintenance or enhancement of treatment gains or as contributory factors to lack of progress or relapse. (The influences on treatment and outcome will be considered more fully later in the book.)

Key points

- Cultural and subcultural differences in the perception of pain and response to it need to be understood in terms of the underlying socialisation mechanisms and how they affect the individual
- Social learning influences the meaning and significance ascribed to pain, communication about it, response to treatment and the development of pain coping
- Evaluation of pain and disability, and consideration for pain management need to recognise the influence of age
- Differences in pain perception and response to treatment may be considered both in terms of biologically based sex differences as well as socially developed gender differences. In matters of general pain management, the latter appear to be of more importance
- There may be a complex and significant role for the patient's family and social network in understanding of pain and perpetuation of disability
- Anger and over-solicitousness among members of patients' families may represent powerful obstacles to recovery if not addressed therapeutically
- The socio-psychological factors involved in professional–patient communication need to be identified, understood and managed appropriately
- Communication needs to be considered both in terms of the technical aspects of communication as well as from a therapeutic perspective
- Potential influences on professional judgement need to be recognised
- Patient factors affecting self-disclosure also need to be addressed
- Special features of different types of professional encounters may need to be recognised.

References

Allison T R, Symmons D P, Brammah T et al 2002 Musculoskeletal pain is more generalised among people from ethnic minorities than among white people in Greater Manchester. Annals of the Rheumatic Diseases 61:151–156

Anderson R T 1984 An orthopaedic ethnography in rural Nepal. Medical Anthropology 8:46–59 (reported in Waddell 1998, p. 5)

Atri J, Falshaw M, Livingstone A et al 1996 Fair shares in health care? Ethnic and socioeconomic influences on recording of preventive care in selected inner London general practices. British Medical Journal 312:614–617

Balarajan R, Raleigh V S, Yuen P 1991 Hospital care among ethnic minorities in Britain. Health Trends 23:90–93

Bhopal R, Donaldson L 1998 White, European, Western, Caucasian or what? Inappropriate labeling in research on race, ethnicity, and health. American Journal of Public Health 88:1303–1307

Burton A K, Tillotson K M, Main C J et al 1995 Psychosocial predictors of outcome in acute and subchronic low back trouble. Spine 20:722–728

Chesterton L S, Barlas P, Foster N E et al 2003 Gender differences in pressure pain threshold in healthy humans. Pain 101:259–266

Consumer's Association 1985 Back pain survey. Consumer's Association, London

Cost B13 Working Group on Guidelines for Chronic Low Back Pain 2004 European guidelines for the management of chronic non-specific low back pain

Craig K D 2002 Pediatric pain: sociodevelopmental aspects. In: Giamberardino M A Pain 2002 – an updated review: refresher course syllabus D, IASP Press, Seattle, ch 31, pp 305–314

Craig K D, Prkatchin K M, Gruneau R V E 1992 The facial expression of pain. In: Turk D C, Melzack R (eds) Handbook of pain assessment. Guilford Press, New York, ch 15, pp 257–276

Croft P, Joseph S, Cosgrove S et al 1994 Low back pain in the community and in hospitals. A report to the Clinical Standards Advisory Group of the Dept of Health. Arthritis and Rheumatism Council Epidemiology Research Unit, University of Manchester

Crook J 1993 Comparative experiences of men and women who have sustained a work-related musculoskeletal injury (Abstract). Proceedings of the 7th World Congress on Pain. IASP Press, Seattle, pp 293–294

CSAG 1994 Clinical Standards Advisory Group report on back pain. HMSO Publications, London

Eccleston C, Malleson P 2003 Managing chronic pain in children and adolescents. British Medical Journal 326:1408–1409

Eccleston C, Crombez G, Scotford A et al 2004 Adolescent chronic pain: patterns and predictors of emotional distress in adolescents with chronic pain and their parents. 108:221–229

Eccleston C, Jordan A, McCracken L M et al 2005 The Bath Adolescent Pain Questionnaire (BAPQ): development and preliminary psychometric evaluation of an instrument to assess the impact of chronic pain on adolescents. Pain 118:263–270

Eden L, Ejlertsson G, Lamberger B et al 1994 Immigration and socio-economy as predictors of early retirement pensions. Scandinavian Journal of Social Medicine 22:187–193

Edwards C L, Fillingim R B, Keefe F J 2001 Race, ethnicity and pain. Pain 94:133–137

Farrell M J, Gibson M J 2004 Pain in older people. In: Dworkin R H, Brietbart W S (eds) Psychosocial aspects of pain: a handbook for health care providers. Progress in pain research and management vol 27. IASP Press, Seattle, ch 22, pp 495–518

Fillingim R B, Maixner W 1995 Gender differences in the responses to noxious stimuli. Pain Forum 4:209–221

Folkman S, Lazarus R 1980 An analysis of coping in a middle-aged community sample. Journal of Health and Social Behaviour 21:219–240

Gask L, Usherwood T 2003 The consultation. In: Mayou R, Sharpe M, Carson A (eds) ABC of psychological medicine. BMJ Books, London, ch 1, pp 1–3

Gibson S J, Helme R D 2001 Pain management in the elderly: age related differences in pain perception and report. In: Ferrell B A (ed) Clinics in geriatric medicine, vol 17. W B Saunders, Philadelphia, PA, pp 433–456

Gillam S, Jarman B, White P et al 1989 Ethnic differences in consultation rates in urban general practice. British Medical Journal 299:953–957

Goodman J E, McGrath P J 1991 The epidemiology of pain in children and adolescents: a review. Pain 46:247–264

Green C, Anderson K O, Baker T A et al 2003 The unequal burden of pain: confronting racial and ethnic disparities in pain. Pain Medicine 4:277–294

Gruneau R V E, Craig K D 1990 Facial activity as a measure of neonatal pain expression. In: Tyler D C, Krane E J (eds) Advances in pain research and therapy, vol 15. Raven Press, New York, pp 147–155

Hadjistavropoulos T, Craig K 2002 A theoretical framework for understanding self-report and observational measures of pain: a communication model. Behaviour Research and Therapy 40:551–570

Hays R D, Kravitz R L, Mazel R M et al 1994 The impact of patient adherence on health outcomes for patients with chronic disease in the medical outcomes study. Journal of Behavioral Medicine 17:347–360

Helme R D, Gibson S J 2001 Pain management in the elderly: the epidemiology of pain in elderly people. In: Ferrell B A (ed) Clinics in geriatric medicine, vol 17. W B Saunders, Philadelphia, PA, pp 417–431

Honeyman P T, Jacobs E A 1996 Effects of culture on back pain in Australian aboriginals. Spine 21:841–843

Hrobjartsson A, Gotzsche P C 2006 Placebo interventions for all clinical conditions. Cochrane database of Systematic Reviews 2006, Issue 3. The Cochrane Collaboration. John Wiley, Chichester

IASP 1997 The curriculum on pain for students in psychology. IASP Press, Seattle

Jones G J, Macfarlane G J 2005 Epidemiology of pain in older persons. In: Gibson S J, Weiner D J (eds) Pain in older persons. Progress in pain research and management, vol 35. IASP Press, Seattle, ch 1, pp 3–22

Keefe F J, Caldwell D S, Baucom D 1996 Spouse-assisted coping skills training in the management of osteoarthritic knee pain. Arthritis Care Research 9:279–291

Keefe F J, Caldwell D S, Baucom D 2001 Spouse-assisted coping skills training in the management of osteoarthritic knee pain: longterm follow-up results. Arthritis Care Research 12:101–111

Klonoff E A, Landrine H, Brown M A 1993 Appraisal and response to pain may be a function of its bodily function. Journal of Psychosomatic Research 37:661–670

Lazarus R, Folkman S 1984 Stress, appraisal and coping. Springer, New York

LeResche L 2000 Epidemiologic perspectives on sex differences in pain. In: Fillingim R B (ed) Sex, gender and pain. Progress in pain research and management, vol 17. IASP Press, Seattle, ch 12, pp 233–249

McCracken L M, Matthews A K, Tang T S et al 2001 A comparison of blacks and whites seeking treatment for chronic pain. Clinical Journal of Pain 17:49–55

McGrath P A, Gillespie J 2001 Pain assessment in children and adolescents. In: Turk D C, Melzack R (eds) Handbook of pain and assessment, 2nd edn. Guilford Press, New York, ch 6, pp 97–118

Magni G, Caldieron C, Rigatti-Luchini S et al 1990 Chronic musculoskeletal pain and depressive symptoms in the general population. An analysis of the 1st National Health and Nutrition Examination Survey data. Pain 43:299–307

Main C J, Waddell G 1998 Behavioural responses to examination: a re-appraisal of the interpretation of 'non-organic signs'. Spine 23:2367–2371

Miaskowski C, Levine J D 2004 Sex differences in pain perceptions, response to treatment and clinical management. In: Dworkin R H, Breitbart W B (eds) Psychosocial aspects of pain: a handbook for health care providers. Progress in pain research and management, vol 27. IASP Press, Seattle, ch 27, pp 607–621

National Statistics Office 2001 Census 2001. London

Nazroo J Y 2003 The structuring of ethnic inequalities in health: economic position, racial discrimination, and racism. American Journal of Public Health 93:277–284

Njobvu P, Hunt I M, Pope D et al 1999 Pain amongst ethnic minority groups of South Asian origin in the United Kingdom: a review. Rheumatology 38:1184–1187

Polleri A 1992 Pain and sex steroids. In: Sicuteri F (ed) Advances in pain research and therapy, vol 20. Raven Press, New York, pp 253–259

Richardson P H 1994 Placebo effects in pain management. Pain Reviews 1:15–32

Riley J L, Robinson M E, Wise E A et al 1998 Sex differences in the perception of experimental pain stimuli. Pain 74:181–187

Riley J L, Robinson M E, Wise E A et al 1999 A meta-analytic review of pain perception across the menstrual cycle. Pain 81:225–235

Riley J L 3rd, Wade J B, Myers C D et al 2002 Racial/ethnic differences in the experience of chronic pain. Pain 100:291–298

Robinson M E, Riley J L III, Myers C D 2004 Psychosocial contributions to sex-related differences in pain responses. In: Fillingim R B (ed) Sex, gender and pain. Progress in pain research and management, vol 17. IASP Press, Seattle, ch 4, pp 41–68

Rudy T, Kerns R D, Turk D C 1988 Chronic pain and depression: a cognitive-mediation model. Pain 35:129–140

Shaya F T, Blume S 2005 Prescriptions for cyclo-oxygenase2 inhibitors and other non-steroidal anti-inflamatory agents in a medicaid managed care population: African Americans versus Caucasians. Pain Medicine 6:11–17

Skevington S 1997 Psychology of pain. John Wiley, Chichester

Thomas E, Peat G, Harris L et al 2004 The prevalence of pain in a general population of older adults: cross-sectional findings from the North Staffordshire Osteoarthritis Project (NORSTOP). Pain 110:361–368

Todd K H, Samaroo N, Hoffman J R 1997 Ethnicity as a risk factor for inadequate emergency department analgesia. Journal of the American Medical Association, 269:1537–1539

Todd K H, Deaton C, D'Adamo A P et al 2000 Ethnicity and analgesic practice. Annals of Emergency Medicine 35:11–16

Turk D C 1996 Clinicians' attitudes about prolonged use of opioids and the issue of patient heterogeneity. Journal of Pain and Symptom Management 11:218–230

Unruh A 1996 Review article: Gender variations in clinical pain experience. Pain 65:123–167

Waddell G 1998 The back pain revolution. Churchill Livingstone, Edinburgh

Waddell G, Main C J 1984 Assessment of severity in low back disorders. Spine 9:204–208

Webb R, Brammah T, Lunt M et al 2003 Prevalence and predictors of intense, chronic, and disabling neck and back pain in the UK general population. Spine 28:1195–202

Zborowski M 1952 Cultural components in responses to pain. Journal of Social Issues 8:16–30

Zborowski M 1969 People in pain, San Franscisco, Jossey-Bass

Chapter Five

5

Risk identification and screening

CHAPTER CONTENTS

Introduction

The context of risk identification and screening

There are a wide range of pain conditions in which there is evidence of significant dysfunction but no evidence of disease or nerve damage. They range from fairly localised pain problems such as visceral pains, pain in joints and headache, to more regional pains in areas of the body, to syndromes with labels such as chronic widespread pain (Croft et al 1993, Hunt et al 1999) and fibromyalgia (Wolfe et al 1995). There are widespread debates not only about possible pain mechanism, but even about classification (Wolfe et al 1990). These issues are neither merely academic nor trivial. The costs of non-specific pain conditions are considerable and there is now widespread recognition in Western societies that such problems need to be tackled. However, since a clearly identifiable 'pain generator' is often not apparent, promise of a complete cure seems improbable. What then can be done? Two major strategies have emerged:

1 Prevention of chronic pain becoming unnecessarily disabling
2 Prevention of the development of chronic pain/disability in patients with acute/subacute pain.

Clarification of terms

Inconsistencies in the literature in the use of terms such as risk factors, predictive factors and prognostic factors can be somewhat confusing, in that they are sometimes used interchangeably, and so it might be helpful to attempt some clarification of terms, at least in so far as they are used in this chapter.

Predictive factors simply are those which are associated statistically with some sort of outcome in the future. Whether or not they are predictive therefore is a matter of statistical association, using whatever criteria are appropriate. They make no assumptions about the relationship, or lack of, between the two sets of events. In practice, they can be divided into risk factors and prognostic factors.

Risk factors should be used to refer to factors associated with the future development or occurrence of an event such as a disease of some sort. They may or may not be implicated causally in the development of the disease, but the disease is not present at the time of risk estimation. Further investigations may be able to demonstrate a direct causal relationship, but the relationship may be indirect (possibly mediated by other factors) or, in so far as can be investigated, may turn out to be a chance association.

Prognostic factors properly refer to factors predictive of outcome of a disease or condition already in progress.

Frequently the distinction is unimportant, but it should be borne in mind.

Implications for understanding outcome in pain management

To confuse matters still further, in understanding the development of pain, chronic pain and pain-associated incapacity, predictors may turn out to be both risk factors and prognostic factors. Thus psychological distress may be a risk factor for the development of pain, a prognostic factor in terms of the development of chronic pain, a risk factor for the development of disability and a prognostic factor for further change in disability. Similarly, pain severity may be both a risk factor for sickness absence and a prognostic factor for recovery.

Modifiable and unmodifiable risk factors

Finally, a distinction can be made between modifiable and unmodifiable predictive factors (whether risk factors or prognostic factors).

Analytic strategy

We propose to review the scientific evidence using the framework outlined in Box 5.1. As a precursor we

Box 5.1

Framework for the investigation of predictive factors

- Risk factors for the development of pain
- Prognostic factors for the persistence of pain
- Risk factors for the development of pain-associated limitations and disability
- Prognostic factors for the persistence of pain-associated limitations and disability.

offer a conceptual overview of concepts of risk and the nature of screening.

Concepts of risk and risk identification

Concepts of risk

Concepts of risk have usually been based on identification of factors associated with poor outcome, but there are different types of predictors of outcome, and not all are potential targets for intervention. *Epidemiological* studies are primarily descriptive, rather than explanatory and are population based. Although a further distinction between population epidemiology (as in public health or population surveys) and clinical epidemiology (in which the population is defined by a symptom, a sign, an illness, a diagnostic procedure or a treatment) can be made, they present similar methodological challenges and the difference primarily is generalisability of findings. Statistically significant associations may serve as a foundation for major clinical initiatives (such as immunisation) or social policy decisions involving the redirection of resources, but such risk factors are usually not sufficiently powerful to be useful for decision making on an individual basis.

The *clinical* perspective on risk tends to focus primarily on factors associated with health-care outcome. Clinical studies are often more narrowly focused than epidemiological investigations, and therefore provide a better basis for clinical intervention. Thus the incorporation of demographic and educational factors, for example, may be helpful in targeting certain groups, in suggesting particular therapeutic targets or in assisting the design of preventative intervention (although, as discussed below, important issues of sensitivity and specificity need to be evaluated prior to their use for clinical decision making on individuals).

Occupational risk factors tend to be wide-ranging, and may be very different from clinical risk factors but equally may be of help in the targeting or design of preventative interventions. It may be helpful to base prevention not on risk as such, but to refocus attention on modifiable risk factors as potential *obstacles to recovery* suggesting possible opportunities for change.

Accuracy of risk identification

Despite the advances in our knowledge about the nature of pain and its impact, and the development of treatment approaches which appear to be promising, we are still a long way from being able to predict outcome of treatment accurately for an individual patient. This is a consequence in part of the fact that much of our research evidence has been gathered from aggregated data. Thus we may have established in general terms that treatment X is more effective than treatment Y, an issue which may be of considerable importance in terms of health-care planning, policy and funding, but yet find ourselves unable to make confident predictions in the individual case. Indeed current clinical guidelines often require the clinician, when offering a course of treatment, to give the patient specific estimates of the probability of different outcomes, including of course poor outcomes and adverse side-effects. This is illustrated graphically in the caveats which now have to accompany claims of benefit from the advertising of commercially available products, including treatments for particular conditions or symptoms.

The significance and costs of risk estimation

Risk estimation, however, is an imprecise science and its worth cannot be gauged in absolute terms. Thus the value of a system of risk identification, or the use of a particular assessment tool, has to be evaluated against its accuracy. In clinical medicine this often translates into consideration of *sensitivity* and *specificity*. Since risk identification can be extremely costly in terms of necessary resources, decisions are made in terms of the probable additional benefit likely to accrue from various degrees of effort in improving overall accuracy. Thus if it was decided to try to identify those needing treatment for clinical depression, it would be relevant to examine the improved 'hit-rate' from including a clinical interview, over and above a simple screening questionnaire or a simple question as part of a population census.

From public health strategies to management of pain in the individual

Reasons for attempting prediction

There is a wide range of information potentially available about individuals, but we are a long way from being able to determine with precision either natural history or response to a clinical intervention. As previously stated, the costs of chronic pain and pain-associated incapacity are considerable, whether viewed from an individual, or a societal perspective. We have a range of treatments which are effective to an extent, but not everyone benefits from intervention. We live in a cost-constrained health-care system; interventions are costly and therefore, considered from a health-economic perspective, there is an imperative to improve the success rate of our interventions.

Many reasons have been put forward for our relative lack of success. The strongest contenders as possible explanations seem to be inherent limitation in the therapeutic power of our treatments or the lack of appropriateness of the treatment for a particular set of individuals (or indeed a combination of both). It may be of course that treatment response is only partly determined by either the nature of the treatment or characteristics of the individual receiving it. Thus, outcome may be influenced strongly by external factors, such as economic and occupational factors or by reactivity of the treatment process, in which initial response to treatment, although not itself predictable at time of initial assessment, may have a significant bearing on longer-term outcome.

Given the above scenario, it is necessary to have a way of evaluating the success of prediction. The identification of predictors of outcome may enable us to select subgroups, whether in terms of possible benefit from treatment ('screening in') or failure to benefit from treatment ('screening out'). Furthermore, identification of predictors may lead to the identification of new and different approaches to treatment for patients with differing presenting characteristics, or at different stages of pain chronicity.

Population studies and the public health perspective

Epidemiological studies in the general population can inform us about the prevalence of symptoms of pain in the community, using a variety of prevalence estimates. It is possible to determine the incidence of new pain episodes, and longitudinal studies begin to inform us about the various exposures (risk factors) associated with harm (pain). We can construct a map of the context of pain and its future development, enabling identification of predictors of chronicity as well as recovery at a population level. Thus demographic and ethnicity variables may lead to public health initiatives focused on particular subgroups or delivered in a variety of ways. At a population level even relatively weak levels of prediction may be of considerable importance in terms of informing public health policy, in terms of prioritising initiatives or in optimising use of resources.

There are two principal reasons why population predictors are unhelpful in the management of individual patients. Firstly population predictors are insufficiently robust in terms of sensitivity and specificity for use in the individual patient, and secondly individual management has to be based on *modifiable* risk factors, which many population predictors are not.

From populations to subpopulations

Population epidemiology has, however, provided an important launch pad for clinical epidemiology and studies of pain patients in which much stronger predictors of natural history and treatment outcome have been identified. There have been many studies of treatment outcome for specific neurogenic, neuroplastic and 'benign' pain conditions. Given the importance of curing pain, wherever possible, there has been a major emphasis on the biomedical parameters associated with outcome of acute pain conditions. Unfortunately a significant proportion of patients develop chronic pain syndromes in which initial biomedical parameters seem to be less predictive, while, in contrast, psychosocial predictors appear to be of increasing importance. In such clinical groups, the potential for screening for predictors appears to merit attention.

A number of approaches to screening, however, have been developed on a variety of clinical populations and it is important to appraise their utility as a part of overall clinical management. Prior to examining their utility for the identification of risk and prognostic factors for pain and pain-associated limitations (disability), the nature of screening will be addressed.

Nature of screening

Principles

The investigation of associations between diseases, as indicators of harm with various sorts of environmental

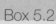

Box 5.2

Criteria for appraising screening from Wilson & Jungner (1968)

- The condition sought should be an important health problem
- There should be an accepted treatment for patients with recognisable disease
- Facilities for diagnosis and treatment should be available
- There should be a recognisable or early latent stage
- There should be a suitable test or examination
- This test should be acceptable to the population
- The natural history of the condition, including development from latent to declared disease, should be adequately understood
- There should be an agreed policy on whom to treat as patients
- The cost of case finding (including diagnosis and treatment of patients diagnosed) should be economically balanced in relation to possible expenditure on medical care as a whole
- Case finding should be a continuing process and not a 'once and for all' project.

variables as potential causal factors (as measures of risk), has led to significant advances in the early detection (and ensuing morbidity/mortality) of a whole range of diseases. The concept of risk factors has entered common parlance, although not infrequently seems to be confused in the media with relative risk, sometimes leading to unnecessary levels of concern and anxiety.

Screening was developed initially in the context of the development of screening programmes for particular diseases. According to Muir Gray (2004), the original criteria for the appraisal for screening, shown in Box 5.2, 'have stood the test of time very well', but need adaptation in the light of concerns about potential harm of screening (and potential litigation), insufficient evidence to justify the supposed benefit, and the rising challenges posed by an ageing population, new technology and rising demand. The National Screening Committee developed more detailed criteria for evaluation of the natural history of the disease, the accuracy of the screening test, the effectiveness of treatment and the acceptability of the screening programme to the general population. Full details are given in Muir Gray (2004, p. 293) as is a list of features common to all national screening programmes (p. 296).

Muir Gray (2004) offers further discussion on new concepts in management, emphasising particularly the need for careful evaluation of both the benefits and harm of screening as well as quality assurance, in an economically constrained health-care system.

The concept of health-care screening, a direct consequence of the identification of the precursors of disease, has led to an emphasis on screening with a view to early intervention. Not all diseases of course are either predictable or preventable, but in those in which early detection is clinically beneficial, significant health gains can accrue. In addition to clinical benefit, the costs of early detection may have to be viewed against competing demands for a limited health-care budget. In such circumstances, not only does clinical benefit of early intervention become an issue, but also the costs of detection in terms of the sensitivity and specificity of the screening.

The concept of screening on the basis of possible risk factors therefore is linked intimately both with the strength of the predictors (whether individually or in combination) and with the prognosis of the disease with or without the early detection and intervention. There are two obvious implications of this analysis. Firstly, if there are no known predictors of outcome for a condition, then there are no risk factors to be detected, and no point in putting effort into screening. Secondly, if neither the morbidity nor mortality is improved as a consequence of early detection, then the costs of screening cannot be justified. Considered another way, unless *modifiable* risk factors can be identified, examination of the sensitivity/specificity of screening is irrelevant.

Purposes

The importance of clarifying the *purpose* of screening, emphasised by Waddell et al (2003) in consideration of screening for long-term incapacity, identified a number of different purposes for screening. They are shown in Box 5.3.

Classically, as highlighted in the last section, screening is carried out at a population level with a view to identifying factors associated with future development of morbidity or mortality.

Methodological issues

There are number of important conclusions which can be learned from the evidence-based review (Waddell et al 2003).

Methods of screening

The value of screening depends not only on the content of the items, but the manner in which the information

> ### Box 5.3
>
> **Some purposes for screening**
>
> - Identifying people at higher risk of long-term incapacity versus those likely to return to work
> - Predicting likely duration of sickness absence
> - Identifying people who need extra therapeutic or rehabilitation help
> - Identifying obstacles to coming off benefit and returning to work that may be appropriate for intervention
> - Identifying people likely to respond to (an) intervention versus those likely not to respond
> - Informing a rehabilitation programme or other work-focused intervention
> - Informing the decision making processes and case management.
>
> From Waddell, Burton & Main (2003, p. 5)

is collected and the way the information is integrated. Different methods may be required to elicit different sorts of information (as outlined in Box 5.3). Routinely available administrative data may be useful at a population, insurance system or organisational level, but usually it has been designed for different purposes such as audit or population risk estimates. More individualised and clinically relevant information may be collected using questionnaire, telephone or face-to-face interview. The additional potential value has to be offset against much greater cost and practical difficulties in eliciting and interpreting the information obtained. As has been illustrated, use of clinical or disability prediction rules has some utility as a 'middle-way' but is extremely context dependent, is based on an averaging of scores across individuals and in assuming a fixed relationship amongst the items effectively is restricted to a 'snapshot' derived at a particular point in time.

Timing

A more worrying problem is that different predictors emerge at different stages of illness or disability. Thus *when* the screening is undertaken has a major influence on the accuracy of the screening. Furthermore there may be different challenges facing screening at different times. Waddell et al (2003) illustrate this in consideration of the prediction of incapacity whereby, at the time of initial presentation, the task for a screening tool may be to identify the 1–2% of individuals who will go on to develop long-term incapacity from amongst the

98–99% with relatively simple problems, most of whom are likely to return to work quite rapidly, more or less irrespective of any intervention. However, with benefit claimants identified only at 26% the task may be to identify the 40% likely to continue on long-term benefit from those who might (or could) be returned to work.

Accuracy

In practice, no screening tool will ever be 100% accurate, and a decision has to be made about the relative costs of 'false positives' and 'false negatives'. Thus if it is extremely important to identify all possible cases of a particular condition, it may be considered justifiable to also include a large number of those who do not have the condition. Conversely, if the costs of screening are prohibitively expensive, a lower hit-rate in terms of identifying those with the condition may be considered acceptable, since a lot of unnecessary costs (false positives) will have been saved. Judgements of acceptability in screening therefore may involve political and ethical considerations as well as statistical computations.

Implications for pain management

Unfortunately the nature and development of pain are insufficiently understood to match up well against Wilson and Jungner's stringent criteria for screening policy, and further advances in the *primary* prevention of pain (in terms of health education and ergonomics) would seem to be improbable. The major focus in the rest of this chapter therefore will be on screening in the context of decision making in clinical and occupational settings, those who are already symptomatic, and therefore can be viewed as a facet of assessment. However, since the prevention of *chronic* pain and *preventable* pain-associated disability in clinical populations has become a major focus of endeavour within clinical populations (whether in primary-care or secondary/tertiary-care populations), this also will be addressed.

A broad overview of possible purposes for screening in the context of pain management is offered in Box 5.4. For the sake of illustration the purposes are grouped in the first instance according to the duration of pain, as is often done in the context of health-care policy, but it is clear from the box that both pain and pain-associated limitations are equally important in terms of screening. It is not possible within the remit of this chapter to give detailed consideration to each of these purposes for screening.

Box 5.4

Overview of purposes of screening in the context of pain management

Pre-onset of symptoms (the public health agenda)
- Primary prevention of accidents and injury
- Reducing the societal burden of unnecessary health-care costs.

Subacute pain (4–12 weeks) (secondary prevention: Stage 1)
- Identifying yellow and blue flags
- Preventing the transition from subacute to persistent pain
- Prevention of unnecessary pain-associated restrictions
- Reducing number and length of work absences.

Subchronic pain (13–26 weeks) (secondary prevention: Stage 2)
- Preventing short-term absence from becoming long-term absence
- Identifying those at risk of developing persistent pain or significant pain-associated limitations:
  - screening in: identifying those likely to benefit from a clinical intervention (modifiable risk factors)
  - screening out: identifying those *not* likely to benefit from a clinical intervention (unsuitable for pain management).

Chronic pain or recurrent pain
- Identifying orange flags
- Minimising pain-associated restrictions
- Preventing unhelpful/damaging health-care use
- Preventing the development of long-term absence
- Identifying black flags
- Identifying those at risk of developing progressive pain-associated limitations
  - screening in: identifying those likely to benefit from a clinical intervention (modifiable risk factors)
  - screening out: identifying those *not* likely to benefit from a clinical intervention (unsuitable for pain management).

General approaches to screening

As previously stated, the term 'screening' encompasses a wide range of approaches to risk identification, from population screening to clinical decision making at the

Box 5.5

Some requirements for a system for screening

- Identify items of information that predict the outcome of interest
- Develop a practical and usable method of collecting the information
- Develop a method of combining the information or scoring the instrument
- Measure the accuracy of prediction.

Adapted from Waddell et al (2003, p. 7)

Box 5.6

Strengths and limitations of the actuarial model

Strengths
- Accurate data
- Maximises use of available data
- Can quantify the precise relationship between individual risk factors and future status
- Can be used to construct algorithms and prediction rules applicable to large populations.

Limitations
- No room for individual differences
- Critically important salient data may not have been collected
- Utility limited when the ceiling for predictive accuracy is relatively low, and when the underlying evidence is weak
- Generalisability of such statistical prediction models to other populations and contexts is often unknown
- Modifiability of the risk factors may be of secondary importance.

time of an individual assessment. However, there are a number of general requirements for a system for screening, as shown in Box 5.5.

Accepting the reality of financially constrained healthcare and security systems, a comprehensive evaluation on an individual basis, however desirable, is never likely to be fundable, or even acceptable. It is likely that there will always be a need for some sort of filtering or screening as a precursor to intervention, but before considering screening per se, it is appropriate to reflect upon the process of clinical decision making, We offer the view that at the heart of the *process* of clinical decision making are probabilistic judgements and in this respect, arrival at a decision involves risk estimation in the context of risk of good and poor outcome (and by implication, whether to offer pain management, and what to offer).

Actuarial methods

A central issue in screening is the accuracy of predicting future ill-health or disability based on various initial data sets. In clinical practice, treatment recommendations are usually based on implicit outcome predictions made by a practitioner. An alternative is to adopt a statistical approach based on population statistics, such that each individual is compared with a wider group in terms of a number of characteristics and a risk profile thus obtained from data often gathered for administrative rather than clinical purposes. Setting of car insurance premiums is an example of this approach. Thus the overall risk of a car accident may be estimated in part from age and a geographical code, as well as accident history. Private health insurance works in a similar manner. The overall risk estimation, seldom disclosed, can range from simple demographic information to more

sophisticated classification using multidimensional cutoffs or mathematical formulas. This empirical approach has been called actuarial and is based on research evidence that allows the predictors to be quantified and combined following a set of empirically supported rules, thus offering the promise of improved accuracy (Dawes et al 1989, Garb 1998, Groth-Marnat 2000).

Such an approach lends itself to wide administrative applications. The exact nature of the predictors is relatively unimportant, but their strength in terms of accuracy of prediction is critical. There is no inherent ordering of variables in terms of the significance and many different types of predictors may end up as part of the optimal algorithm, as the selection is based on each variable's contribution to the prediction of outcomes, such as duration of disability, return to work, or costs.

Some strengths and limitations associated with the empirically based actuarial approach are shown in Box 5.6.

Firstly, it assumes that the variables are stable and static (Groth-Marnat 2003). Secondly, it is not possible to accommodate individual differences as the same statistical formula is always used, leading to misclassifications. Thirdly, important clinical data often are not collected. Fourthly, the utility of a strictly actuarial model is limited when the ceiling for predictive accuracy is relatively low (Lanyon & Goodstein 1997) and when the underlying evidence is weak. Fifthly, the generalisability of such statistical prediction models to other populations and contexts is often unknown. Finally, since prediction is the driving factor, the modifiability of the risk factors may be of secondary importance. Therefore, actuarial models may not be easily translated into secondary prevention applications.

Clinical decision making

In narrowing focus from the population to the individual, it is necessary to reflect upon the process of clinical decision making, which in terms of its general purpose is straightforward, but considered further leads to a number of further questions (as shown in Box 5.7).

At the heart of clinical decision making is a judgement matching the needs of the patient with the possible benefits from our intervention. Given the wide range of information which may be available to us on an individual patient, clinical decision making can be a complex task. We know in clinical practice that there are at times different opinions expressed, both in terms of clinical formulation (and diagnosis) and about what treatment is appropriate for a particular patient. Indeed as will be discussed in Chapter 11, by the time patients find a place on a tertiary pain management programme, they may have been offered a plethora of diagnoses and recommendations, such that they may have become confused and distressed about the nature of their condition; it may be a major task initially for the physician in the team to clarify these issues for the patient.

In deciding about suitability for pain management, it is sometimes helpful to try to 'unpack' our clinical decisions. (Indeed this should be an important feature of clinical training.)

Appraisal of suitability for treatment

A number of important facets of clinical appraisal are shown in Box 5.8. They will be discussed only briefly.

Aspects of clinical history. In addition to the clinical history offered by the patient, the clinician may have available a wide range of additional information. If clinical records are available, attention should be paid not only to the 'facts of the matter' but also the interpretation placed by the clinicians on clinical symptoms and responses to treatment. The patient's understanding and interpretation also should be elicited, since mismatches may be illuminating.

Characteristics of presenting symptomatology. It is important to take proper account of all facets of clinical history, but not be unduly influenced by certain factors. Thus, identification of a psychiatric history or forensic involvement does not mean that the patient does not deserve to be taken seriously (Ch. 3), although either may turn out to be a contra-indication to straightforward pain management, or indicate the need for triage to a mental health professional.

Psychological 'morbidity' (and comorbidity). Ongoing significant psychological problems constitute orange flags for poor outcome, and need to be managed as such (Chs 8, 10 and 11).

Physical comorbidity. Other health problems may contra-indicate a straightforward reactivation programme. Medication needs also to be appraised in terms of its possible influence on the patients' cognitions and performance.

Family and social circumstances. Occasionally a patient may be considered suitable but a set of family circumstances may preclude attendance, either on practical grounds (such as the burden of significant caring responsibilities), because of other significant life stresses requiring attention, or because of disagreement by a family member about the appropriateness of pain management.

Box 5.7

The clinical decision-making process

Basis of clinical decision making

- A prediction of how an individual will respond to a clinical intervention.

Key questions

- How do we arrive at our prediction?
- What is our evidence base?
- What is an appropriate outcome measure?
- What are our criteria for a satisfactory outcome?

Box 5.8

Important facets of clinical appraisal

- Aspects of clinical history
- Characteristics of presenting symptomatology
- Psychological 'morbidity' (and comorbidity)
- Physical comorbidity
- Family circumstances
- Economic factors (incl. compensation).

Economic factors (including compensation). Finally, economic factors may have powerful influences on both the decision to consult and the response to treatment. Deciding whether or not to offer a patient pain management will depend on whether such factors are considered to be an obstacle to treatment (Chs 10, 11 and 12). There are some clinics which consider involvement in litigation to be a absolute obstacle to pain management but in our view, although such factors should always be viewed as potential obstacles to treatment, their precise significance should be weighed up on an individual basis. The role of economic factors is discussed in more detail in Chapter 12.

A number of the more important influences on clinical decision making are shown in Box 5.9. The first three of these are fairly straightforward, and perhaps, in these days of evidence-based medicine, uncontroversial. Any competent treating clinician might reasonably be expected to be familiar with the nature of the condition, the treatment options and risks of treatment. However, as previously stated, two clinicians, assessing the same patient, and presented therefore with a very similar set of clinical data (and having access to the same scientific literature) may arrive at different conclusions. There may of course be no single clearcut solution, but a number of alternatives of comparable merit. As previously discussed, the difference in opinion may be a consequence of differences in elicitation of information, or in the weighing-up of integrating the various elements, but differences in appraisal of suitability may be a consequence also of prejudices or biases against particular approaches to treatment, or against particular types of patient. Such biases may be conscious or unconscious and may become apparent only by external evaluation or audit. Systems of peer review and clinical audit are designed to identify such shortfalls in professional competence. One can be optimistic or pessimistic about the strength of such systems of governance, but it needs to be accepted that all clinical decision making can and may be subject to influences undermining their successful implementation.

Difficulties in appraisal of suitability

A number of technical difficulties underpinning clinical decision making offer a further challenge, and may go some way to explain inconsistencies in diagnosis and in the offer of treatment. They are shown in Box 5.10. A comprehensive analysis of the process of clinical decision making would require an accurate appraisal of each of these factors; a daunting task.

Finally, a summary of the strengths and weaknesses of clinical decision making in the appraisal of risk is shown in Box 5.11.

Box 5.10

Technical difficulties in appraisal of suitability for treatment

- Accuracy of identification of relevant factors
- Estimation of the relative importance of different factors
- Differential weighting
- Integration of specific factors into the clinical decision.

Box 5.11

Strengths and weaknesses of clinical decision making in the appraisal of risk

Strengths

- Based principally on information obtained directly or indirectly from the patient
- Opportunity to maximise gathering of relevant data
- Allows individual weighting of the data
- Permits inclusion of the patient' perceptions of their condition, thus enabling a more accurate overall appraisal
- Potentially offers basis for an immediate risk estimate at the time the patient is seen.

Limitations

- Still only probabilistic
- Potentially subject to biases and prejudices
- Costly (in requiring an individual assessment)
- Not practical for large groups or populations.

Box 5.9

Important influences on clinical decision making

- Epidemiology or natural history of the condition with or without treatment
- Evidence base for treatment outcomes
- Perceived risks of treatment
- Biases and prejudices.

Presurgical screening

In this chapter the primary focus is on psychosocial screening in patients with low-back pain (LBP) in the context of consideration for surgery. (Specific *surgical* indications are beyond the remit of this chapter.)

Costs of surgical interventions

In studies of back pain, 10–15% of the patients account for 80–90% of the cost with the 1–2% who undergo surgery being the most expensive group (Waddell et al 2000). Surgery is expensive and costs of failure are high, in terms of further patient suffering, further health-care costs and work loss. Ten per cent of those who undergo laminectomy or discectomy will go on to further surgery (Hoffman et al 1993), as will 23% of those undergoing spinal fusion (Franklin et al 1994). There has been a growing interest therefore in identifying those chronic pain patients who are unlikely to benefit from surgery, thereby considerably reducing health-care costs and the emotional trauma of failed surgery.

Purposes of presurgical screening

Gatchel & Main (2004) identified four distinct purposes of presurgical evaluation. They are shown in Box 5.12.

Clearly the precise purpose will depend on the specific health-care context and configuration of services, and availability of psychological resources clearly is necessary if positive selection for psychological intervention can be considered. Unfortunately in many clinics, without psychologically oriented rehabilitation, a major use of psychological evaluation has been to 'select out', i.e. identify 'poor bets' for good surgical outcome. While it might be argued that it is actually in the patients' interests to avoid failed surgery, there seem to be ethical concerns in using evaluation only for that purpose.

Box 5.12

Purposes of pre-surgical psychological evaluation

- Identifying contra-indications to surgery
- Selecting for prior psychological intervention
- Identifying need for conjoint psychological therapy
- Flagging for post-surgical psychological management.

Typically patients of a nervous disposition, with low pain tolerance, with poor pain coping skills and unrealistic expectations have a worse prognosis. It might be argued that it is precisely such patients who might require a pain management approach.

Types of assessment

Presurgical psychological screening typically will include both a clinical interview and a psychometric evaluation (Robinson & Riley 2002).

Clinical interview

Studies of outcomes of surgery have clearly demonstrated that the strongest predictors of poor surgical outcome are psychosocial factors (Block 1999). The purpose of the interview is to identify psychosocial factors which may influence the probable outcome of surgery, not in technical terms but in the recovery of optimal function and the optimising of psychological adaptation to any residual pain and pain-associated limitations. Since optimal recovery requires active participation in the rehabilitative phase, it is necessary to appraise the patient's ability to accept this responsibility. Ideally the evaluation will be in the form of a structured interview, as recommended by Gatchel et al (1995) with the objective not only to identify major obstacles to treatment, but also identify psychopathology which may need treatment in its own right (Chs 3 and 10). A less dramatic but equally import aspect of the interview is to identify levels of distress, misunderstandings, unrealistic expectations or maladaptive coping strategies which can be addressed prior to surgery, during the recovery phase, or in the context of post-surgery rehabilitation. Block (1999) considers that the interview should include in particular the history of past psychological treatment, physical abuse, sexual abuse, abandonment and substance abuse as risk factors for poor outcome of treatment. It would seem important, however, to treat every patient as an individual and it should only be if such factors seemed likely to compromise outcome that they should play a major part in the decision making.

Psychometric evaluations

Questionnaires have been used widely in presurgical screening and indeed are an identified part of the costs of assessment in some North American clinics. As might be expected, by far the most widely used test is the Minnesota Multiphasic Personality Inventory 2 (MMPI-2) (Hathaway et al 1989), and group studies have consistently shown that certain MMPI profiles, associated in particular with the Hs (Hypochondriasis), D (Depression) and Hy (Hysteria) scales, are predictors of poorer surgical outcome (Robinson & Riley 2002, Block 1999) but MMPI enthusiasts have identified associations with other scales. The MMPI, however, is cumbersome to administer, and not particularly sensitive in the individual case.

In general, it would seem that the same sort of appraisal of cognitive, emotional and behavioural factors associated with the persistence of pain and development of prolonged disability should be evaluated, in terms of possible targets for treatment or as significant obstacles to recovery.

The profiling or 'scorecard' approach

Finally, Robinson & Riley (2002) have recommended the use of a scorecard approach to presurgical psychological screening (PPS), based on summation of risk factors from the medical domain (chronicity, previous surgeries, destructiveness of proposed surgery, non-organic signs, non-spine-related treatments, smoking status and obesity), clinical interview data (litigation and compensation status, job dissatisfaction, heavy-lifting job, substance abuse, family reinforcement of pain behaviour, marital dissatisfaction, physical and sexual abuse, pre-injury psychopathology) and test results (MMPI, Coping Strategies Questionnaire (CSQ)) (Block 1999) since it has been reported to have some predictive validity. Much as the concept of a scorecard is an attractive one, without considerable more developmental work, it is not possible to recommend it for usage, and it appears cumbersome in any event.

Risk factors for the development of pain

How common is pain?

Pain is common in the community. According to McBeth & Macfarlane (2002), prevalence (in terms of lifetime estimates) vary between 50% and 84% in various studies; 20–60% of the general population report experiencing symptoms in the previous 12 months; and there is a point prevalence (on the day of interview) of 26–35%. Overall, McBeth & Macfarlane found lower estimates for shoulder pain, but still with significant variation across studies. Wide differences in the definition of pain, its classification criteria and its severity are probably responsible for a large proportion of the

variation in these estimates, but clearly pain (however defined) is common. The Manchester group therefore decided to study a more clearly defined subgroup of pain conditions, and decided to focus on chronic widespread pain and fibromyalgia (for which in criteria there is a significant overlap). The limited number of available population studies (mainly over the last 12 months) suggest an average period prevalence of around 12% using the American College of Rheumatology (ACR) criteria (Wolfe et al 1990) with an estimate of around 4.7% using the more stringent Manchester criteria (Macfarlane et al 1996). The prevalence of fibromyalgia in the general population varies between 1% and 11% across studies with an overall rate of around 2% (estimates of primary-care consulters).

As a precursor to consideration of development of the persistence of pain and pain-associated disability later in this chapter it is relevant to offer a brief review of what is known about risk factors for pain *onset*. In this brief review we are heavily indebted to Waddell (2004, pp. 91–113), using back pain as an example, and making the broad distinction between *individual* risk factors and *environmental* risk factors.

Individual risk factors for pain onset

In one study (Adams et al 1999) personal risk factors accounted for about 12% of variance in new back pain onset. As Waddell (2004) points out, however, there are a considerable number of studies of risk factors in back pain, and of course they may interact within the individual. In summarising the evidence on risk factors for back pain, he classifies them under the headings of *individual risk factors*, *environmental physical risk factors* and *environmental psychosocial risk factors*. His analysis of the strength of evidence and effect size are shown in Table 5.1.

Of the individual risk factors there appears to be most compelling evidence for previous history for back pain with consistent evidence, but of various strengths for age and gender. No clear evidence emerges regarding anthropomorphic factors. There is a strong, although variable, effect of social class in men and strong evidence of a weak effect of psychological distress.

Environmental risk factors for pain onset

Physical risk factors

Perhaps unsurprisingly there is strong evidence for a number of biomechanical factors, although the effect size is variable.

Table 5.1 Summary of the evidence on risk factors for back pain

Risk factor	Strength of evidence	Effect size
Individual risk factors		
Previous history of back pain	Strong	Large – the overwhelming risk factor
Genetic/familial	Moderate/strong?	Variable
Gender	Strong	Variable
Age	Strong	Variable
Body build: height, weight, leg length inequality	Strong	No effect
Physical fitness	Moderate	No effect
Smoking	Inconsistent	Small
Social class, education	Strong (men)	Variable
Emotional distress	Strong	Small
Environmental risk factors: physical		
Manual handling/lifting	Strong	Moderate (variable)
Bending and twisting	Strong	Small–moderate
Repetitive movements	Inconsistent	Unproven
Static work postures and sitting	Strong	No effect
Driving and whole-body vibration	Strong	Moderate–small[a]
Leisure activities and sports	Moderate	Most have no effect
Environmental risk factors: psychosocial aspects of work		
Job satisfaction	Strong	Small
Work 'stress'	Limited	Small
High job demands and pace	Inconsistent	No effect
Poor job content	Inconsistent	No effect
Low social support	Strong	Small
Job 'strain'	Inconsistent	Unproven

[a] Probably small on modern damped seats.

From Waddell (2004, Table 6.5, p. 109), with permission of Elsevier Ltd.

Psychosocial risk factors

Psychosocial aspects of work such as job satisfaction and low social support appear to have strong evidence but with small effect sizes. In general the strength of evidence appears to be inconsistent and the effect sizes small or unimportant.

Risk factors for the persistence of pain, pain-associated limitations and work compromise

Risk factors for the persistence of pain

Understanding natural history

For many purposes it is convenient to assume that either acute pain resolves, or it does not, and in the latter event there is a smooth and clearly identifiable trajectory into chronic pain. This assumption, however, would appear to be unsafe. Burton et al (2004b), in a prospective cohort study of 252 LBP patients attending for manipulative care, were able to follow up 60% of the sample 4 years later. The occurrence of pain episodes over those 4 years is shown in Table 5.2. It can be seen that of those attending initially with acute LBP, 60.9% have further episodes, with 50% identifying between 1 and 5 episodes over the ensuing 4 years, and 10.9% identifying more than 6 episodes or persistent pain.

The comparable figures for the subacute group are 70.6%, 32.3% and 38.2%. For the chronic group, the comparable figures are 88.9%, 33.3% and 55.6%. Admittedly the actual numbers in this study are relatively small, but they suggest firstly that most back pain is recurrent and secondly that the future course is influenced by the clinical history at the time of initial consultation.

Symptom variability; periodicity

Conventionally, the development of chronicity is viewed along a continuous timeline, with pragmatic cut-off points devised primarily as a way of deciding about resource allocation. As can be inferred from some of the previous discussion, however, there is significant variation in the clinical course of back pain. Von Korff & Miglioretti (2006) have suggested a new approach to the definition of pain, by classifying it in terms of the probability of the likelihood of significant pain being present one or more years in the future; making a further distinction between *possible* chronic back pain (with a likelihood of occurrence of 50%+) and *probable* chronic back pain (with a likelihood of occurrence of 80%+). They based their estimation on three variables, shown in Box 5.13.

Using a baseline score, with cut-offs as a basis for risk estimation, they found that 58.7% of possible and 82.1% of probable chronic back pain patients had a Chronic Pain Grade of 2–4 one year later, and the classification also strongly predicted the presence of clinically significant back pain at years 2 and 5. Furthermore, of those with probable chronic back pain at year 1, 90.9% and 76.5% had clinically significant back pain at years 2 and 5 respectively. This prognostic approach would seem

Table 5.2 Future back pain episodes

Initial LBP		None	1	2–5	6+	Persistent	Total (n)
Acute (<3/52)	n	18	4	19	4	1	46
	%	39.1	8.7	41.3	8.7	2.2	
Subacute (3/52–6/12)	n	10	1	10	12	1	34
	%	29.4	2.9	29.4	35.3	2.9	
Chronic (>6/12)	n	1	1	2	5	0	9
	%	11.1	11.1	22.2	55.6	0	
Total	n	29	6	31	21	2	89
	%	32.6	6.7	34.8	23.6	2.1	

Box 5.13

Prognostic variables for chronicity

- Symptom Check List (SCL-90) Depression Scale (Derogatis 1983)
- Number of days with back pain in the previous 6 months (Von Korff et al 1992)
- Number of other pain sites.

From Von Korff & Miglioretti (2006)

Box 5.14

Recommendations for treatment of acute non-specific low-back pain

- Give adequate information and reassure the patient
- Do not prescribe bed rest as a treatment
- Advise patients to stay active and continue normal daily activities including work if possible
- Prescribe medication, if necessary for pain relief; preferably to be taken at regular intervals; first choice paracetamol, second choice NSAIDs
- Consider adding a short course of muscle relaxants on its own or added to NSAIDs, if paracetamol or NSAIDs have failed to reduce pain
- Consider (referral for) spinal manipulation for patients who are failing to return to normal activities
- Multidisciplinary treatment programmes in occupational settings may be an option for workers with subacute low-back pain and sick leave for more than 4–8 weeks.

Van Tulder et al (2005)

Box 5.15

Concepts of prevention and overarching comments (extracts)

- There is limited scope for preventing its incidence (first-time onset)
- Prevention in the context of this guideline is focused primarily on reduction of the impact and consequences of LBP
- Primary causative mechanisms remain largely undetermined: risk factor modification will not necessarily achieve prevention
- There is considerable scope, in principle, for prevention of the *consequences* of LBP
- Different interventions and outcomes will be appropriate for different populations
- There is evidence suggesting that prevention of various consequences of LBP is feasible
- The most promising approaches seem to involve physical activity/exercise and appropriate (biopsychosocial) education, at least for adults
- But, no single intervention is likely to be effective to prevent the overall problem of LBP, owing to its multidimensional nature
- Optimal progress on prevention in LBP will likely require a cultural shift in the way LBP is viewed, its relation with activity and work, how it may best be tackled and just what is reasonable to expect from preventive strategies
- It is important to get all the players onside, but innovative studies are required to understand better the mechanisms and delivery of prevention in LBP.

From Burton et al (2004b)

to merit further investigation since potentially it offers an opportunity for screening and targeting (see below).

It is difficult, however, to differentiate clearly between persistence of pain and pain-associated disability because in many studies a single outcome measure is used. Also, the two are not independent since arguably, one of the most appealing, and to an extent effective, ways of controlling pain is to diminish activities. It might be argued also that an exclusive focus on pain, although consistent with a specific biomedical focus on pain nociception, is important particularly in the management of neoplastic and neurogenic pain and becomes somewhat more problematic in the management of 'non-specific' musculoskeletal pain. Most evidence for the efficacy of treatment for acute pain problems lies in pharmacological trials, but there have recently been a number of trials published on the Cochrane website (Cochrane) of a range of other sorts of treatment. The European Commission, under the Cost B13 funding initiative, established three working groups charged with developing LBP guidelines for acute pain, chronic pain and prevention, respectively.

The acute non-specific LBP guidelines (Van Tulder et al 2005) are shown in Box 5.14. It can be seen that these are targeted primarily on the management of pain, although there is recognition that with the passage of time a broader approach might be considered. A parallel working group (Burton et al 2004a) considered prevention. It has extensive specific evidence-based recommendation which can be found on the website but it offers also a summary of the concepts of prevention accompanied by some overarching comments, some of which are shown in Box 5.15.

Risk factors for persistent pain and pain-associated limitations (including work)

As far as risk factors for long-term work disability are concerned, in terms of individual factors, Sullivan et al (2005) in their review found evidence for fear, beliefs in severity of health conditions, catastrophising (yellow flags), and also poor problem solving, low return-to-work (RTW) expectancies and lack of confidence in performing work-related activities (blue flags). They also found evidence of pain severity and level of depressive symptoms contributing to the transition to chronicity. In terms of workplace factors, they found further evidence for job stress, co-worker support, job dissatisfaction, employer attitudes, job autonomy and availability of modified work as factors influencing duration of work disability and RTW outcomes.

Their findings are consistent with the earlier more widespread review by Waddell et al (2003) in their review of predictors of chronic pain and disability. Although the original remit of the review specifically was on 'long-term incapacity for work' (or work disability in North American parlance), as aforementioned not only are pain and functional limitations often used as single outcomes, they are often interpreted in effect as if they were equivalent to each other. Similar problems arise in trying to distinguish clinical outcomes such as increase in activity or postural tolerance from occupational variables such as RTW rates or indices of work capability.

In fact the Cost 13B prevention guidelines (Burton et al 2004a) offered a distinction between the general population and workers. Despite some variation in the level of evidence available, the similarity among the recommendations is striking.

The guidelines for workers obviously contain a number of recommendations specific to work settings, but otherwise, in terms of the usefulness of information or educational approaches, the lack of support for traditional biomechanical and biomedical approaches, and traditional clinical interventions is similar.

In fact, over the last decade, with the exception of a series of reviews in the Cochrane Library synthesising the findings of earlier conservative management, and studies of outcome of surgery (which are beyond the remit of this chapter), there appears to have been relatively little new research with clinical outcomes as a primary focus.

Waddell et al (2003) appraised the evidence for different sorts of predictors of chronic pain and disability. In their first set of evidence tables they summarise the findings from published studies of clinical and psychosocial predictors (Table 5.3) where the strength of evidence and strength of predictors are shown along with a tentative flag assignment in the right-hand column.

Aggregation of such a large set of data, with such a wide variety of specific variables is by nature imprecise, as are the 27 variables under which the predictors have been gathered. Accepting these strictures, it can be seen that there is evidence for an influence of both socio-demographic and personal history variables, but the strongest influences appear to be from yellow or blue flags (most of which are potentially modifiable) and black flags (which are more immutable, although may present opportunities for a 'systems solution'; equivalent to Sullivan et al (2005) Type-I (individually centred) and Type-II (workplace or system-based) solutions, as discussed in Chapters 14 and 15).

Classification, clustering and screening

Use of prediction rules

As aforementioned, risk assessment at a population level, whether for public health or insurance purposes (frequently disability management) often adopts developed mathematical models for classification and predictive purposes. Examples include the German Social Insurance Screening Tool (Biefang et al 1998), a screening tool based on predictors of long-term incapacity in LBP social security claimants (Van der Giezen et al 2000) and the well-known Vocational Rehabilitation Index (Cornes 1990). Other occupationally focused tools include the Finnish Work Ability Index (Tuomi et al 1998), essentially a structured occupational health assessment based on a self-report questionnaire.

There has in general been a move to developing models with more detailed clinical content, in terms of both physical and psychological parameters. Hicks et al (2005) developed a clinical prediction tool for response to spinal stabilisation exercises. The yellow-flag model (Kendall et al 1997), widely referenced elsewhere in this book (Schultz et al 2002), for example developed an occupational LBP disability predictive model incorporating five groups of variables: sociodemographic, medical, psychosocial, pain behaviour and workplace-related factors. Interestingly, they found that 'cognitions dominated the integrated model'.

Ultimately, there appears to be a continuum of predictive decision rules ranging from gut feelings in the clinic to advanced statistical algorithms. Different models may have varying degrees of empirical support

Table 5.3 Individual clinic and psychosocial predictors of chronic pain and disability

	Strength of evidence	Strength of predictor	Type of variable	Flag assignment
Age	***	***	Demog.	
Gender	*	Variable	Demog.	
Ethnicity	**	Not signif.		
Marital status	*	Variable	Demog.	
Education	*	*	Demog.	
Clinical history	*** (LBP)	***	Clinical	?Red?Yellow
Clinical exam	*	*	Clinical	?Red
Comorbidity	***	*	Clinical	?Red
Alcohol or substance abuse	*	*	Clinical	Orange
Personality	*	*		Orange
Psychological hist.	*	*		?Orange
Anxiety	*	*		?Orange
Stressful life events	*	*		?Orange
Pain intensity, funct. disability	***	**	Clinical	?
Poor perceptions of general health	***	**	Clinical	Yellow
Psychological distress	***	***	Clinical	Yellow/orange
Depression	***	**	Clinical	Orange/yellow
Fear avoidance	**	**	Clinical	Yellow
Maladaptive coping (Catastrophising)	***	**	Clinical	Yellow
Pain behaviour	***	**	Clinical	Yellow
Duration sickness absence	***	***	Clin./Occ.	Yellow/blue?Black
Employment status	***	***	Occ.	Blue/black
Job dissatisfaction	***	***	Occ.	Blue
Expectations re RTW	***	***		Blue
Physical demands of work	***	*	Occ.	Black
Financial incentives	***	***	Occ.	Black
Unemployment rates	**	***	Occ.	Black

*** Strong
** Moderate
* Weak

as well as varying balances between sensitivity and specificity, and different relevance for application. Any variable may be a valuable predictor, so the first stage of model building may include a broad epidemiological sweep. The identification of predictors, however, is only a first step. For risk assessment in the context of clinical application, there is a need to be able to apply the model on an individual level with a view on utilising the screening technique to improve the results of intervention.

Classification and clustering

It is important, pragmatically as well as conceptually, to identify similarities amongst individuals at the time of initial presentation. According to Bouter et al (1998), lack of effectiveness in early intervention may be the lack of a method for subgrouping or classifying patients as a precursor to clinical decision making, yet most clinicians seem to accept that subgroups exist (Kent & Keating 2004). The distinction between measurement of specific characteristics, patient description and patient classification or clustering is somewhat arbitrary, since measurement instruments frequently are employed for purposes for which they were not designed. There are also a vast number of available measurement instruments (Turk & Melzack 2001), some of which are described in Chapter 8. In this chapter a number of different types of clinical classification are described, with examples of different assessment measures used, primarily for illustrative purposes.

Clinical signs and symptoms

There has been particular interest in classifying or grouping patients prior to physical therapy interventions. Typically patients are classified according to the clinical signs and symptoms identified at initial assessment (Delitto et al 1995). Improved outcomes from subgrouping have been reported (Delitto et al 1993, Erhard et al 1994, Fritz et al 2003). In the Fritz et al (2003) study, patients were randomised to either guideline-based treatment (low-stress aerobic exercise and advice to remain active) with no attempt at subgrouping, or to classification-based treatment (manipulation, specific exercise, stabilisation exercise or traction) based on patterns of signs and symptoms suggesting a particular clinical approach. The 'classification group' had significantly better outcomes in terms of cost, disability and RTW at 4 weeks, and also at 1 year. According to Brennan et al (2006), however, the improved outcomes may have been the result of being assigned to more efficacious treatments rather than a consequence of the classification process per se. Brennan et al (2006) therefore compared assignment to treatment (manipulation, specific exercise or stabilisation exercise) based on classification with randomisation to one of the three treatment groups. They found that patients receiving matched treatment experienced greater short-term and long-term reductions in disability than those receiving unmatched treatments.

Specific clinical (physical) characteristics

There have also been other attempts to subgroup on the basis of specific clinical characteristics. Rowbotham et al (1998) identified three distinct subtypes of patients with post-herpetic neuralgia; Smart et al (1997) offered a classification of fibromyalgia based on mechanisms of T-cell activation; Dworkin & LeResche (1992) offered eight subtypes of temporomandibular joint patients based on physical examination of muscles and joints; and Spitzer et al (1995) developed their well-known classification of whiplash disorders based on presenting clinical characteristics.

Pain characteristics

The McGill Pain Questionnaire (Melzack 1975, 1987) has been used to identify both the sensory and emotional characteristics of pain from the use of pain vocabulary, but has not been developed specifically for patient clustering or classification. Pain drawings, however, have been used in a number of ways. As mentioned above, they have proved to be a useful epidemiological tool but they are often also included in clinical assessment, perhaps in part because patients usually show no reluctance to complete them, and indeed sometimes do so with relish. There have been a number of variants of mannekins (or drawings) but commonly they give indication of location of pain, permit some sort of quantification and can also be used to capture some of the qualitative features of pain. Ransford et al (1976) originally attempted to classify patients as 'nonorganic' from 'psychogenic' pain on the basis of drawings. Drawings were evaluated for the extent to which they appear to correspond to a clear anatomical pathway. Widespread patterns, with non-anatomical distributions and use of all sorts of additional emphasis are considered indicative of 'psychological overlay' or distress. A clearly abnormal pain drawing is almost always indicative of pain-associated distress and should alert the clinician to the need for a more careful psychosocial assessment. However, as emphasised in Chapter 7, they should not be overinterpreted, as the test is insufficiently sensitive to be recommended as a single screening procedure to identify distress. (A more comprehensive discussion on pain measures is offered in Ch. 7.)

Personality type

There have been attempts to identify clusters of patients on the basis of their MMPI profiles, such as the four-part P-A-I-N classification (Robinson et al 1989) with some evidence of an association of the cluster types with pain coping strategies and treatment outcome (Swimmer et al 1992), and the SCL-90 (Derogatis 1983) has also been used in association with lumbar dynamometry to predict treatment outcome (Hutten et al 2001), but recently classification and screening pain has come to focus on more specific factors such as pain cognition, emotional responses and pain behaviour.

Pain behaviours

There is little in the literature in terms of the development of specific behaviour typologies or classifications. Historically, experimental analysis of behaviour, and the derivation of the principles of learning theory (Ch. 2) led to the crucial distinction between operant and respondent behaviour in terms of the circumstances of its occurrence, but although the importance of the distinction as the bedrock from which modern pain management developed cannot be underestimated, specific classification systems have not been developed as such. There are a number of rating scales which include pain behaviours, but the most widely used are probably the Behavioural Observation Test (Keefe et al 1990), used primarily as a research tool and the Behavioural Signs Test (Waddell et al 1980), an assessment of pain behaviour using physical examination. It was developed originally as a research and clinical tool as a first-stage identification of 'nonorganic influences'. The test has been misused clinically as a measure of contra-indication to surgery per se (rather than as a screening for the need for psychological assessment) and misused also as an indicator of malingering (Main & Waddell 1998).

Distress

There are several self-report questionnaires such as the General Health Questionnaire, or GHQ (Goldberg & Williams 1998) and SF-36 (Ware et al 1994) available in a range of forms, which can be used as screening tools for the identification of distress, and 'caseness' in psychiatric parlance (Chs 3 and 8), but they have not been used specifically for the development of typologies among pain patients. However the Distress Risk

Box 5.16

Distress Risk Assessment Method (DRAM)

Classification

N	Modified Zung score <17
R	Modified Zung score 17–33 *and* MSPQ score LE 12
DD	Modified Zung score >33
DS	Modified Zung score 17–33 *and* MSPQ score GE 13

Recommendations for use

- Recommended in secondary and tertiary care clinics as a screening tool to aid clinical appraisal of the patient
- Particularly recommended in problem back clinics and pain clinics
- Should be viewed as a first stage screener, *not* as a complete psychological assessment or as a test of malingering
- Distress and its management should always be considered as part of decisions about surgery
- Distress patients not requiring surgery require pain management.

Adapted from Main et al (1992, p. 52)

Assessment Method, or DRAM (Main et al 1992) was developed specifically as a screening tool for the identification of distress in LBP patients. It comprises a somatic awareness scale and a depressive symptoms inventory. The items and their scoring are shown in Appendices 5.1 and 5.2. The DRAM classification is shown in Box 5.16.

The DRAM classification had both concurrent and predictive validity in identifying patients who require a patient-centred pain management approach. In patients with significantly troublesome pain problems, a patient-centred approach to evaluation is always appropriate and it is certainly not appropriate to view distress as a contra-indication to treatment with good surgical indications (Hobby et al 2001).

Pain- and disability-specific psychological content

Boersma & Linton (2005), in a study of 185 patients, selected four of the items (pain intensity, fear-avoidance beliefs, depressed mood and functional ability) from the Örebro Screening Questionnaire for Pain, and employing cluster-analytic techniques, using a sequence of procedures, finally identified four clusters of patients, shown in Box 5.17.

Box 5.17

Psychological clusters

- Low risk on all variables: 'Low Risk' cluster (83/185)
- High score on all variables: 'Distressed–Fear Avoidant' cluster (29/185)
- High pain, fear-avoidance and functional problems: 'Fear Avoidant' cluster (45/185)
- High scores of pain and depressed mood: 'Low-risk–Depressed Mood' cluster (28/185).

Boersma and Linton (2005)

They then replicated the clusters on a second sample of 178 patients. According to the authors, their analyses identified two low-risk profiles and two higher-risk profiles, raising the possibility of targeting interventions consistent with the fear-avoidance model (Vlaeyen et al 1995, Vlaeyen & Linton 2002). In a further exploration of the fear-avoidance model (Boersma & Linton 2006) identified five clusters, described as 'pain-related fear', 'pain-related fear + depressed mood', 'medium pain-related fear', 'depressed mood' and 'low risk'. Patients in the 'pain-related fear' and 'pain-related fear + depressed mood' groups reported more long-term sick leave during follow-up, and the patients in the 'depressed mood' group reported most health-care usage.

Multifaceted instruments

Differentiation of types of self-report instruments on the basis of their specific content to an extent is somewhat arbitrary since the content is variable, but one of the best-known examples of a multidimensional, yet reasonably practical, instrument is the Multiphasic Pain Inventory, or MPI (Kerns et al 1985).

Multidimensional pain inventory

As Turk (2005) has observed, while the 'patient uniformity myth' has been exploded, many of the attempts at patient classification have been based on single factors. There is, however, widespread evidence that outcome of treatment is multifactorial and therefore attempt to derive a somewhat broader approach to classification would seem to have appeal. In a landmark publication, Turk & Rudy (1988), using the West Haven–Yale Multidimensional Pain Inventory, initially referred to as the WHYMPI and later the MPI (Kerns et al 1985), used the empirically derived scales to develop a patient

Box 5.18

MPI scales and patient classification

MPI scales
- Pain severity
- Interference with family and marital functioning
- Support received from significant others
- Life control (including perceived ability to solve problems and feelings of personal mastery and competence)
- Affective distress
- Performance of activities.

Patient types
- *Dysfunctional (DYS)*:
  - Severity of their pain perceived as high
  - High pain interference
  - High distress
  - Low levels of activity.
- *Interpersonally distressed (IP)*:
  - Significant others perceived as unsupportive.
- *Active copers (AC)*:
  - High levels of social support
  - Relatively low levels of pain intensity and interference
  - Relatively high levels of activity.

classification using cluster analysis. (The scales and patient classification are shown in Box 5.18.)

This classification has been widely used and replicated in several countries. Interestingly the groups do not seem to differ on specific indices of physical functioning or prevalence of various symptoms, and according to Turk (2005) 'The results reinforce the suggestion that the psychosocial dimension of chronic pain syndromes may be independent of physical pathology' (p. 47).

The general taxonomy of the MPI has been replicated in different pain conditions. Turk (2005) offers a candid view of the strengths and limitations of the MPI. They are summarised in Box 5.19.

Despite its impressive pedigree, the classification has a number of limitations. Nonetheless not all patients can be assigned unambiguously to one of the three groups, and in some studies up to 20% cannot be satisfactorily classified. Missing data can be problematic, particularly on questions referring to 'significant others'. A number of recent studies have failed to identify differential responses of the subgroups to standard treatment (Bergstrom et al 2001, Walen et al 2002, Gatchel et al 2002). There are a wide range of potential confounders

Box 5.19

Strengths and limitations of the MPI

Strengths

- High face validity and concurrent validity
- Widely used in research studies and clinical practice
- Apparently fairly robust structurally across clinical settings and cultures
- Offers a simple patient classification
- Potentially useful as a first-stage screener.

Limitations

- Not all patients can be assigned unambiguously to the clusters
- Missing data can be problematic (particularly with reference to 'significant others')
- Variation across results in intervention studies, possibly as a consequence of confounders
- Some studies have failed to demonstrate anticipated outcomes of treatment for the different clusters
- As yet few attempts to use the typology specifically to target treatment.

in terms of presenting patient characteristics and in the nature of interventions which might explain different results in different studies, but as a first-stage system of classification, the MPI would seem to have general utility.

To date there have been relatively few attempts to customise treatment on the basis of presenting psychosocial characteristics. Turk (2005) considers that although the results have not been uniformly consistent, there are now a number of studies supporting the potential value of treatment matching and he advocates further clinical investigations to determine the relative utility of different treatment modalities matched to presenting characteristics.

The use of the MPI as a first-stage screening instrument, to be possibly supplemented by the collection of additional information may also have merit, and as such the utility of the instrument can be compared directly with other 'screeners'. (Clearly no classification system will ever be able to incorporate all patient influences on outcome.) Similarly the value of the MPI subgroups as 'prototypes with significant room for variability within the subgroups' as Turk suggests, can be compared directly with alternative approaches such specific targeting of psychosocial risk factors (as discussed below).

Clinical and occupational screening instruments

There are a wide range of assessment tools, potentially available for screening, which have been developed for patient or assessment and classification. A description and evaluation of these many instruments is offered in Waddell et al (2003, Appendix B). These include complex multifaceted insurance and social screening tools highlighted by Bloch & Prins (2001) in their six-nation comparison, including the Vocational Rehabilitation Index, or VRI (Cornes 1990), a fairly simple scale based on administrative data; and the Finnish Work Ability Index, essentially a structured occupational health assessment (Tuomi et al 1998) and a number of more specific instruments.

The recent impetus towards early identification with a view to secondary prevention, however, requires an instrument which is reasonably broad in scope, is reasonably simple to administer and offers a way of integrating the information in a straightforward manner. A number of such tools have been developed.

The Vermont Disability Prediction Questionnaire (Hazard et al 1996)

This simple questionnaire comprises 11 items: a mixture of self-report items, including five clinical items (including attribution of blame), a pain intensity rating, four occupational items (including not only physical demand but also items on relationship with co-workers and future work expectation) and a question about the number of times the person has been married (perhaps indicative of the North American origins of the questionnaire!). Each item is scored on a 0–5 scale, and the scores are summed and presented as a fraction of the total possible score. The authors reported a sensitivity of 0.94 and a specificity of 0.84 for the prediction of RTW at 3 months for workers filing injury claims. However, the structural validity has not been reported in detail, and the results do not appear to have been replicated and so it cannot as yet be recommended.

Obstacles to Return-to-Work Questionnaire or ORQ (Marhold et al 2002)

Marhold et al (2002) produced a 55-item questionnaire which after factor analysis yielded nine subscales, of 'satisfactory reliability' according to the authors and of comparable predictive validity to the MPI and the

Disability Rating Index (Salen et al 1994), significantly predicting sick leave and correctly classifying 79% of the patients, but with the advantage of including items specifically concerning work.

However, the questionnaire was developed originally in a study of 154 patients and since there are 55 items on the scale, there have to be concerns about factor stability because of the low subject–variable ratio. Thus, while the ORQ certainly seems to merit further investigation, it would not as yet appear to be sufficiently validated for screening purposes.

Örebro Screening Questionnaire for Pain (OSQP)

Linton & Hallden (1998) developed a screening tool, primarily for psychosocial risk factors for chronic pain and chronicity. Although not offering clustering as such, the widespread clinical use of cut-off scores to identify the presence of significant psychosocial risk factors enable patient screening. It was included in the New Zealand Screening Instrument (Kendall et al 1997) and was published later in a slightly modified form as the Örebro Screening Questionnaire for Pain (Boersma & Linton 2002).

The final version comprises 25 items of which six deal with background factors, and 19 deal with a variety of background factors. There are extremely minor differences in the precise descriptors between the New Zealand and Swedish versions and the way in which employment status is coded (featuring as an additional numbered item) but in all important respects the versions seem to be equivalent. The content of the questionnaire is shown in Appendix 5.3. The scored layout and scoring instructions are shown in Appendix 5.4.

The authors state that in order to give all items equal weight, they were scaled from 0 to 10 (with some items reversed) and the scores summated to form a total score. Since the background items (1–4) were not found to contribute statistically, they were not included in the calculation of the total score. A scoring system was provided such that a total score could be obtained.

In the earlier publication (Linton & Hallden 1998), it was stated that a cut-off of 105 enabled 75% correct identification of those not needing modification to ongoing management, 86% correct identification of those who would have between 1 and 30 days off work in the next year and 83% correct identification of those who would have more than 30 days off work.

Hurley et al (2000), in an investigation of the instrument's utility in predicting RTW after physical therapy, found that a cut-off of 112 correctly identified 80% of patients failing to RTW at the end of treatment (sensitivity) and 59% of those who did RTW (specificity). In further analysis of the same cohort of patients (Hurley et al 2001) they found that scores on the instrument (labelled the ALBPSQ) were correlated with the patients' level of pain and reported disability at 1-year follow-up and 'correctly identified all patients reporting some degree of work loss but had minimal predictive strength for the other patient-centred variables evaluated'.

In the more recent publication (Boersma & Linton 2002), the authors report satisfactory test–retest reliability (0.83), using a cut-off of 105 (the maximum is 210), and a specificity of 0.75 with a sensitivity of 0.88 in the prediction of future absenteeism, and examine the utility of various cut-off scores in the prediction of sick listing (ranging from 90 to 120) and for functional ability (ranging from 80 to 110) in terms of sensitivity and specificity. As they point out, decisions about the trade-off between sensitivity and specificity may be different in relation to differing goals among health-care professionals.

Comment on OSQP

The questionnaire has considerable appeal as a general psychosocial screener, and is now fairly widely used in clinical practice. Some of its strengths and limitations are shown in Box 5.20. The questionnaire targets important predictors of long-term pain-associated functional limitations and also occupational outcomes such as duration of sick leave and RTW, but on the evidence currently available would seem to function best in relation to occupational outcomes. As a *screener* therefore it is to be recommended.

It is clear that very different clinical and occupational profiles can yield similar scores on the questionnaire. This may not be critical in terms of first-level screening, but, as mentioned earlier in this chapter, screening should only be undertaken with specific purposes in mind. As the properties of the questionnaire become clearer with its use in a range of settings, it will be possible hopefully to examine its utility as a stand-alone screener, and also, possibly linking with more detailed and specific evaluations, to identify individuals likely to benefit from targeted interventions of various types.

It is to be hoped that as part of its further development, there will be further appraisal of its structural properties with the development of more sensitive scoring systems. As things stand it represents an extremely worthwhile addition to the psychometric armamentarium.

Box 5.20

Strengths and limitations of the OSQP

Strengths

- High face validity and concurrent validity
- Predominantly based on psychosocial risk factors
- Has an intuitive appeal to clinicians
- Fairly straightforward to administer and score
- Particularly useful in content of secondary prevention
- Strongest predictive validity for occupational outcomes
- Useful as a first-stage psychosocial screener and possibly as part of a process of treatment targeting.

Limitations

- Relatively little information on the reliability, stability or sensitivity of change of individual items
- Structurally underdeveloped
- Restricting its use to the production of a simple cut-off score may hide important heterogeneity amongst patients with similar scores
- Influence of possible confounders on the relationship between cut-offs and outcomes would merit further investigation
- As yet few attempts to use the typology specifically to target treatment.

Box 5.21

Important features of the flag system in the context of risk identification

- Highlights the importance of a 'systems perspective'
- Contains both clinical and occupational elements
- Distinguishes individual perceptions from objective features.

types of specifically targeted interventions based on modifiable risk. An attempted mapping of the flags onto the individual predictors of chronic pain and disability was illustrated in Table 5.3. Different flags, and combinations of flags, require different types of interventions, and a multiflag approach appears to lend itself flexibly to both individual clinical decision making and widescale system applications (Main et al 2005). However, its predictive accuracy in administrative applications will likely be lower than one arising from a purely statistical or 'actuarial' approach and will likely result in overidentification of individuals at risk. Further reflections on the linking of screening with targeting are offered below.

Screening and targeting

Turk (1990) has been a long advocate of customising patients for treatment on the basis of their initial presenting characteristics. Screening has to be understood *in context*, not only in terms of the specific purposes of screening and the stage in illness, but also in terms of the base rates of the characteristic of interest in the particular group being screened. Most screening, however, can be described in terms of 'screening in', 'screening out' and 'screening with targeting' and the sensitivities/specificities need to be examined in relationship to the specific purpose of screening. Screening out from one treatment does not necessary imply screening in for another sort of treatment. In this final section of the chapter, five examples of screening and targeting are described: two examples of general targeting and three examples of more specific targeting.

Flags as a method of risk identification

It is possible also to consider the flag system (Kendall et al 1997, Main & Spanswick 2000) as a method of risk identification, and it has been described as a methodological compromise between the inflexibilities of a purely actuarial model and a purely subjective approach based on clinical judgement (Linton et al 2005). In this context there are three important features (Box 5.21). Firstly, it offers a 'systems perspective' and assumes that an adequate understanding of the problem requires consideration of both the injured worker and the individual's social and occupational context. Secondly, it contains both clinical and occupational elements. Thirdly, it makes an important distinction between the individual's perception of the situation and the objective features.

Flagging systems may be useful therefore as a conceptual framework capable of including both actuarial data and individually assessed risk factors informing different

General targeting for prolonged disability

Gatchel et al (2003) developed a statistical algorithm for differentiating acute LBP patients who were designated as either high or low risk for developing chronic disability. In one study, 'high-risk' acute patients were randomly assigned to one of two groups: an early functional restoration group with a cognitive–behavioural approach or a treatment-as-usual group. Results showed that, relative to the treatment-as-usual group, the functional restoration group displayed significantly fewer indices of chronic pain disability on a wide range of work, health-care utilisation, medication use and self-reported pain variables.

Linton & Andersson (2000) also used a risk-screening procedure to select patients for a secondary prevention intervention. They compared the effects of a 6-week cognitive–behavioural group intervention to two information-provision comparison groups, for individuals who were identified as higher risk based on their scores on the Örebro Screening Questionnaire for Pain. All groups showed comparable improvements in pain severity, mood and activity level. However, follow-up analyses showed that the cognitive–behavioural intervention led to a significantly lower probability of being on long-term sick leave compared to the two information groups.

Targeting of specific risk factors

Pain-related fears

A programme of intervention developed by Vlaeyen and his colleagues (Vlaeyen et al 2002) proceeds from the view that disability results from the development of high levels of pain-related fears. Individuals with high levels of pain-related fears are gradually exposed to activities that have been avoided with an approach similar to that which would be used for the treatment of phobic conditions. A recent clinical trial has shown that this type of intervention can be effective in reducing levels of fear, pain and pain-related disability (George et al 2003).

Other investigations have pointed to the potential benefit of matching intervention approaches to specific psychosocial risk profiles.

Psychosocial risk factors

Community-based intervention programmes, such as the Pain-Disability Prevention (PDP) Program, have also been developed to specifically target certain psychosocial risk factors (Sullivan & Stanish 2003). They are described in more detail in Chapter 14, but it is relevant to allude to them in the context of screening and targeting. Individuals are selected for treatment if they obtain elevated scores (above the 50th percentile) on risk factors addressed by the intervention programme (pain catastrophising, fear of movement/re-injury,

perceived disability and depression). The PDP Program then uses structured activity-scheduling strategies and graded activity involvement to target risk factors such as fear of movements/re-injury and perceived disability. Thought monitoring and cognitive restructuring strategies are used to target catastrophic thinking and depression. A preliminary study yielded encouraging results with 60% of PDP-treated clients returning to work, as compared to an 18% base rate of return. A recent study showed that, in a sample of 215 injured workers who completed the PDP Program, treatment-related reductions in pain catastrophising significantly predicted RTW (Sullivan et al 2005). As a further step, the Progressive Goal Attainment Program (PGAP) has been developed for front-line rehabilitation professionals such as physiotherapists and occupational therapists (Sullivan et al 2006). The PGAP also aims to reduce risk factors for prolonged work disability such as pain catastrophising, fear of movement and re-injury and perceived disability and, as with the PDP Program, individuals are selected for the intervention based on elevated scores on measures of psychosocial risk factors targeted by the intervention. In a recent clinical trial with a sample of individuals who had been work disabled due to whiplash symptoms, 75% of individuals in the PGAP group returned to work compared to 50% who followed usual treatment (Sullivan et al 2006).

Screening and targeting in primary-care settings

Most assessment tools have been developed for and validated on patients attending specialist care, but the screening and targeting approach pioneered by Sullivan et al (2006) has now been developed in primary care. Hill et al (2007), at Keele University, have developed a screening tool, the STarT Back Decision Tool (SBDT), as the basis of a system of triaging and targeting LBP patients presenting with modifiable physical and psychosocial prognostic indicators for persistent pain at the time of consultation to their general practitioner in primary care. An initial set of items was selected on the basis of secondary analysis of pre-existing data on 1200 LBP consulters to primary care, an extensive literature review and input from an expert panel of clinicians. All items for the tool were developed from validated primary-care measurement tools. For prognostic indicators measured using composite instruments, individual questions were chosen using receiver operator curves with high sensitivity and at least moderate specificity for identifying patients above the median on full scores of their composite measures. The clinical validity of the items was confirmed following appraisal by a consensus

STarT Back Decision Tool

For this first set of questions, please think about your back pain over the **past two weeks.**

*1. Overall, how **bothersome** has your back pain been in the **last 2 weeks**?

Not at all	Slightly	Moderately	Very much	Extremely
☐	☐	☐	☐	☐

For each of the following, please cross one box to show whether you agree or disagree with the statement, thinking about the last **2 weeks.**

2. My back pain has **spread down my legs** at some time in the last 2 weeks.

Agree ☐   Disagree ☐

3. I have had back pain in the **shoulder** or **neck** at some time in the last 2 weeks.

Agree ☐   Disagree ☐

*4. It's really not safe for a person with a condition like mine to be physically active.

Agree ☐   Disagree ☐

5. In the last 2 weeks, I have **dressed more slowly** than usual because of my back pain.

Agree ☐   Disagree ☐

6. In the last 2 weeks, I have only **walked short distances** because of my back pain.

Agree ☐   Disagree ☐

*7. **Worrying thoughts** have been going through my mind a lot of the time in the last 2 weeks.

Agree ☐   Disagree ☐

*8. I feel that **my back pain is terrible** and that **it's never going to get any better**.

Agree ☐   Disagree ☐

*9. In general in the last 2 weeks, I have **not enjoyed** all the things I used to enjoy.

Agree ☐   Disagree ☐

SBDT total score 0–3 = 'low risk group'; 4–9 'medium risk group'
Psychosocial subscale 4 or 5 = 'high risk group'
(item 1 is positive with 'very much' or extremely' bothered)

Figure 5.1 • STarT Decision Tool (or SBDT) from Hill et al (2007).

Screening for primary care back pain

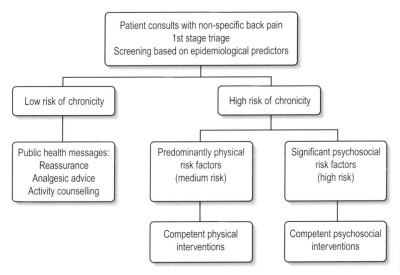

Figure 5.2 • SBDT triage and targeting pathway.

group of some 40 GPs and clinical physiotherapists, and blinded ratings of 12 videotaped 20-minute interviews of patients who had independently completed the SBDT. The tool was then tested for feasibility, repeatability and validity on a consecutive series of 244 patients consulting with LBP in eight GP practices. The SBDT is shown in Figure 5.1. The logic of the triaging system is depicted in Figure 5.2.

Following examination of the distribution of SBDT scores, optimal cut-offs, based on the prognostic indicators included were derived, to allocate patients into one of three groups. An SBDT score of 0–3 was determined to be low risk; a score of four or more of the five psychosocial items (items 1, 4, 7, 8 and 9, starred in figure), allocates patients to the high-risk group. The remainder (SBDT score of more than 3, but less than four of the five psychosocial items) allocates patients to the medium-risk group. This procedure led to an allocation of 40% into the low-risk group with 35% into the medium-risk group, with predominantly physical indicators and 25% into the high-risk group with a higher proportion of psychological indicators.

The external validity of the tool was examined in an independent observational sample of 500 LBP primary-care consulters. SBDT scores were similar and recommended cut-offs for allocation to the three subgroups validated. The SBDT also demonstrated high predictive abilities with medium- and high-risk groups having relative risks of 3.0 and 4.5 respectively, compared to the low-risk group for high disability (RMDQ = 7) at 6-month follow-up. An intensive training programme is

also being developed by the STarT Back research team at Keele University to equip primary-care health professionals to appropriately target and manage prognostic indicators identified by the SBDT.

Conclusions re risk identification and screening

A number of the important issues for pain management have been identified in this chapter (summarised in the Key Points). They are discussed below.

Need for an overarching conceptual framework

Risk identification and screening has a long tradition in public health, and with the advent of evidence-based medicine the focus and 'outcome' has required a new way of thinking about the possibilities for pain management. The biomedical and biomechanical models of pain and function to an extent have served us well, but newer understandings of the influences on and effects of pain have required a broader perspective, and the biopsychosocial model has served as a vehicle for this. We have, however, moved beyond descriptions, classifications and model building to a focus not only on treatment but towards prevention. In our view we now need a conceptual framework which allows us to understand the pain patient in context.

Table 5.4 Methodological issues isolated in the prognosis research field

Issue	Recommendation
Design	Prospective, inception cohorts required
Sampling	Strictly outline inclusion/exclusion criteria
	State enrolment time point clearly
	For many questions, clear, early enrolment is necessary (<3 weeks following onset)
	Representative sampling techniques (random selection or consecutive cases)
Prognostic indicators	Strictly define constructs of measure
	Selection should flow from conceptual framework, recognising the multifactorial nature of the problem
	Use standardised, psychometrically sound instruments
Analysis	Multivariable techniques to adjust for all potential confounders
	Avoid overfitting the data (too many covariates for sample size)
	Prospective validation in homogenous cohorts required
Follow-up	Strictly define outcome(s) of interest
	Adequate duration of follow-up (years)
	Strive for >80% follow-up rate
	Patterns of attrition should be investigated to determine if it is random or systematic
	Blinded outcome measurement with standardised, psychometrically sound instruments
Conceptual framework	Strictly define the construct of the problem being studied
	Account for the recurrent and multifactorial nature of back pain disability
	Overarching theory needed identifying specific hypothesised relationships between variables
	Broaden the view to include factors over the usual professional/discipline boundaries

Linton et al (2005, Table 1, p. 460).

Screening with a purpose

When viewed from a public health perspective, it is important to identify all potential risk factors which may be of relevance. We have drawn a distinction between actuarial screening, based principally on administrative data, and individual screening in the context of consideration for pain management. We have emphasised the need for clarity in terms of purpose for screening, since predictors are, to an extent, outcome specific, and may highlight the potential value of different types of interventions.

Understanding the context

We have made a clear distinction in the first instance between clinical and occupational outcomes, although of course many patients consult health-care practitioners as a consequence specifically of pain-related work compromise. When we adopt a patient- or employee-centred approach we can identify not only targets for intervention but potential obstacles to recovery of optimal function.

Uses and abuses of screening

It is important to understand the difference between the strengths and the limitations of a screening tool. The worth of the screening tool will depend on its accuracy, and different criteria for success in terms of accuracy need to be considered both in terms of the costs of being mistaken and the costs of the screening itself. There are different purposes for screening: screening in, screening out and highlighting the areas in which further evaluation may be required.

Link with clinical decision making

In our view, screening has to be linked with appraisal and management of the individual in pain. Tools such as the DRAM, the MPI and the OSQP appear to be of assistance and can be used in clinic scheduling and in highlighting patients requiring a more comprehensive assessment. With significant pain problems, this will need to include a clinical assessment by a competent health-care professional and may require further expertise to evaluate and address specific occupational problems. You cannot weigh an elephant on a set of kitchen scales.

Potential for screening and targeting

It is our firm opinion that, in consideration of the needs of the pain patient, we need to link our assessments with specific targeting of obstacles to recovery as well as pain and pain-associated limitations in function. We may be assisted in this regard by adopting the flag framework, with its primary emphasis on psychosocial risk factors for persistent pain and prolonged work compromise, its strong influence on the individual's

perception of their pain and pain-associated limitations, leading in occupational settings to the design of both worker-centred and workplace- or system-centred interventions.

Need for better research

Finally we need to accept responsibility for improving the focus and quality of our interventions within an evidence-based framework and with a clear focus on outcomes. The Hopkinton Think Tank meeting in 2005 led to a number of methodological recommendations for improvement in disability research (Linton et al 2005). They are shown in Table 5.4.

Linton et al (2005) concluded by recommending adoption of a broader conceptual framework as a canvas for the identification of predictive and prognostic factors. They advocated the inclusion of employer behaviour within this model and improved methodology research design and data analysis. Such a broadening of perspective has considerable implications for the development of screening linked with targeted interventions in clinical and occupational settings, but seems to offer a worthwhile development for risk identification, screening and targeting for pain management in clinical as well as occupational settings.

Key points

- **Need for an overarching conceptual framework**
- **Screening with a purpose**
- **Understanding the context**
- **Uses and abuses of screening**
- **Link with clinical decision making**
- **Potential for screening and targeting**
- **Need for better research.**

References

Adams M A, Mannion A F, Dolan P 1999 Personal risk factors for first time low back pain. Spine 24:2497

Bergstrom G, Bodin L, Jensen I B et al 2001 Long-term, non-specific spinal pain: reliable and valid sub-groups of patients. Behavior Research and Therapy 39:75–87

Biefang S, Potthoff P, Bellach B-M et al 1998 Predictors of early retirement and rehabilitation for use in a screening to detect workers in need of rehabilitation. International Journal of Rehabilitation Research 21:13–28

Bloch F S, Prins R 2001 Who returns to work and why? Transaction Publishers, New Brunswick

Block A R 1999 Presurgical psychological screening in chronic pain syndromes: psychosocial risk factors for poor surgical results. In: Gatchel R J, Turk D C (eds) Psychosocial factors in pain: critical perspectives. The Guilford Press, New York, ch 24, pp 390–400

Boersma K, Linton S J 2002 Early assessment of psychological factors: the Örebro Screening Questionnaire for Pain.

In: Linton S J (ed) New avenues for the prevention of chronic musculoskeletal pain and disability. Pain Research and Clinical Management, Elsevier Ltd, Amsterdam, 12:205–213

Boersma K, Linton S J 2005 Screening to identify patients at risk: profiles of psychological risk factors for early intervention. Clinical Journal of Pain 21:38–44

Boersma K, Linton S J 2006 Psychological processes underlying the development of a chronic pain problem: a prospective study of the relationship between profiles in the fear-avoidance model and disability. Clinical Journal of Pain 22:160–166

Bouter L, van Tulder M W, Koes B W 1998 Methodological issues in low back pain research in primary care. Spine 23:2014–2020

Brennan G P, Fritz J M, Hunter S J et al 2006 Identifying subgroups of patients with acute/subacute 'non-specific' low back pain. Spine 31:623–631

Burton A K, Balague F, Cardon G et al 2004a European guidelines for prevention in low back pain. www.backpaineurope.org

Burton A K, McClune T D, Clarke R D et al 2004b Long-term follow-up of patients with low back pain attending for manipulative care: outcomes and predictors. Manual Therapy 9:30–35

Cochrane. Website: http//www.cochrane.org

Cornes P 1990 Vocational Rehabilitation Index: a guide to accident victims' requirements for return-to-work assistance. International Disability Studies 12:32–36

Croft P R, Rigby A S, Boswell R et al 1993 The prevalence of chronic widespread pain in the general population. Journal of Rheumatology 20:710–713

Dawes R M, Faust D, Meehl P E 1989 Clinical versus actuarial judgment. Science 243:1668–1674

Delitto A, Cibulka M T, Erhard R E et al 1993 Evidence for the use of an extension-mobilization category in acute low back syndrome: a prescriptive validation pilot study. Physical Therapy 73:216–218

Delitto A, Erhard R E, Bowling R W 1995 A treatment-based classification approach to low back syndrome: identifying and staging patients for conservative management. Physical Therapy 75:470–489

Derogatis L R 1983 SCL-90–R: Administration, scoring and procedures manual for the revised version. Clinical Psychometric Research, Towson, MD

Dworkin S F, LeResche L 1992 Research diagnostic criteria for temporomandibular joint disorders: review, criteria, examination and specifications, critique. Journal of Craniomandibular Disorders 6:301–355

Erhard R E, Delitto A, Cibulka M T 1994 Relative effectiveness of an extension program and a combined program of manipulation and flexion and extension exercises in patients with acute low back syndrome. Physical Therapy 74:1093–1100

Franklin G M, Haug J, Heter N J et al 1994 Outcome of lumbar fusion in Washington State's workers' compensation. Spine 19:1897–1904

Fritz J M, Delitto A, Erhard R E 2003 Comparison of a classification-based approach to physical therapy and therapy based on clinical practice guidelines for patients with acute low back pain: a randomised clinical trial. Spine 28:1363–1372

Garb H N 1998 Studying the clinician: judgment research and psychological assessment. American Psychological Association, Washington, DC

Gatchell R J, Main C J 2004 Psychological approaches to the management of failed surgery and revision surgery. In: Herkowitz H J, Dvorak G, Bell M, Nordin Grob D (eds) The lumbar spine, 3rd edn. Lippincott Williams and Wilkins, Philadelphia, pp 859–866

Gatchel R J, Polatin P B, Kinney R K 1995 Predicting outcome of chronic low back pain using clinical predictors of psychopathology. A prospective analysis. Health Psychology 14:415–420

Gatchel R J, Noe C E, Pulliam C 2002 A preliminary study of MPI profile differences in predicting treatment outcome in a heterogeneous chronic pain patient cohort. Clinical Journal of Pain 18:139–143

Gatchel R J, Polatin P B, Noe C E et al 2003 Treatment- and cost-effectiveness of early intervention for acute low back pain patients: a one-year prospective study. Journal of Occupational Rehabilitation 13:1–9

George Z S, Fritz M J, Bialosky J et al 2003 The effect of a fear avoidance based physical therapy intervention for patients with acute low back pain: a randomised controlled trial. Spine 28:2551–2560

Goldberg D, Williams P 1998 A user's guide to the General Health Questionnaire. NFER-Nelson, Windsor

Groth-Marnat G 2000 Visions of clinical assessment: then, now, and a brief history of the future. Journal of Clinical Psychology 56:349–365

Groth-Marnat G (ed) 2003 Handbook of psychological assessment, 4th edn. John Wiley, Hoboken, NJ

Hathaway S R, McKinley J C, Butcher J N et al 1989 Minnesota multiphasic personality inventory – 2: Manual for administration. University of Minnesota Press, Minneapolis

Hazard R G, Haugh L D, Reid S et al 1996 Early prediction of chronic disability after occupational low back injury. Spine 21:945–951

Hicks G E, Fritz J M, Delitto A et al 2005 Preliminary development of a clinical prediction rule for determining which patients with low back pain will respond to a stabilization programme. Archives of Physical Medicine and Rehabilitation 86:1753–1762

Hill J C, Dunn K M, Mullis R et al 2007 The STarT Back Decision Tool (SBDT): an evaluation of a simple assessment of prognostic indicators to subgroup patients with back pain in primary care. Arthritis Care and Research (Submitted)

Hobby J L, Lutchman L N, Powell J M et al 2001 The Distress Risk Assessment Method (DRAM): failure to predict the outcome of lumbar discectomy. Journal of Bone and Joint Surgery 83B(1):19–21

Hoffman R M, Wheeler K J, Deyo R A 1993 Surgery for herniated lumbar disks. A literature synthesis. Journal of General Internal Medicine 8:487–496

Hunt I M, Silman A J, Benjamin S et al 1999 The prevalence and associated features of chronic widespread pain in the community using the 'Manchester' definition of chronic widespread pain. Rheumatology 38:275–279

Hurley D A, Dusoir T, McDonough S et al 2000 Biopsychosocial screening questionnaire for patients with low back pain: preliminary report of utility in physiotherapy practice in N Ireland. Clinical Journal of Pain 16:214–228

Hurley D A, Dusoir T, McDonough S et al 2001 How effective is the Acute Low Back Screening Questionnaire for predicting one-year follow-up in patients with low back pain? Clinical Journal of Pain 17:256–263

Hutten M M R, Hermens H J, Zilvold G 2001 Differences in treatment outcome between subgroups of patients with chronic low back pain using lumbar dynamometry and psychological aspects Clinical Rehabilitation 15:479–488

Keefe F J, Bradley L A, Crisson J E 1990 Behavioural assessment of low back pain: identification of pain behaviour subgroups. Pain 40:153–160

Kendall N, Linton S L, Main C J 1997 Guide to assessing psychological yellow flags in acute low back pain: risk factors for long term disability and work loss. Accident Rehabilitation and Compensation Insurance Corporation of New Zealand and the National Health Committee. Wellington, NZ

Kent P, Keating J L 2004 Do primary care clinicians think that non-specific low back pain is one condition? Spine 29:1022–1031

Kerns R D, Turk D C, Rudy T E 1985 The West Haven Yale Multidimensional Pain Inventory (WHYMPI). Pain 23:345–356

Lanyon R I, Goodstein L D (eds) 1997 Personality assessment, 3rd edn. John Wiley, New York

Linton S J, Andersson T 2000 Can chronic disability be prevented? A randomized trial of a cognitive-behavioural intervention and two forms of information for patients with spinal pain. Spine 25:2825–2831

Linton S J, Hallden K 1998 Can we screen for problematic back pain? A screening questionnaire for predicting outcome in acute and subacute back pain: Clinical Journal of Pain 14:209–215

Linton S J, Gross D, Schultz I Z et al 2005 Prognosis and the identification of workers risking disability: research issues and directions for future research. Journal of Occupational Rehabilitation 15:457–474

Macfarlane G J, Croft P R, Schollum J et al 1996 Widespread pain: is an improved classification possible? Journal of Rheumatology 23:1628–1632

McBeth J, Macfarlane G J 2002 The prevalence of regional and widespread musculoskeletal pain symptoms. In: Linton S J (ed) New avenues for the prevention of chronic musculoskeletal pain and disability. Pain research and clinical management, vol 12. Elsevier, Amsterdam, ch 2, pp 7–22

Main C J, Spanswick C C 2000 Pain management: an interdisciplinary approach. Churchill Livingstone, Edinburgh

Main C J, Waddell G 1998 Behavioural responses to examination: a reappraisal of the interpretation of 'Nonorganic Signs'. Spine 23(21):2367–2371

Main C J, Wood P L R, Hollis S et al 1992 The distress assessment method: a simple patient classification to identify distress and evaluate risk of poor outcome. Spine 17:42–50

Main C J, Phillips C J, Watson P J 2005 Secondary prevention in health care and occupational settings in musculoskeletal conditions focusing on low back pain. In: Schultz I Z, Gatchel R J (eds) Handbook of complex occupational disability claims: early risk identification, intervention and prevention. Springer, New York, pp 387–404

Marhold C, Linton S J, Melin L 2002 Identification of obstacles for chronic pain patients to return to work: evaluation of a questionnaire. Journal of Occupational Rehabilitation 12:65–75

Melzack R 1975 The McGill Pain Questionnaire: major properties and scoring methods. Pain 1:277–299

Melzack R 1987 The Short-Form McGill Pain Questionnaire. Pain 30:191–197

Muir Gray J A 2004 New concepts of screening. British Journal of General Practice 54:292–298

Ransford A O, Cairns D, Mooney V 1976 The pain drawing as an aid to the psychological evaluation of patients with low back pain. Spine 1:127–134

Robinson M E, Riley J L III 2002 Presurgical psychological screening. In: Turk D C, Melzack R 2002 Handbook of pain assessment, 2nd edn. The Guilford Press, New York, ch 20, pp 385–399

Robinson M E, Swimmer G I, Railof D 1989 The PAIN MMPI classification system: a critical review. Pain 37:211–214

Rowbotham M C, Petersen K L, Fields H L 1998 Is postherpetic neuralgia more than one disorder? Pain Forum 7:231–237

Salen B A, Spangfort E V, Nygren A L et al 1994 The Disability Rating Index: an instrument for the assessment of disability in clinical settings. Journal of Clinical Epidemiology 47:1423–1435

Schultz I Z, Crook J M, Berkowitz J et al 2002 Biopsychosocial multivariate predictive model of occupational low back disability. Spine 27:2720–2725

Smart P A, Waylonis G W, Hacksha K V 1997 Immunologic profile for patients with fibromyalgia. American Journal of Physiology and Medical Rehabilitation 76:231–234

Spitzer W O, Skovron M L, Salmi L R et al 1995 Scientific monograph of the Quebec Task Force on Whiplash-Associated Disorders: redefining 'whiplash' and its management. Spine 20(suppl):1S–73S

Sullivan M J L, Stanish W D 2003 Psychologically based occupational rehabilitation: The Pain-Disability Prevention Program. Clinical Journal of Pain 19:97–104

Sullivan M J L, Ward L C, Tripp D et al 2005 Secondary prevention of work disability: community-based psychosocial intervention for musculoskeletal disorders. Journal of Occupational Rehabilitation 15:377–392

Sullivan M J L, Adams H, Rhodenizer T et al 2006 A psychosocial risk factor targeted intervention for the prevention of chronic pain and disability following whiplash injury. Physical Therapy 86:8–18

Swimmer G I, Robinson M E, Geisser M E 1992 Relationship of MMPI cluster types, pain coping strategy and treatment outcome. Clinical Journal of Pain 8:131–137

Tuomi K, Ilmarinen J, Jahkola A 1998 Work ability index. Finnish Institute of Occupational Health, Helsinki

Turk D C 1990 Customising treatment for chronic pain patients; who, what, and why. Clinical Journal of Pain 6:255–270

Turk D C 2005 The potential of treatment matching for subgroups of patients with chronic pain: lumping versus splitting. Clinical Journal of Pain 21:44–55

Turk D C, Melzack R 2001 Handbook of pain assessment, 2nd edn. Guilford, New York

Turk D C, Rudy T E 1988 Towards an empirically derived taxonomy of chronic pain patients: integration of psychological assessment data. Journal of Consulting and Clinical Psychology 56:233–238

Van der Giezen A M, Bouter L M, Nijhuis F J N 2000 Prediction of return-to-work of low back pain patients sicklisted for 3–4 months. Pain 87:285–294

Van Tulder M, Becker A, Bekkering T et al on behalf of the COST B13 Working Group on Guidelines for the management of Acute Low Back pain in Primary Care 2005 www.backpaineurope.org

Vlaeyen J W S, Linton S J 2002 Pain-related fear and its consequences in chronic musculoskeletal pain. In: Linton S J (ed) New avenues for the prevention of chronic musculoskeletal pain and disability. Elsevier Science, Amsterdam, pp 81–103

Vlaeyen J W S, Kole-Snijders A M J, Beren R B G et al 1995 Fear of movement/re-injury in chronic low back pain and its relation to behavioural performance. Pain 62:363–372

Vlaeyen J W, De Jong J R, Onghena P et al 2002 Can pain-related fear be reduced? The application of cognitive-behavioral exposure in vivo. Pain Research and Management 7:144–153

Von Korff M, Miglioretti D L 2006 A prospective approach to defining chronic pain. In: Flor H, Kalso E, Dostrovsky J O (eds) Proceedings of the 11th World Congress on Pain. IASP Press, Seattle, ch 66, pp 761–769

Von Korff M, Ormel J, Keefe F et al 1992 Grading the severity of chronic pain. Pain 50:133–149

Waddell G 2004 The back pain revolution, 2nd edn. Churchill Livingstone, Edinburgh

Waddell G, McCulloch J A, Kummell E et al 1980 Nonorganic physical signs in low back pain. Spine 5:117–125

Waddell G, Gibson J N A, Grant I 2000 Surgical treatment of lumbar disk prolapse and degenerative lumbar disk disease. In: Nachemson A, Jonsson E (eds) Neck and back pain: the scientific evidence of causes, diagnoses and treatments. Williams & Wilkins, Philadelphia, ch 13, pp 305–325

Waddell G, Burton A K, Main C J 2003 Screening of DWP clients for risk of long-term incapacity: a conceptual and scientific review. Royal Society of Medicine Monograph; Royal Society of Medicine Press, London

Walen H R, Cronan T A, Serber E R et al 2002 Subgroups of fibromyalgia patients: evidence for heterogeneity and examination of differential effects following a community-based intervention. Journal of Musculoskeletal Medicine 10:9–32

Ware J, Kosinski M, Keller S D 1994 Physical and mental health summary scales: a user's manual. Health Assessment Lab, Boston

Wilson J M G, Jungner J J 1968 Principles and practice of screening for disease. World Health Organisation, Geneva

Wolfe F, Smythe H A, Yunus M B et al 1990 The American College of Rheumatology 1990 criteria for the classification of fibromyalgia. Arthritis and Rheumatism 33:160–172

Wolfe F, Ross K, Anderson J et al 1995 The prevalence and characteristics of fibromyalgia in the general population. Arthritis and Rheumatism 38:19–28

APPENDIX 5.1

Modified Somatic Perception Questionnaire

Please describe how you have felt during the PAST WEEK by making a check mark (✓) in the appropriate box. Please answer all questions. Do not think too long before answering.

	Not at all	A little, slightly	A great deal, quite a bit	Extremely, could not have been worse
Heart rate increase				
Feeling hot all over	0	1	2	3
Sweating all over	0	1	2	3
Sweating in a particular part of the body				
Pulse in neck				
Pounding in head				
Dizziness	0	1	2	3
Blurring of vision	0	1	2	3
Feeling faint	0	1	2	3
Everything appearing unreal				
Nausea	0	1	2	3
Butterflies in stomach				
Pain or ache in stomach	0	1	2	3
Stomach churning	0	1	2	3
Desire to pass water				
Mouth becoming dry	0	1	2	3
Difficulty swallowing				
Muscles in neck aching	0	1	2	3
Legs feeling weak	0	1	2	3
Muscles twitching or jumping	0	1	2	3
Tense feeling across forehead	0	1	2	3
Tense feeling in jaw muscles				

From Main et al (1992, p. 51).

APPENDIX 5.2

Modified Zung Depression Index

Please indicate for each of these questions which answer best describes how you have been feeling recently

	Rarely or none of the time (less than 1 day per week)	Some or little of the time (1–2 days per week)	A moderate amount of time (3–4 days per week)	Most of the time (5–7 days per week)
1. I feel downhearted and sad	0	1	2	3
2. Morning is when I feel best	3	2	1	0
3. I have crying spells or feel like it	0	1	2	3
4. I have trouble getting to sleep at night	0	1	2	3
5. I feel that nobody cares	0	1	2	3
6. I eat as much as I used to	3	2	1	0
7. I still enjoy sex	3	2	1	0
8. I notice I am losing weight	0	1	2	3
9. I have trouble with constipation	0	1	2	3
10. My heart beats faster than usual	0	1	2	3
11. I get tired for no reason	0	1	2	3
12. My mind is as clear as it used to be	3	2	1	0
13. I tend to wake up too early	0	1	2	3
14. I find it easy to do the things I used to	3	2	1	0
15. I am restless and can't keep still	0	1	2	3
16. I feel hopeful about the future	3	2	1	0
17. I am more irritable than usual	0	1	2	3
18. I find it easy to make a decision	3	2	1	0
19. I feel quite guilty	0	1	2	3
20. I feel that I am useful and needed	3	2	1	0
21. My life is pretty full	3	2	1	0
22. I feel that others would be better off if I were dead	0	1	2	3
23. I am still able to enjoy the things I used to	3	2	1	0

From Main et al (1992, p. 52).

APPENDIX 5.3

Örebro Screening Questionnaire for Pain: Content

Question		Variable name
1 What year were you born?	Fill in blank	Age
2 Are you	Male/Female	Gender
3 What is your current employment status?	Categories	Employed
4 Are you born in Sweden?	Yes/No	Nationality
5 Where do you have pain?	Categories	Pain site
6 How many days of work have you missed (sick leave) because of pain during the past 12 months?	Categories	Sick leave
7 How many weeks have you suffered from your current pain problem?	Categories	Duration
8 Is your work heavy or monotonous?	0–10	Heavy work
9 How would you rate the pain you have had during the past week?	0–10	Current pain
10 In the past 3 months, on average, how intense was your pain?	0–10	Average pain
11 How often would you say that you have experienced pain episodes, on average, during the past 3 months?	0–10	Frequency
12 Based on all things you do to cope or deal with your pain, on an average day, how much are you able to decrease it?	0–10	Coping
13 How tense or anxious have you felt in the past week?	0–10	Stress
14 How much have you been bothered by feeling depressed in the past week?	0–10	Depression
15 In your view, how large is the risk that your current pain may become persistent (may not go away)?	0–10	Risk chronic
16 In your estimation, what are the chances that you will be working in 6 months?	0–10	Chance working
17 If you take into consideration your work routines, management, salary, promotion possibilities, and work mates, how satisfied are you with your job?	0–10	Job satisfaction
18 Physical activity makes my pain worse.	0–10	Belief: increase
19 An increase in pain is an indication that I should stop what I am doing until the pain decreases.	0–10	Belief: stop
20 I should not do my normal work with my present pain.	0–10	Belief: not work

(Continued)

Örebro Screening Questionnaire for Pain: content *(Continued)*

Question		Variable name
21 I can do light work for an hour.	0–10	Light work
22 I can walk for an hour.	0–10	Walk
23 I can do ordinary household chores.	0–10	Household work
24 I can do the weekly shopping.	0–10	Shopping
25 I can sleep at night.	0–10	Sleep

From Boersma & Linton (2002, Table 1, p. 208), with permission from Elsevier Ltd.

APPENDIX 5.4

Örebro Screening Questionnaire for Pain: Layout and Scoring

Today's Date __/__/__

Name _____ ACC Claim Number _____

Address _____ Telephone (__)_____ (home)

_____ (__)_____ (work)

Job Title (occupation) _____ Date stopped work for this episode __/__/__

These questions and statements apply if you have aches or pains, such as back, shoulder or neck pain. Please read and answer each question carefully. Do not take too long to answer the questions. However, it is important that you answer every question. There is always a response for your particular situation.

1 What year were you born? 19__

2 Are you: ☐ male ☐ female

3 Were you born in New Zealand? ☐ Yes ☐ No

4 Where do you have pain? Place a ✓ for all the appropriate sites.

2x count ☐

☐ neck ☐ shoulders ☐ upper back ☐ lower back ☐ leg

5 How many days of work have you missed because of pain during the past 18 months? Tick (✓) one.

☐ 0 days [1] ☐ 1–2 days [2] ☐ 3–7 days [3] ☐ 8–14 days [4] ☐ 15–30 days [5]
☐ 1 month [8] ☐ 2 months [7] ☐ 3–6 months [8] ☐ 6–12 months [9] ☐ over 1 year [10]

☐

6 How long have you had your current pain problem? Tick (✓) one.

☐ 0–1 weeks [1] ☐ 1–2 weeks [2] ☐ 3–4 weeks [3] ☐ 4–5 weeks [4] ☐ 5–8 weeks [5]
☐ 9–11 weeks [6] ☐ 3–6 months [7] ☐ 6–9 months [8] ☐ 9–12 months [9] ☐ over 1 year [10]

☐

7 Is your work heavy or monotonous? Circle the best alternative.

0   1   2   3   4   5   6   7   8   9   10
Not at all   *Extremely*

☐

(Continued)

Örebro Screening Questionnaire for Pain: Layout and Scoring (*Continued*)

8 How would you rate the pain that you have had during the past week? Circle one.

    0   1   2   3   4   5   6   7   8   9   10
No pain   *Pain as bad*
                                    as it could be

9 In the past 3 months, on average, how bad was your pain? Circle one.

    0   1   2   3   4   5   6   7   8   9   10
No pain   *Pain as bad*
                                    as it could be

10 How often would you say that you have experienced pain episodes, on average, during the past 3 months? Circle one.

    0   1   2   3   4   5   6   7   8   9   10
Never   *Always*

11 Based on all the things you do to cope, or deal with your pain, on an average day, how much are you able to decrease it? Circle one.

    0   1   2   3   4   5   6   7   8   9   10
Can't decrease   *Can decrease it*   **10-x**
it at all   *completely*

12 How tense or anxious have you felt in the past week? Circle one.

    0   1   2   3   4   5   6   7   8   9   10
Absolutely calm   *As tense and anxious*
and relaxed   *as I've ever felt*

13 How much have you been bothered by feeling depressed in the past week? Circle one.

    0   1   2   3   4   5   6   7   8   9   10
Not at all   *Extremely*

14 In your view, how large is the risk that your current pain may become persistent? Circle one.

    0   1   2   3   4   5   6   7   8   9   10
No risk   *Very large risk*

15 In your estimation, what are the chances that you will be working in 6 months? Circle one.

    0   1   2   3   4   5   6   7   8   9   10   **10-x**
No chance   *Very large chance*

16 If you take into consideration your work routines, management, salary, promotion possibilities and work mates, how satisfied are you with your job? Circle one.

    0   1   2   3   4   5   6   7   8   9   10
Not at all   *Completely*   **10-x**
satisfied   *satisfied*

Here are some of the things which other people have told us about their back pain. For each statement please circle one number from 0 to 10 to say how much physical activities, such as bending, lifting, walking or driving would affect your back.

17 Physical activity makes my pain worse.

    0   1   2   3   4   5   6   7   8   9   10
Completely   *Completely*
disagree   *agree*

(*Continued*)

Örebro Screening Questionnaire for Pain: Layout and Scoring (*Continued*)

18 An increase in pain is an indication that I should stop what I am doing until the pain decreases.

    0   1   2   3   4   5   6   7   8   9   10

Completely   *Completely*

disagree   *agree* ☐

19 I should not do my normal work with my present pain.

    0   1   2   3   4   5   6   7   8   9   10

Completely   *Completely*

disagree   *agree* ☐

Here is a list of 5 activities. Please circle the one number which best describes your current ability to participate in each of these activities.

20 I can do light work for an hour.

    0   1   2   3   4   5   6   7   8   9   10

Can't do it   *Can do it*

because of pain   *without pain*   10-x

problem   *being a problem* ☐

21 I can walk for an hour.

    0   1   2   3   4   5   6   7   8   9   10

Can't do it   *Can do it*

because of pain   *without pain*   10-x

problem   *being a problem* ☐

22 I can do ordinary household chores.

    0   1   2   3   4   5   6   7   8   9   10

Can't do it   *Can do it*

because of pain   *without pain*   10-x

problem   *being a problem* ☐

23 I can go shopping.

    0   1   2   3   4   5   6   7   8   9   10

Can't do it   *Can do it*

because of pain   *without pain*

problem   *being a problem*   10-x ☐

24 I can sleep at night.

    0   1   2   3   4   5   6   7   8   9   10

Can't do it   *Can do it*

because of pain   *without pain*   10-x

problem   *being a problem*   Sum ☐

Adapted from Waddell (2004, Box 7.4, pp. 131–132 and Box 7.5, p. 133), with permission of Elsevier Ltd.

Section **Two**

Assessment

In Chapter 6 the use of nature and purpose of biomedical and pain assessment in secondary- and tertiary-care settings is outlined. There is a specific focus on physical examination, medication management and the importance of communication.

In Chapter 7 the context and nature of pain assessment is followed by identification of some important issues in measurement. There is then a detailed appraisal of the nature and utility of measures of physical functioning, impairment and disability. The chapter concludes with a brief consideration of occupational outcomes.

In Chapter 8, the focus is on psychological assessment, including both the clinical interview and formal psychometric assessment in the determination of suitability for pain management. Following discussion of the identification of psychopathology, there is detailed consideration of possible mental health targets for intervention. The chapter concludes with a specific focus on the identification of psychological risk factors for persisting pain and disability.

Chapter Six

Biomedical and pain assessment in secondary- and tertiary-care settings

Bengt Sjölund

CHAPTER CONTENTS

Introduction

The role of the GP in early pain management is discussed in Chapter 9. The focus of this chapter is on the role of the physician in secondary and tertiary care where most patients will present with persistent pain of a severity considered to merit specialist referral. Frequently the pain will have become chronic and require careful assessment.

Arguably, the most common mistake with regard to management of chronic pain is to consider chronic pain as if it were acute. Unfortunately, this holds not only for the lay public (i.e. the patients and their relatives) but also for many health professionals. Generally, the training of physicians as well as that of nurses and of paramedical staff mostly includes pain as a sign of acute disease or injury, both in diagnosis and treatment. The consequences are that the immediate interpretation of as well as the communication about the painful condition usually contain components of 'injury' or 'harm'. This is also reflected in the desire of the patient to receive a conventional medical 'cure' for his/her problem, explaining the multitude of doctors consulted by any single patient. The time perspective on relief measures is likewise grossly inadequate in that, especially with 'severe' pain, local anaesthetics or short-acting opioids are commonly given through injections or indwelling catheters with little attention given to long-term management.

A further misconception is that the cause of long-standing pain can be identified by visualisation of minor deviations in body structure using imaging techniques such as computerised tomography or magnetic resonance imaging (MRI) techniques. On the other hand, in order for a rehabilitation programme of patients with chronic pain to be credible, it is necessary prior to therapy that any major pathology has been excluded and that any concurrent disease has been identified by conventional medical screening. It should be realised that those patients with circumscribed pain conditions and only a 6–12-month history carry an extra risk of having an undetected malignancy as the cause of their pain, usually a metastasis, a process in the retroperitoneal space or a soft-tissue tumour. It is therefore vital that any pain management procedure should be preceded by a medical assessment of high quality by a sufficiently skilled physician. Depending on the local organisation of health care, this may be either the referring physician or the pain clinic physician (who may be of one of several medical disciplines).

Role of the physician

In patients with significant pain problems, the physician thus is an essential member of the team not only or even mainly for general medical screening but for analysing and treating the biological aspects of pain and also for facilitating the implementation of a biopsychosocial approach to pain management.

The range of medical disciplines

There is a range of medical disciplines which are appropriate for general medical screening, from general practitioners (see Ch. 7) to specialists on the musculoskeletal system (rheumatology, orthopaedics), on the nervous system (neurology, neurosurgery) or on the gastroenterological system (gastroenterology, surgery). In some countries there is a specific physical and rehabilitation medicine (PRM) specialty (physiatry) which would seem to have a particularly relevant range of skills applicable to the chronic patient. Such physicians are well suited to this type of setting, since he/she is 'concerned with the promotion of physical and cognitive functioning, activities (including behaviour), participation (including quality of life) and modifying personal and environmental factors' as defined by the PRM Section of the Union Europeénne Medecin Specialistes (UEMS 2004). Additionally, the PRM specialist is trained in multi- or interdisciplinary team work and in physical medicine, and has a special focus on the assessment of impairments and functions (ICF 2001). Here, it should be noted that pain in itself, not only its motor

consequences, constitutes an impairment, one of sensory nature (Sjölund 2003). In many countries, PRM specialists take on an increasingly large role in pain management. Facets of this expertise are evident in specialisms with an interest in rehabilitation, although much rehabilitation in the UK is approached more from a neurorehabilitation perspective with a very strong biomedical emphasis rather than from the somewhat broader pain management perspective. In practice, in the UK most pain management programmes are led medically by anaesthetists specialising in pain management (or pain medicine), although a number of rehabilitation physicians and rheumatologists also become involved in pain management programmes (PMPs).

Historically, anaesthetists would typically be the attending physicians in pain management programs, since their therapeutic arsenal is well fitted for the relief of acute and cancer-related pain conditions. However, John J Bonica, in creating the world's first multidisciplinary pain clinic, opened up the link with the local departments of rehabilitation medicine and neurosurgery (Bonica 1990). In many countries, such as the UK, anaesthetists still dominate the pain clinic field, with the advantage of having experience from evaluating general medical conditions in the emergency perspective, but with the disadvantages of (i) applying therapeutic modalities more suited for acute pain and (ii) not having the experience of following up patients with longstanding impairments and disabilities. In the UK, during the last 20 years the burgeoning of pain management programmes, often as derivatives from the pain service, has facilitated broadening of the role of pain clinic anaesthetists ranging from initial diagnostics and biomedical treatments to active participation within multi- and interdisciplinary pain management programmes (Ch. 11).

However, perhaps of more importance than a physician's specific medical accreditation is their clinical perspective and whether they recognise chronic pain as a biopsychosocial phenomenon requiring interdisciplinary pain management.

For any attending physician, however, additional training is necessary in the neurobiology of long-standing pain as well as in the principles (attitudes, communication, assessment, therapies) of management of non-malignant chronic pain. Some European countries and some states in the USA recognise *pain management* as a separate or an add-on medical speciality. The International Association for the Study of Pain has developed curricula in pain management that can be obtained from its home page (IASP).

A number of distinct functions are provided by the physician (Box 6.1).

Box 6.1

Role of the physician

- Medical screening and diagnostics
- Screening for disease
- Identification and evaluation of comorbidity
- Selling the biopsychosocial model
- Prevention of iatrogenically worsened pain.

Box 6.2

Key features of neuropathic pain

- A history indicating injury or disturbed function in the nervous system
- Projected pain from one or several neuroanatomically defined nervous system lesions
- Signs indicating injury to or dysfunction in the peripheral or the central nervous system, as evident from assessments demonstrating an abnormal sensory function of the skin.

Medical diagnostics

A major role for the attending physician in the assessment process is to double-check that no underlying pathology to the painful condition is actually present. This may involve additional referrals to organ specialists inside or outside the unit, to additional laboratory blood tests, e.g. to rule out inflammatory or other systemic conditions, or to laboratory examinations like electromyography or MRI.

A second major role is appraisal of the biological mechanism of the pain condition (Woolf et al 1998). For the nervous system, this should involve a systematic assessment of sensory nervous function and for the musculoskeletal system (ideally in conjunction with a physiotherapist), a functional analysis of relevant regions. In abdominal pain and in chest pain a corresponding dialogue may be necessary with a gastroenterologist and with a cardiologist, respectively. The key purpose of this initial evaluation is to categorise the pain condition in general terms as nociceptive, neuropathic, psychogenic, of unknown origin or a mixture. These fundamental distinctions are the bedrock of subsequent clinical management. Key features in arriving at this classification are shown in Box 6.2.

A careful description of the diagnostic findings, supported where necessary by reference to the scientific literature, must then be communicated to the patient and any significant others, using language they understand, as a precursor to discussing therapeutic options, with realistic expectations of probable benefit.

Screening for disease

As previously indicated, it is necessary with all patients seeking medical assistance for chronic pain to perform a general medical screening initially by checking the previous clinical history and clarify self-reports with confirmation of clinical records. This may also lead to a more extensive physical examination and to referrals for specialist investigations if indicated.

Identification and evaluation of comorbidity

Comorbidity, such as hypertension, cardiovascular disease, diabetes, respiratory insufficiency, obesity, alcoholism and drug abuse, should be identified and be addressed as possible complicating factors for pain management. Such conditions may influence both physical performance and the side-effects of analgesic drugs. Simple screening for psychological problems requiring specialist attention is also necessary, although in multidisciplinary teams a more detailed evaluation should be undertaken by a specialist mental health practitioner (such as a psychologist or psychiatrist).

Selling the biopsychosocial model

Many patients in chronic pain consulting a pain clinic question the need to be assessed by a team, especially if it includes a consultation by a psychiatrist or a psychologist ('I am not mentally ill'). It is therefore essential that the assessment includes a thorough physical component to meet the patient's expectations regarding the physical pain mechanisms. However, it is important also that the physician explains the need for a psychological assessment as an important part of the overall analysis of pain and its impact if the patient appears to find it difficult to move from the narrow somatic model. The importance of taking into account the patient's beliefs, emotional responses and pain coping strategies, as aspects of normal reactions to pain needs be distinguished from appraisal of possible mental illness or orange flags (Ch. 3) The elicitation of a detailed socioeconomic and occupational history, whether this is done by a social worker, by the psychologist or by the physician, needs to be handled with equal care and sensitivity.

Prevention of iatrogenically worsened pain

Patients have usually consulted many doctors for their chronic pain problems, and in patients with significant persistent pain, a degree of iatrogenic confusion and distress is to be expected. The patients may have received contradictory explanations and been disappointed at promised benefit from treatment. They may feel the legitimacy of their symptoms has been questioned. Furthermore, they may have been offered multiple surgical or other interventional therapies, such as neuro-destructive blocks without effect and perhaps even been left with additional impairments secondary to treatment, sometimes including worsened pain.

It is important ethically and clinically to offer an honest evaluation, based on best available scientific evidence, of the long-term effectiveness as well as the risk of side-effects before new interventions are instituted. (Indeed in some countries there is a legal obligation to do so.) In fact it can be helpful sometimes, in establishing realistic expectations of probable therapeutic benefit, to 'immunise' the patients against further interventions by sharing with them the relevant scientific data and probabilities of various outcomes. Indeed they should be counselled not to accept just any procedure haphazardly proposed by an intervention-oriented physician in the hope of pain relief.

Pain evaluation

Facets of initial pain evaluation are summarised in Box 6.3.

Present pain characteristics: location, character and aggravating factors

When a patient is referred for management of chronic pain, the referral letter is often sparse as regards the extent and character of pain. It is wise to ask the patient to complete a careful pain drawing as one part of a questionnaire on basic demographic information as well as on information on the pain condition, to be filled out before the visit. Such data improve the dialogue with the assessment team and avoid repetition of data. The interview with the patient should start with present pain: its location with maxima, depth, radiation, character, time pattern (periodicity) and aggravating and alleviating factors. The patient may be asked to carefully outline the body area(s) in pain with one index finger, thus assisting the physician in locating the affected organ part, structure or pathway.

A brief appraisal should be made of the impact of pain on function and activities of daily living (including sleep pattern). Some clinics ask patients to complete a diary for the day or week prior to their clinic attendance. Analysis of variation of pain levels, relationship with activity and sleep and medication use can be a helpful precursor to the initial clinical evaluation. More detailed evaluations may be conducted by other members of the interdisciplinary team. (A more detailed appraisal certainly will be necessary in consideration of establishment of possible treatment goals for a pain management programme, as discussed in Ch. 11.)

Circumstances of pain onset

From present pain it is usually easy to shift focus to the circumstances at the time of pain onset and if applicable, at the time of aggravation. Here, it is important to detect residual physical effects of previous trauma or disease as well as if the patient or his/her family were particularly vulnerable in any respect at the time of onset of pain. Attention should be paid not only in terms of the nature of the onset and possible painful injuries but also in terms of the patient's psychological reaction. The possibility of the development of post-traumatic stress disorder may require specific appraisal by a mental health specialist.

Pain treatment history

The history of previous pain treatments is important, not only in terms of what was done, but also in terms of its clinical competence, in that the treatment may be revisited as a therapeutic option. This finding is not uncommon with physical modalities such as TENS (transcutaneous electrical nerve stimulation), acupuncture or with various forms of physiotherapy. However, treatment should not be repeated without a strong probability of benefit. It should be remembered also that the side-effects of interventional pain therapy are

---

Box 6.3

Initial pain evaluation

- Present pain: location, radiation, character and aggravating factors
- Circumstances of pain onset
- Pain treatment history.

sometimes in themselves considerable and irreversible, including aggravated pain or the precipitation of other forms of (usually neuropathic) pain. This holds especially for procedures where sensory nervous tissue is intentionally or unintentionally injured. To get a full picture, a retrieval of old medical records is usually necessary to compare with the story recalled and told by the patient.

Medication

A most important part of the treatment history is the current and previous use of medications. Almost all patients have tried analgesic drugs, at least paracetamol and/or NSAIDs (non-steroidal anti-inflammatory drugs). In addition, many have tried the weaker opioid agonists such as codeine and tramadol. Usually these drugs have been prescribed as needed (PRN) instead of at specific time points (time-contingent) and often in inadequate dosages. Drug monitoring has often been less than adequate, both regarding effect and dose adjustment. Frequently the drugs have not been effective, at least not over longer time periods, and the patient has stopped taking them. Occasionally, drug addiction is detected, most commonly with overconsumption of over-the-counter preparations containing weak opioids like codeine. If the patient manipulates drug prescriptions, e.g. by consulting several physicians in parallel, this may also occur with strong opioid agonists, usually in oral preparations.

Sometimes antidepressants have been prescribed, either to alleviate pain or to help restore the sleep pattern. Here, the tricyclic antidepressants are to be preferred due to demonstrated effectiveness in contrast to the more recently developed selective serotonin reuptake inhibitors. It is important to determine whether the antidepressant has been prescribed in an analgesic dose or in a psychotropic dose. Specific inquiry of the patient as to whether the drug was given to help sleep/pain or to help their mood may illuminate the issue. Hypnotics such as benzodiazepines should be avoided because of the well-known risks of tolerance and addiction. A number of newer antiepileptics have shown hypoalgesic properties in neuropathic pain conditions but they have rarely been tried outside pain clinic settings.

Substance use and abuse

Substance abuse may also occur with excessive alcohol or tobacco use and with the use of cannabinoids that have recently been advocated against pain related to malignancy. A particular pain-specific problem relates to the ability of ethanol to influence the sensory transmission

Box 6.4

Evaluation of impact of past and present pain

- Brief appraisal of social economic and occupational factors
- Primary focus on pain-associated limitations
- Decision about whether more detailed evaluation required by another member of the team.

by interfering with NMDA receptor function, thereby substantiating the claim that it may act as an analgesic and thereby provoke an increased consumption.

Impact of past and present pain

Key issues in evaluation of the impact of past and present pain are summarised in Box 6.4. To evaluate the impact of past and present pain on the individual, it is necessary to include an assessment of social, economic and occupational factors. A brief screening evaluation of the patient's social and family situation including educational level and occupational status with a special emphasis on physical demands is helpful. The primary focus should be on pain-associated limitations, i.e. the impact of pain on work. Enquiries about sick certification, about work loss and danger of job loss should be made and the impact on economic circumstances ('costs of illness') be estimated. An ongoing litigation should be detected; it may not necessarily be an obstacle to recovery but often an additional burden and could form a potential obstacle to rehabilitation. A decision needs to be taken about whether a more detailed evaluation is required during assessment by others in the team.

Physical examination

For the majority of patients presenting with chronic pain, it is sufficient to make a focused examination based on key elements from the history. For example, it is not appropriate to conduct a complete neurological examination unless major nervous system pathology is suspected. On the other hand, a focused neurological examination may need to be very detailed, e.g. by examining different sensory modalities very carefully in the painful area and expressing the results in a correct nomenclature (Appendix 6.1) and by drawing on body schemes.

Box 6.5

Important aspects of physical examination

- Decide on need for full neurological examination
- Musculoskeletal appraisal of appearance and function of structures around the painful area
- Likewise, a focused examination of the musculoskeletal system does not involve assessment of, e.g., all body joints but of the visual and palpable appearance and function of all structures in and around the painful region
- Investigate concordance between signs and symptoms
- Identify the behavioural responses to examination.

Box 6.6

Common medications in the treatment of pain problems

- NSAIDs
- Opioids and opioid-containing medicines including co-compounds
- Paracetamol
- Muscle relaxants and hypnotics (benzodiazepines)
- Antidepressants (tricyclic antidepressants, newer antidepressants, selective serotonin reuptake inhibitors (SSRIs))
- Hypnotics
- Anticonvulsants.

Box 6.7

Rationalising medication use

- Clarify current medication use:
  - distinguish prescription from usage
  - evaluate use of non-prescribed drugs.
- Identify any medical contra-indications to use of particular drugs or combinations
- Evaluate history of medication use (and abuse)
- Elicit beliefs about, and expectations of, medicines
- Provide advice and safe and appropriate long-term and short-term use of medicines for pain control.

Likewise, a focused examination of the musculoskeletal system does not involve assessment of, e.g. all body joints but of the visual and palpable appearance and function of all structures in and around the painful region. During the examination, it is important to investigate the concordance between signs and symptoms and to identify the behavioural responses to examination, such as noticing a coactivation of antagonistic muscle groups when testing muscle strength or a non-organic variation of responses depending on body posture. Some key aspects of the physical examination are shown in Box 6.5.

In the UK, the importance of physical examination is recognised and medical students are now taught to use GALS (gait, arms, legs, spine) screening examination method adopted by the Arthritis Research Campaign (ARC on-line). It is available both on-line and in DVD format, and perhaps the next generation of medical practitioners will have a better grounding in musculoskeletal examination.

Appraisal and rationalisation of medication use

As previously stated, by the time patients consult doctors they may already have tried a range of common over-the-counter pain remedies, such as NSAIDS, mild analgesics and a range of holistic and herbal products. Presumably these have been partially beneficial at best or they would not be consulting. A list of the more common medicines used in pain management are shown in Box 6.6.

Rationalisation of medication use

The steps in rationalising medication use are shown in Box 6.7. Prior to taking any action, there are four preparatory stages.

Firstly, it is important to clarify the patient's current medication use. A surprising number of patients are not clear about the drugs they are taking or why and so ask for sight of their list of prescriptions if it is available. It is important also to distinguish what has been prescribed and what is actually being taken. Check also whether the medication is being taken appropriately (as instructed), identify whether medication is being obtained from other family members and evaluate use of non-prescribed drugs.

Secondly, prior to offering any specific recommendations about increasing, decreasing or changing drug use, it is important to check whether there are any medical contra-indications to particular types of medication.

Thirdly, it is important to supplement the evaluation of current drug use with an evaluation of previous medication use (and abuse) to identify those who might have difficulty in managing their medication appropriately.

Finally, elicit the patient's beliefs about, and expectations of, the use of medicines, and correct any misunderstandings.

It is then possible to provide advice on safe and appropriate long-term and short-term use of medicines for pain control. (More detail on medication management for patients presenting with high levels of use of pain medication are presented in Ch. 11.)

Communicating with the patient

The initial diagnostic formulation should be formulated with appropriate degree of specificity and a 'non-specific diagnosis' should be explained carefully. It should be remembered that the patient needs an explanation of what causes the pain, i.e. the probable mechanisms, and that a clear 'non-specific' diagnosis is better than no diagnosis at all. Generally speaking, the conventional diagnostic manual (ICD-10 1997) is far from adequate when it comes to describing sensory nervous system dysfunction, as is the present IASP taxonomy of pain (Merskey and Bogduk 1994). The new International Classification of Function (ICF 2001) offers some promise as a more relevant instrument to describe sensory impairments such as pain as well as the resulting disabilities (Sjölund 2003). However, a lot of new neurobiological information and its clinical implications needs to be gathered before this goal is reached.

It is usually helpful to involve family members as co-carriers of information, sometimes even as potential therapeutic agents. However, it may be that they present obstacles to engagement and therefore one should look out for negativity and oversolicitousness by family members.

It is usually an advantage if they are available for interview and are present at the end of the assessment. The patient's understanding should be checked in response to the diagnostic (mechanistic) clarification given by the physician. Some important aspects in the provision of information are shown in Box 6.8.

Communicating with colleagues

With subacute, recurrent and chronic problems, however, the care of the patient may be shared, either simultaneously, or sequentially with other health-care professionals. It is important therefore that the details of the medical management plan are clearly and simply communicated not only to the patient but also to other health-care professionals who may become involved with the patient.

This is particularly important within pain management programmes, where there may be complex sequential scheduling and concurrent advice about treatment. With non-trivial pain patients, team conferences are highly desirable. At such times as many team members as possible should be present and the key medical features should be integrated into the team evaluation prior to the feedback to the patient and family.

In the presentation of the results of the evaluation, it is usually best to highlight key medical features prior to other assessments. The summary provided should be clear, concise and in lay language to be understandable for all interested parties. Finally, the patient's understanding should be checked.

Box 6.8

Provision of information

- Give clear explanation to the patient (including respectability of a 'non-specific' diagnosis)
- Clarify if necessary the reasons for requiring further information
- Involve family members in consultation and note their contribution
- Check the patient's understanding at the end of the consultation.

Key points

- **The physician has a pivotal role in pain management**
- **Competent medical screening and pain diagnostics is the foundation of assessment**
- **Provision of optimal pain relief and rationalisation of use of medication either as a precursor to pain management or in conjunction with it**
- **The physician also has an important educational role in selling the biopsycho-social perspective and, where appropriate, serving as a conduit to other health-care professionals.**

References

ARC (on-line) Clinical assessment of the musculoskeletal system: a handbook for medical students. http://www.arc.org.uk/about_arth/othrpubs.htm

Bonica J J (ed) 1990 The management of pain, 2nd edn. Lea and Febiger, Philadelphia

IASP: International Association for the Study of Pain. Homepage: www.iasp.org

ICD-10 1997 The international classification of diseases, 10th edn. World Health Organisation, Geneva

ICF 2001 International classification of functioning, disability and health. World Health Organization, Geneva, pp 1–299

Merskey H, Bogduk N (eds) 1994 Classification of chronic pain. Descriptions of chronic pain syndromes and definitions of pain terms, 2nd edn. IASP Press, Seattle, pp 1–212

Sjölund B H 2003 Current and future treatment strategies for chronic pain. In: Soroker N, Ring H (eds) Advances in physical and rehabilitation medicine. Monduzzi Editore, Bologna, pp 307–313

UEMS 2004 PRM section home page. http://www.euro-prm.org/

Woolf C J, Bennett G J et al 1998 Towards a mechanism-based classification of pain? Pain 77(3):227–229

APPENDIX 6.1

Nomenclature of pain terms (modified from Merskey & Bogduk 1994)

Allodynia

Pain due to a stimulus which does not normally provoke pain.

Note: The term allodynia was originally introduced to distinguish the condition from hyperalgesia and hyperaesthesia, which are seen in patients with lesions of the nervous system where touch, light pressure, or moderate cold or warmth evoke pain when applied to apparently normal skin. *Allo* means 'other' in Greek and is a common prefix for medical conditions that diverge from the expected. Odynia is derived from the Greek word *odune* or *odyne*, which is used in 'pleurodynia' and 'coccydynia'.

Anaesthesia dolorosa

Pain in an area or region which is anaesthetic.

Analgesia

Absence of pain in response to stimulation which would normally be painful.

Causalgia

A syndrome of sustained burning pain, allodynia, and hyperpathia after a traumatic nerve lesion, often combined with vasomotor and sudomotor dysfunction and later trophic changes.

Central pain

Pain initiated or caused by a primary lesion or dysfunction in the central nervous system.

Dysaesthesia

An unpleasant abnormal sensation, whether spontaneous or evoked.

Note: Special cases of dysaesthesia include hyperalgesia and allodynia. It should always be specified whether the sensations are spontaneous or evoked.

Hyperalgesia

An increased response to a stimulus which is normally painful.

Note: Hyperalgesia reflects increased pain on suprathreshold stimulation. For pain evoked by stimuli that usually are not painful, the term allodynia is preferred, while hyperalgesia is more appropriately used for cases with an increased response at a normal threshold, or at an increased threshold, e.g., in patients with neuropathy.

Hyperaesthesia

Increased sensitivity to stimulation, excluding the special senses.

Note: The stimulus and locus should be specified. Hyperaesthesia may refer to various modes of cutaneous sensibility including touch and thermal sensation without pain, as well as to pain. The word is used to indicate both diminished threshold to any stimulus and an increased response to stimuli that are normally recognised.

Allodynia is suggested for pain after stimulation which is not normally painful. Hyperaesthesia includes both allodynia and hyperalgesia, but the more specific terms should be used wherever they are applicable.

Hyperpathia

A syndrome characterised by an abnormally painful reaction to a stimulus, especially a repetitive stimulus, as well as an increased threshold.

Note: It may occur with allodynia, hyperaesthesia, hyperalgesia or dysaesthesia. Faulty identification and localization of the stimulus, delay, radiating sensation, and after-sensation may be present, and the pain is often explosive in character.

Hypoaesthesia

Decreased sensitivity to stimulation, excluding the special senses.

Note: Stimulation and locus to be specified.

Hypoalgesia

Diminished pain in response to a normally painful stimulus.

Note: Hypoalgesia was formerly defined as diminished sensitivity to noxious stimulation, making it a particular case of hypoaesthesia. However, it now refers only to the occurrence of relatively less pain in response to stimulation that produces pain. Hypoaesthesia covers the case of diminished sensitivity to stimulation that is normally painful.

Neuralgia

Pain in the distribution of a nerve or nerves.

Note: Common usage, especially in Europe, often implies a paroxysmal quality, but neuralgia should not be reserved for paroxysmal pains.

Neuritis

Inflammation of a nerve or nerves.

Neurogenic pain

Pain initiated or caused by a primary lesion, dysfunction, or transitory perturbation in the peripheral or central nervous system.

Neuropathic pain

Pain initiated or caused by a primary lesion or dysfunction in the nervous system.

Nociceptor

A receptor preferentially sensitive to a noxious stimulus or to a stimulus which would become noxious if prolonged.

Note: Avoid use of terms like pain receptor, pain pathway, etc.

Noxious stimulus

A stimulus which is damaging to normal tissues.

Pain threshold

The least experience of pain which a subject can recognise.

Pain tolerance level

The greatest level of pain which a subject is prepared to tolerate.

Paraesthesia

An abnormal sensation, whether spontaneous or evoked.

Chapter Seven

7

The assessment of pain and function

Introduction

The aims of a pain intervention programme vary according to the setting and the intended outcome. When considering what to assess one must start with the intended aim of the programme; if the programme focuses on return to work then work status and duration of absence are key. Most programmes in the acute/subacute stage focus on reduction of pain, increase in physical function and reduction in self-reported disability; chronic pain management programmes often focus more on reducing psychological distress and increasing active coping. A further consideration concerns the use of the data. Managers may require certain activity information and funders or referring agents may require information which may or may not be of interest to the clinician, and of course the clinician has a desire to measure his or her effectiveness.

Before one embarks on a whole series of measures one must consider the amount of administrative effort that is required to score, collate, enter on to a database and analyse the data. There is little point in collecting large amounts of data if it is destined to be housed in a cupboard until some one can get it onto a database and analyse it. For this reason one must be clear what is essential to collect, what is desirable and what is exceptional, or what one would like to collect if time and resources were not an issue. A suggested hierarchy of outcomes to consider when choosing what might be measured on a clinical programme is shown in Box 7.1.

Good clinical practice requires not only clarity regarding the intended outcome of treatment but also careful choice of assessment measures. As a precursor to the appraisal of elements of the assessment of

Box 7.1

Suggested hierarchy of outcomes

- *Essential*:
  - directly related to aims of programme
  - resource implications if not collected.
- *Desirable*:
  - useful information – defines population
  - allows comparisons with others
  - monitor changes in patient population over years.
- *Exceptional*:
  - research driven.

pain and disability, it is perhaps worth reminding our-selves of the advantages of a systematic assessment in the context of an evidence-based approach as outlined by Peat (2000) in the previous edition of this textbook. These are reproduced (with only minor amendments) below.

Despite methodological problems, routine, systematic and comprehensive assessment of treatment outcome has several advantages over clinical judgement alone.

1. Criteria for successful outcome can begin to be clearly expressed. *This has been a neglected area in pain management outcome studies … and yet it is essential to the process of defining clinically significant improvements and of measuring individual patient outcomes.*
2. Comparisons of treatment outcome (and baseline) can be made between patients. *This is a process that is intuitively performed by clinicians when rating outcome (or initial severity) but is made more explicit by a systematic approach.*
3. Comparisons with treatments in other settings can be made. *This includes comparison with pain management programmes run in pain centres elsewhere in the country or even abroad. This is likely to be a major consideration for purchasers. It requires consensus between different centres on which measures to use.*
4. They can provide a candid appraisal of the adverse effects of treatment. *Most treatments, even placebos, carry the risk of adverse or detrimental effects. Pain management programmes are no exception. Some of the*

effects of failed treatments (discussed in chronic pain centres with the benefit of hindsight) also apply to failed pain management. Patients and clinicians alike may be reluctant or unwilling to identify these in the usual clinical setting.

5. Clearer formulation of hypotheses. *By examining outcome in a systematic and comprehensive way clinicians can begin to look for patterns in outcome and to speculate on associations. Hypotheses can later be formally tested using appropriate methodological frameworks.*
6. The information can be used for patient feedback to reinforce change. *Evidence on the changes made following treatment can be used for feedback. This includes identifying individual priorities for further (self-)management. In some circumstances, measures can be administered during the course of treatment to provide individual 'progress reports'. The information can then be used to direct individual intervention or reinforce patient change (p. 365).*

There are few who would disagree with the aforementioned objectives. The challenge is how to do it. In this chapter we shall explore these perspectives as applied to the assessment of pain and disability.

The context of pain assessment

Adequate pain relief is essential for all patients. This does not always mean the elimination of pain, but optimisation of analgesia should form part of all interventions. Although a reduction in the patient's pain report following intervention is reported by many pain management rehabilitation programmes, it is not one of the declared primary aims of pain management. Patients are not encouraged to expect a reduction in their level of pain and the focus is on the management of the pain and disability, thereby helping them to manage the intrusive nature of their pain. Nevertheless, a reduction in the level of pain is a desirable characteristic of pain rehabilitation and so measurement of pain should be conducted. Measurement of the level of pain also describes the patient population. It allows comparison between programmes for audit and research purposes. It is not intended to give a detailed account of the measurement of pain in its various forms in this chapter; the reader is directed to specific texts on the subject such as the excellent book by Turk & Melzack (2001). A brief review based on the observations by Jensen & Karoly (2001) and others is given in Appendix 7.1.

Pain characteristics

Pain may be described by its intensity, affective component, and location. Each requires investigation. Other pain states such as hyperalgesia or allodynia may be evident only on testing and would not be amenable to most self-report measures. The assessment of such states will not be addressed in this chapter and the reader should investigate specialist texts on this subject (e.g. Boivie et al 1994).

Pain intensity

Classically, pain intensity has been assessed in three domains, as shown in Box 7.2. They comprise: the effect on the autonomic nervous system (an increase in heart rate, skin sweating and blood pressure), effect on the motor or musculoskeletal system (in terms of reflexive responses, adoption of pain-relieving postures or alteration in movement), and effect on the verbal domain or the patients' self-report or their verbal expression including groaning.

Assessment of the autonomic responses to pain (heart rate, skin sweating and blood pressure) is difficult to perform accurately outside of the laboratory and so is of little use in clinical practice and will not be addressed here. The assessment of motor activity (including reflexive responses, adoption of pain-relieving postures or alterations in movement) can be monitored by surface electromyography in the laboratory or the clinic setting. In the clinic the systematic observation of pain-associated motor behaviours is more useful and this is discussed later under the assessment of pain behaviours. The most popular method, and perhaps the most valid measure of pain, is patients' own self-report. This is the easiest information to collect but can be the most misunderstood and misused.

Those with chronic pain almost invariably report that their pain, although continuous, is of a variable quality and intensity. It varies throughout the day and changes depending on whether the patient is active or at rest. This makes the snapshot of the pain that we measure on initial assessment and at follow-up rather a blunt instrument in pain assessment. Our assessment needs to reflect different dimensions of the pain experience. However, we first must identify the criteria for good

Box 7.2

The three domains of pain intensity

- *The autonomic responses to pain*:
  - e.g. heart rate, skin sweating and blood pressure.
- *The motor domain*:
  - reflexive responses
  - adoption of pain-relieving postures
  - alterations in movement.
- *The verbal domain*:
  - self-report
  - numerical measures
  - graphical measures.

Box 7.3

Key criteria for pain measures (Price et al 2001)

- Have ratio scale properties
- Be relatively free of biases inherent in different methods
- Provide immediate information about the accuracy and reliability of the subject's performance of the scaling responses
- Be useful for both experimental and clinical pain and allow for reliable comparison between both types of pain
- Be reliable and generalisable
- Be sensitive to changes in pain intensity
- Be simple and easy to use in pain patients in both clinical and non-clinical settings
- Separately assess the sensory intensive and affective dimensions of pain.

pain measures. Price et al (2001) identified nine key criteria for pain measures (Box 7.3).

Almost all commonly used pain measures in fact fail to satisfy all of these fairly stringent criteria, but an understanding of why they fail can help in the evaluation of the relative usefulness of different measurement instruments. For the purposes of this chapter it is not essential that all the above points are considered in detail, and only those aspects that are most important in the clinical setting will be dealt with here.

Examples of some commonly used rating scales are shown in Figure 7.1. The strengths and weakness of such scales are shown in Table 7.1.

Visual analogue scale

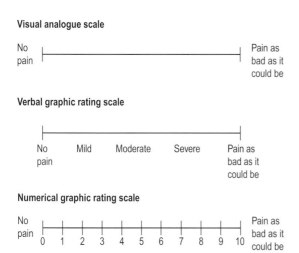

Verbal graphic rating scale

Numerical graphic rating scale

Figure 7.1 • Common numerical and graphical scales. From Jensen & Karoly in Turk & Melzack, 2001, reproduced with permission of Guilford Press, New York.

Pain affect (the emotional component of pain)

Pain has been described as a sensory and an emotional experience. Patients in pain not only make some judgement about the intensity of the signal but also respond to the sensation with differing degrees of emotional reaction, affording it a degree of unpleasantness or intrusiveness. This is termed the 'affective dimension' of the pain experience. However, an assessment of intensity does not necessarily address the intrusive nature of the pain. People may endure pain and not allow it to intrude into their lives to the point of limiting their activity. A reduction in the intensity of the pain following a pain management programme may not be achievable but a reduction in the intrusive nature or unpleasantness of the pain *is* a realistic aim of pain management programmes. Pain affect is normally assessed by asking the patient to rate the pain using a number of descriptors

Table 7.1 Strengths and weaknesses of commonly used pain intensity measures

Scale	Strengths	Weaknesses
Verbal rating scale (VRS)	Easy to administer Easy to score Good evidence for construct validity Compliance with measurement task is high May approximate ratio scaling if cross-modality matching methods (or scores developed from such methods) are used	• Can be difficult for persons with limited vocabulary • Relatively few response categories compared to the VAS or 101-point NRS[a] • If scored via the ranking method, the scores do not necessarily have ratio qualities • People are forced to choose one word, even if no word on the scale adequately describes their pain intensity
Visual analogue scale (VAS)	Easy to administer Many ('infinite') response categories Scores can be treated as ratio data Good evidence for construct validity	• Extra step in scoring the paper-and-pencil version can take more time and adds an additional source of error
Numerical rating scale (NRS)	Easy to administer Many response categories if 101-point NRS is chosen Easy to score Good evidence for construct validity	• Limited number of response categories if 11-point NRS is used • Compliance with measurement task is high • Scores cannot necessarily be treated as ratio data
Picture or face scale	Easy to administer Easy to score	• No evidence regarding relative compliance rates • Limited number of response categories • Scores cannot necessarily be treated as ratio data
Descriptor differential scale (DDS-I)	Because the scale has several items, it may be more reliable than single-item rating scales Allows for estimates of the consistency with which people complete the measure	• Some patients may have difficulty comprehending the measure • Limited research on the validity and sensitivity of the measure • Completion of the scale takes more time than other measures

[a]There is no evidence to suggest that VRSs with 15 or more items are less sensitive to treatment effects than VASs or NRSs, but evidence does suggest that VRSs with 5 or fewer categories may be less sensitive in some situations.

Adapted from Jensen & Karoly, in Turk & Melzack (2001, Table 2.3, p. 25).

such as on the McGill Pain Questionnaire (Melzack 1975), but later developed into a shorter more useable clinical tool. Short form, while certainly a significant improvement on the long and unwieldy longer form (Melzack 1975), although useable in a self-report format is more safely given using prompts. It is shown in Figure 7.2.

The FACES scale (Bieri et al 1990), mainly used in the evaluation of pain in children, is not reliant on verbal content, and has a simple clinical utility. Although the tool has not been used extensively with adults it has utility in assessing the elderly and people with difficulty understanding other measures. Pictorial depictions of pain have also been used with both children and adults. The FACES scale consists of a series of simple drawings of facial expressions illustrating degrees of pain intensity or emotional impact ranging from untroubled to intense (Fig. 7.3).

A simpler way of rating affect is to ask the patient to rate the 'bothersomeness' of the pain (Cherkin et al 1996). This has an attractive simplicity and is increasingly used as a research in epidemiological studies (Dunn & Croft 2005). Although it would appear to have use as a screening tool it cannot be recommended as a clinical measure with chronic pain patients without further validation.

Pain location

The localisation of pain can be ascertained by use of a pain drawing; the patient simply indicates the area of pain on a printed mannequin. A typical scoring template for pain drawings (Margolis et al 1986) is shown in Figure 7.4.

This can be scored up using a body chart to give an approximation of the surface affected, and compared with post-treatment scores. There have been a number of variants on this theme, including the pain mannequin used in epidemiological studies to define criteria for various regional pain syndromes and chronic widespread pain. In fact this type of pain quantification is rarely used in clinical practice.

Pain drawings which demonstrate large areas of pain or complex patterns also have been associated with psychological distress. Ransford et al (1976) developed a scoring system designed to identify distress. The nature of this 'overlay' has been debated over the years. Examples of two pain drawings completed by patients with low-back pain and sciatica with similar clinical histories are shown in Figure 7.5. It can be seen that drawing B contains much more embellishment and is illustrative of a much higher level of pain preoccupation, suggesting that the depiction of pain may be influenced by a number of factors.

Pain drawings have an intuitive appeal, patients show no hesitation in completing them, and the drawing can be a useful starting point for a clinical interview. They can be a useful 'screener' highlighting the need for a broader assessment, but they need to be interpreted with care since 50% of distressed patients produce 'normal' pain drawings (Parker et al 1995). Distress needs to be evaluated using appropriate assessment (as described in Ch. 8).

Statistical properties

In assessing pain a number of specific statistical considerations need to be borne in mind. They are shown in Box 7.4.

Scaling properties

Pain measures ideally should have ratio scale properties. A pain measure should start at zero, and the distance between each of the points on the pain scale should be equal; the change in intensity between one and three should be equal to the change in intensity between three and five, five and seven, and so on. This confers a linear relationship between an increasing intensity and an increase in pain report. Experimental evidence suggests, however, that the relationship between increasing scores on pain instruments or verbal report for pain is non-linear. A fall in pain rating from nine to seven may represent a different reduction in intensity than from five to three. Verbal rating scales relying on adjectives describing the pain are particularly prone to this phenomenon of non-linearity. The data collected on such scales are categorical and do not have ratio scale properties. The difference in intensity between 'mild pain' and 'moderate pain' may not be the same as the perceived difference between 'moderate pain' and 'severe pain'. This is very important when dealing with the data statistically and makes nonsense of statements such as 'The patient group reported a mean reduction of 30% in their pain'. Categorical scales such as these can only tell us that the pain increased or decreased; they cannot give meaningful information about the magnitude of the change in pain. Experimental evidence suggests that scoring systems such as visual analogue scales (VASs) are less prone to this phenomenon. However, they can be used as ratio data only if they have a zero starting point (i.e. are anchored by 'no pain' at one end). Verbal rating or verbal descriptor scales are particularly prone to distorted scaling.

A further distortion can arise if attempts are made to quantify responses to descriptive scales by converting them into numerical ratings and assigning them the

Patient's name: _____   Date: _____

Throbbing	0) _____	1) _____	2) _____	3) _____
Shooting	0) _____	1) _____	2) _____	3) _____
Stabbing	0) _____	1) _____	2) _____	3) _____
Sharp	0) _____	1) _____	2) _____	3) _____
Cramping	0) _____	1) _____	2) _____	3) _____
Gnawing	0) _____	1) _____	2) _____	3) _____
Hot-burning	0) _____	1) _____	2) _____	3) _____
Aching	0) _____	1) _____	2) _____	3) _____
Heavy	0) _____	1) _____	2) _____	3) _____
Tender	0) _____	1) _____	2) _____	3) _____
Splitting	0) _____	1) _____	2) _____	3) _____
Tiring-exhausting	0) _____	1) _____	2) _____	3) _____
Sickening	0) _____	1) _____	2) _____	3) _____
Fearful	0) _____	1) _____	2) _____	3) _____
Punishing-cruel	0) _____	1) _____	2) _____	3) _____

No pain |———————————————————————————————————| Worst possible pain

PPI

0	No pain	_____
1	Mild	_____
2	Discomforting	_____
3.	Distressing	_____
4	Horrible	_____
5	Excruciating	_____

Figure 7.2 • Short-form McGill Pain Questionnaire (SF-MPQ). Descriptors 1–11 represent the sensory dimension of pain experience, and 12–15 represent the affective dimension. Each descriptor is ranked on an intensity scale of 0 = 'none', 1 = 'mild', 2 = 'moderate', 3 = 'severe'. The PPI of the standard MPQ and the VAS are also included to provide overall pain intensity scores. From Melzack & Katz in Turk & Melzack (2001, p. 46), reproduced with permission.

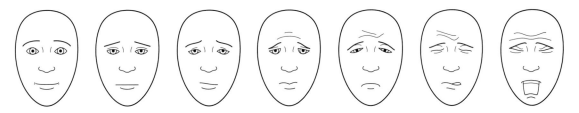

Figure 7.3 • FACES Pain Scale scored 0–6 (Bieri et al 1990, reproduced with permission of the International Association for the Study of Pain).

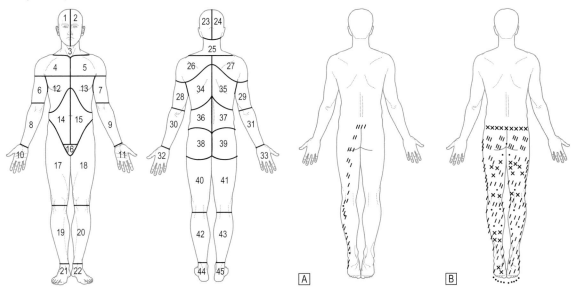

Figure 7.4 • Pain drawing template (after Margolis et al 1986). From Jensen & Karoly in Turk & Melzack (2001, p. 29, Figure 2.3).

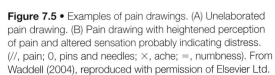

Figure 7.5 • Examples of pain drawings. (A) Unelaborated pain drawing. (B) Pain drawing with heightened perception of pain and altered sensation probably indicating distress. (//, pain; 0, pins and needles; ×, ache; =, numbness). From Waddell (2004), reproduced with permission of Elsevier Ltd.

status of ratio or interval data. The Short-Form McGill Pain Questionnaire, or SF-MPQ (Melzack 1987) requires subjects to report the level of intensity of different descriptors of pain in both the sensory and affective domains. This is then ascribed a number and the sensory component is assumed to give an indication of the intensity of the pain. It may be argued that this is a qualitative measure of pain rather than a quantitative measure. A patient may only describe their pain as having only one descriptive sensory component (e.g. throbbing) but report it as being severe, while another patient may report mild pain on more than three descriptors and the scores would be the same.

Sensitivity to change

The scaling of the measure determines its sensitivity to change. The most popular pain measures utilise scales from five (Present Pain Intensity, or PPI; Melzack 1987)

> ### Box 7.4
>
> **Statistical considerations in the use of scales**
>
> - Scaling properties
> - Sensitivity to change
> - Problem of non-linearity
> - Validity across patient groups.

to 101 (VAS) reference points. The more choices patients have the more likely the scale is to detect change. Scales relying on fewer points, such as four-point scales of no pain, mild, moderate, and severe pain, are less discriminative than those with a greater number of points. Patients may have moderate pain at the beginning of the programme and may report a reduction in pain on direct questioning but may still class their pain as 'moderate'. Hence, the pain measure has failed to detect the change.

Problem of non-linearity

It has been demonstrated in experimental research that there may not be a direct relationship between the stimulus intensity and report of pain when using conventional clinical pain measures. If the relationship between the rise in the stimulus and the increase in pain report is variable then the sensitivity to change of the measure used will vary also. It is therefore highly likely that this is also the case in clinical pain. This means that changes, for example, in the upper intensity scores may be easier to detect than those at lower levels of intensity.

Validity across patient groups

It would be advantageous to have pain measures that could be used to describe mixed groups of patients. Pain management programmes take patients with a variety of conditions, some of which are better represented in numbers than others. The validity and generalisability of pain measures determine the relative confidence in the measure to produce the same results for a given intensity within individuals as well as within and between different patient groups. Can we assume that the intensity of the pain and the affective component are generally the same in different pain populations? This is probably not the case. Differences in the magnitude of the affective and sensory components have been demonstrated between different pain conditions. Well-established measures such as the VAS and the MPQ have demonstrated differences in report of pain in the intensity and affective scales in patients with different medical diagnoses (Jensen & Karoly 2001).

Influences on pain rating

A number of the important influences on pain ratings are shown in Box 7.5. The way in which the measure is introduced to the patient can unwittingly introduce a bias in the measure. Social desirability in a patient wishing to demonstrate to a clinician that a treatment is having an effect may influence the reporting of pain. It is very difficult to control for this. Similarly, subjects on initial presentation with painful conditions are unlikely to make light of their pains for fear that the clinician may not take their conditions seriously.

The presentation of the instrument to the patient by the clinician can similarly influence the results.

Box 7.5

Influences on pain ratings

- Influences of language
- Practical considerations
- Pain relief
- Satisfaction with symptoms
- Importance of the affective component.

A measure that requires minimal explanation to the patient is desirable. Scales such as the VAS may require significant explanation for some people. Despite this, even with appropriate explanation some subjects still find them difficult to understand.

Influences of language

Many self-report measures depend upon the use of descriptive words. Patients are presented with a list of words and are required to choose a word or words that best describe their pain. Such measurement instruments are biased against those who have poor educational attainment or whose first language is not the same as the language of the questionnaire. Communication problems such as those occurring following stroke likewise threaten the validity of such questionnaires.

Some patients find their pain hard to describe. Patients with chronic regional pain syndromes in particular have been demonstrated to have difficulty in identifying their pain with the words on commonly used standardised pain questionnaires.

Practical considerations

Pain measures used in the clinical setting should be relatively simple to administer and to score, especially if patients are expected to complete them regularly. Few pain management centres will have research assistants to administer and check all the responses. Complex measures with complicated scoring systems are more susceptible to scoring errors. This presents us with the age-old problem of looking for measures that are simple but give sufficient information to allow us to represent patients' pain and monitor change adequately.

Pain relief

In addition to an assessment of pain, pain relief can also be measured and many composite measures of pain contain such a measure. Most simply ask the patient to rate the percentage improvement the treatment or medication provides. (See the section on the Brief Pain Inventory for an example of such a measure.)

Satisfaction with symptoms

As has been stated earlier, people with chronic pain are unlikely to get complete relief from their symptoms and many continue to report relatively high levels of pain after interventions. Some patients might report similar levels of pain but have a higher level of function; in effect they are physically active within a range of pain that they find 'acceptable'. In order to account for this Haythornthwaite & Fauerbach (2001) recommend a satisfaction-with-symptoms assessment. This simply asks the patient to rate how satisfied they would be if they had to continue to live with their current level of symptoms.

Importance of the affective component

In pain management, a change in the intensity of the pain is not the focus of treatment but a reduction in the intrusiveness or the emotional component of the pain should be expected. For this reason it is recommended that the affective component of pain (as discussed above) is evaluated. A simpler method is the affective VAS. (A brief, more specific account of these measures is given at the end of this chapter.)

More general measurement considerations

Although studies have failed to demonstrate a strong relationship between measures of physical function, functional limitation (impairment) and disability in the broadest context, the assessment of physical and functional measures serves several different functions in chronic pain management other than simply that of attempting to infer cause and effect. The main purposes of assessment are shown in Box 7.6.

Despite significant limitations these measures are useful. They will help in describing the population being observed. Such data may be used for research purposes provided the measures are standardised. The performance of physical tests can serve as a behavioural assessment. They can be used to corroborate self-report measures, and can also serve as a baseline, which will aid goal setting with individual patients. Finally, they may be used as outcome measures for audit.

In appraising further the available measurement tools, however, it is necessary to consider other aspects of measurement. These are shown in Box 7.7.

Box 7.6

Purposes of assessment of physical incapacity, functional limitation and disability

- Population description (case mix)
- Pretreatment baseline for goal setting (treatment)
- Potential outcome measures (audit).

Box 7.7

Additional methodological considerations

- Reproducibility
- Responsiveness
- Validity
- Control over the test environment
- The importance of clinical relevance
- Relationship with outcome.

Reproducibility

All measures have some random error. In patients whose condition is unchanged the extent to which scores vary will indicate the reproducibility of the measure. In a sense this can be regarded as background 'noise'.

In measurements that require the rating of an observer, the scores obtained by different examiners of the same stable patient will be important (inter-rater reliability).

Responsiveness

Over and above the 'noise' of random measurement error it is important to identify the signal that indicates a true change in the patient. Measures with poor responsiveness may fail to detect clinically important change. It may be reproducible but it fails to detect improvements in the patients' status. There are many statistical ways of summarising how well a measure can detect clinically important change including standardised effect sizes and standardised response means. Almost all are based on this concept of the ratio of signal to noise. A more detailed account of measurement responsiveness is provided by Guyatt et al (1992) and Stratford et al (1996).

In assessing response to treatment, it is important to distinguish between clinically important change that has resulted from the treatment and naturally occurring variability. Chronic pain is a very variable condition with respect to disability and pain. Two single snap-shots in time may demonstrate a change but this may be purely as a result in this variability, i.e. a result of testing the subject on a 'bad' day (when they are most likely to consult) and a 'good' day when the pain is less troublesome.

Care must also be taken when selecting the test. Activities which are used as part of a rehabilitation pro-gramme (e.g. step-ups and speed walking) are likely to improve solely through practice. Repeated performance will result in improvements which are not attributable to the treatment, only to the testing, a learning effect.

Validity

Measures are never in themselves valid or invalid. They are judged to be valid *for a stated purpose*. Validity can be assessed in a number of ways:

- Look at the content of the measure (e.g. items in a self-report questionnaire). Does it cover all the important points? Does it contain many irrelevant items?
- Does it show changes in predictable circumstances? For example, a measure of disability should show reductions in acute cases that largely resolve by themselves.
- Do changes in the measure correlate with other observed changes in the expected way? For example, improvements in physical tests should correlate negatively with changes in reported functional limitation.

Control over the test environment

Care must be taken to control the environment during testing. Environmental factors influencing performance and test results include:

- The instructions given (e.g. Matheson et al 1992)
- The level of feedback and encouragement given (e.g. Guyatt et al 1984)
- The presence of other parties – especially the spouse (Paulsen & Altmaier 1995)
- The gender interaction between patients and observers (e.g. Levine & De Simone 1991)
- The time of testing – especially flexibility and strength (Ensink et al 1996).

Minimise bias in outcome evaluation by using staff unconnected with the treatment.

The importance of clinical relevance

The measures should ideally be generalisable to every-day function. Changes in a physical performance meas-ure should, therefore, reflect an increase in levels of physical activity. Not only should the measures relate to function but they should also be sensitive to changes that may occur following a rehabilitation programme.

Relationship with outcome

The relative usefulness of physical function measures at outcome is a poorly researched area. Many reported rehabilitation schemes rely on self-report of pain and disability as outcome measures rather than physical function measures. The relationship between measures of physical function and self-report of physical activity, however, has not been adequately established.

Assessment of physical functioning

The conceptual basis

The key aims of interventions for painful conditions are reduction of incapacity and an increase in physical function to the maximum achievable. As a declared outcome it becomes incumbent upon the clinician to monitor and measure the level of function and dis-ability. It is worthwhile to define the terms used in the measurement of patient performance and discuss their relevance to the various measurements that may be employed in pain management.

The concept and classification of impairment, disabil-ity and handicap is outlined in the 1980 World Health Organisation's International Classification of Impair-ments, Disabilities and Handicaps (ICIDH). It has more recently evolved into the International Classi-fication of Functioning, or ICF (WHO 2000) in which the distinction has been made between bodily impair-ments, activity limitations and participation restric-tions. Interestingly, this maps reasonably well onto the biopsychosocial model of low-back pain disability, as illustrated in Figure 7.6.

The ICIDH model starts with the assumption that there is an initial disease or dysfunction as the root cause of the handicap; this may be due to a disease process, trauma, or a congenital abnormality. Impairment is defined as the loss or abnormality of the anatomical, psychological, or physiological function of the body. Disability refers to the restriction of ability to perform

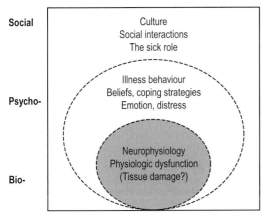

Social	Culture Social interactions The sick role	ICF (WHO 2000) Participation (restrictions)
Psycho-	Illness behaviour Beliefs, coping strategies Emotion, distress	Activity (limitations) Personal factors
Bio-	Neurophysiology Physiologic dysfunction (Tissue damage?)	Impairments Body structure and functions

Figure 7.6 • ICF and the biopsychosocial model. From Waddell (2004), reproduced with permission of Elsevier Ltd.

functions as a result of that impairment. The handicap is the disadvantage resulting from the inability to perform those functional tasks to a level considered normal for a person of the same age, sex and culture. In this respect the handicap refers to the socially defined roles rather than the individual's function. In this model the handicap may be related to the social environment. It cannot be adequately evaluated without reference to external factors, for example the attitudes of employers to those with a long history of work loss due to musculoskeletal pain.

Impairment

The relationship between a disease process and the resulting physical impairment is clearly not as linear as the above model suggests. In many persistently painful conditions, especially those arising from the musculoskeletal system, the precise diagnosis of a causal pathology may be very difficult or even impossible. This has proved to be particularly true in chronic low-back pain where there may be no obvious cause of the pain. Patients may report extreme pain and demonstrate gross physical impairment, loss of range of movement and weakness of muscle action, with little actual identifiable pathology. Pain-free subjects may demonstrate evidence of considerable abnormality (e.g. degenerative changes on X-ray of the spine) but have excellent measurable function. Main et al (2005) offer a review of the relationship between incapacity and disability, in the context of rehabilitation for pain patients.

Influence of restriction

Continued restriction of activity and function, which frequently accompanies chronic painful conditions, may further complicate matters by producing a varying degree of secondary physical impairment. These include physical deconditioning and loss of cardiovascular fitness, reduced exercise tolerance, muscle wasting, restricted range of joint motion and loss of extensibility of soft tissues through the development of guarded movements. These in themselves may also contribute to the painful condition. Reduced paraspinal muscle endurance and elevated resting muscle action in the back have both been implicated in the possible generation of musculoskeletal pain. This demonstrates that the development of disability is not linear but a dynamic process, which is interrelated to other factors.

Quantification of impairment

All of the above discrepancies become even more apparent when attempting to quantify the physical impairment. When measuring physical capacity in this context it should be understood that the measurement is one of *physical performance* rather than *physical capacity*.

Physical capacity and physical performance

Physical capacity refers to the actual performance that would be predicted by the physiological parameters. The maximal force developed by the contraction of a muscle would be predicted by, amongst other factors, the length–tension relationship of the muscle, the coordination, type and size of motor units recruited, the cross-sectional diameter of the muscle, fibre arrangement, the type of contraction and the velocity of the contraction (Rothwell 1987).

Influence of psychological factors

When assessing the pain patient the performance of a test is modified by motivational and cognitive factors, which render the assessment of true capacity difficult if not impossible. Measures of physical impairment cannot be seen as true measures of physical capacity; they are psychophysiological measurements and should be interpreted as such. All performance measures are likely to be perceived by patients in terms of their relationship with the immediate or anticipated environment, for example access to treatment or anticipated pain (Watson 1999).

A summary of the key features of physical capacity and physical function is shown in Box 7.8.

Disability

The measurement of disability relies on the assessment of performance, particularly performance of social roles. It is at this point that the relatively weak relationship between the organic basis, the pain and performance becomes apparent. Research into various painful conditions has repeatedly commented on the lack of a direct relationship.

Psychological influences

Internal processes may be described as psychological attributes and coping styles adopted by individuals in response to the disease state. Those who develop low self-efficacy beliefs or who are very fearful of activity because of distorted beliefs about the nature of their condition are more likely to demonstrate poor function and higher levels of disability. (They are discussed in detail in Ch. 2.)

Social and environmental influences

External influences include a large number of factors from the social and physical environment. The role of the family or significant others can serve to reinforce or reduce disability. Those with oversolicitous partners

are more prone to reducing their social role than those with non-solicitous partners. Access to employment is frequently limited for persons with chronic pain, and retraining or work experience placements for such people are rarely if ever available.

Handicap occurs when individuals interact with their environment. For example, people in wheelchairs may be able to perform all the functions of daily living in a home environment that has been adapted for their needs. They are not disabled in this environment. Once they go outside of their homes, however, access to transport and into buildings, requiring the provision of ramps, lifts and disabled toilets, handicaps them from participating in society to a full extent. The environment, not the condition, is the limiting factor. Patients with back pain may be unable to remain at work because there is no provision in the work task for changing position regularly, chairs are unsuitable for them or work stations are badly designed to meet their needs.

Measures of physical function and impairment

Measures of physical function used in pain management should be easy to use, acceptable to the patient, familiar to the patient (to offset the effect of learning), require a minimum of equipment and reflect activities that would be performed in everyday life. A whole industry has developed in testing the physical function of people with chronic pain. This is seen in the development of functional capacity assessments, which are marketed as tests that inform about a worker's suitability to do their job. Testing methods simple and complex will be discussed here, but simple, cheap measures are often the best and often need no more equipment than a mat, a stopwatch and a trained observer.

Range of motion

The range of motion of the affected area can be measured by goniometry, or other means such as the modified Schoeber's test for spinal movement using a tape measure. The reliability, reproducibility and validity are generally good for most measures if careful attention is paid to the isolation of the particular joint action. Many measures of range of motion fail to be valid, however, because they are composites of different joint ranges. This is exemplified in the measurement of lumbar spinal movement. Fingertip distance from the floor for the lumbar spine is often used. This is an inaccurate measure of lumbar spinal movement as it is a composite of lumbar spine and hip motion. Similarly the angle of the humerus in relation to the trunk as a measure of the shoulder activity is a composite of all the shoulder girdle complex not the glenohumeral joint alone.

The importance of normative data

Many of the normal values for range of motion are for general populations and there are few modified for age and gender. It is insufficient for those measuring range of motion to assume that a particular measure is repeatable and reliable in their clinic before they have established the fact. All clinicians who intend to rely on such measurements must satisfy themselves of this before they can draw conclusions on outcomes.

The influence of psychological factors

Ranges of joint motion rarely appear to be related, in chronic low-back pain, to the degree of disability (Gronblad et al 1997, Al Obaidi et al 2000) and have been reported as being significantly influenced by exaggerated illness behaviour and fear of movement. It is therefore important to be aware of the other factors that may influence these measurements by having measures of the other factors.

Muscle strength

Objective measures

Objective measures of muscle strength usually require the use of sophisticated machines such as isokinetic or isometric muscle-testing machines. These require training and expertise to give meaningful results. They usually have a known level of reliability, reproducibility and validity and have been used extensively in clinical research. Most have published normative databases for comparison but these are on a normal general population and not specifically matched to a sedentary group. Databases do exist for chronic pain patients, in particular for the most tested group – low-back pain. They are expensive and, for the average clinical setting, give no better additional data on the function of the patient than simpler measures.

Limitations of objective measures

Such machines have a number of disadvantages in the pain clinic or pain management programme. They are expensive to purchase and to maintain. The machines are designed to test specific joint and muscles necessitating

the purchase of different machines if different joints or range of motion measurements are required. There is a considerable learning effect with repeated testing and this is greater in patients than in controls (Newton et al 1993). Patients may be daunted by the machine; the machines by their nature are large and look very threatening. The context in which the measurement takes place may represent a great challenge to the patient and the potential confounds of fear of injury should not be underestimated. Patients who are fearful with low self-efficacy beliefs perform less well than do those who are more confident about their ability to perform the task required (Estlander et al 1994, Lackner et al 1996, Al Obaidi et al 2000). Results from such machines therefore should be interpreted with considerable caution.

Muscular endurance

In recent years the role of the endurance or 'fatigability' of muscles in the maintenance or generation of painful conditions has received attention. The evaluation of muscle endurance as a measure of physical performance or limitation has, therefore, been established.

The nature of muscle endurance

Muscle endurance can be termed central (as a result of the subject's willingness to maintain the contraction as identified by the number of action potentials recorded from the muscle on electromyography) or peripheral. The changes in the type of muscle fibre activity (a reduction in fast-twitch activity and an increase in slow-twitch activity) within the muscle, which occurs as a result of physiological fatigue, may be recorded by electromyography.

The role of endurance

The role of endurance in chronic low-back pain is, at present, the only area with sufficient data to establish cause and effect. The reliability and repeatability for the most sophisticated methodologies appear to be very good (Roy et al 1997). Recent studies (Koumentakis et al 2005) have found no relationship between paraspinal endurance measures and a reduction in pain and incapacity and more fundamental research on fibre type has called into question whether there is a relationship at all (Crossman et al 2004). This type of assessment requires sophisticated equipment and a high level of expertise to operate reliably and is unlikely to be appropriate for the average clinic.

Clinical measures

A simple measure of general, non-specific, activity endurance without electromyography, holding the arms aloft at 90 degrees to the body, has been used and found to be reliable, reproducible and sensitive to change following pain management (Harding et al 1994). Other endurance measures that may be used are sitting and standing tolerance and the Sorenson test (Biering-Sorensen 1984). These performance measures are highly correlated with measures of pain behaviour and are interpreted as such by some authors (Vlaeyen 1991). No statements can be made about physiological muscular endurance from these tests.

Cardiovascular fitness

Utility

Cardiovascular fitness is commonly measured in chronic pain management programmes. The notion of deconditioning in chronic pain – that people with chronic pain problems become less fit – has been challenged (Crossman et al 2004, Wittink et al 2000, Verbunt et al 2001), and recent evidence suggests that such patients are not physiologically deconditioned compared to healthy controls, presumably because healthy controls are not fit. Some patients with chronic pain do suffer secondary deconditioning as a result of limited activity but these people were probably physically active prior to the onset of their problem (Verbunt et al 2005). The message is that those who were fit before the onset of the pain become deconditioned; for those who were inactive and unfit prior to onset, the pain does not impact on their fitness levels. An assessment of cardiovascular fitness can help to quantify the degree of fitness and may be used to monitor progress. The utility of cardiovascular fitness testing in assessing adherence to an exercise regimen and to monitor increased fitness at follow-up appears an attractive proposition. There is a considerable database on normal, healthy age- and sex-grouped cardiovascular responses to exercise testing for use as a comparator. Despite these considerations there is good evidence that an increase in physical fitness is associated with reduced disability, but the causal effect is unclear.

Assessment

Cardiovascular testing may be performed using treadmill or bicycle ergometers. There is no physiological advantage in either method of testing. The ability to tolerate each test may depend upon the specific functional limitation (i.e. location of the pain problem). It has been reported that patients with chronic low-back pain, particularly those with spinal stenosis, tolerate the bicycle ergometer much better than the treadmill. Improvements in ergometer tolerance times and increases in physical fitness have been reported following pain management programmes.

Submaximal testing

Submaximal testing should be used for considerations of safety and standardised protocols for cardiovascular testing exist. A target rate of age-related maximal heart rate (usually 75 or 85%) is predetermined, and the work rate is increased gradually until the target rate is achieved. The baseline heart rate, the time taken to reach the target, work performed during the test and the target (or maximum rate achieved) is recorded. Anticipation of the exercise task and its performance may be psychologically stressful for some subjects and cause a stress/anxiety-related tachycardia, thus affecting the reliability of the results. Desensitisation through familiarisation with the task and a low-level practice run with the equipment may assist in the establishment of a more representative baseline.

Timed tests

A number of studies have described using timed physical function measures. Many of the timed measures have good reliability, reproducibility and have been shown to be sensitive to change in back pain and general pain groups (Gronblad et al 1997, Harding et al 1994, Simmonds et al 1998) and above all are low cost and simple to perform. The correlation between each of these measures appears to be very high. It is debatable, therefore, whether they individually contribute anything unique to the assessment of the patient or may be substituted by a single measure alone. Investigations on general pain populations have not usually attempted to identify differences in performance by site of pain other than by upper- and lower-body pain. Efforts to construct meaningful indexes of physical tests have had little success – there is simply no consensus on how to weight and amalgamate them.

Timed walk

The time taken to walk a fixed distance, or the distance walked in a set time has been used in many pain management studies. These vary in length from a 20-metre timed test to a measure of the distance walked in a fixed time from 1 to 10 minutes. A timed 20-metre walk test has the advantage of being relatively quick to perform. A distance is marked out on a flat corridor and the patient is asked to walk the distance as fast as possible and is timed over the course. Normally this is performed without walking aids. The reliability, repeatability and sensitivity to change of the 20-metre, 10-minute and 5-minute walk tests have been demonstrated to be very good. These tests appear to correlate highly with each other, so the assessor should decide if the extra length of assessment time is necessary, particularly if many physical measures are to be tested in a short time. One disadvantage of the shorter walk test is that there is likely to be an uneven distribution of the scores, particularly in the less-disabled patient group. This results in a 'floor effect' and a skewed distribution of data, particularly after successful treatment. There is a limit to how fast a person can walk a 20-metre distance. Most fit people can walk the 20 metres in about 9 seconds; any faster and they must run. Longer walk distances give a more even distribution of performance scores. Differences in performance should also be expected between patients with upper- and those with lower-body pain.

Stair climbing

The subject is asked to climb up and down a set of stairs as many times as possible in 1 minute. The measure demonstrates excellent inter-rater reliability and is sensitive to change. A highly significant correlation has been demonstrated between tests of differing length, suggesting that 1 minute is sufficient to give good data and will tire the person less when performing multiple tests.

Sit-ups

The performance of sit-ups in a timed period has been suggested by some authors, but the skewed distribution of performances in task performance has been shown to be a problem. In a study by Harding et al (1994), 52% of subjects scored zero prior to pain management, suggesting poor patient compliance and low acceptability of the test. Nonetheless it has been demonstrated to have moderate test–retest reliability and is sensitive to changes following interventions. One minute is the recommended test period (it correlates highly with longer test periods).

Other physical measurements

A whole battery of physical assessment measures has been used in research but these are generally poorly described. This has not allowed standardisation amongst research projects. Grip strength, peak flow and performance of a general exercise or functional task circuit have all been employed. Subjects are often required

---

Box 7.9

Key points: using physical function tests

- Is the test a valid measure?
- Has the reliability and validity of the test been established for this group of patients?
- Is there a reliable and comparable, normative database?
- Is the test acceptable to the patients – will they comply?
- What may be the effect of performing large batteries of physical tests on the performance of the patient?
- Establish which tests are to be used as outcome measures and which are to be used for goal setting.
- Determine, and periodically check, your own intra- and inter-rater reliability.

---

to complete an exercise circuit, and the time taken to perform the whole circuit or the number of exercises performed (or both) is recorded. Generally the reliability of these measures has been mixed, and they have not proved to be particularly sensitive to change. This may be due to the variability inherent in broad-ranging exercises or the mixed nature of the groups studied.

A reminder of some of the key considerations in the use of physical function tests are presented in Box 7.9.

Functional capacity assessments

Background

Functional capacity assessments (FCAs) are particularly common in North America, indeed around half a million are conducted each year in the USA, mainly at the behest of insurance companies or third-party payers for health care, and are supported by a whole industry of companies competing to provide testing. They range from simple timed tasks involving moving weights and performing simple tasks and covering distances walked to the use of complex machines used to test maximum force, range of motion or endurance in a variety of planes of motion.

The nature of FCAs

Functional capacity assessments are a detailed examination and evaluation that purport to offer an objective measurement of a client's current level of function in terms of the demands of competitive employment

(American Physical Therapy Association 1997). They have been used extensively in the United States, in particular to assess readiness to return to work and as outcome evaluations from rehabilitation programmes. There are many different systems of FCA, some of which are extensively marketed and promoted. Typically FCAs comprise a number of physical tests which are designed to represent the physical demands of a job. Successful achievement or exceeding preset targets is purported to be an indication of suitability to return to work. They are also used to monitor the progress of the injured worker to guide treatment progression (King et al 1998, Mooney 2002).

Reliability and face validity

Some FCAs have acceptable test–retest ability and many also have acceptable inter-rater reliability provided those who administer the test have receive the appropriate training in the use of the system. Many require the use of test equipment which is specific to the test and thus requires considerable capital investment so are rarely used as clinical tools alone. Depending on the complexity and comprehensiveness of the test they can take from a minimum of a few hours to more than one day to complete. Although FCAs have been demonstrated to have acceptable reliability for some of the measures employed, commercially available FCAs are not interchangeable and performance in one cannot be translated to another, nor can one mix and match different testing regimes.

There is some evidence that performance on FCA is related to self-report of disability on self-report assessment measures, but as most of these self-report measures rarely contain items relating to the demands of the job one must be cautious in taking this as evidence of construct validity.

The face validity of FCAs very much depends on the demands of the worker's occupation and the tasks selected which should closely match those demands. It should be remembered that testing within a controlled environment may demonstrate that the injured person can perform the maximum lift required for the job or even perform repeated tasks demonstrating endurance. As most of this takes place on one occasion, rather than over a working day or week, the face validity of the assessment as representing the stress and strain of the job is suspect.

Interpretation and utility of FCA results

As stated earlier in this chapter, FCAs are, like all other measures, tests of physical performance and not

physical capacity, and stable test–retest values are better seen as a stable psychophysiological state (Kaplan et al 1996, Watson 1999, Gross 2004).

The main purpose of performing an FCA is to determine a person's suitability to return to work; if we are to take the FCA as valid, adequate performance on the appropriate tests should predict successful, sustained return to work without recurrence of the condition. Some proponents have suggested that FCAs actually protect the worker because they can confirm when it is safe for the worker to return to their job. The latter is a particular problem in that chronic low-back pain, for example, is a recurrent condition and about 18–22% of people who have absented from work will get a second episode within a year. Gross et al (2004) found that although only 4% of workers tested passed all elements of the FCA, most returned to work, demonstrating a poor predictive ability for that series of tests. Although better performance on the tests was related to a quicker return to work, the amount of variance explained was only 7%. In a previous report by the same group, 20% of people who had an episode of back pain and work absence absented from work again within a year. In contrast to expectations, better performance on the FCA was related to increased risk of a recurrence.

Implications for pain management

In conclusion, although a lot of time and money have been invested in the development of FCA, there is still only poor evidence that FCA can be used to predict safe and sustainable return to work. It can offer a measure of the level of performance that an individual is willing or able to undertake, but its apparent objectivity is illusory since the interpretation of performance, particularly in the context of fearful patients with significant pain problems, is significantly problematic; it is therefore of extremely limited usefulness in the context of routine pain management.

Measures of disability

There are a number of self-report disability scales from which the clinician can choose. However, many are disorder specific. The Roland and Morris Disability Questionnaire (Roland & Morris 1983), for example, is designed for the assessment of low-back-pain-associated disability, although later versions have been adapted for use in general pain populations. Others have been used in a wide variety of chronic pain conditions and therefore will be briefly reviewed here. They vary greatly in length, a factor that may be important if there are constraints in terms of time or patient compliance (as when patients are requested to complete large numbers of questionnaires). The obvious advantage of the longer questionnaires, however, is that they give a more comprehensive appraisal of the chronic pain problem (and often incorporate measures of pain, coping and adaptation into their structure), though these may be less sensitive and reliable than instruments designed specifically to look at these constructs. The same considerations with regard to reliability, validity and reproducibility discussed earlier of course still apply. A careful review of the literature is recommended before the clinician opts for one instrument over another.

Composite measures

A number of self-report measures have been developed that contain several scales to represent multifactorial outcomes of interest such as health, the impact of pain or the pain experience itself. These have been reported in outcome studies of pain management and musculoskeletal pain and so have a good track record. Their wide appeal makes them suitable for comparing different treatment centres. Some can be quite time consuming to complete (e.g. the SIP contains 136 questions). In contrast, shorter indices have constructed scales from very few items (e.g. the role-emotional scale of the SF-36) and it is unlikely that such scales act as good indicators for individual change. Calculating scores on some of these indices can be complicated and time consuming. Despite their drawbacks, they remain a substantial improvement over the many poorly validated unidimensional measures. Efforts to construct meaningful indexes of physical tests have had little success – there is simply no consensus on how to weight and amalgamate them.

Sickness impact profile (SIP)

The Sickness Impact Profile (Bergner et al 1981) is a well-researched, wide-ranging and comprehensive assessment of disability, physical and social functioning. It is split into three major sections covering all areas of activity including physical activity, psychosocial, recreational and work activities and has 12 specific category scores. Normative data is available for healthy controls and subject groups with differing conditions including chronic pain groups. It was developed for use with people with chronic illness and not specifically for those with chronic pain. It has been demonstrated to have good reliability in chronic pain patients and correlates with avoidance of activity in low-back pain subjects. It has been demonstrated to be sensitive to changes following

cognitive–behavioural interventions in a group of general chronic pain patients and low-back pain patients (Follick et al 1985, Harding et al 1994, Williams et al 1996). Some observers have suggested (Deyo & Inui 1984) that it may be a more appropriate measure of deteriorating health rather than improvement. The major disadvantage of the SIP is its length (136 items), making it possibly the longest disability measure. Other workers have produced shortened disability measures based on the SIP categories for specific patient groups (e.g. Roland & Morris 1983).

Short Form 36 (SF-36)

The Short Form 36 (Ware & Sherbourne 1992) has eight subcategories covering the areas of physical functioning, role-physical, role-emotional, bodily pain, general health, vitality, social functioning and mental health. These scales can be summarised into physical and mental health scales. Normative data sets graded by age and sex are available and population norms have been developed for chronic pain and chronic illness groups. It must be pointed out that the inclusion and exclusion criteria for the subjects in these population norms are very broad and rather vague. They relied heavily on patients' reports of physician diagnoses. The SF-36 has an advantage of being relatively short and easy to score when compared with other measures. It has demonstrated very good reliability and repeatability in both normal population and chronic illness groups. It has been recommended as a generic outcome measure for use in a variety of conditions. It has been translated into a number of different languages, and shorter versions for use in different clinical and research settings have been developed. It and shorter derivatives are promoted though a well-maintained website (SF-36).

Chronic Illness Problem Inventory (CIPI)

The Chronic Illness Problem Inventory (Kames et al 1984) addresses all problem areas associated with chronic illness. It has 19 individual scales, including scales for physical limitation, psychosocial functioning, healthcare usage and marital changes. It is still a formidable length (65 items) but is shorter and more easily scored than the SIP. It has been demonstrated to be reliable in a variety of chronic diseases, including chronic respiratory and chronic pain patients (Kames et al 1984) and differentiates these groups from healthy controls. The responses are graded from 0 (not at all) to 4 (very much) allowing an insight into the degree of perceived disability as well as the perception of the existence of a problem. This is not possible with some of the dichotomous 'yes/no' responses in some disability questionnaires. In a study by Romano et al (1992) the CIPI was sensitive to changes following a pain management programme and it correlated highly with the SIP in chronic low-back pain patients and was demonstrated to correlate with pain report, reclining time and overt pain behaviours. However, the group in this study were moderately disabled and demonstrated low levels of overt pain behaviour and the relationships between the variables may be different in a more disabled group. To date few studies have reported using the CIPI to judge its usefulness in a wide variety of pain conditions.

Pain Disability Index (PDI)

The Pain and Disability Index (Pollard 1984) was designed to be a short and quick-to-use multidimensional measure of disability. It is divided into seven categories requiring the respondent to chose responses on a Likert scale scored from 0 to 10. The test–retest reliability was demonstrated to be only modest in a relatively small group of chronic pain patients. It has been seen to correlated highly with other limited measures (also Likert scales) of self-report of disability (downtime, stopping activity) but did not correlate significantly with observed downtime (Tait et al 1990). Interestingly the scores for the PDI were significantly correlated with patients self-scoring their own pain behaviour, suggesting that the scores on the PDI are related to the communication of pain behaviour. Comparisons with a wide variety of observed physical activity data are not available to confirm this, however. Although the PDI is short and easy to score it has not been compared with other more established measures of dysfunction and disability to assess its validity.

Multidimensional Pain Inventory (MPI)

Developed by Kerns et al. (1985) as the West Haven–Yale Multidimensional Pain Inventory, this was an attempt to identify not only the impact of patients' pain on their function but also the response of others to this pain, the level of distress associated with the pain and a gross assessment of the coping style (adaptive coping subgroup) and perceived control. As such it is not purely a measure of disability or functional interference. It was developed from a cognitive–behavioural view of disability, hence the assessment of factors that influence disability as well as measures of functional interference. Responses to the questionnaire have been clustered into three groups (dysfunctional, interpersonally distressed and adaptive copers). It is a relatively brief instrument; it has been used widely

in a broad range of pain-associated conditions and has demonstrated excellent reproducibility since its original development.

Brief Pain Inventory

As its name suggests, this is a short and simple instrument which assesses the three dimensions of pain report, pain relief through medication and pain interference in daily life, including sleep. Originally developed for use in cancer pain, its brevity has made it popular in pain clinics (Cleeland & Ryan 1994). It repeatedly has been demonstrated to be robust and have good face and internal validity on its two main scales of pain intensity and pain interference. The pain relief scale seems less well researched and rarely reported. It has an added advantage in that it has been translated into many different languages, although there are insufficient comparisons between languages to justify combining the results from different language groups into one data set.

Occupational outcome

Assessment of outcome is difficult not only because of the wide range of possible measures (such as pain severity, impaired functioning, distress, health-care usage and return to work) but because different stakeholders may differ in the importance they give to the alternative outcome measures.

The pre-eminence of occupational variables as outcome measures for pain management in North America, for example, is a direct consequence of the socioeconomics of health care where there is an important relationship between the provision of health insurance, the workplace and employer through the Workmen's Compensation Board schemes. Satisfactory return to work in this situation is considered to be the main criterion of success of treatment programmes since they are usually established and funded with the specific aim of enabling people to return to work.

Treatment programmes in the UK, however, frequently include patients who are unemployed and may have been so for a considerable time. Richardson et al (1994) reported that in a group of general pain patients recruited onto a pain management programme 74% of the subjects were unemployed. Waddell et al (2003) reported that 46% of persons claiming sickness and invalidity benefit for back pain were not employed at the commencement of benefit. Unemployed people with pain face unique additional problems in returning to work which cannot be addressed through medical intervention

Box 7.10

Appropriateness to undertake active job seeking or return to work

- Level of fitness
- Strength
- Range of movement
- Tolerance for exercise or sustained posture
- Vigilance and concentration
- Medication use
- Psychological obstacles to return to work (yellow and blue flags).

Box 7.11

Occupational outcome following rehabilitation

1 Full return to previous job at long-term follow-up (1–2 years?)
2 Obtaining new job and remaining at work at long-term follow-up (1–2 years?)
3 Returning to old job (temporarily on a part-time basis)
4 Returning to old job (but with restricted duties)
5 Return to only part-time work
6 Sheltered work (on a full- or part-time basis)
7 Not working (assuming availability of work)
8 Medically retired.

alone (Watson & Patel 2006). Such patients frequently do not feature in North American programmes. These issues are explored in more detail in Chapters 14 and 15 where issues of work retention and work rehabilitation are explored in a lot more detail. Some considerations concerning work are shown in Box 7.10.

Outcome data in terms of work status may not therefore be comparable. It has to be recognised that post-treatment work status is determined not only by response to pain management but also by the availability of work and marketable job skills. Nonetheless, as far as many patients are concerned, staying at work or returning to it is of prime importance and, although traditionally this has not been targeted as the principal objective of rehabilitation, recent initiatives by the UK government specifically encourage partnerships between employers, the Department of Health (DoH) and the Department of Work and Pensions (DWP 2006). Fundamental to evaluation of the impact of any such changes will be the assessment of work status and movement towards employment.

Work status

The impact of rehabilitation on work has to be considered in the context of *previous* work status, and also in the context of job availability. High levels of unemployment make it particularly difficult for individuals with a history of musculoskeletal pain or injury to obtain work. Increase in litigation requires consideration of the degree of risk of further injury facing a potential employer in considering employing or re-employing someone with a history of injury. Studies into the success of rehabilitation have varied in their definition of successful outcome. Outcome has to be measured against the goals for the individual and the objectives of the programme. There may be several 'stakeholders' all having different criteria for successful outcome. For those not intending

to adopt paid employment following treatment (such as housewives, the elderly or schoolchildren) working status may not be an appropriate outcome measure.

Suggestions for classification in terms of occupational outcome following rehabilitation are shown in Box 7.11. (Work retention and rehabilitation and the varying stakeholder perspectives are discussed in more detail in Chs 14 and 15.)

Conclusion

At the beginning of this chapter we revisited the challenge put by Peat (2000) to adopt a systematic approach to assessment. However, a systematic approach is important not only for research but for individual clinical management since without careful assessment, it is impossible to arrive at a competent clinical decision about treatment. However complex the ultimate formulation of a patient's set of problems, it is important to recognise that the patient presented initially with pain and pain-associated incapacities and it is sensible therefore to use a number of measures of differing types in order to ensure a broad and accurate assessment of the patient group.

As we have illustrated, the assessment of pain, disability and physical function is fraught with pitfalls and there is a wide range of options in terms of what to measure and how to measure it. We have stressed that it is essential to use measures that are clinically relevant and suitable for the purpose. Thus, in the evaluation of clinical treatment, measurement of outcome must be made with a tool that is not only sensitive to change but must also describe the population being treated

Box 7.12

Clinical reasons for systematic assessment of pain, disability and physical functioning

- Initial evaluation of the significance of the pain problem
- Appraisal of the relative importance of various aspects of the patient's difficulties
- Correcting any iatrogenic confusion or misunderstanding
- Alleviation of iatrogenic distress and anger
- Identification of possible treatment objectives
- Decision about specific treatment strategies
- Monitoring of change
- Evaluation of outcome.

accurately. Assessment of pain, reported disability and physical functioning is therefore absolutely fundamental.

We conclude by highlighting the principal clinical reasons for systematic assessment, shown in Box 7.12. (The specific assessment of the psychological factors

that influence pain, disability and physical functioning is addressed in the next chapter.)

Key points

- **Measurements of pain, disability and physical function should conform to minimum scientific criteria**
- **There are clear distinctions amongst impairment, physical capacity, physical performance and disability**
- **Measurement tools should be chosen with care and be dependent upon their intended use**
- **Self-report measures have significant limitations and should be chosen according to their intended use (e.g. case mix, outcome measures)**
- **Occupational outcome may be of particular importance but has been shown to be difficult to quantify**
- **The context of the measurement of pain behaviour will dictate which measure should be used.**

References

Al Obaidi S M, Nelson R M, Al-Alwadhi S et al 2000 The role of anticipation and fear of pain in the persistence of avoidance behavior in patients with chronic low back pain. Spine 25:1125–1131

American Physical Therapy Association 1997 Occupational health guidelines: evaluating functional capacity. American Physical Therapy Association, Alexandria, VA

Bergner M, Bobbitt R A, Carter W B et al 1981 The Sickness Impact Profile: development and final revision of a health status measure. Medical Care 19:787–805

Bieri D, Reeve R A, Champion G D et al 1990 The Faces Pain Scale for the self-assessment of the severity of pain experienced by children: development, initial validation, and preliminary investigation for ratio scale properties. Pain 41(2):139–150

Biering-Sorensen F 1984 Physical measurements as risk factors for low-back trouble over a one-year period. Spine 9:106–109

Boivie J, Hansson P, Lindblom U (eds) 1994 Progress in pain research and management, vol 3. Touch, temperature and pain in health and disease mechanisms and assessments IASP, Seattle

Cherkin D C, Deyo R A, Street J H et al 1996 Predicting poor outcomes for back pain seen in primary care using patients' own criteria. Spine 21(24):2900–2907

Cleeland C S, Ryan K M 1994 Pain assessment: global use of the Brief Pain Inventory. Annals of the Academy of Medicine Singapore 23(2):129–138

Crossman K, Mahon M, Watson P J et al 2004 Chronic low back pain-associated paraspinal muscle dysfunction is not the result of a constitutionally determined adverse fiber-type composition. Spine, 29: 628–634

Deyo R A, Inui T S 1984 Towards clinical applications of health status measures: sensitivity of scales to clinically important changes. Health Services Research 19:275–289

Dunn K, Croft P R 2005 Classification of low back pain in primary care: using 'Bothersomeness' to identify the most severe case. Spine 30:1887–1992

DWP (Department of Work and Pensions) 2006 A new deal for welfare: empowering people to work. HMSO, Norwich

Ensink F-B M, Saur P M M, Frese K et al 1996 Lumbar range of motion: influence of time of day and individual factors on measurements. Spine 21:1339–1343

Estlander A M, Vanharanta H, Moneta G B et al 1994 Anthropometric variables, self-efficacy beliefs and pain and disability ratings on the isokinetic performance of low back pain patients. Spine 19:941–947

Follick M J, Smith T W, Ahern D K 1985 The Sickness Impact Profile: a global measure of disability in chronic low back pain. Pain 21:67–75

Gronblad M, Hurri H, Kouri J-K 1997 Relationships between spinal mobility, physical performance tests, pain intensity and disability assessments in chronic low back pain patients. Scandinavian Journal of Rehabilitation Medicine 29:17–24

Gross D F 2004 Measurement properties of performance bases assessments of functional capacity. Journal of Occupational Rehabilitation 3:165–174

Gross D F, Battie M C, Cassidy J D 2004 The prognostic value of functional capacity evaluations in patients with chronic low back pain: Part 1. Timely return to work. Spine 29:914–919

Guyatt G H, Kirschner B, Jaeschke R 1992 Measuring health status: what are the necessary measurement properties? Journal of Clinical Epidemiology 45:1341–1345

Guyatt G H, Pugsley S O, Sullivan M J et al 1984 Effect of encouragement on walking test performance. Thorax 39:818–822

Harding V R, Williams A C, Richardson P H et al 1994 The development of a battery of measures for assessing physical functioning of chronic pain patients. Pain 58(3):367–375

Haythornthwaite J A, Fauerbach J A 2001 Assessment of acute pain, pain relief and patient satisfaction. In: Turk D C, Melzack R (eds) Handbook of pain assessment, 2nd edn. Guilford Press, New York, pp 417–431

Jensen M P, Karoly P 2001 Self report scales and procedures for assessing pain in adults. In: Turk D C, Melzack R (eds) Handbook of pain assessment, 2nd edn. Guilford Press, New York, pp 15–34

Kames L D, Naliboff B D, Heinrich R L et al 1984 The Chronic Illness Problem Inventory: problem-oriented psychosocial assessment of patients with chronic illness. International Journal of Psychiatry in Medicine 14:65–69

Kaplan G M, Wurtele S K, Gillis D 1996 Maximal effort during functional capacity evaluations: an examination of psychological factors. Archives of Physical Medicine and Rehabilitation 77:161–4

Kerns R D, Turk D C, Rudy T E 1985 The West-Haven Yale Multidimensional Pain Inventory (WHYMPI). Pain 23:345–356

King P M, Tuckwell N, Barrett T E 1998 A critical review of functional capacity evaluations. Physical Therapy 78:852–866

Koumentakis G A, Watson P J Oldham J A 2005 Supplementation of general endurance exercise with stabilisation training versus general exercise only. Physiological and functional outcomes of a randomised controlled trial of patients with recurrent low back pain. Clinical Biomechanics 20:474–482

Lackner J M, Carosella A M, Feuerstein M 1996 Pain expectancies, pain and functional self-efficacy expectancies as determinants of disability in patients with chronic low back disorders. Journal of Consulting and Clinical Psychology 64(1):212–220

Levine F M, De Simone L L 1991 The effects of experimenter gender on pain report in male and female subjects. Pain 44:69–72

Main C J, Robinson J P, Watson P J 2005 Disability, incapacity and rehabilitation for pain patients. In: Justins D M (ed) Pain 2005 – an updated review: Refresher course syllabus. Seattle, IASP Press, ch 34, pp 331–340

Margolis R B, Tait R C, Krause S J 1986 A rating system for use with patient pain drawings. Pain 24:57–65

Matheson L, Mooney V, Caiozzi V et al 1992 Effect of instructions on isokinetic trunk strength testing variability, reliability, absolute value, and predictive validity. Spine 17:914–921

Melzack R 1975 The McGill Pain Questionnaire: major properties and scoring methods. Pain 1:277–299

Melzack R 1987 The Short-Form McGill Pain Questionnaire. Pain 30:191–197

Mooney V 2002 Functional capacity evaluation. Orthopedics 25:1094–1099

Newton M, Thow M, Sommerville D et al 1993 Trunk strength testing with iso-machines, part 2: experimental evaluation of the Cybex II back testing machine in normal subjects and patients with chronic low back pain. Spine 18:812–824

Parker H, Wood P L R, Main C J 1995 The use of the pain drawing as a screening measure to predict psychological distress in chronic low back pain. Spine 20:236–243

Paulsen J S, Altmaier E M 1995 The effects of perceived versus enacted social support on the discriminative cue function of spouses for pain behaviors. Pain 60:103–110

Peat G M 2000 Evaluation of outcome. In: Main C J, Spanswick C C (eds) Pain management: an interdisciplinary approach. Churchill Livingstone, Edinburgh, ch 17, pp 363–385

Pollard C A 1984 Preliminary validity study of the Pain Disability Index. Perceptual and Motor Skills 59:974

Price D D, Harkins S W 1992 Psychophysiological approaches to pain measurement and assessment. In: Turk D C, Melzack R (eds) Handbook of pain assessment, 1st edn. Guilford Press, New York, pp 111–134

Price D D, Riley J L III, Wade J B 2001 Psychophysical approaches to pain measurement of the dimensions and stages of pain. In: Turk D C, Melzack R (eds) Handbook of pain assessment, 2nd edn. Guilford Press, New York, pp 53–75

Ransford A O, Cairns D, Mooney V 1976 The pain drawing as an aid to the psychological evaluation of patients with low back pain. Spine 1:27–134

Richardson I H, Richardson P H, Williams A C et al 1994 The effects of a cognitive-behavioural pain management programme on the quality of work and employment status of severely impaired chronic pain patients. Disability and Rehabilitation 16:26–34

Roland M, Morris R 1983 A study in the natural history of back pain. Part I: development of a reliable and sensitive measure of disability in low-back pain. Spine 8(2): 141–144

Romano J M, Turner J A, Freidman L S et al 1992 Sequential analysis of chronic pain behaviours and spouse responses. Journal of Consulting and Clinical Psychology 60: 777–782

Rothwell J C 1987 Control of human voluntary movement. Croom Helm, London

Roy S H, DeLuca C J, Emley M et al 1997 Classification of back muscle impairment based on the surface electro-myographic signal. Journal of Rehabilitation Research and Development 34:405–414

SF-36 website. www.sf-36.com

Simmonds M J, Olson S L, Jones S et al 1998 Psychometric characteristics and clinical usefulness of physical performance test in patients with low back pain. Spine 23:2412–2421

Stratford P W, Binkley F M, Riddle D M 1996 Health status measures: strategies and analytic methods for assessing change scores. Physical Therapy 76:1109–1123

Tait R C, Chibnall J T, Krause S 1990 The Pain Disability Index; psychometric properties. Pain 40:171–182

Turk D C, Melzack R (eds) 2001 Handbook of pain assess-ment, 2nd edn. Guilford Press, New York

Verbunt J A, Westerterp K R, van der Heijden G J et al 2001 Physical activity in daily life in patients with chronic low back pain. Archives of Physical Medicine and Rehabilitation 82:726–730

Verbunt J A, Sieben J M, Seelen H A et al 2005 Decline in physical activity, disability and pain-related fear in sub-acute low back pain. European Journal of Pain 9(4):417–425

Vlaeyen J W S 1991 Chronic low back pain: assessment and treatment from a behavioural rehabilitation perspective. Swets & Zeitlinger, Amsterdam

Waddell G (ed.) 2004 The back pain revolution, 2nd edn. Churchill Livingstone, Edinburgh

Waddell G, Aylward M, Sawney P 2003 Back pain, incap-acity for work and social security benefits Royal Society of Medicine, London

Ware J E, Sherbourne C D 1992 The MOS 36-item short-form health survey (SF-36). I Conceptual framework and item selection. Medical Care 30(6):473–483

Watson P J 1999 Non-physiological determinants of phys-ical performance in musculoskeletal pain. Pain 1999 – an updated review. IASP, Seattle, pp 153–159

Watson P J, Patel S 2006 Chronic pain and the benefits system: obstacles to returning to work for unemployed people. Topical issues in pain, vol 5. CNS Press, Falmouth, pp 175–194

WHO 2000 International classification of functioning disabil-ity and health (ICF). Geneva, World Health Organization

Williams A C, Richardson P H, Nicholas M K et al 1996 Inpatient vs. outpatient pain management: results of a randomised controlled trial. Pain 66(1):13–22

Wittink H, Hoskins-Michel T, Wagner A et al 2000 Deconditioning in patients with chronic low back pain: fact or fiction? Spine 25:2221–2228

APPENDIX 7.1

A brief review based on the observations by Price & Harkins (1992)

Measure	Description	Comments
Visual Analogue Scale	Patients mark a point on a 10-cm line indicating their level of pain between two 'anchors' such as 'no pain' to 'pain as bad as it could be' for intensity and 'not at all bad' to 'the most unpleasant feeling possible' for affective assessment. Operator measures the distance from the zero anchor in millimetres.	Can be considered to have ratio scale properties. Scored quickly to give feedback to clinician. Sensitive to treatment effects. Good evidence for reliability and repeatability for both affective and intensity scales. Good evidence for discrimination between affective and intensity domains. Explanations to patient need to be clear and may influence rating. Elderly people, drowsy patients, and people of low intelligence find them less easy to use than other measures.
Numerical Rating Scale	Patients are asked to verbally rate their pain on a scale of either 1–10 (NRS 11) or 1–100 (NRS 101) between two anchor points as described in the VAS.	Can be considered to have ratio scale properties. Rating is instant and does not have the potential for measurement error in the VAS. NRS 101 offers a large number of response categories and so is sensitive to change. NRS 11 is not as sensitive to change as the VAS. NRS for affective change is poorly researched, requires explanation and may still not be understood by elderly or drowsy patients.
Verbal Rating Scales	Lists of words are presented to the patient to assess either the intensity or the affective domain. Patients are asked to choose from the list one that best describes the intensity or the affective component of their pain. Scores are assigned to the words in increasing levels of intensity or affect. Current scales use 5, 6 or 15 points.	Represents ordinal data. Rating is instant. Requires a level of understanding and reading ability not necessary in other measures. Allows a choice of only one word which may not fit the patients own description. Reliability may not be as good as other measures.
Picture Scale (Pain Faces scale)	Line drawings of eight faces representing a person experiencing different levels of pain intensity are presented to the patient and they choose the one which best represents their pain. The response is scored from 0 to 7.	Data is ordinal. Intended for the assessment of intensity but may more closely represent the affective domain. Easy to use and score. Useful in those who are unable to understand other measures (does not rely on understanding written instructions). Little data on the validity. Limited evidence for sensitivity to treatment. Limited 8-point scale.

(Continued)

A brief review based on the observations by Price & Harkins (1992) (Continued)

Measure	Description	Comments
McGill Pain Questionnaire (MPQ)	Consists of 20 subclasses of grouped words; a categorical evaluation of the pain (the PPI) which uses a no pain anchor and 5 affective descriptive words and a pain drawing with description of the nature of the pain. The responses from the 20 subclasses are scored, based on their ranked value in the subgroup, into sensory, affective, evaluative and miscellaneous domains and summed to give a total score. A PPI categorical evaluation provides an additional score. The number of words chosen is also recorded.	Multidimensional instrument assessing all areas of pain response and intensity. Frequently used as ratio data but may be more representative of ordinal data. Complex scoring does not give immediate feedback and may result in errors. Widely used with very good evidence on validity repeatability and reliability in a wide range of conditions. Sensitive to change in affect and sensory components. Discriminates the affective and sensory components. Reliance on descriptive words, some of which may be unfamiliar to many patients. Unsuitable for use in those with difficulty reading or low educational level. Responses differ between clinical groups.
Short-form MPQ (SF-MPQ)	Patients are required to choose from 15 descriptive words (11 sensory and 4 affective) those that best describe their pain, and rank the intensity of that word from none to severe. A VAS scale for intensity and the PPI scale are also included.	Assesses the multidimensional aspects of pain. Frequently used as ratio data but may be more representative of ordinal data. Less complex than the MPQ. Scoring errors may occur. Evidence for reliability, repeatability and validity in wide number of conditions. Some evidence for differential responses from different clinical groups. Unsuitable for use in those with difficulty reading or low educational level. Demonstrates sensitivity to changes in the affective, sensory and intensity domains.

Chapter Eight

8

Psychological assessment

CHAPTER CONTENTS

Introduction

The purpose and content of a psychological evaluation will depend on whether the assessment is 'stand-alone' or part of a multidisciplinary assessment, and in the latter case on the scheduling of the psychological component within the rest of the assessment clinic. Nonetheless, there are a number of general issues common to all such assessments. The distinction between psychological factors requiring independent specialised management (characterised as orange flags) instead of, or as a precursor to, pain management has already been discussed in Chapter 3. The detection of psychosocial risk factors for the development of chronicity (yellow flags) has been discussed in Chapter 5, and will be discussed later in terms of clinical management in Chapter 10.

In this chapter, the focus will be on the identification of mental health problems as possible targets for psychological intervention and on the psychological risk factors for pain and disability.

General context

Historically, psychological assessments have been used for a variety of purposes such as the identification of psychological disorders, screening in the context of treatment planning, in providing descriptions of the psychological characteristics of groups of patients (whether in the context or research or clinical audit) and in the evaluation of outcome of treatment, but it is perhaps useful to begin with consideration of them in terms of a number of general objectives, shown in Box 8.1.

Box 8.1

General objectives of initial psychological assessment

- Determining general suitability for pain management
- Identifying specific psychological targets for treatment
- Identifying specific psychological obstacles to reactivation.

Box 8.2

Specific aims of the initial psychological assessment

- Assessment of psychopathology, primarily in the context of whether or not patients are likely to benefit from a pain management approach
- Assessment of specific mental health problems as specific targets for intervention, whether within the pain management service or as a precursor to it
- Assessment of psychological factors, specifically as risk factors for pain persistence or chronicity.

Box 8.3

Primary sources of psychological information

- Clinical documentation and history
- Clinical interview
- Psychometric assessment.

In the context of pain management, however, there has been a move away from the general assessment of psychological factors, of which there are many, and from using specific psychometric tools, of which there are a huge number, towards more targeted psychological assessments focused on clinical decision making.

This chapter will focus on a number of specific objectives as outlined in Box 8.2. (This chapter in turn will map on to the nature of psychological techniques (Ch. 10) and to the content of interdisciplinary pain management (Ch. 11).) As a precursor to the discussion of the content of these specific applications, the nature of psychological assessments will be reviewed.

Methods of assessment

At the time of initial clinical presentation, there may be wide variation in the amount of information accompanying the referral. Direct access clinics, particularly in North America, may require little more than patient assent and guarantee of reimbursement. In contrast, tertiary-care clinics in other parts of the world may require not only medical referral, but the supply of all relevant clinical documentation and a range of self-report schedules completed by the patient. Consequently, there may be a wide range of potentially relevant information, which may be illuminating in its own right, or may serve to shape the content and emphasis of the initial psychological evaluation. The primary sources of information are shown in Box 8.3.

Whenever possible, the assessment of psychological factors should not rely on information obtained from a single source, but should be the product of a combination of the methods above.

Clinical documentation and history

As previously mentioned, the amount of clinical history that 'accompanies' the patient can vary widely in practice. However, even a small amount of information can be illuminating. Particular attention should be paid to the patient's prior history of pain problems and treatment received, and to the patient's response to these experiences. Most of the information will be provided by third parties whose opinion may or may not have been biased or inaccurate and must, therefore, be considered as provisional, and requiring confirmation from the patient. Nonetheless, if one has the opportunity to evaluate material prior to the assessment of the patient, one may be able to identify a number of key features in the patient's clinical history, which can be useful both as a focal point for the subsequent interview, and as a means of comparing the treating clinician's account with the patient's own perspective. Significant discrepancies between the two should alert the assessor to iatrogenic confusion or distress as possible influences on the patient's self-disclosure. When reaching discussion of possible objectives for a pain management approach, detailed documentation on what has previously been offered in the way of treatment can facilitate discussion of the specific benefits of further pain management.

Finally, an appraisal of other aspects of clinical history may provide a more general picture of how the patient has previously responded to symptoms, illness and various approaches to treatment. A patient's clinical history may also indicate pre-existing psychological vulnerabilities in terms of psychological difficulties, thereby alerting the assessor to the possibility of an ongoing psychiatric disorder that might compromise a patient's likely benefit from pain management, and suggest the need for an orange flag triage.

The clinical interview: general issues

The clinical interview should be carried out by a clinical psychologist experienced in working with patients with chronic pain using a cognitive–behavioural approach. It is strongly recommended that a semi-structured interview is used to make sure that all relevant areas are covered in the interview, but also to ensure a degree of consistency in information gathering across patients, whether for the purpose of audits or research.

The precise format of the interview will depend on factors such as the type of pain problem being evaluated and the need to consider which areas are being addressed by other members of the team, since unnecessary duplication (i.e. beyond the issue of clarification) is not only wasteful but also irritating to the patient and should be avoided, if possible.

If the psychological interview occurs as part of the initial assessment process, patients may still be wedded fairly firmly to a dualistic concept of pain, and may be concerned that the role of the psychologist is to somehow 'prove' that they are either mentally ill or that their pain is 'all in the mind'. Thus, a small proportion of patients may be overtly hostile at the start of the assessment. It is therefore vital that in the early stages of the interview the psychologist attempts to explain, in terms that can be easily understood by the patient, the purpose of the interview. It may be useful to stress that the psychological interview is a *routine* part of the assessment process, that the patient's pain is being taken seriously, and that no one believes the patient's pain is 'all in their mind'. It can also be of great value to stress the 'normality' of distress in individuals with chronic pain.

Psychometric assessment

There are a number of key points to consider when selecting psychometric tests. These are shown in Box 8.4.

In this section a brief overview will be given of the more important aspects of psychometric assessment. The issues are presented in much more depth

Box 8.4

Overall considerations in the use of psychometric tests

- What is the purpose for which I wish to use the test?
- Has this test been standardised for use with the particular patient population that I wish to employ it with?
- Is the test both reliable and valid for the purposes for which I wish to use the test?
- Are there adequate norms for the test?
- If selecting a test battery: how many different measures can I reasonably expect the patient to complete?
- Who will administer the tests, where will they be administered and who will score the tests?
- Who will interpret the test results?

in sources such as Nunnally & Bernstein (1994) and Groth-Marnat (2003).

The importance of reliability and validity in measurement

It is of great importance that any psychological measures selected should be reliable and valid and that they have been standardised for use with the patient population. Thus a measure standardised for use with chronic low-back pain may well not be appropriate for use with neck pain. In order to evaluate whether the psychometric measures chosen meet the above criteria, it will be necessary for the clinician to refer to the relevant research literature (Groth-Marnat 2003). The following section provides an overview of the concepts of reliability and validity. The major types of reliability and validity are shown in Box 8.5.

Reliability of measures

Within the assessment of chronic pain, there are three main types of reliability measures that will be of concern to the clinician in the selection of appropriate assessments: the coefficient of stability, the coefficient of internal consistency, and inter-rater reliability.

Coefficient of stability

Also known as test–retest reliability, this measure assesses the stability of the results of a test over time. The test is administered to the same group of individuals

Box 8.5

Major types of reliability and validity

Reliability of measures
- Coefficient of stability
- Coefficient of internal consistency
- Inter-rater reliability.

Validity of measures
- Face validity
- Content validity
- Criterion-related validity
- Construct validity
- Discriminant and convergent validity.

on two separate occasions and the results are correlated. The closer the correlation coefficient approaches to a score of 1, the more reliable the measure can be said to be. Williams (1988) indicates that reliability coefficients above 0.85 are generally regarded as high and those between 0.6 to 0.85 as being moderate.

When selecting measures, consideration should be given to the size of the test–retest interval (in general, the shorter the interval, the higher the reliability coefficient). Very short intervals give some cause for concern, as it is probable that those taking the test for the second time will recall their previous answers and these memories will influence their new responses. A further consideration is that for a number of measures it is probable that the construct being measured will not be stable over time and that this will lead to lowered test–retest reliability levels. For example, coping strategy use may alter with the passage of time, which would lead to a reduction in test–retest reliability. Changes in the underlying disorder giving rise to pain may also lead to the reduction of test–retest reliability. For example, if a measure of depressive symptomatology is assessed in the context of a disorder such as rheumatoid arthritis (in which pain levels can fluctuate over time) a low test–retest reliability coefficient may be a reflection of changes in pain levels, rather than any inadequacies of the measure being used.

Coefficient of internal consistency

This is a measure of the consistency of content sampling, and it examines whether any single item in a particular scale measures the same thing as the other scale items. The most common method of assessing internal consistency is Cronbach's alpha coefficient. Generally, coefficient sizes range from 0 to 1, and the higher the

coefficient, the higher the internal consistency of the scale. Todd & Bradley (1996) indicate that for a scale with 10 items or more, coefficients of 0.7–0.8 are acceptable. Excessively high values (e.g. 0.9 and above) generally indicate the redundancy of scale items, and those lower than 0.7 indicate that the scale is too diffuse.

Inter-rater reliability

Within pain assessment, this type of reliability is most commonly used in the evaluation of behavioural observation methods. The most appropriate method for assessing inter-rater reliability is Cohen's Kappa statistic. Simple percentage agreement figures are a poor substitute for the Kappa statistic, as they can lead to overinflated estimates of reliability. Values of Kappa can range from -1 to $+1$ with higher ratings indicating increased agreement. Landis & Koch (1977) indicate that values of 0.41–0.60 can be considered moderate, values of 0.61–0.80 can be considered substantial, and values of 0.81–1 can be considered almost perfect.

Validity of measures

The validity of a test gives an indication of how well a particular test measures what it claims to measure. For example, does a test of depressive symptomatology actually measure this area, or does it measure symptoms that are related to pain? Four types of validity are important with respect to the evaluation of measures: face validity, content validity, criterion-related validity and construct validity (including discriminant and convergent validity).

Face validity

Face validity is not validity in the true sense of the word, but refers to what a test appears to be measuring. Face validity can be of particular importance in assuring patient cooperation and motivation to complete tests. This is of particular importance when questionnaires are sent by mail, so that the clinician does not have the opportunity to explain the reason for the use of certain tests. The higher the face validity, the more likely the patient will cooperate in the completion of the test. Measures such as the McGill Pain Questionnaire will have high face validity for the majority of pain patients.

Content validity

This will determine whether the items of a particular test cover a representative sample of the area that is being measured. For example, a measure of depression should not be limited to questions relating only to appetite and sleep, nor should a measure of pain behaviour be limited to the evaluation of only facial expressions.

Criterion-related validity

Criterion-related validity will indicate how well a test is able to predict a person's behaviour in specific situations (predictive validity), or its ability to diagnose an existing state (concurrent validity). When concurrent validity is being evaluated, the test will generally be compared with a 'gold standard' (i.e. the best currently available method for assessing the particular area); thus, for example, a measure of depressive symptomatology may be compared with a DSM-IV diagnosis of depressive disorders.

Construct validity

Construct validity refers to the extent to which a test measures hypothetical constructs or traits, such as, for example, beliefs about the understandability of pain. There are a number of methods used to examine this aspect of validity. Factor analysis is often used with multi-scale tests (e.g. Pain Beliefs and Perceptions Inventory) (Williams & Thorn 1989) to confirm the presence of discrete subscales.

Both discriminant and convergent validity are forms of construct validity. In discriminant validity, the aim is to demonstrate that the test does not correlate with other measures of dissimilar constructs, and in convergent validity the aim is to demonstrate that the measure correlates well with other measures of similar or identical constructs.

Common problems encountered in the use of psychometric measures

The common problems encountered in the use of psychological tests are shown in Box 8.6.

Inadequate psychometric properties

The reliability and validity of the test may not have been adequately investigated for the patient population for which the test is used. In certain cases, while investigators report reliability and validity information on a test, the sample used is either inadequately described and/or is heterogeneous for types of pain. For example, the sample may comprise patients suffering cancer pain, headache and low-back pain.

Confusion between psychological symptoms and physical limitations

This problem is most commonly encountered when measures originally developed for use with, and standardised on, psychiatric populations are used to assess

Box 8.6

Common problems in use of psychometric measures

- Inadequate psychometric properties
- Confusion between psychological symptoms and physical limitations
- Lack of comparability between groups of patients studied
- Lack of normative data.

patients with chronic pain, since a number of the symptoms of certain psychiatric disorders and pain are common to both groups. The most commonly encountered tests that fall under this category are: personality tests such as the Minnesota Multiphasic Personality Inventory (Hathaway et al 1989), screening tests for psychopathology such as the Symptom Checklist, or SCL-90 (Derogatis 1983), General Health Questionnaire, or GHQ (Goldberg & Williams 1988), and measures such as the Beck Depression Inventory (Beck et al 1996) and Anxiety Inventory (Beck & Steer 1990). Such tests frequently include items relating to physical factors that may lead to the production of 'false positive' errors as patients may endorse such items as a consequence of their pain, and not as a consequence of any underlying psychopathology. For example, the SCL-90 Psychoticism Scale contains the following item: 'The idea that something serious is wrong with your body.' Obviously this item may well be endorsed by a patient with chronic pain as a consequence of his or her medical problems (or their beliefs about what is wrong with them), in which case the endorsement would not be indicative of psychotic thinking.

Lack of comparability between groups of patients studied

Even if adequate psychometric properties have been demonstrated for one type of pain, it cannot be assumed that the test will be reliable and valid for another pain type. For example, it cannot be assumed that a test developed and standardised for patients with arthritic pain will be either reliable and/or valid for patients with chronic low-back pain.

Lack of normative data

A surprising number of articles describing the development of tests specific for pain patients fail to give basic statistical information regarding the means and standard deviations of scores obtained. This lack makes it impossible to evaluate the significance of an individual's score.

Issues in the administration of psychometric measures

The purpose of the assessment will dictate to a large degree the type of tests selected. Each test must have a specific role to play in the evaluation process. There is little use in administering a large battery of tests only to have these languishing, unscored and unevaluated, in the back of the patient's notes. A number of considerations in the administration of psychometric measures are highlighted in Box 8.7.

In practice, patients rarely object to completing psychometric tests once they have understood their importance; indeed, they may regard such tests as an indication that their problems are being taken 'seriously'. Refusal to complete tests may be an initial indicator of the patient's ambivalence about the entire assessment process.

Problems may be encountered if patients possess limited intellectual abilities and/or have problems with reading. The clinician should be alerted to these possibilities by any of the following scenarios: the patient frequently inquires about the meanings of words/phrases used on the measure; the patient writes the answers rather than checking the appropriate place on the questionnaire; the patient asks the clinician what to put for his or her answers. In these circumstances, the clinician should use his or her experience to decide whether to continue with the assessment. Problems with reading

may be overcome by reading the questions aloud to the patient, although it must be noted that this may have an effect on the psychometric properties of the test and the clinician must resist the attempt to 'prompt' or answer for the patient.

A number of clinics elect to send a limited number of psychometric measures to the patient prior to the triage process in order to decide whether the patient is suitable for assessment and, if so, the type of assessment required. This method of administration has the advantage that the patient can complete the measures without feeling like they are under time pressure or being flustered by the stress of the initial assessment, which they may have invested with considerable significance. However, there are a number of disadvantages to this method. Patients may omit (either intentionally or unintentionally) questionnaire items (if too many items are omitted this will mean that it is not possible to score the test or to obtain much meaningful information from it); they may ask for help from family members in completing the assessments; and it is not possible to ascertain whether patients have completely understood the questionnaire instructions.

If patients complete psychometric assessments in the clinic, however, the importance of the measures can be stressed, any misconceptions cleared up, completed questionnaires can be checked for omitted items, and one can ensure that the questionnaires have been

Box 8.8

General aims and specific objectives of the initial psychological assessment

General aims

- Evaluation of presenting psychological characteristics
- Evaluation of mechanisms influencing the perception of pain and disability
- Identification of any psychological barriers to treatment
- Identification of whether further psychological treatment is required prior to embarking on pain management.

Specific objectives

- Determination of general suitability for pain management
- Identification of specific psychological targets for treatment
- Identification of specific psychological obstacles to reactivation.

Box 8.7

Reflections on the administration of psychometric measures

- Patients need to be persuaded of the relevance of the tests
- Reluctance to complete the tests may be indicative of a wider ambivalence about the whole assessment process
- It is important to be aware of potential linguistic or intellectual difficulties
- Sending out questionnaires in advance has some advantages but can also have drawbacks
- Except in very specific circumstances such as screening, formal psychometric assessment should constitute only part of the assessment.

completed with no outside assistance. The disadvantage to this process is that the patient will have to attend for a longer period of time.

There are obvious practical (and research/audit) advantages to the computerised administration and scoring of questionnaires if this is a practical possibility in the clinic concerned.

Overview of psychological assessment

The general aims of psychological assessment with three additional specific objectives are shown in Box 8.8.

Further consideration now will be given to the three specific objectives.

Determination of general suitability for pain management

In terms of general suitability, there is a wide range of psychosocial factors that may preclude active participation in pain management, and specific psychological factors are only one component of these. At the time of assessment, of course, patients do not normally specifically select which information they wish to disclose to health professionals, although they may have expectation about the range of topics likely to be addressed in the assessment by a particular health care professional. Nonetheless, the primary purpose of the psychological assessment is to focus on psychological issues.

Assessment of contra-indication to acceptance for pain management on specifically psychological grounds is effectively an orange flag assessment. This topic has already been addressed in Chapter 3, but, for the sake of convenience, the summary table is reproduced as Box 8.9.

Evidence of major personality disorders, substance abuse disorders, or current forensic involvement are all contra-indications likely to benefit from pain management. However, an ongoing psychiatric disorder should also be considered a temporary contra-indication; if the patient otherwise seems to be a good candidate for pain management, then it is reasonable to suggest a reassessment at a later date.

Similarly, difficulties in comprehension attributable to medication indicate a temporary obstacle to full participation in pain management, and again suggest a temporary deferment with a re-evaluation at a later date.

Difficulties in comprehension as a consequence of post-traumatic cognitive impairment, or other neuropsychological difficulties of a severity likely to compromise participation in the programme suggest the need for

an individualised clinical approach rather than a full pain management programme. Similarly, major communication problems resulting from illiteracy or the inability to communicate in the language of the programme

Box 8.9

Major types of orange flag

Flags indicative of unsuitability for pain management

Major personality disorder:

- evidence of aggressive or disruptive behaviour
- clear evidence of unwillingness to take any personal responsibility
- marked irritation at having to 'share treatment' (i.e. be part of a group).

Substance abuse disorder:

- concentration, cooperation or participation likely to be compromised by major recent or ongoing illicit drug use or markedly excessive alcohol use.

Current forensic involvement:

- scheduling of treatment or negotiation of reasonable rehabilitation goals not possible until resolution of ongoing forensic involvement.

Flags indicative of need for specialist referral

Active psychiatric disorder:

- showing evidence of psychotic symptoms such as disordered thinking, marked agitation
- under psychiatric management for ongoing psychiatric illness
- experiencing significant cognitive side-effects from medication.

Difficulties in comprehension (apart from medication side-effects):

- post-traumatic cognitive impairment
- other neuropsychological difficulties of a severity likely to compromise participation in programme.

Very high level of distress:

- unable to fully participate in assessment because of distress
- not able to participate in the establishment of treatment goals because of distress.

Major communication problems:

- illiteracy
- unable to communicate in the language of the programme.

represent obvious contra-indications, although these may be matters that the pain service needs to address more generally in terms of its overall service provision.

Finally, if the level of distress is compromising the patient's ability to fully participate in assessment or to identify appropriate treatment goals, their distress should be viewed as a temporary obstacle to participation in a full pain management programme. In that event, individual psychological therapy (whether 'in-house' or from mental health services) should be pursued prior to the reassessment of suitability for the pain management programme.

General issues in the assessment of psychopathology

The sort of assessment appropriate for a particular clinic will depend in part on whether there has been any 'filtering' of the patients who have been referred to the clinic. With open access to health care, particularly with a 'fee-for-service system' such as that which used to be the norm in the USA, there may have been no clinical decision as to the suitability of the patient for pain management. In the newer system of managed care, treatment is rationed. Treatment providers must pay careful attention to the selection of patients, since treatment outcome is used in marketing to attract new business. Since the screening carried out by HMOs (health maintenance organisations) is arguably more financially than clinically based, many treatment providers will carry out some sort of psychological screening.

In consideration for pain management, screening focuses primarily on the identification of primary psychological disorder (or psychiatric illness), defined in terms of either Axis I clinical disorders or Axis II personality (character) disorders.

Proper psychiatric diagnosis requires formal assessment according to established criteria such as that described in the Diagnostic and Statistical Manual of Mental Disorders, or DSM-IV (1994). There are two structured psychiatric interviews that produce reliable and valid psychiatric diagnoses based on the DSM-IV criteria. These are the Diagnostic Interview Schedule, or DIS (Eaton et al 1997) and the Structured Clinical Interview for DSM-IV, or SCID (Spitzer et al 1992). The DIS has some advantages in that there is computer software available that allow patients to self-administer the interview in the clinician's office. This software also allows the clinician to assess the patient's responses according to DSM-IV criteria and thus obtain a record

of the patient's lifetime psychiatric history. It is not appropriate at this juncture to consider psychiatric diagnosis in detail, but a brief comment will be made on each of the major categories highlighted above.

DSM-IV distinguishes clinical disorders (Axis I) from personality disorders (Axis II). Although the distinction is not absolutely clear-cut, with respect to the assessment of pain patients, the presence of Axis I disorders principally affects decisions related to the type of treatment that is likely to be most appropriate. The presence of Axis II disorders has a greater bearing on *whether* to offer treatment at all.

Axis I psychiatric disorders

The most common psychiatric diagnoses among pain patients are found in Box 8.10, and the most common DSM-IV diagnostic criteria are shown in Appendix 8.1.

Anxiety and depression seem to be the most relevant of the distinct psychiatric Axis I disorders in patients with chronic pain problems. The identification of *clinically significant* anxiety or depression may be important factors to consider in relation to primary or conjoint psychiatric treatment. In the context of chronic pain, however, anxiety is usually characterised by specific fears or concerns, and depression is usually secondary to pain and its disabling effects (and as such is most appropriately 'treated' with pain management techniques).

If a patient presents with a clinical history suggestive of long-standing ill-health affecting a variety of symptoms, then the assessment of a somatisation disorder may be indicated. If the patient has been injured in an

Box 8.10

Axis I diagnoses most commonly ascribed to pain patients

- Generalised anxiety disorder
- Anxiety due to a general medical condition
- Adjustment disorders
- Somatoform disorders
- Conversion disorder
- Hypochondriasis
- Depression
- Post-traumatic stress disorder
- Pain disorder.

How effective does the patient believe their coping strategies to be?

accident, however, then an assessment of post-traumatic stress disorder should be considered.

Identification of Axis II personality or character disorders

A personality disorder is defined as:

> an enduring pattern of inner experiences and behaviour that deviates markedly from the expectations of the individual's culture, is pervasive and inflexible, has an onset in adolescence or early adulthood, is stable over time and leads to distress or impairment (DSM-IV 1994, p. 629).

The major types of personality disorder are shown in Box 8A.11 (Appendix 8.1). A much fuller description of each of these syndromes is presented in DSM-IV (1994).

The ascription of personality disorder is not without controversy. It could be argued that the concept of personality disorder is as much a cultural as a clinical concept. In the prospective Boeing study into the development of chronic low-back pain (Bigos et al 1991), no *specific* personality disorder was found to predict chronic incapacity, but whether or not an individual had *any* personality disorder was found to be predictive. Since a major characteristic of such individuals is their (arguably) poor coping styles and strategies, in practical terms, it would seem more useful to consider the influence of personality in terms of behaviours or attitudes likely to compromise the individual's suitability for treatment, their likelihood of benefiting from treatment, and their likelihood of compromising the treatment of others.

According to Dersh et al (2002), personality disorders are thought to have their origin in childhood; hence, they usually antedate chronic pain and may be implicated in its development. Furthermore, an Axis II disorder may coexist with Axis I disorders such as anxiety or depression. Although specific personality disorders appear to be higher in groups of pain patients than in the general population, there is little consistency among the research groups. Gatchel et al (1995) suggest plausibly that Axis II disorders may be associated with coping skills deficits linked with chronic disability. According to Weisberg & Keefe (1999), personality patterns that are associated with marginally adaptive coping styles normally decompensate under the stress of injury, disability and pain; therefore, they can be thought of as a type of vulnerability factor.

In practice, it is difficult to make a clear distinction between personality disorders and other formal mental disorders, and even more difficult to reliably differentiate one personality from another (Zimmerman 1994). It may be important to identify certain types of personality disorders, such as alcohol abuse, substance abuse, or pathological lying, which might confound assessment or serve as a contra-indication to acceptance for treatment. This issue is particularly relevant within health systems offering direct access to care. Where the system requires a medical gatekeeper such as a general practitioner for referral, the need for a formal assessment may be unnecessary. A competent clinical history and review of medical notes should make MMPI screening unnecessary. Such characteristics are perhaps best considered as potential obstacles to rehabilitation or as orange flags (see below).

In conclusion, Gatchel (1996) has observed that when patients reach the more chronic stages of pain, there is usually some significant psychopathology that needs to be addressed. It might be argued that in terms of distress, fear, mistaken beliefs and dysfunctional coping strategies, psychopathology is an inherent component of the chronic pain syndrome. Indeed, the management and modification of such features is at the heart of interdisciplinary pain management. Alone, high rates of psychopathology in pain patients do not necessarily interfere significantly with their rehabilitation (Gatchel et al 1994). While recognising, therefore, that the adoption of a psychiatric perspective may be appropriate for the identification of primary psychiatric disorders and personality disorders, most patients should be evaluated from a psychological perspective.

Use of psychiatric taxonomy in the assessment of personal injury

As highlighted in Chapter 3, the persistence of pain and pain-associated incapacity frequently has an adverse psychological impact on patients. This may be evident in negative beliefs/expectation about pain and treatment, in emotional reactions and in pain coping strategies. This syndrome has been previously described as a 'psychologically mediated chronic pain syndrome' (Main 1999).

In the context of patients seeking redress for personal injury, the extent to which a psychologically mediated chronic pain syndrome should be classified as a psychiatric injury or not has been the subject of some debate. Historically, 'psychological injury' was defined in terms of identifiable psychiatric disorder, and although 'pain and suffering' were explicitly identified in terms of grounds for compensation, they were

Box 8.11

Criteria for psychological factors affecting a general medical condition

- A general medical condition is present
- Psychological factors adversely affect the medical condition in one of the following ways:
  - the factors have influenced the course of the general medical condition as shown by a close temporal association between the psychological factors and the development or exacerbation of, or delayed recovery from, the general medical condition
  - the factors interfere with the treatment of the general medical condition
  - the factors constitute additional health risks for the individual
  - stress-related physiological responses precipitate or exacerbate symptoms of the general medical condition.

Shapiro & Teasell (1998, p. 26)

not recognised as an injury as such. The DSM-IV recommends differentiation of *somatoform disorder* from *pain disorder*, and states:

> An additional diagnosis of Pain Disorder should be considered only if the pain is an independent focus of clinical attention, leads to clinically significant distress or impairment, and is in excess of that usually associated with the other mental disorder (DSM-IV 1994, p. 461).

In fact most cases of personal injury in which an expert psychological opinion is sought, claimants would be considered to have a pain disorder rather than a non-pain-related mental illness (Main 2003).

According to Shapiro & Teasell (1998) there already exists a diagnosis in DSM-IV which is not considered as a mental disorder but is consistent with a biopsychosocial conceptualisation of chronic pain, i.e. *psychological factors affecting a general medical condition*, the criteria of which are shown in Box 8.11.

In summary, psychiatric diagnostic criteria are not particularly helpful specifically in elucidating the psychological features associated with chronic pain. However, these problems are of more than academic significance. If chronic pain and pain-associated incapacity cannot be explained in terms of physical signs or structural damage, and if the presenting problem is a

chronic pain syndrome rather than a diagnosable mental illness, it could be argued that the claimant has not sustained a recognised injury.

Mental health problems as psychological targets for intervention

The assessment of mental health problems is a critical aspect of providing adequate care for the pain patient. It is important to distinguish between mental health problems assessed by structured interview and symptoms of mental health problems assessed by questionnaire. A mental health diagnosis can only be advanced on the basis of a clinical interview conducted by a professional who has received specialised training in diagnostic interviewing. A score on a self-report questionnaire cannot be used to diagnose a mental health condition. Methods of conducting diagnostic interviews will be described in this chapter, but should only be used by individuals who have been trained to administer them. The following section only addresses methods of assessing the most common mental health problems observed in patients with persistent pain. These include depression, post-traumatic stress disorder (PTSD), other anxiety disorders, and somatoform disorders.

Depression

According to DSM-IV (1994) criteria, a diagnosis of Major Depressive Disorder (MDD) requires the presence of at least five depressive symptoms (from a list of nine possible symptoms) that have persisted over a 2-week period, and represent a change from the previous level functioning. Depressed mood and a markedly diminished interest in pleasure are considered essential symptoms of MDD such that at least one of these must be present in order to consider a diagnosis. Other depressive symptoms considered for a diagnosis of MDD include: significant weight loss when not dieting or weight gain or decrease or increase in appetite, insomnia or hypersomnia, observable psychomotor agitation or retardation, fatigue or loss of energy, feelings of worthlessness or excessive or inappropriate guilt, diminished ability to think or concentrate, or indecisiveness, and recurrent thoughts of death with or without a specific plan, or a suicide attempt.

For a diagnosis of MDD, presenting symptoms must cause clinically significant distress or impairment in social, occupational or other areas of functioning, and must not be due to the direct physiological effects of a substance or a general medical condition. The symptoms must not be better accounted for by bereavement, and they must not meet the criteria for a mixed episode.

Symptoms of chronic pain and depression overlap to some degree. For example, symptoms of appetite and sleep disturbance, psychomotor retardation, fatigue or reduced energy are common to both chronic pain and depression. Therefore, criterion contamination complicates the assessment of depression in the chronic pain population (Dersh et al 2002). There have been numerous discussions of strategies that might minimise the potential for false positive diagnoses of depression (due to symptom overlap) in patients with chronic pain (Banks & Kerns 1996, Rodin et al 1991, Sullivan et al 1992, Wilson et al 2002). It has become clear that the probability of false positive diagnoses will vary significantly as a function of the method used to deal with symptom overlap (Wilson et al 2002). Given the difficulty of reliably determining whether a particular symptom should be attributed to chronic pain or to depression, several clinical researchers have suggested that current diagnostic symptoms should be used in a standard fashion with patients suffering from chronic pain (Banks & Kerns 1996, Rodin et al 1991, Sullivan et al 1992).

Although current diagnostic approaches might be associated with higher risk of false positive diagnoses when used with chronic pain patients, the elimination of overlapping symptoms, or symptom substitution, risks increasing the rate of false negative diagnoses. The clinical inconvenience of offering treatment to someone who is not clinically depressed (i.e. the consequence of false positive diagnosis) is preferable to not offering treatment to someone who is depressed (i.e. the consequence of false negative diagnosis).

Numerous self-report measures have also been developed to facilitate the assessment of depressive symptoms. Although self-report measures of depression are not well suited as diagnostic instruments, they can be very useful as screening measures or as measures of improvement associated with treatment (Bishop et al 1993, Burns et al 2003, Vowles et al 2004). The Beck Depression Inventory (Beck et al 1996) is a self-report measure of depression that is being used with increasing frequency with chronic pain patients (Burns et al 2003, Sullivan & Stanish 2003). The BDI-II consists of 21 items describing various symptoms of depression. The BDI-II has been shown to be a reliable and valid index of depressive symptoms in chronic pain patients and primary care medical patients (Arnau et al 2001, Bishop et al 1993, Morley et al 2002). Other self-report measures of depression that have been used with chronic pain include the Centre for Epidemiological

Studies Depression Scale, or CES-D (Radloff 1977), the Zung Self Rating Depression Scale (Zung et al 1965) and the Hamilton Rating Scale for Depression (Hamilton 1960). Although these different self-report measures share similar psychometric properties, several investigators have discussed the advantages of the BDI due to its relatively low proportion of somatic items (Rodin et al 1991, Sullivan et al 1992).

Post-traumatic stress disorder

The diagnosis of PTSD is one of the few mental health diagnoses that requires, as an essential symptom, the occurrence of an external event. The majority of mental health diagnoses are based on symptom profiles that exist within the individual. PTSD, on the other hand, requires that an individual be exposed to an event (i.e. a stressor) that is 'outside the usual range of human experience' (DSM-IV 1994). Criminal acts, wars, natural disasters and motor vehicle accidents are some examples of traumatic events that would satisfy the stressor criterion (Criterion A). The DSM-IV also notes that the individuals' reaction to the stressor must have been one that included intense fear, horror or helplessness.

The symptom domains considered for a diagnosis of PTSD include (1) re-experiencing phenomena, (2) cognitive or behavioural avoidance and (3) physiological hyper-reactivity. Re-experiencing phenomena may include intrusive and recurrent recollections of the event, nightmares, and behaving or feeling as though one is reliving the traumatic situation. Avoidance phenomena might include efforts to avoid thoughts of the trauma, and persistent avoidance of stimuli associated with the trauma. Avoidance phenomena also include a diminished interest in activities, a feeling of detachment from others, a restricted range of affect and a sense of a foreshortened future. Symptoms of physiological hyper-reactivity might include increased arousal, difficulty falling or staying asleep, irritability, difficulty concentrating and hypervigilance. For a diagnosis of PTSD to be considered, the above symptoms must not have been present before the traumatic event. The duration of the post-traumatic symptoms must be greater than 1 month, and must be associated with an observable disturbance in social, personal or occupational functioning.

As with depression, symptom overlap might also contribute to false positive diagnoses of PTSD. Symptoms of appetite and sleep disturbance, psychomotor retardation, fatigue or reduced energy, and activity avoidance are common to both chronic pain and PTSD. The dangers associated with the exclusion of overlapping symptoms, or with the substitution of symptoms are the same for PTSD as they are with depression. As such, adherence to standard diagnostic guidelines with particular attention to differential diagnosis probably constitutes the best clinical practice.

Litigation and compensation might also play a role in increasing the probability of false positive diagnoses of PTSD. Since a diagnosis of PTSD requires the experience of a traumatic event, questions of liability with regard to the traumatic event might engender litigation or compensation for losses (Ferrari & Russell 1997, Mayou et al 2002, Rainville et al 1997). If PTSD symptoms arise from a motor vehicle accident, the individual 'at fault' for the accident would be liable not only for the distress and disability associated with pain symptoms, but also for the distress and disability associated with PTSD symptoms (Mayou et al 2002).

In recent years, there has been a dramatic rise in the number of claims for PTSD made to insurers following motor vehicle accidents. Part of this increase might be the result of the increased sensitivity of health professionals to the potential emotional consequences of exposure to a traumatic incident involving injury. This sensitivity, however, might also take the form of excessively liberal diagnostic practices where symptoms associated with normal adjustment to trauma are misinterpreted as being consistent with a diagnosis of PTSD (Bryant & Harvey 1997, Wakefield 1992). It is beyond the scope of this chapter to review normal and pathological processes of adaptation. However, recollections of trauma, intrusive thoughts and nightmares are part of the natural process of adaptation to trauma (Horowitz 1986, Lazarus 1983, Roth & Cohen 1986). These symptoms become pathological only when they persist intensely over time and lead to disruptions in functioning (Foa et al 1989, McNally 1999). Unfortunately, health professionals who are not well versed in the distinguishing features of normal and pathological adjustment to trauma may erroneously make a diagnosis of PTSD for what is essentially a normal pattern of adjustment. Once a diagnosis appears on paper, it has a tendency to take on a life of its own, and the client may eventually begin to believe in the truth of the diagnosis as well. Careful adherence to standards of practice and respect for the limits of expertise cannot be overemphasised as they pertain to the diagnosis of PTSD.

Clinician ratings scales that yield both a continuous index of PTSD symptom severity and a categorical measure of diagnostic classification have also been developed (Blake et al 1990). A number of self-report instruments have been developed to assess the severity of symptoms associated with PTSD (Asmundson et al 1998, Davidson et al 1997, Falsetti et al 1993). Although these scales should not be viewed as diagnostic tools, they can

be very useful as screening instruments for potential cases of PTSD, and for monitoring changes in symptom severity. Commonly used measures of PTSD symptom severity include the Impact of Events Scale (Horowitz et al 1979), the Davidson Trauma Scale (Davidson et al 1997), the PTSD Checklist (Andrykowski et al 1998) and the Post-traumatic Stress Diagnostic Scale (Foa et al 1997). Changes in symptom severity can also be examined using domain-specific measures that assess the severity of depressive (e.g., BDI; Beck et al 1996), anxious (STAI; Spielberger et al 1970) or avoidance symptoms.

Anxiety disorders

According to the DSM-IV (1994), fears are considered phobias when 'the avoidance, fear, or anxious anticipation of encountering the phobic stimulus interferes significantly with the person's daily routine, occupational functioning, or social life, or if the person is markedly distressed about having the phobia'.

Social phobias may be characterised by a generalised fear of most social situations, or a fear of circumscribed social situations such as speaking in public or eating in public. Specific phobias observed in pain patients might include fears of driving subsequent to a motor vehicle accident, or fears of places or activities associated with an occupational injury (Kuch et al 1994, Taylor & Koch 1995). Generalised anxiety disorder is characterised by excessive and uncontrollable worry about a number of life events or activities, and by its extension over a long period of time.

Structured diagnostic interviews based on DSM-IV criteria are considered the most valid approach to diagnosing anxiety disorders associated with pain. Self-report instruments can be useful tools for screening or for monitoring progress in treatment. Commonly used self-report measures of fears or phobias associated with pain include the Fear Survey Schedule (Wolpe & Lang 1964), the Social Phobia and Anxiety Inventory (Biedel et al 1989) and the Fear Questionnaire (Cox et al 1993).

Somatoform disorders

According to the DSM-IV, most chronic pain conditions would meet the criteria for a diagnosis of a 'Pain Disorder associated with a medical condition'. Pain Disorder is classified as one of the somatoform disorders. The essential feature of somatoform disorders is that psychological conflicts have been transformed into physical symptoms. The DSM-IV (1994) considers several potential diagnoses within the category of somatoform disorders, including somatisation disorder, hypochondriasis, undifferentiated somatoform disorder, conversion disorder, body dysmorphic disorder and pain disorder. Among these, somatoform pain disorder is the most frequently applied diagnosis in chronic pain patients. Pain disorder is characterised notably by pain in one or more anatomical sites and of sufficient severity to warrant clinical attention (Criterion A). The pain must cause clinically significant distress or impairment in social, occupational or other important areas of functioning (Criterion B). Furthermore, psychological factors must have been judged to have an important role in the onset, severity, exacerbation or maintenance of the pain (Criterion C). The final two criteria are that the symptoms must not be intentionally produced (Criterion D) and cannot better be explained by affective or anxiety disorders, or by psychotic disorder (Criterion E).

The inclusion of chronic pain phenomena within the taxonomy of psychiatric disorders perpetuates the view that mental health issues are at the root of, as opposed to the consequence of, chronic pain and encourages the undesirable clinical practice of diagnosis by exclusion (Weintraub 1988). Requiring that the clinician judge whether psychological factors are causally related to the onset of pain implies that a knowledge base exists to accurately discern physical and psychological contributions to the aetiology of pain (Ciamarella et al 2004, Howell et al 2003). Given that such a knowledge base does not currently exist, the diagnosis of pain-related somatoform disorders necessarily proceeds solely on the basis of clinical intuition.

Psychological risk factors for persisting pain and disability

Psychosocial risk factors for chronic pain and disability are not mental disorders, nor would they necessarily be considered indices of dysfunction (in the absence of musculoskeletal symptoms). Nevertheless, their presence contributes to a higher probability that a pain condition will persist over time. Unlike mental health disorders, which can only be assessed through diagnostic interview, psychological risk factors for chronic pain and disability are assessed primarily with self-report questionnaires. The following section addresses only methods of assessing the psychological risk factors that have shown robust relations with pain-related outcomes. These include pain catastrophising, pain-related fears, self-efficacy and disability beliefs.

Pain catastrophising

The two most widely used self-report measures of catastrophising are the catastrophising subscale of the Coping Strategies Questionnaire (CSQ; Rosenstiel & Keefe 1983) and the Pain Catastrophising Scale (PCS; Sullivan et al 1995). Both scales have been shown to have good psychometric properties and to be related to negative outcomes in response to acute and chronic pain experience (Rosenstiel & Keefe 1983, Sullivan et al 1995).

An advantage of using the CSQ is that it includes six coping subscales in addition to the catastrophising subscale. The catastrophising subscale of the CSQ contains six items that are rated in relation to their frequency of occurrence on six-point scales with the endpoints (0) never and (5) almost always (Rosenstiel & Keefe 1983). The CSQ allows the clinician to examine a comprehensive profile of a patient's repertoire of adaptive and maladaptive cognitions associated with pain experience.

The PCS was developed specifically in order to assess catastrophic thinking associated with pain. The PCS yields subscale scores on three different dimensions of catastrophising: rumination ('I can't stop thinking about how much it hurts') magnification ('I worry that something serious may happen') and helplessness ('There is nothing I can do to reduce the intensity of my pain'). The three-factor structure of the PCS has been replicated in clinical and non-clinical samples (Sullivan et al 1995, 2000, Osman et al 1997).

The PCS total score and subscale scores are computed as the algebraic sum of the ratings for each item. PCS items are rated in relation to their frequency of occurrence on five-point scales with the endpoints (0) never and (4) almost always. The PCS is a 13-item self-report measure that can be completed and scored in less than 5 minutes, and thus is easily amenable to inclusion in standard clinical practice.

Pain-related fears

Three of the most frequently used self-report measures of fear of pain are the Pain Anxiety Symptom Scale (PASS; McCracken et al 1992), the Tampa Scale for Kinesiophobia (TSK; Kori et al 1990) and the Fear-Avoidance Beliefs Questionnaire (FABQ; Waddell et al 1993). The PASS assesses pain-related fear appraisals, cognitive symptoms of anxiety and physiological symptoms of anxiety. The TSK assesses respondents' beliefs about the potential for harm associated with physical activity (Kori et al 1990, Vlaeyen et al 1995). The FABQ assesses fear-avoidance beliefs about physical and work-related activities. Each of these measures has been shown to predict pain-related disability better than medical status variables (Asmundson et al 1999).

Self-efficacy

Self-efficacy judgements are considered to be most predictive of proximal behaviour (Bandura 1977). As such, the bulk of research on self-efficacy and behavioural outcomes has made use of single-item scales worded in a fashion directly relevant to the behaviour of interest. In pain research, several single-item scales have been developed to assess self-efficacy in relation to specific aspects of experimental paradigms. A two-item subscale of the CSQ (Rosenstiel & Keefe 1983) has often been used to assess coping efficacy in relation to pain.

A number of scales have also been developed to assess a 'generalised' self-efficacy orientation to dealing with pain and illness-related symptoms. The Arthritis Self-Efficacy Scale (Lorig et al 1989) has been used in numerous studies to assess individuals' confidence in their ability to perform various behaviours aimed at controlling pain and arthritis symptoms. This instrument yields three subscales that assess pain management, physical function and other arthritis symptoms. A similar measure was developed to assess self-efficacy beliefs in chronic pain patients not restricted to arthritis (Anderson et al 1995). The Chronic Pain Self-Efficacy Scale is a 22-item questionnaire that generates scores on three subscales: pain management, coping and physical function. A measure of functional self-efficacy was developed by Barry et al (2003). On this scale, respondents are asked to rate their confidence in their ability to carry out ten different activities of daily living.

Coping styles and strategies

The assessment of coping styles and strategies dominated much of the research on the psychology of pain in the 1980s. This work emerged from the view that pain symptoms could be viewed as physical and psychological stressors, and that the manner in which individuals coped with their pain would have implications for physical and emotional outcomes. Numerous investigations have used the CSQ (Rosenstiel & Keefe 1983) to assess coping strategies for pain. The CSQ consists of seven coping subscales: coping self-statements, praying or hoping, ignoring pain sensations, reinterpreting pain sensations, increasing behavioural activities and catastrophising. Subscale scores have been used in research examining the correlates of coping, as well as in clinical practice as a means of identifying targets of intervention.

The Vanderbilt Pain Management Inventory (VPMI) was developed based on a two-dimensional conceptualisation of coping (Brown & Nicassio 1987). The VPMI yields two scales that assess passive and active coping. Research has shown that passive coping is associated with poor adaptational outcomes (Brown & Nicassio 1987).

A different approach to the assessment of coping and adaptation is reflected in the Multidimensional Pain Inventory (MPI) developed by Kerns and his colleagues (Kerns et al 1985). The instrument is based on Turk and Rudy's Multiaxial Assessment of Pain, which integrates medical, psychosocial and behavioural data. The MPI addresses coping and adaptation in relation to an empirically derived typology where individuals are classified as (1) adaptive copers, (2) interpersonally distressed or (3) dysfunctional. The MPI has been used as a tool to predict health outcomes in patients with persistent pain conditions and to match patients with appropriate interventions (Turk & Rudy 1990).

Pain behaviour

Fordyce (1976) first drew attention to the study of pain behaviour. Fordyce and his colleagues applied the concepts of learning theory to the problem of chronic pain with a particular focus on the behaviours associated with pain (Fordyce 1976). The results of several studies revealed that the manipulation of reinforcement contingencies could exert a powerful influence on the frequency of display of pain behaviours (Fordyce et al 1985).

Keefe & Block (1982) developed the first systematic approach to the coding of pain behaviours. In this system, pain patients were asked to engage in a variety of physical manoeuvres, which were videotaped and later coded for the presence and duration of pain behaviour. Patients typically performed the required physical manoeuvres as part of a standardised physical examination. The physical manoeuvres included 2-minute periods of standing, sitting and walking. The pain behaviours assessed by the Keefe & Block (1982) system included guarding, bracing, rubbing, sighing and grimacing. Within this system, pain behaviours had to be present for at least 3 seconds to be coded. Investigations revealed that the assessment of pain behaviour could reliably distinguish pain patients from non-patient controls (Labus et al 2003).

More recently, Prkachin et al (2002) elaborated on the Keefe & Block (1982) system by incorporating greater focus on facial displays of pain. Prkachin et al (2002) argued that a limitation of the Keefe & Block (1982) pain behaviour coding system was it did not permit a thorough analysis of communicative dimensions of pain behaviour such as facial responses or vocalisations. Since most facial displays and vocalisations are expressed for periods less than 3 seconds, they would not be effectively captured by a system that requires a minimum duration of expression in order to be coded as a pain behaviour. In addition, Prkachin et al (2002) noted that the Keefe & Block (1982) was a binary coding system (present vs absent) and thus could not address questions concerning the intensity of pain behaviour displays.

The pain behaviour coping system proposed by Prkachin et al (2002) retained most of the coding classifications of the Keefe & Block (1982) system, but altered the duration criterion for classification, provided a more precise method of assessing facial displays, and included a rating of behaviour intensity. As in the Keefe & Block (1982) system, pain behaviour is coded in the context of a standardised physical examination. Research has shown that the pain behaviours assessed through the Prkachin et al (2002) system show good psychometric properties and test–retest reliability. Pain behaviours assessed with this system have also been shown to prospectively predict which injured workers will return to work and which will remain disabled (Schultz et al 2002).

Self-reported functional limitations

To date, several self-report measures of functional limitations have been developed (Bergner et al 1981, Fairbank et al 1980, Tait et al 1987, 1990). The format is similar across measures. Essentially, respondents are asked to rate their level of disability for different types of life activities. Respondents' ratings are calculated to yield a composite score, the magnitude of which is intended to reflect the severity of pain-related functional limitations.

There are several advantages to the use of self-report questionnaires of functional limitations. They are relatively easy to administer and score, thus facilitating their inclusion in clinical assessment protocols. In addition, self-ratings of functional limitations permit the examination of variations in disability when objective indices such as return to work are not available, or not relevant (i.e., as in post-retirement populations). One major limitation of self-report questionnaires is that they are susceptible to wilful distortion, which can have a significant drawback if the questionnaires are administered under conditions where there might be incentives (e.g. compensation) for certain forms of self-presentation (e.g. disability).

There are factors other than wilful distortion that are likely to influence how an individual will respond to a subjective measure of functional limitations. An individual's rating of his or her ability can be construed as an 'appraisal'. In other words, the rating of disability consists of a judgement of one's ability to successfully execute certain tasks or behaviours.

The most commonly used self-report measures of functional limitations include the Roland and Morris Disability Questionnaire (Roland & Morris 1983), the Oswestry Disability Questionnaire (Fairbank et al 1980) and the Pain Disability Index (Tait et al 1987, 1990). On these questionnaires, respondents are asked to make judgements about their ability to successfully complete various domestic, recreational or occupational tasks.

Conclusions

It is now accepted that chronic pain and pain-associated limitations have a significant impact on patients' general well-being and on their mental health. When patients present with chronic pain problems to pain clinics, their symptomatic presentation is frequently accompanied by significant levels of distress, confusion about the nature and prognosis of their condition, and evidence of failure to cope. In assessing the significance of such psychological factors, the clinician can be confronted with a difficult task regarding recommendations for treatment. Dealing with the psychological impact of pain is a key facet of most pain management programmes, but adverse psychological factors of sufficient intensity may compromise the patient's response to pain management and may indeed indicate the need for referral to a mental health specialist for consideration of specific psychological or psychiatric treatment.

In this chapter, some recommendations have been made for the identification of both patients unlikely to benefit from pain management at all, and of those with an identifiable mental health problem who might merit reassessment for pain management following an appropriate mental health intervention.

A plethora of helpful assessment tools are currently available, but a specialist in mental health assessment is required to determine the need for psychological/psychiatric treatment and the core of this process is the focused clinical interview, which may be supplemented by psychometric evaluation.

In addition to orange flag triage, it is appropriate to identify the psychological factors that can be targeted with a pain management approach. It is recommended that primary attention should be directed at the identification and assessment of modifiable risk factors for persistent pain and disability since these can become primary objectives for the pain management intervention.

There has been a clear intent to shift perspective from mapping the psychological backdrop in general to focusing on key issues related to clinical decision making and management. In reviewing the available literature, we have attempted to identify psychometric tools which may be of assistance, but we would wish to emphasise our conviction that the clinical interview (whether for purposes of orange flag triage or in terms of yellow flag management) should remain a foundation that can be supplemented by clinical records and former psychometric evaluation. Our intention in reviewing the assessment of the specific mental health conditions to be found in the chronic pain population is not only to provide general guidance for orange flag triage to non-mental health professionals, but also to provide guidance for the management of mental health conditions (from appropriately qualified professionals) and the management of modifiable psychological risk factors for persistent pain and chronicity within the pain management approach.

Key points

- Historically, psychological assessment has been employed for a wide variety of purposes
- It is important to distinguish assessment of general suitability for pain management, from identification of targets for treatment and from obstacles to reactivation

(Continued)

- The core assessment usually should be a structured clinical interview but formal psychometric assessment can offer useful additional information
- Choice of assessment measures requires understanding of their psychometric properties, and a clear understanding both of the utility and limitations of psychometric assessment
- Consideration of general suitability for pain management should include an appraisal of orange flags and a competent assessment of mental health be undertaken
- It is useful to distinguish Axis I psychiatric disorders, Axis II psychiatric disorders and chronic pain disorders (particularly in the context of medicolegal assessment)
- The major psychiatric disorders requiring identification among chronic pain patients are depression, post-traumatic stress disorder, anxiety disorders and somatisation disorders
- Risk factors for the persistence of chronic pain and disability should also be appraised. The most important features of assessment are pain catastrophising, pain-related fears, self-efficacy beliefs, coping styles and strategies and pain behaviour and self-reported functional limitations
- The overall message is that competent and relevant psychological assessment is of critical importance to the practice of pain management, but the assessment requires clear objectives and a clear focus on clinical decision making and interventions with clearly identified outcomes (such as removal of obstacles to re-engagement or changes in functional activities).

References

Anderson K O, Dowds B N, Pelletz R E et al 1995 Development and initial validation of a scale to measure self-efficacy beliefs in patients with chronic pain. Pain 63:77–83

Andrykowski M A, Cordova M J, Studts J L et al 1998 PTSD after treatment for breast cancer: prevalence of diagnosis, and use of the PTSD Checklist – Civilian Version (PCL-CV) as a screening instrument. Journal of Consulting and Clinical Psychology 66:586–590

Arnau R C, Meagher M W, Norris M P et al 2001 Psychometric properties of the Beck Depression Inventory II with primary care medical patients. Health Psychology 20:112–119

Asmundson G J G, Norton G R, Allerdings M D et al 1998 Post-traumatic stress disorder and work related injury. Journal of Anxiety Disorders 12:57–69

Asmundson G J G, Norton P J, Norton G R 1999 Beyond pain: the role of fear and avoidance in chronicity. Clinical Psychology Review 19:97–119

Bandura A 1977 Self-efficacy: the exercise of control. Freeman, New York

Banks S M, Kerns R D 1996 Explaining high rates of depression in chronic pain: a diathesis-stress framework. Psychology Bulletin 119:95–110

Barry L C, Guo Z, Kerns R D et al 2003 Functional self-efficacy and pain-related disability among older veterans with chronic pain in a primary care setting. Pain 104:131–137

Beck A T, Steer R A 1990 The Beck anxiety inventory manual. Psychological Corporation San Antonio, TX

Beck A T, Steer R A, Brown G K 1996 Manual for the Beck depression inventory – II. Psychological Corporation, San Antonio, TX

Bergner M, Bobbitt R A, Carter W B et al 1981 The sickness impact profile: development and final revision of a health status measure. Medical Care 8:787–805

Biedel D C, Turner S M, Stanley M A et al 1989 The social phobic and anxiety inventory: concurrent and external validity. Behavioral Therapy 20:417–427

Bigos S J Battie M C, Spengler D M et al 1991 A prospective study of work perceptions and psychosocial factors affecting the report of back injury. Spine 16:1–6

Bishop S, Edgley K, Fisher R et al 1993 Screening for depression in chronic low back pain with the Beck depression inventory. Canadian Journal of Rehabilitation 7:143–148

Blake D D, Nagy L M, Kaloupek D G et al 1990 A clinician rating scale for assessing current and lifetime PTSD: the CAPS-1. The behaviour therapist 13:187–188

Brown G K, Nicassio P M 1987 The development of a questionnaire for the assessment of active and passive coping strategies in chronic pain patients. Pain 31:53–64

Bryant R A, Harvey A G 1997 Acute stress disorder: a critical review of diagnostic issues. Clinical Psychology Review 17:757–773

Burns J Kubilus A, Bruehl S et al 2003 Do changes in cognitive factors influence outcome following multidisciplinary treatment of chronic pain? A crossed-lagged panel analysis. Journal of Consulting and Clinical Psychology 71:81–91

Ciamarella A, Grosso S, Poli P, Gioia A et al 2004 When pain is not fully explained by organic lesion: a psychiatric perspective on chronic pain patients. European Journal of Pain 8:13–22

Cox B J, Swinson R P, Parker J D A et al 1993 Confirmatory factor analysis of the fear questionnaire in panic disorder with agoraphobia. Psychological Assessment 5:235–237

Davidson J R, Book S W, Colket J T 1997 Assessment of a new self-rating scale for post-traumatic stress disorder. Psychological Medicine 27:153–160

Derogatis R 1983 The SCL-90R manual – II. Administration, scoring and procedures. Clinical Psychometric Research, Towson MD

Dersh J, Polatin P, Gatchel R 2002 Chronic pain and psychopathology: research findings and theoretical considerations. Psychosomatic Medicine 64:773–786

DSM-IV 1994 Diagnostic and statistical manual of mental disorders, 4th edn. American Psychiatric Association, Washington, DC

Eaton W W, Gallo J A, Cai A et al 1997 Natural history of diagnostic interview schedule/DSM-IV major depression. The Baltimore epidemiologic catchment area follow-up. Archives of General Psychiatry 54:993–999

Fairbank J C, Davies T, Couper J B et al 1980 The Oswestry low-back pain disability questionnaire. Physiotherapy 66:271–273

Falsetti S A, Resnick H S, Resnick P A et al 1993 The modified PTSD symptom scale: A brief self-report of post-traumatic stress disorder. Behavioral Therapist 16:161–162

Ferrari R, Russell A S 1997 The whiplash syndrome – common sense revisited. Rheumatology 24:618–622

Foa E B, Stekete G, Rothbaum B O 1989 Behavioral/cognitive conceptualizations of post-traumatic stress disorder. Behavioral Therapy 20:155–176

Foa E B, Cashman L, Jaycox L et al 1997 The validation of a self-report measure of posttraumatic stress disorder: the Posttraumatic Diagnostic Scale. Psychological Assessment 9(4):445–451

Fordyce W 1976 Behavioral methods in chronic pain and illness. CV Mosby, St Louis

Fordyce W E, Roberts A H, Sternbach R A 1985 The behavioral management of chronic pain: a response to critics. Pain 22:113–125

Gatchel R J 1996 Psychological disorders and chronic pain: cause and effect relationships. In: Gatchel R J, Turk D C (eds) Psychological approaches to pain management: a practitioner's handbook. Guilford Press, New York, pp 33–54

Gatchel R, Polatin P, Mayer T et al 1994 Psychopathology and the rehabilitation of patients with chronic low back pain disability. Archives of Physical Medicine and Rehabilitation 75:95–103

Gatchel R, Polatin P, Mayer R 1995 The dominant role of psychosocial risk factors in the development of chronic low back pain. Spine 20:2701–2709

Goldberg D, Williams P 1988 A user's guide to the general health questionnaire (GHQ). NFER-Nelson, Windsor

Groth-Marnat G 2003 Handbook of psychological assessment. Wiley, New York

Hamilton M A 1960 A rating scale for depression. Journal of Neurology and Neurosurgical Psychiatry 23:56–62

Hathaway S R, McKinley J C, Butcher J N et al 1989 Minnesota multiphasic personality inventory – 2: manual for administration. University of Minnesota Press, Minneapolis

Horowitz M J 1986 Stress response syndromes, 2nd edn. Jason Aronson, New York

Horowitz M J, Wilner N, Alvarez W 1979 Impact of event scale: a measure of subjective stress. Psychosomatic Medicine 41:209–218

Howell S, Poulton R, Caspi A et al 2003 Relationship between abdominal pain subgroups in the community and psychiatric diagnosis and personality. A birth cohort. Journal of Psychosomatic Research 55:179–187

Keefe F, Block A 1982 Development of an observational method for assessing pain behavior in chronic pain patients. Behavioral Therapy 13:363–375

Kerns R D, Turk D C, Rudy T E 1985 The West Haven Yale Multidimensional Pain Inventory (WHYMPI). Pain 23:345–356

Kori S, Miller R, Todd D 1990 Kinesiophobia: a new view of chronic pain behavior. Pain Management Jan:35–43

Kuch K, Cox B J, Evans R et al 1994 Phobias, panic, and pain in survivors of road vehicle accidents. Journal of Anxiety Disorders 8:181–187

Labus J S, Keefe F J, Jensen M P 2003 Self-reports of pain intensity and direct observations of pain behavior: when are they correlated? Pain 102:109–24

Landis J R, Koch G G 1977 The measurement of observer agreement for categorical data. Biometrics 33:159–174

Lazarus R S 1983 The cost and benefits of denial. In: Breznitz S (ed) The denial of stress. International Universities Press, New York, pp 1–30

Lorig K, Chastain R I, Ung F et al 1989 Development and evaluation of a scale to measure perceived self-efficacy in people with arthritis. Arthritis and Rheumatism 32: 37–44

Main C J 1999 Medicolegal aspects of pain: the nature of psychological opinion in cases of personal injury. In: Gatchel R J, Turk D C (eds) Psychosocial aspects of pain. Guilford Press, New York, pp 132–147

Main C J 2003 The nature of chronic pain: a clinical and legal challenge. In: Halligan P, Bass C, Oakley D (eds) Malingering and illness deception. Oxford University Press, Oxford, ch 13, pp 171–183

Mayou R A, Ehlers A, Bryant B 2002 Posttraumatic stress disorder after motor vehicle accidents: 3-year follow-up of a prospective longitudinal study. Behavioral Research and Therapy 40:665–675

McCracken L M, Zayfert C, Gross R T 1992 The pain anxiety scale: development and validation of a scale to measure fear of pain. Pain 50:67–73

McNally R 1999 Post-traumatic stress disorder. In: Millon T, Blaney P H, Davis R D (eds) Oxford textbook of psychopathology. Oxford University Press, Oxford, pp 144–165

Morley S, Williams A C de C, Black S 2002 A confirmatory factor analysis of the Beck depression inventory in chronic pain. Pain 99:157–165

Nunnally J C, Bernstein I H 1994 Psychometric theory. McGraw-Hill, New York

Osman A, Barrios F X, Kopper B A et al 1997 Factor structure, reliability, and validity of the pain catastrophizing scale. Journal of Behavioral Medicine 20:589–605

Prkachin K, Schultz I, Berkowitz J et al 2002 Assessing pain behavior of low back pain patients in real time: concurrent validity and examiner sensitivity. Behaviour Research and Therapy 2002 40:595–607

Radloff L S 1977 The CES-D Scale: a self-reported depression scale for research in the general population. Applied Psychology Measures 1:385–401

Rainville J, Sobel J B, Hartigan C et al 1997 The effect of compensation involvement on the reporting of pain and disability by patients referred for rehabilitation of chronic low back pain. Spine 26:2016–2024

Rodin G, Craven J, Littlefield C 1991 Depression in the medically ill: an integrated approach. Bruner/Mazel, New York

Roland M, Morris R A 1983 study of the natural history of back pain Part I: development of a reliable and sensitive measure of disability in low-back pain. Spine 8:141–144

Rosenstiel A K, Keefe F J 1983 The use of coping strategies in chronic low back pain patients: relationship to patient characteristics and current adjustment. Pain 17:33–44

Roth S, Cohen L J 1986 Approach avoidance and coping with stress. American Psychologist 41:813–819

Schultz I Z, Prkachin K M, Hughes E et al 2002 A system for observing pain behaviour during physical examination: reliability of components and their relation to return to work. Presented at the Meeting of the International Association for the Study of Pain, Seattle

Shapiro A P, Teasell R W 1998 Misdiagnosis of chronic pain as hysteria and malingering. Current Review of Pain 2:19–28

Spielberger C D, Gorsuch R L, Lushen R E 1970 Manual for the state trait anxiety inventory. Counselling Psychologists Press, Palo Alto, CA

Spitzer R L, Williams J B, Gibbon M et al 1992 The structured clinical interview for DSM-III-R (SCID), I: history, rationale and description. Archives of General Psychiatry 49:624–629

Sullivan M J L, Stanish W D 2003 Psychologically based occupational rehabilitation: the pain-disability prevention program. Clinical Journal of Pain 19:97–104

Sullivan M J L, Reesor K, Mikail S et al 1992 The treatment of depression in chronic low back pain: review and recommendations. Pain 5:5–13

Sullivan M J L, Bishop S, Pivik J 1995 The pain catastrophizing scale: development and validation. Psychological Assessment 7:524–532

Sullivan M J L, Tripp D, Rodgers W et al 2000 Catastrophizing and pain perception in sports participants. Journal of Applied Sports Psychology 12:151–167

Tait R C, Pollard C A, Margolis R B et al 1987 The pain disability index: psychometric and validity data. Archives of Physical Medicine and Rehabilitation 68:438–441

Tait R C, Chibnall J T, Krause S 1990 The pain disability index; psychometric properties. Pain 40:171–182

Taylor S, Koch W J 1995 Anxiety disorders due to motor vehicle accidents: nature and treatment. Clinical Psychology Review 15:721–738

Todd C, Bradley C 1996 Evaluating the design and development of psychological scales. In: Bradley C (ed) Handbook of psychology and diabetes. Harwood Academic Publishers, The Netherlands, ch 2, pp 15–42

Turk D C, Rudy T E 1990 The robustness of an empirically derived taxonomy of chronic pain patients. Pain 43:27–35

Vlaeyen J W S, Kole-Snijders A M J, Rotteveel A et al 1995 The role of fear of movement/(re)injury in pain disability. Journal of Occupational Rehabilitation 5:235–252

Vowles K E, Gross R T, Sorrell J T 2004 Predicting work status following interdisciplinary treatment for chronic pain. European Journal of Pain 8:351–358

Waddell G, Newton M, Henderson I et al 1993 Fear-avoidance beliefs questionnaire (FABQ) and the role of fear-avoidance beliefs in chronic low back pain and disability. Pain 52:157–168

Wakefield J C 1992 Disorder as harmful dysfunction: a conceptual critique of DSM-III-R's definition of mental disorder. Psychology Review 99:232–247

Weintraub M I 1988 Regional pain is usually hysterical. Archives of Neurology 44:914–915

Weisberg J, Keefe F 1999 Personality, individual differences and psychopathology in chronic pain. In: Gatchel R, Turk D (eds) Psychosocial factors in pain. Guilford Press, New York, pp 56–73

Williams R C 1988 Toward a set of reliable and valid measures for chronic pain assessment and outcome research. Pain 35:239–251

Williams D A, Thorn B E 1989 An empirical assessment of pain beliefs. Pain 36:351–358

Wilson K G, Eriksson M Y, D'Eon J L et al 2002 Major depression and insomnia in chronic pain. Clinical Journal of Pain 18:77–83

Wolpe J, Lang P J 1964 A fear schedule for use in behaviour therapy. Behavioral Research and Therapy 2:7–30

Zimmerman M 1994 Diagnosing personality disorders: a review of issues and research methods. Archives of General Psychiatry 51:225–245

Zung W W, Richards C B, Short M J 1965 Self-rating depression scale in an outpatient clinic. Further validation of the SDS. Archives of General Psychiatry 13(6):508–515

APPENDIX 8.1

The assessment of psychiatric disorder

It has been estimated that a significant proportion of chronic pain patients have identifiable psychiatric illness. In the majority of chronic pain patients there is evidence of emotional disturbance such as anxiety, depression or anger. Frequently the emotional intensity is not sufficient to indicate the need for formal psychiatric evaluation. Psychiatric disorder may antedate the development of pain, coexist with the presence of a pain syndrome or develop as a consequence of it. In patients in whom the reason for their distress is not associated with their pain, or in whom the severity of their distress is an obstacle to pain management, a formal assessment of the need for primary psychiatric treatment should be undertaken.

The most commonly used assessment systems are the International Classification of Diseases and Related Health Problems, now in its 10th edition (ICD-10), and the Diagnostic and Statistical Manual of Mental Disorders (DSM), now in its fourth edition (DSM-IV 1994). Currently the most commonly used system (certainly in the UK) appears to be the DSM-IV. Assessment of psychiatric disorder requires specialised training but for those not familiar with it a brief description of a number of the more commonly found diagnoses in pain patients is offered here. The actual diagnostic criteria from DSM-IV, together with their classification numbers, are also reproduced.

Generalised anxiety disorder

Generalised anxiety disorder is characterised by excessive anxiety and worry on more days than not for the previous 6 months; it is associated with a number of other symptoms such as restlessness, fatigue, difficulty concentrating, sleep disturbance and muscle tension, and the anxiety itself causes significant distress or impairment. Pain patients are normally focused on *specific* concerns about pain, its effects and its significance. The major characteristics for generalised disorder are:

- Excessive anxiety and worry occurring more days than not for at least 6 months, about a number of events and activities
- Difficulty in controlling the worry
- Associated with three or more of the following symptoms:
  - restlessness or feeling keyed-up or on edge
  - being easily fatigued
  - difficulty in concentrating or the mind going blank
  - irritability
  - muscle tension
  - sleep disturbance.
- Focus not confined to features of another axis I disorder

- Anxiety, worry or physical symptoms causing clinically significant distress or impairment in functioning
- Not due to direct physiological effects of a substance.

The full diagnostic criteria for generalised anxiety disorder (classified as 300.02 in the DSM-IV) are presented in Box 8A.1.

Box 8A.1

Diagnostic criteria for generalised anxiety disorder

A. Excessive anxiety and worry (apprehensive expectation), occurring more days than not for at least 6 months, about a number of events or activities (such as work or school performance).
B. The person finds it difficult to control the worry.
C. The anxiety and worry are associated with three (or more) of the following six symptoms (with at least some symptoms present for more days than not for the past 6 months). **Note:** Only one item is required in children.
   (1) restlessness or feeling keyed up or on edge
   (2) being easily fatigued
   (3) difficulty concentrating or mind going blank
   (4) irritability
   (5) muscle tension
   (6) sleep disturbance (difficulty falling or staying asleep, or restless unsatisfying sleep).
D. The focus of the anxiety and worry is not confined to features of an Axis I disorder, e.g. the anxiety or worry is not about having a panic attack (as in panic disorder), being embarrassed in public (as in social phobia), being contaminated (as in obsessive–compulsive disorder), being away from home or close relatives (as in separation anxiety disorder), gaining weight (as in anorexia nervosa), having multiple physical complaints (as in somatisation disorder), or having a serious illness (as in hypochondriasis), and the anxiety and worry do not occur exclusively during post-traumatic stress disorder.
E. The anxiety, worry, or physical symptoms cause clinically significant distress or impairment in social, occupational, or other important areas of functioning.
F. The disturbance is not due to the direct physiological effects of a substance (e.g. a drug of abuse, a medication) or a general medical condition (e.g. hyperthyroidism) and does not occur exclusively during a mood disorder, a psychotic disorder, or a pervasive developmental disorder.

Anxiety due to a general medical condition

Anxiety due to a general medical condition is clinically significant anxiety judged to be due to the *direct physiological effects* of a general medical condition. In a sense the physiological effects mimic primary psychological symptoms (such as tachycardia). Such features can usually be diagnosed only if a disorder other than a pain syndrome is present. The full diagnostic criteria for an anxiety disorder secondary to a medical condition (classified as 293.84 in the DSM-IV) are shown in Box 8A.2.

Depression

The importance of depression has been discussed at length in Chapter 3. As previously discussed, although history

Box 8A.2

Diagnostic criteria for anxiety disorder due to … [indicate the general medical condition]

A. Prominent anxiety, panic attacks, or obsessions or compulsions predominate in the clinical picture.
B. There is evidence from the history, physical examination, or laboratory findings that the disturbance is the direct physiological consequence of a general medical condition.
C. The disturbance is not better accounted for by another mental disorder (e.g. adjustment disorder with anxiety in which the stressor is a serious general medical condition).
D. The disturbance does not occur exclusively during the course of a delirium.
E. The disturbance causes clinically significant distress or impairment in social, occupational, or other important areas of functioning.

Specify if:

with generalised anxiety: if excessive anxiety or worry about a number of events or activities predominates in the clinical presentation
with panic attacks: if panic attacks predominate in the clinical presentation
with obsessive–compulsive symptoms: if obsessions or compulsions predominate in the clinical presentation.

  Coding note: include the name of the general medical condition on Axis I, e.g. 293.84 anxiety disorder due to phaeochromocytoma. With generalised anxiety, also code the general medical condition on Axis III.

of depression constitutes an increased risk for the development of chronic pain, pain is a stronger predictor of depression. The depression observed in many pain patients would not be sufficiently intense to constitute the basis for a diagnosable psychiatric illness. In fact pain management is arguably the preferred treatment option for depression secondary to pain-associated incapacity.

The principal features of clinical depression are shown below. Five of the following nine symptoms must be continuously present over a 2-week period:

- Depressed mood
- Loss of pleasure or interest in most activities
- Weight or appetite changes
- Increased or decreased sleep
- Increased or decreased psychomotor activity
- Fatigue
- Feelings of guilt or worthlessness
- Reduced ability to concentrate/make decisions
- Recurrent thoughts of death or suicide.

Criteria for a major depressive episode are presented in Box 8A.3.

Somatoform disorders

The term 'somatoform disorder' is used to cover a variety of disorders in which physical symptoms suggesting a physical condition cause significant distress or impairment, but are not fully explained by a general medical condition. The major types are shown in Box 8A.4.

Box 8A.3

Criteria for major depressive episode

A. Five (or more) of the following symptoms have been present during the same 2-week period and represent a change from previous functioning; at least one of the symptoms is either (1) depressed mood or (2) loss of interest or pleasure.

   Note: Do not include symptoms that are clearly due to a general medical condition, or mood-incongruent delusions or hallucinations.

   (1) depressed mood most of the day, nearly every day, as indicated by either subjective report (e.g. feels sad or empty) or observation made by others (e.g. appears tearful). **Note:** In children and adolescents, can be irritable mood

   (2) markedly diminished interest or pleasure in all, or almost all, activities most of the day, nearly every day (as indicated by either subjective account or observation made by others)

   (Continued)

Criteria for major depressive episode (*Continued*)

   (3) significant weight loss when not dieting or weight gain (e.g. a change of more than 5% of body weight in a month), or decrease or increase in appetite nearly every day. **Note:** In children, consider failure to make expected weight gains

   (4) insomnia or hypersomnia nearly every day

   (5) psychomotor agitation or retardation nearly every day (observable by others, not merely subjective feelings of restlessness or being slowed down)

   (6) fatigue or loss of energy nearly every day

   (7) feelings of worthlessness or excessive or inappropriate guilt (which may be delusional) nearly every day (not merely self-reproach or guilt about being sick)

   (8) diminished ability to think or concentrate, or indecisiveness, nearly every day (either by subjective account or as observed by others)

   (9) recurrent thoughts of death (not just fear of dying), recurrent suicidal ideation without a specific plan, or a suicide attempt or a specific plan for committing suicide.

B. The symptoms do not meet criteria for a mixed episode.

C. The symptoms cause clinically significant distress or impairment in social, occupational, or other important areas of functioning.

D. The symptoms are not due to the direct physiological effects of a substance (e.g. a drug of abuse, a medication) or a general medical condition (e.g. hypothyroidism).

E. The symptoms are not better accounted for by bereavement, i.e., after the loss of a loved one, the symptoms persist for longer than 2 months or are characterised by marked functional impairment, morbid preoccupation with worthlessness, suicidal ideation, psychotic symptoms, or psychomotor retardation.

Box 8A.4

Types of somatoform disorder

- Somatisation disorder
- Undifferentiated somatoform disorder
- Conversion disorder
- Pain disorder
- Hypochondriasis
- Body dysmorphic disorder
- Somatoform disorder not otherwise specified.

Box 8A.5

Diagnostic criteria for somatisation disorder

A. A history of many physical complaints beginning before age 30 years that occur over a period of several years and result in treatment being sought or significant impairment in social, occupational, or other important areas of functioning.

B. Each of the following criteria must have been met, with individual symptoms occurring at any time during the course of the disturbance:

   (1) *four pain symptoms:* a history of pain related to at least four different sites or functions (e.g. head, abdomen, back, joints, extremities, chest, rectum, during menstruation, during sexual intercourse, or during urination)

   (2) *two gastrointestinal symptoms:* a history of at least two gastrointestinal symptoms other than pain (e.g. nausea, bloating, vomiting other than during pregnancy, diarrhoea or intolerance of several different foods)

   (3) *one sexual symptom:* a history of at least one sexual or reproductive symptom other than pain (e.g. sexual indifference, erectile or ejaculatory dysfunction, irregular menses, excessive menstrual bleeding, vomiting throughout pregnancy)

   (4) *one pseudoneurological symptom:* a history of at least one symptom or deficit suggesting a neurological condition not limited to pain (conversion symptoms such as impaired coordination or balance, paralysis or localised weakness, difficulty swallowing or lump in throat, aphonia, urinary retention, hallucinations, loss of touch or pain sensation, double vision, blindness, deafness, seizures; dissociative symptoms such as amnesia; or loss of consciousness other than fainting).

C. Either (1) or (2):

   (1) after appropriate investigation, each of the symptoms in criterion B cannot be fully explained by a known general medical condition or the direct effects of a substance (e.g., a drug of abuse, a medication)

   (2) when there is a related general medical condition, the physical complaints or resulting social or occupational impairment are in excess of what would be expected from the history, physical examination, or laboratory findings.

D. The symptoms are not intentionally produced or feigned (as in factitious disorder or malingering).

Recently, the term 'somatisation' has become popular. Somatisation disorders (formerly described as hysteria, or Briquet's syndrome) are characterised by multiple symptoms, beginning before the age of 30 years, extending over many years and including a combination of pain, gastrointestinal, sexual and pseudoneurological symptoms. They differ from 'psychological factors affecting medical condition' in that there is no diagnosable general medical condition to account for the physical symptoms. A lesser variant (undifferentiated somatoform disorder) has been evoked to classify patients not quite fulfilling the criteria for a somatisation disorder. The major criteria for somatisation disorder (classified as 300.81 in the DSM-IV) are shown in Box 8A.5.

Conversion disorder

Conversion disorder is characterised by unexplained symptoms or deficits affecting voluntary motor or sensory function that suggest a neurological or other general medical condition. Psychological factors are judged to be associated with the symptoms or deficits. Such a diagnosis should be made with extreme caution, since it may lead to complacency in proper investigation of the physical basis of a complaint, and lead to the patient being labelled pejoratively and taken less than seriously. The diagnosis is usually unhelpful in the context of chronic pain since it is safe to assume (unless proved otherwise) that there *is* a physical basis for the complaint. Although less fashionable than formerly, patients will sometimes be given such a diagnosis. The full diagnostic criteria (classified as 300.11 in the DSM-IV) are shown in Box 8A.6.

Hypochondriasis

The essential feature of hypochondriasis is preoccupation with the fear of having, or the idea that one has, a serious disease based on one's misinterpretation of bodily symptoms. In the context of chronic pain, a primary diagnosis of hypochondriasis (as with conversion hysteria) should be made only with considerable caution after a comprehensive cognitive and behavioural evaluation has been undertaken. Diagnostic criteria for hypochondriasis (classified as 300.7 in the DSM-IV) are shown in Box 8A.7.

Adjustment disorders

An adjustment disorder is characterised by clinically significant emotional or behavioural symptoms in response to an identifiable psychosocial stress or stressor. The symptoms must develop within 3 months of

Box 8A.6

Diagnostic criteria for conversion disorder

A. One or more symptoms or deficits affecting voluntary motor or sensory function that suggest a neurological or other general medical condition.

B. Psychological factors are judged to be associated with the symptom or deficit because the initiation or exacerbation of the symptom or deficit is preceded by conflicts or other stressors.

C. The symptom or deficit is not intentionally produced or feigned (as in factitious disorder or malingering).

D. The symptom or deficit cannot, after appropriate investigation, be fully explained by a general medical condition, or by the direct effects of a substance, or as a culturally sanctioned behaviour or experience.

E. The symptom or deficit causes clinically significant distress or impairment in social, occupational, or other important areas of functioning or warrants medical evaluation.

F. The symptom or deficit is not limited to pain or sexual dysfunction, does not occur exclusively during the course of somatisation disorder, and is not better accounted for by another mental disorder.

Specify type of symptom or deficit:

**with motor symptom or deficit
with sensory symptom or deficit
with seizures or convulsions
with mixed presentation.**

Box 8A.7

Diagnostic criteria for hypochondriasis

A. Preoccupation with fears of having, or the idea that one has, a serious disease based on the person's misinterpretation of bodily symptoms.

B. The preoccupation persists despite appropriate medical evaluation and reassurance.

C. The belief in criterion A is not of delusional intensity (as in delusional disorder, somatic type) and is not restricted to a circumscribed concern about appearance (as in body dysmorphic disorder).

D. The preoccupation causes clinically significant distress or impairment in social, occupational, or other important areas of functioning.

E. The duration of the disturbance is at least 6 months.

F. The preoccupation is not better accounted for by generalised anxiety disorder, obsessive–compulsive disorder, panic disorder, a major depressive episode, separation anxiety or another somatoform disorder.

Specify if:

with poor insight: if, for most of the time during the current episode, the person does not recognise that the concern about having a serious illness is excessive or unreasonable.

disorder, the person must persistently re-experience the event in a number of ways, demonstrate persistent avoidance of stimuli associated with the trauma and experience persistent symptoms of increased arousal. If the individual demonstrates sufficient evidence of features in each of these categories, and if the duration of the symptoms is greater than 1 month, then the individual may be considered to be suffering from a diagnosable PTSD. The specific criteria (classified as 309.81 in the DSM-IV) are shown in Box 8A.9.

Pain disorder

The DSM-IV classification of pain disorder is unhelpful. It purports to distinguish three subtypes, depending on the relative importance of the psychological factors in comparison with the general medical condition. It is wise to assume that all significant pain problems have both a physiological and a psychological component (Chs 1 and 2) unless there is overwhelming evidence to the contrary. The diagnostic criteria for pain disorder are shown in Box 8A.10.

the stressor and resolve within 6 months of its termination, although it may persist for a prolonged period (i.e. longer than 6 months) if occurring in response to a chronic stressor (e.g. a chronic disabling medical condition). Almost all patients could be considered to fall within this category, and therefore the diagnosis does appear to be particularly helpful. The diagnostic criteria for adjustment disorders (classified as 309.0 to 309.9 in the DSM-IV) are shown in Box 8A.8.

Post-traumatic stress disorder

The essential characteristics of post-traumatic stress disorder (PTSD) are the development of a set of psychological and physiological symptoms following a traumatic event (such as a serious road traffic accident). Assuming the event can be considered of such an nature as potentially to fulfil criteria for the basis of such a

Box 8A.8

Diagnostic criteria for adjustment disorders

A. The development of emotional or behavioural symptoms in response to an identifiable stressor(s) occurring within 3 months of the onset of the stressor(s).

B. These symptoms or behaviours are clinically significant as evidenced by either of the following:
   (1) marked distress that is in excess of what would be expected from exposure to the stressor
   (2) significant impairment in social or occupational (academic) functioning.

C. The stress-related disturbance does not meet the criteria for another specific Axis I disorder and is not merely an exacerbation of a pre-existing Axis I or Axis II disorder.

D. The symptoms do not represent bereavement.

E. Once the stressor (or its consequences) has terminated, the symptoms do not persist for more than an additional 6 months.

Specify if:
acute: if the disturbance lasts less than 6 months

chronic: if the disturbance lasts for 6 months or longer.

Adjustment disorders are coded based on the subtype, which is selected according to the predominant symptoms. The specific stressor(s) can be specified on Axis IV.

309.0	with depressed mood
309.24	with anxiety
309.28	with mixed anxiety and depressed mood
309.3	with disturbance of conduct
309.4	with mixed disturbance of emotions and conduct
309.9	unspecified

Personality or character disorder

In addition to the identification of psychiatric disease, DSM-IV offers an appraisal of various types of personality disorder or character disorder, the identification of which is considered by clinicians to indicate a poor prognosis for outcome from pain management, or even be a contraindication to acceptance for treatment. The major types of personality disorder are illustrated in Box 8A.11.

Box 8A.9

Diagnostic criteria for post-traumatic stress disorder

A. The person has been exposed to a traumatic event in which both of the following were present:
   (1) the person experienced, witnessed, or was confronted with an event or events that involved actual or threatened death or serious injury, or a threat to the physical integrity of self or others
   (2) the person's response involved intense fear, helplessness, or horror. **Note:** In children, this may be expressed instead by disorganised or agitated behaviour.

B. The traumatic event is persistently re-experienced in one (or more) of the following ways:
   (1) recurrent and intrusive distressing recollections of the event, including images, thoughts, or perceptions. **Note:** In young children, repetitive play may occur in which themes or aspects of the trauma are expressed
   (2) recurrent distressing dreams of the event. **Note:** In children, there may be frightening dreams without recognisable content
   (3) acting or feeling as if the traumatic event were recurring (includes a sense of reliving the experience, illusions, hallucinations, and dissociative flashback episodes, including those that occur on awakening or when intoxicated). **Note:** In young children, trauma-specific re-enactment may occur
   (4) intense psychological distress at exposure to internal or external cues that symbolise or resemble an aspect of the traumatic event
   (5) physiological reactivity on exposure to internal or external cues that symbolise or resemble an aspect of the traumatic event.

C. Persistent avoidance of stimuli associated with the trauma and numbing of general responsiveness (not present before the trauma), as indicated by three (or more) of the following:
   (1) efforts to avoid thoughts, feelings, or conversations associated with the trauma
   (2) efforts to avoid activities, places, or people that arouse recollections of the trauma
   (3) inability to recall an important aspect of the trauma
   (4) markedly diminished interest or participation in significant activities

(Continued)

Diagnostic criteria for post-traumatic stress disorder (*Continued*)

   (5) feeling of detachment or estrangement from others
   (6) restricted range of affect (e.g. unable to have loving feelings)
   (7) sense of a foreshortened future (e.g. does not expect to have a career, marriage, children, or a normal life span).
D. Persistent symptoms of increased arousal (not present before the trauma), as indicated by two (or more) of the following:
   (1) difficulty falling or staying asleep
   (2) irritability or outbursts of anger
   (3) difficulty concentrating
   (4) hypervigilance
   (5) exaggerated startle response.
E. Duration of the disturbance (symptoms in criteria B, C, and D) is more than 1 month.
F. The disturbance causes clinically significant distress or impairment in social, occupational, or other important areas of functioning.

Specify if:

acute: if duration of symptoms is less than 3 months
chronic: if duration of symptoms is 3 months or more.

Specify if:

with delayed onset: if onset of symptoms is at least 6 months after the stressor.

Box 8A.10

Diagnostic criteria for pain disorder

A. Pain in one or more anatomical sites is the predominant focus of the clinical presentation and is of sufficient severity to warrant clinical attention.
B. The pain causes clinically significant distress or impairment in social, occupational or other important areas of functioning.
C. Psychological factors are judged to have an important role in the onset, severity, exacerbation or maintenance of the pain.
D. The symptom or deficit is not intentionally produced or feigned (as in factitious disorder or malingering).
E. The pain is not better accounted for by a mood, anxiety, or psychotic disorder and does not meet criteria for dyspareunia.

(Continued)

Diagnostic criteria for pain disorder (*Continued*)

Code as follows:

307.80 pain disorder associated with psychological factors: psychological factors are judged to have the major role in the onset, severity, exacerbation, or maintenance of the pain. (If a general medical condition is present, it does not have a major role in the onset, severity, exacerbation, or maintenance of the pain.) This type of pain disorder is not diagnosed if criteria are also met for somatisation disorder.

Specify if:

acute: duration of less than 6 months
chronic: duration of 6 months or longer

307.89 pain disorder associated with both psychological factors and a general medical condition: both psychological factors and a general medical condition are judged to have important roles in the onset, severity, exacerbation, or maintenance of the pain. The associated general medical condition or anatomical site of the pain (see below) is coded on axis III.

Specify if:

acute: duration of less than 6 months
chronic: duration of 6 months or longer.

   Note: The following is not considered to be a mental disorder and is included here to facilitate differential diagnosis.

pain disorder associated with a general medical condition: a general medical condition has a major role in the onset, severity, exacerbation, or maintenance of the pain. (If psychological factors are present, they are not judged to have a major role in the onset, severity, exacerbation, or maintenance of the pain.) The diagnostic code for the pain is selected based on the associated general medical condition if one has been established or on the anatomical location of the pain if the underlying general medical condition is not yet clearly established – for example, low back (724.2), sciatic (724.3), pelvic (625.9), headache (784.0), facial (784.0), chest (786.50), joint (719.4), bone (733.90), abdominal (789.0), breast (611.71), renal (788.0), ear (388.70), eye (379.91), throat (784.1), tooth (525.9) and urinary (788.0).

In general clinical practice, however, such classifications are seldom helpful and, as Gatchel et al (1995) have indicated, the scientific evidence for such disorders being contraindications for treatment is not clearly established.

Box 8A.11

Major types of personality disorder

- *Paranoid personality disorder* is a pattern of distrust and suspiciousness such that others' motives are interpreted as malevolent
- *Schizoid personality disorder* is a pattern of detachment from social relationships and a restricted range of emotional expression
- *Schizotypal personality disorder* is a pattern of acute discomfort in close relationships, cognitive or perceptual distortions, and eccentricities of behaviour
- *Antisocial personality disorder* is a pattern of disregard for, and violation of, the rights of others
- *Borderline personality disorder* is a pattern of instability in interpersonal relationships, self-image and affects, and marked impulsivity
- *Histrionic personality disorder* is a pattern of excessive emotionality and attention seeking
- *Narcissistic personality disorder* is a pattern of grandiosity, need for admiration and lack of empathy
- *Avoidant personality disorder* is a pattern of social inhibition, feelings of inadequacy and hypersensitivity to negative evaluation
- *Dependent personality disorder* is a pattern of submissive and clinging behaviour related to an excessive need to be taken care of
- *Obsessive–compulsive personality disorder* is a pattern of preoccupation with orderliness, perfectionism and control.

References

DSM-IV 1994 Diagnostic and statistical manual of mental disorders, 4th edn. American Psychiatric Association, Washington DC

Gatchel R J, Polatin P B, Kinney R K 1995 Predicting outcome of chronic back pain using clinical predictors of psychopathology: a prospective analysis. Health Psychology 14:415–420

ICD-10 1994 International statistical classification of diseases and related health problems, 10th edn. World Health Organisation, Geneva

Section **Three**

Psychosocial interventions

In Chapter 9, the nature of psychosocial interventions is considered. The case for early intervention precedes a discussion of the nature of early interventions, ranging from simple information giving and advice to variants of the cognitive–behavioural approach. There is a specific focus on the importance of communication and dealing with distress within GP and therapist consultations in primary care settings. The chapter concludes with a summary of lessons learned from recent trials, including the importance of competencies and the need for targeted interventions.

In Chapter 10, pain management intervention models and techniques are reviewed, initially from a historical perspective, and then specific consideration is given to educational approaches (such as back schools), behavioural interventions, cognitive–behavioural programmes, stress management programmes before more recent risk-factor-targeted interventions are reviewed. In the second part of the chapter, specific applications of specific pain management techniques such as disclosure, cognitive restructuring, activity scheduling, relaxation, biofeedback, hypnosis and exposure are addressed in detail.

Chapter Nine

9

The nature of psychosocial interventions

CHAPTER CONTENTS

Introduction

In earlier chapters we have offered a view on the nature of pain and the development of pain-associated limitations in function. We have considered the nature of pain in terms of its cognitive, emotional and behavioural aspects and offered a contextual view blending consideration of both the timeline (from antecedents to future expectations) and the current context (in terms of symptom experience and presentation in its social and occupational context). Much has been learned from the assessment and management of the chronic pain patients (discussed further in Ch. 10) but of course by the time patients present with chronic pain problems, they are likely already to have had a significant amount of treatment. In practice, interventions range in complexity from simple verbal advice to highly specific cognitive–behavioural interventions, but complex interventions are relatively costly and require a level of specific professional competency not always available in a routine clinic. It could be argued in any event that complex and costly interventions are only necessary if the pain problem has 'got out of hand'. In this chapter we offer therefore an appraisal of approaches to early psychosocial intervention.

A detailed comparison of the nature of the psychosocial interactions and influences on outcome across such a wide variety of therapeutic approaches is far beyond the remit of this textbook, but it would seem necessary to move at least one stage beyond the initial GP consultation.

Guidelines for the management of both low-back pain and whiplash disorder recommend early intervention. Waddell & Watson (2004) report that the evidence for intervening sooner rather than later is overwhelming. The problem presented to us is what type of intervention should be delivered? The natural history of most musculoskeletal conditions demonstrates a significant improvement in disability and symptoms and a reduction in consulting in the first 6 to 8 weeks. Many people remain symptomatic but they cope well with their symptoms and do not consult. Complex interventions with those who will go on to improve and cope well with their pain anyway are unlikely to prove cost effective.

The case for early intervention

Most reviews have focused on low-back pain and the consensus of opinion is that it is easier to intervene early with simple low-cost approaches to treatment than to expend considerable time and resources on rehabilitating a person who has become incapacitated by chronic pain. Early interventions are not only more effective they are also more cost effective in the long run. There is most evidence in treatment of musculoskeletal pain (particularly neck and back pain). Von Korff & Moore (2001) offer a straightforward stepped care approach to the management of low-back pain, but this approach could be usefully applied in other musculoskeletal pain conditions. The interventions start with simple advice and reassurance and increase in complexity (and of course cost) as time progresses.

The term 'early intervention', however, can be something of a misnomer, since most musculoskeletal pain is recurrent in nature and true acute episodes are not often seen in the clinic; patients often try and self-manage their pain and only consult if the pain continues or if it interferes with their activities – usually their work. Furthermore, most people with chronic pain do not habitually consult; most are employed and working and only consult when the pain affects function.

The nature of interventions

Information and advice

Patients consulting general practitioners arrive with a range of beliefs derived from a range of sources. Some sources of beliefs about back pain, and the potentially detrimental characteristics that can influence their accuracy as shown in Table 9.1. Unfortunately such beliefs are not always either accurate or helpful. This was illustrated some years ago in Deyo's (1998) depiction of seven myths about back pain, as illustrated in Table 9.2.

Information therefore needs to begin with accurate and up-to-date information. Modern guidelines for the management of back pain all state that the person should be given early advice to remain as active as possible and return to normal activities, including work as soon as feasible. A number of research studies and a systematic review have concluded that such advice is useful in speeding up return to activity, reducing fear about injury and may reduce consulting (Staal et al 2003). However, the guidelines do not address the way in which advice is delivered, by whom and whether it has resulted in adaptive–behavioural change.

There is a consensus, however, within the guidelines that rest is acceptable for a day or two but no more. This can be a difficult rule to apply in practice since patients may have different concepts of 'rest' and they vary in the physical demands required of them in their work. It is important that the clinician has an appreciation of the type of tasks the patient normally undertakes in order to advise on how to resume them without unmanageable increases in pain. Blanket advice to 'take it

Table 9.1 Sources and accuracy of information

Source	Characteristics potentially contributing to inaccuracy
Family	Tendency to be overconcerned and overprotective
Medical professionals	Unreliable – different health professionals give different information and advice
Culture	Inherently inaccurate, being contaminated by outdated notions and information
Media	Sensational presentations, owing more to the need to entertain than impart information
Legislation	Inappropriate messages about health and safety, with a stimulus to enter litigation
Science	Inaccessible to most and not universally trusted

From Burton et al (2006, p. 163) (By permission of Oxford University Press)

easy for a couple of days' then get back to normal as soon as possible is at best vague. Rest should be viewed as a period of 'time-out' rather than a treatment as such and rest therefore must be interspersed with periods of moderate activity. Remaining stationary for long periods of time (sitting or lying) is not useful; patients should be encouraged to perform gentle stretches and keep mobile – taking walks and making changes of position regularly. This is particularly important to those who remain seated for long periods in their work.

Giving information in the form of a booklet can help, and in the UK and other countries *The Back Book* (Roland et al 2002), a simple low-cost booklet which informs the patient on self-managing back pain and how to keep active and adopt an active lifestyle, can be used as an aspect of clinical management. The clinician must ensure, however, that the patient reads and understands the information they have been given. In order to do this it is essential that the clinician is sure about what the patient already knows and understands (or misunderstands) about their pain.

Premature reassurance that the pain will resolve in a particular number of days can be a risky strategy since, should the pain not resolve in that time, the patient will not only mistrust the clinician's judgement on this matter but may also consider the attribution that they have been given is suspect too. It has often been said that back pain normally resolves in 4–6 weeks, this is not always the case and many patients still report symptoms a year after the onset of their problem. Most people either stop consulting or return to work after a few weeks but this does not mean that they are symptom free. In a recent follow-up study of patients attending an osteopathic clinic, of those presenting within 3 weeks of onset of back pain, 71% had had 1–5 further attacks over a 1–4-year follow-up period (Burton et al 2004). Most episodes are short-lived, and recurrent rather than chronic, and so it is important to point out that the great majority of acute episodes of pain improve with time and that exercise will assist this process. The clinician can take the opportunity to 'normalise' the episode of back pain which, although painful, is not threatening and can be self-managed.

Table 9.2 Some common myths about back pain

	Myth	Reality
1	If you have a slipped disc you must have surgery: surgeons agree about exactly who needs surgery	The majority of disc problems resolve without surgery. Surgery rates vary dramatically from country to country and surgeon to surgeon
2	X-ray and newer imaging tests (CT and MRI scans) can always identify the cause of pain	Scans cannot determine the source of back pain. Degenerative changes on scans are mostly normal age-related changes
3	If your back hurts, you should take it easy until the pain goes away	Staying active or returning to activity (including work), even if still painful, enhances recovery
4	Most back pain is caused by heavy lifting	The cause is mostly unknown, and the onset does not usually follow a lifting. Back pain is similarly common among sedentary and manual workers
5	Back pain is usually disabling	Most episodes of back pain recover uneventfully within days or weeks. Few patients are disabled beyond a few days
6	Everyone with back pain should have a spine X-ray	Scan findings do not correlate with symptoms, and do not provide a reliable guide to treatment
7	Bed rest is the mainstay of therapy	Bed rest as a treatment is anathema – it interferes with staying active and leads to longer time from work

From Burton, et al (2006, p. 164) (By permission of Oxford University Press)

In their review, Burton & Waddell (2002) concluded:

carefully selected and presented information and advice about back pain in line with current management guidelines can [their emphasis] have a positive effect on patients' beliefs and clinical outcomes. Written material is just one way of achieving this and, whilst its effect size may be small, its very low patient cost may render it highly cost effective. Nevertheless, there is considerable scope for refinement of the messages and their method of delivery within the whole scope of health care and the contribution of innovative educational interventions for back pain deserves further scientific investigation (p. 256).

Recommendations for the design of educational material are shown in Box 9.1.

Approaches to communication

The importance of good communication is a key facet of the overall care of the patient and methods designed to enhance the efficacy of communication skills, and is highlighted in almost all textbooks and training programmes for health-care professionals. Skilled communication is believed to be an important ingredient of therapeutic encounters. Maguire & Pitceathly (2002), on the basis of their studies of therapeutic encounters in more specialised settings such as oncology, have offered an excellent analysis which is of relevance also in primary care settings. The key tasks as identified by them are shown in Box 9.2.

The essence of good communication is the ability to be able to understand patients' problems from their perspective. In order to do this the doctor/therapist must gain the patient's confidence. The patient has to be convinced that the doctor/therapist takes the patient's pain seriously. Only then will patients be willing to give credence to what the doctor/therapist says to them. The converse is perhaps even more true – that is, if patients feel that the doctor/therapist is dismissive or not taking their pain seriously they will not be prepared to reveal sensitive information nor actively comply with treatment suggestions.

A number of practical guidelines for managing the communication process are shown in Box 9.3. (The subject is considered in more detail in Ch. 4.)

In establishing a competent appraisal of a patient, the first and most important principle is to suspend judgement until all facets of the patient's difficulties have been appraised. Clinical decision making is subject to a range of possible biases which can cloud clinical judgement. Clinicians should be prepared to give the patient the benefit of the doubt and listen.

Listening skills are vital. Simply allowing patients to explain how they feel and ask questions can have a significantly beneficial effect. Successfully predicting the impact of the pain will reinforce to patients that doctors or therapists are not out of their depth but understand their problem. This will help to establish the confidence of patients. The clinician should also check the patients' own beliefs about their pain and its causation, correcting any misconceptions at the time if necessary. A number of strategies to assist the development of an appropriate style of communication are presented in Box 9.4.

Box 9.2

Key tasks in communication with patients

- Eliciting a patient's main problems; the patient's perceptions of these; and the physical, emotional and social impact of the patient's problems on the patient and family
- Tailoring information to what the patient wants to know; checking his or her understanding
- Eliciting the patient's reactions to the information given and his/her main concerns
- Determining how much the patient wants to participate in decision making (when treatment options are available)
- Discussing treatment options so that the patient understands the implications
- Maximising the chance that the patient will follow agreed decisions about treatment and advice about changes in lifestyle.

Maguire & Pitceathly (2002, p. 697: Box 1)

Box 9.1

Recommendations for the design of educational material

- Be clear about the core content of the message
- Identify the targeted audience
- Specify learning objectives
- Address style and format as well as content of the material
- Associate learning objectives with recommendations for behavioural change
- Check comprehension and reinforce adherence.

Clinicians need to explain the complexity of chronic pain problems and the impact of pain. They should give reasons for enquiring not only about the pain but also what this has done to patients and how they have been coping with it. They need to observe carefully what patients say and how they say it.

It is important to empathise without colluding. It needs to be explained that the pain is real. The clinician should also check whether others (including doctors and therapists) have implied the pain is imaginary, by enquiring what the patient has been told about the cause of their pain by others. The clinician needs to find out what treatments have been recommended or what they have been told to do or not do. It may be necessary to correct a number of misconceptions. Many patients are confused as a consequence of receiving differing explanations from different professionals. It may be necessary to defuse significant anger about previous assessments and treatments. The clinician should explain potential treatment options with the expected outcome, and explain what cannot be done and why.

Enquiry about sensitive information (e.g. use of alcohol or misuse of medication) will need to be approached in a way that 'allows' the patient to disclose such information without feeling threatened. Judgemental statements, questioning or even body language will not be helpful and are unlikely to reveal the truth, as the patient is then likely to become defensive.

In conclusion, the clinician should make specific enquiry about the patient's pain: its nature, effects and how patients are coping with and managing their pain. It is helpful to emphasise that it is normal for pain to affect mood (irritability, depression and anxiety), sleep, work and relationships with others.

Box 9.3

Important elements of communication

- Develop and apply competent listening skills
- Carefully observe the patient's behaviour
- Attend not only to *what* is said but also *how* it is said
- Attempt to understand how the patient feels
- Offer encouragement to disclose fears and feelings
- Offer reassurance that you accept the 'reality' of the patient's pain
- Correct misunderstandings or miscommunications about the consultation
- Offer appropriate challenge to negative thoughts (such as catastrophising)
- Appraise the general social and economic circumstances
- Include assessment and involvement of the partner/significant other wherever possible.

Box 9.4

Style of communication

- Suspend judgement
- Listen and observe
- Be empathic but not collusive
- Encourage self-disclosure
- Explain what you can do
- Explain what you cannot do
- Re-establish confidence
- 'Kick-start' self-control.

The importance of reassurance

Reassurance is frequently commented on but little understood, either in terms of its nature or its impact on patients. Reassurance is context specific and has to be understood in the context of communication between the therapist and the patient. Some patients may be seeking specific information from or actions by the professional rather than reassurance per se. Although a degree of reassurance regarding fear about the nature or their pain, or its prognosis, may be appropriate, bland reassurance may not only be unhelpful but irritating to the patient.

Gask & Usherwood (2002) describe the *appropriate* use of reassurance:

> *Reassurance is effective only when doctors understand exactly what it is that their patients fear and when they address those fears truthfully and accurately. Often it is not possible to reassure patients about the diagnosis or outcome of disease, but it is always possible to provide support and show personal concern for them (p. 2).*

Reassurance needs to be understood within the context of the overall purpose of the medical consultation, the key pillars of which are building the relationship, collecting relevant information and agreeing a management plan with the patient. A summary of the research evidence is shown in Box 9.5.

More systematic approaches to 'constructing' the consultation are described elsewhere (Gask & Usherwood 2002, Main & Williams 2002, Price & Leaver 2002).

Box 9.5

Evidence based summary on the importance of the consultation

- The style with which a doctor listens to the patient will influence what the patient says
- Effective communication between doctor and patient leads to improved outcome for many common diseases
- Patients' compliance will be improved if the management plan had been negotiated jointly.

Box 9.6

Establishing the distress profile

- Pain
- Limitations in activity
- Sleep
- Quality of life
- Work
- Previous treatments.

Dealing with distress

A more focused approach can be developed for patients who are clearly distressed. Patients frequently show evidence of distress. Given the fact that most patients present primarily with the same symptom (i.e. pain), it is perhaps surprising to find that pain patients differ not only in the intensity of their distress, but also in precisely what they are distressed about. It is very important to establish clearly the specific nature of their distress. This should be appraised systematically and a distress profile obtained, which identifies the key features of their distress. It may be helpful to address the issue under the headings shown in Box 9.6.

In initiating the discussion, it may be helpful to adopt a somewhat indirect approach. Thus, rather than asking whether the patient feels depressed, for example, it may be less threatening to observe that many patients with chronic pain feel helpless and find their mood drifts down, and then to enquire whether this has happened to them. Patients thereby are 'permitted' to disclose feelings that they may feel very sensitive about. It enables the doctor or therapist to gain a more realistic understanding of the impact of the pain.

There are many potential reasons for anger and distress (Ch. 2) and it will be necessary to elucidate the reasons so that they may be tackled. Much anger will revolve around misunderstandings about causation and unfortunately all too commonly about how patients have been treated by their previous doctors and healthcare professionals.

It is normal to become physiologically aroused when faced with an angry patient especially when the anger appears to be directed at oneself. For clinicians to become angry or distressed themselves is not helpful. However, while it is important to empathise with patients and listen to them carefully, it is also vital to remain detached from their anger or distress in order

Box 9.7

Key strategies for the assessment and management of pain-associated distress and anger

- Give patients time
- Signal that it is permitted to be upset
- Find out gently the particular focus of their concern
- Find out *why* they are telling you
- Distinguish *pain- and disability-associated distress* from more general distress
- Identify iatrogenic *misunderstandings*
- Identify mistaken beliefs and fears
- Try to correct misunderstandings
- Identify iatrogenic *distress and anger*
- Listen and empathise
- Do not get angry yourself
- Decide what *you* can deal with and what requires someone else
- Be open about this with them
- If appropriate, offer to help them enlist additional assistance.

to preserve as much objectivity as possible. An overview of the most important strategies in the assessment and management of pain-associated distress and anger is presented in Box 9.7.

Psychosocial interventions and complementary and alternative medicine (CAM)

Since most CAM is offered by the private sector, it is difficult to obtain a clear picture of the nature and extent of uptake of CAM, but CAM has always been the preferred option for some people and the extent of its coverage in the popular press would suggest that it may be becoming increasingly popular.

Matters are complicated further by inclusion within the umbrella term of a wide range of other interventions. Ernst's guide to CAM (Ernst et al 2001) lists a fascinating range of diagnostic methods (such as bioresonance, Kirlian photography and tongue diagnosis), a huge range of therapies (including obscure approaches such Bach flower remedies, chelation therapy and craniosacral therapy, as well as the more widely known Alexander technique, chiropractic, homeopathy and yoga), 44 herbal and non-herbal medicines, and 38 different conditions (including back pain, neck pain, fibromyalgia, insomnia, anxiety and depression). There are major cultural variations in access to and use of CAM, but as early as 2000 the prevalence of use of CAM across 12 studies ranged from 9% to 65%, although because of the uncertain quality of much of the data the 'true prevalence of use in the population remained uncertain' (Ernst 2000a). Unfortunately despite the energy and enthusiasm with which CAM is promoted, the evidence base for its specific effectiveness is meagre, as frequently is their rationale and justification. Does this matter?

Ernst (2000b) offers interesting observations on the possible reasons for trying CAM. They are shown in Box 9.8.

Any consultation involves the establishment of some sort of therapeutic relationship and incorporates to a greater or lesser extent the beliefs and emotions of the patient, and therefore there is a level of 'engagement', and interventions such as yoga and various forms of relaxation require active participation of the patient. Most of the techniques, however, are fairly passive in nature, their mode of action is uncertain and the therapeutic rationale open to question. Without question some patients benefit, whether as a consequence of addressing their emotional/spiritual needs or by satisfying their desire for a certain type of treatment or therapeutic relationship is unclear, but to the sceptical (with the exception perhaps of acupuncture, chiropractic and osteopathy) they do not seem to be offering a systematic way of influencing the physiological or psychological mechanisms which appear to influence pain or the adjustment to it.

Ernst (2000b) suggested:

We should listen less to the opinions of those who either overtly promote or stubbornly reject complementary and alternative medicine without acceptable evidence. The many patients who use complementary and alternative medicine deserve better. Patients and healthcare providers need to know which forms are safe and effective. Its future

---

Box 9.8

Motivations for trying complementary and alternative medicine

Positive motivations
- Perceived effectiveness
- Perceived safety
- Philosophical congruence: 'Zeitgeist'; spiritual dimension; emphasis on holism, embracing all things natural; active role of the patient; explanations intuitively acceptable
- Control over treatment
- 'High touch, low tech'
- Good patient/therapist relationship; enough time available; on equal terms, emotional factors, empathy
- Non-invasive nature
- Accessibility
- Pleasant therapeutic experience
- Affluence.

Negative motivations
- Dissatisfaction with (some aspects of) conventional care; ineffective for certain conditions, serious adverse effects; poor doctor–patient relationship; insufficient time with doctor; waiting lists; 'high tech, low touch'
- Rejection of science and technology
- Rejection of 'the establishment'
- Desperation.

From Ernst (2000b, p. 1134), reproduced with permission

---

should (and hopefully will) be determined by unbiased scientific evaluation (p. 1135).

However, the worth of CAM continues to be hotly debated, as illustrated in Ernst & Cantor (2006) who, in a recent review of the systematic reviews on spinal manipulation in appraised articles published between 2000 and 2005, concluded that:

these data do not demonstrate that spinal manipulation is an effective intervention … except for back pain where it is superior to sham treatments but no better than conventional treatments. Considering the possibility of adverse effects, this review does not suggest that spinal manipulation is a recommendable treatment (p. 189).

This publication generated considerable interest in the British media and provoked some heated correspondence in the *Journal of the Royal Society of Medicine* (1 June 2006).

Thus there is debate not only about the value of CAM but also about the interpretation and synthesis of the scientific evidence. Further discussion of CAM is not possible within the confines of this chapter. In the rest of this chapter more clearly defined and focused interventions will be reviewed.

The cognitive–behavioural approach

The nature of psychological mechanisms has been addressed in detail in Chapter 2, as has their integration into models of pain and disability (Ch. 1). In consideration specifically of psychosocial interventions it is appropriate to attempt to clarify both the development and the current status of the cognitive–behavioural (CB) approach to therapy as applied to pain problems. In terms of an overall perspective, it will be argued that this term encompasses a whole range of approaches from imprecise attention to beliefs, emotions and behaviour to full-blown cognitive–behavioural therapy (CBT) (it is quite clear that many so-called CBT interventions fall far short of a systematic approach). It is relevant, however, to trace the history of the CB approach.

During the last 20 years, there has been increasing interest in cognitive aspects of pain. The arrival of a major textbook on CB approaches to pain (Turk et al 1983) represented a significant phase of conceptual development. It had been observed that there were similarities between chronic pain patients and depressed patients both behaviourally and cognitively. Concepts of the cognitive distortion and learned helplessness (derived from treatment of patients with depression) were blended with training in cognitive coping strategies for pain (derived principally from the hypnosis literature). These cognitive approaches were combined with some of the behavioural methods outlined by Fordyce (1976). Simply put, the behavioural model focuses primarily (and some would say exclusively) on what patients are *doing*. Cognitions, if deemed relevant at all, are seen as being of secondary importance. In contrast to the radical behavioural approach, CBT aims to change the way patients think, challenge their beliefs about their pain and therefore influence how they behave. This blending of cognitive and behavioural approaches therefore characterises CBT.

The assumptions behind the CB approach are illustrated in Box 9.9. These translate into a series of therapeutic objectives for treatment. The nature of

Box 9.9

Key assumptions of the cognitive–behavioural approach

- Individuals are active processors of information and not passive reactors
- Thoughts can influence and be influenced by mood, have social consequences and can serve as an impetus for behaviour
- Behaviour is reciprocally determined by both individual and environmental factors
- Individuals can learn more adaptive ways of thinking, feeling and behaving
- Individuals should be active collaborative agents in changing their maladaptive thoughts, feelings and behaviours.

Adapted from Turk & Okifuji (2003, Table 36.1, p. 534)

Box 9.10

Primary objectives of cognitive–behavioural treatment programmes

- To combat demoralisation by assisting patients to change their view of their pain and suffering from overwhelming to manageable
- To teach patients coping strategies and techniques to help them to adapt and respond to pain and the resultant problems
- To assist patients to reconceptualise themselves as active, resourceful and competent
- To learn the associations between thoughts, feelings and their behaviour, and subsequently to identify and alter automatic, maladaptive patterns
- To utilise these more adaptive responses
- To bolster self-confidence and attribute successful outcomes to their own efforts
- To help patients anticipate problems proactively and generate solutions, thereby facilitating maintenance and generalisation.

Adapted from Turk & Okifuji (2003, Table 36.3, p. 535)

psychological interventions are discussed in more detail in Chapters 10 and 11 but aspects of the approach underpin all modern psychosocial management and so it is important to be aware also of the primary objectives of the approach. They are summarised in Box 9.10.

Efficacy: does the approach work?

The chronic pain patient presenting with a high level of pain and disability may be considered to have developed a psychologically mediated chronic pain syndrome requiring a major therapeutic initiative. 'Full-blown' CBT clearly represents a complex and fairly sophisticated interdisciplinary approach to rehabilitation and in the context of early intervention such a breadth and depth of approach would not normally be required, but both the philosophy of care and the therapeutic approach seem to have an intuitive appeal in the context of patient-centred approaches to health care.

In an early meta-analytic review (Flor et al 1992) CBT programmes were found to be superior to no-treatment controls, waiting-list controls and single-discipline interventions on a range of outcome measures, including pain, mood, physical functioning, return-to-work and health-care utilisation.

Morley et al (1999) later confirmed superiority of CBT over other active treatments on ranges of outcomes and pain syndromes. However, some of the effect sizes were 'quite modest (around 0.50)' and 'there still seems to be ample room for improvement in the efficacy of CBT in chronic pain' (Vlaeyen & Morley 2005, p. 7). Nonetheless, given the chronicity of most of the patients in the studies, and the relative success of CBT in comparison with other approaches, the approach would seem to merit investigation in patients before chronic pain becomes established.

CBT, as a systematic approach to psychological therapy, is a detailed and sophisticated intervention requiring specialist therapeutic skill and training. There has been a progressive tendency, however, to adopt the language of CBT to refer to a wide range of therapeutic interventions. Clearly all therapeutic encounters incorporate, at least to some extent, a focus on cognitions and behaviour, but CBT differs in that the *explicit* focus of intervention is on the modification of thoughts and behaviour, rather than medical or biomechanical abnormality. It is necessary to find a middle way between 'full-blown' CBT as a psychotherapy and physical treatment. In the context of early interventions (usually in terms of secondary prevention) the derivation of simpler psychosocial interventions, containing a specific but narrower focus on pain- or disability-specific cognitions and behaviour, in patients with less entrenched disability, has offered an alternative to 'traditional' physiotherapy, based on manipulation or mobilisation. This more 'patient-centred' approach, inspired by work of Linton and his colleagues and the targeting of psychosocial risk factors as in the yellow-flag initiative (Kendall et al 1997) has now become a major focus of interest both in terms of efficacy of treatment and patient selection.

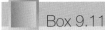

Box 9.11

Implications for the design and delivery of early interventions

- The approach is characterised by an active self-help approach rather than passive treatment delivery
- Successful intervention requires a multifaceted approach
- It may be necessary to identify a range of therapeutic targets
- Successful therapeutic intervention is likely to be beneficial for a range of different outcomes
- The approach offers encouragement for design of a preventative approach, similar in philosophy but less intensive in terms of therapeutic intervention.

It must be emphasised that the psychosocial component is offered within a framework of reactivation and therefore should be viewed more as 'psychologically enhanced physiotherapy' rather than psychotherapy per se, although questions have to be raised concerning therapeutic skill requirements, against a backdrop of accreditation and professional turf wars.

The key implications for the design and delivery of early interventions are highlighted in Box 9.11. The design and delivery of early interventions are dependent, however, not only on the content of the intervention but also on the *context* within which it is delivered. This will be addressed in the next section of the chapter.

Delivery of individualised psychosocial interventions in primary-care and community settings

There are many variations in the configuration of health-care services, both in terms of type of health-care provision and access to it. Interventions differ in their nature focus and degree of complexity. In the UK, historically the major distinction has been primary and secondary/tertiary care, with general practitioner referral as the entry route into specialist care. Access to allied health professionals usually requires medical sanction. More recently, in the UK services the development of community-based physiotherapy, nurse-led clinics and direct GP access to hospital-based physiotherapeutic

Box 9.12

Differences between primary- and secondary-care settings

- Focus of clinical evaluation
- Knowledge of the patient
- Degree of specialisation
- Breadth of service provision
- Role of screening
- Nature of assessment
- Multidisciplinary input
- Sequential vs simultaneous interventions.

services has led to a much wider range of opportunities for early interventions other than by GPs, and of course within the private sector, patients have always been able to purchase care from private practitioners of various disciplines. The major differences are summarised in Box 9.12.

With the exception of emergency service provision, the first important difference is that the GP is normally the first 'port-of-call', and indeed a number of complementary medicine practitioners and allied health practitioners also may find themselves in this role. Patients, however, are registered with their GP and access to specialist services is usually via GP referral. Secondly, many of the patients at the time of consultation will already be known by their GP and the initial evaluation therefore has a historical context. Although GP service provision is increasingly delivered as part of an aggregated service, administered through Primary Care Trusts (PCTs), and in some respect similar to the old 'cottage hospitals', hospital services will usually have a higher level of specialisation, with faster access to sophisticated technology like MRI scanning, on-site biochemistry and fast-track access to other hospital services, incorporating a wider range of health-care professionals. Nonetheless for the vast majority of patients consulting with new pain problems in primary care, hospital referral and access to special provision is not indicated, and so the role of the GP is paramount.

A new role for general practitioners?

The analysis presented in this section focuses primarily on the role of the GP in the UK, working in the context of a National Health Service, rather than on a fee-for-service basis (whether privately or insurance-funded) as in other health-care systems. Nonetheless in terms of clinical decision making, and on the nature of interactions, there are strong similarities in the role of GPs and community physicians in other health-care systems.

In the UK, the picture has been made even more complicated by the development of a new role, described as *General Practitioners with Special Interests (GPwSIs)*. In 2000, the *NHS Plan* (Secretary of State for Health 2000) called for the introduction of 1000 'specialist general practitioners' to establish clinics in community settings for 'carefully selected patients'. Although GPs with special interests of various sorts have existed for many years, sometimes adopting a clinical assistant role at hospital consultant-led clinics, in the UK, a number of policy documents have been produced by bodies such as the Department of Health (2002), in conjunction with the Royal College of General Practitioners and other professional bodies, and the more recent proposals by the NHS Modernisation Agency (2003) have made specific recommendations on a new role for the GP.

The key elements in the new GPwSI role are considered to be clinical, education (and liaison) and leadership. Clearly this potentially represents a much broader role than that of the 'traditional' GP. Interestingly, a set of competencies for those with a special interest in musculoskeletal conditions was also developed. They are summarised in Table 9.3.

The role was further differentiated into *generalist* skills, skills at training health-care professionals, and *special interest* skills, accreditation for which required 'evidence of working under direct supervision with a specialist clinician in relevant clinical areas' or a *personal development* portfolio 'showing evidence of advanced skills and knowledge' and 'evidence of attendance at relevant courses' or 'self-directed learning'. This was illustrated with examples of different evidence of competencies for the service, shown in Box 9.13.

Clearly it is difficult to offer more than general guidelines regarding competencies without understanding the particular context within which the GP works. This was recognised in the delineation of a set of guidelines, shown in Box 9.14.

There is no doubt that a major contributing factor to the success of primary-care management is the development and establishment of effective service pathways, supported by appropriate monitoring and governance. Few would have problems in signing up to such an aspiration but doubts, however, have been expressed about the feasibility of the original NHS Plan recommendations (Rosen et al 2003). A recent UK survey (unpublished) carried out by the Arthritis Research Campaign (ARC), the Primary Care Rheumatological Society and Keele University (Hay 2005) found wide variation

Table 9.3 Recommended competencies for GPwSIs with a special interest in musculoskeletal conditions

Activity of GPwSI musculoskeletal services	Competence
Assessment and treatment of musculoskeletal problems	History taking; examination, investigation of function and disability and formation of management plan
	A good understanding of psychological factors and ability to take a psychosocial history
	A good understanding of further specialist investigations (in line with best practice)
	Able to assess and refer appropriately for exercise management
Injection of joints	Use agreed referral guidelines and protocols
Minor surgery	Supervised training programme from previous local providers under commissioning protocols
Pain control	Good knowledge of relevant interventions, their indications and contra-indications
Education and training	Good knowledge of primary care organisations' training opportunities; good teaching and training skills
Recognising and managing clinically urgent conditions	Understand 'red flag' approach and able to recognise and understand appropriate treatment pathways including inflammatory arthritis
Team work	Able to work with multiprofessional teams

Adapted from Department of Health (2002)

Box 9.14

Local guidelines for use of the service

- Referral pathways
- Communication pathways
- Inclusion and exclusion criteria for patients referred or treated by the service
- Referral pathways for urgent problems.

Box 9.13

Examples of different evidence of competencies for the service

- Demonstration of skills under direct supervision by a senior clinician
- Demonstration of knowledge by personal study supported by appraisal
- Evidence of gained knowledge via attendance at accredited courses or conferences
- Demonstration of ability to work in multidisciplinary teams, to plan and deliver service provision and individual patient care
- Delivering multi- and uni-professional training
- Baseline experience working as a clinical assistance.

across the country in what GPwSIs actually do, with only 34% of those who considered themselves to be a GPwSI having a contract and only 17% having an annual specific appraisal (Hay & Adebajo 2005). They concluded that 'despite the fact that musculoskeletal conditions was one of the ten condition-specific frameworks' and that 'progress was made in terms of agreeing core competencies … Robust evaluation will be required to assess the clinical effectiveness, cost-effectiveness, acceptability and sustainability of such services'.

The role of the GP: lessons from recent research

In practice, for the foreseeable future, the first contact for most patients in primary care will be with non-specialist GPs, and the breadth of assessment and intervention recommended for GPwSIs will not be achieved in the time allowed to consult with a general practitioner – in the UK this may be as little as 10 minutes. A more realistic role would be as outlined in Box 9.15.

The GP may elect also to direct the patient's attention towards simple educational materials such as the *Back Book* (Roland et al 2002), discussed earlier in the chapter. Main & Williams (2002) recently advocated a systematic approach to early intervention, incorporating the identification of yellow flags using 'stem-and-leaf' questions (Main & Watson 2002). Jellema et al (2005b), in a recent randomised controlled trial, compared this approach, described as a 'Minimum Intervention Strategy' (MIS) delivered by GPs who were offered two 2.5-hour training sessions in brief psychosocial interventions for patients consulting with subacute back pain. The MIS consultation took about 20 minutes and consisted of three phases: 'stem-and-leaf' exploration, an information phase about the nature of low-back pain (LBP) and treatment (but including the patients' cognitions, emotions and behaviour) and a self-care phase. The intervention proved no more effective than 'treatment-as-usual' in the level of disability 1 year later. However, according to Main (2005) it was not clear that the GPs had in fact performed the intervention as required by the protocol, and indeed 72% of the patients had no more than one 20-minute consultation, with only 3% offered more than two sessions. The GPs were asked to record the content of their interventions using standardised forms, and the GPs mostly carried out the MIS intervention as intended. However, '18% of the patients in the group reported referral to a therapist even though we explicitly asked the general practitioners in the group not to refer in the first six weeks' (pp. 5–6). In a second paper from the same trial, Jellema et al (2005a) observed that although a high proportion of the participating GPs 'agreed that MIS was a valuable strategy for treatment of LBP' and that the training sessions 'afforded sufficient skills to apply MIS in practice' during the recruitment period their 'orientation regarding LBP hardly changed' and they were only 'moderately successful' in identifying psychosocial factors (p. 354). The authors concluded 'Five hours of training did not lead to sufficient GP competency with regard to the identification of psychosocial factors' (p. 357).

In their conclusions they recommended also reappraisal of the performance of the psychometric tools (both as screening tools and as outcome measures) in general practice settings, consideration of more powerful interventions, and assessing process measures on the level of both care-giver and patient.

The role for the GP in early intervention: concluding observations

Most acute episodes of back pain can be managed effectively and efficiently by the GP at the initial consultation and require no further health-care management. Some suggestions about the structuring and focus of the consultation have been made above.

There is, however, clear evidence that in a minority of patients, psychosocial obstacles (yellow flags) can impede recovery. Some suggestions about how such patients might be identified have already been presented. In such patients it would seem that if the general practitioner cannot dedicate sufficient time to find out what the patient believes about back pain, gain information about the patient's regular activities, give information and allow time for questions and to check that information has indeed been understood and is likely to be acted upon by the patient, then this role should be taken on by another health-care professional such as a practice nurse or physiotherapist. Finally, given that the length of the GP consultation is never likely to be more than 10–20 minutes, it may be that a more appropriate role for the GP consultation should be regarded as a 'first step' in terms of advice, reassurance and screening rather than a psychosocial intervention likely to prevent chronic incapacity in patients with significant psychosocial obstacles to recovery.

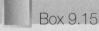

Box 9.15

The first consultation

- 'Red flags' assessment
- Yellow flag screening
- Appraisal of patient's understanding of the problem
- Reassurance about the recurrent nature of back/neck pain, and its essentially 'benign' nature
- Appraisal of habitual activity level and demands of work/housework
- Advice on adequate analgesia
- Advice on rest and resumption of normal activities.

Early pain management: the role of other health-care professionals?

Since pain is the most frequent symptom with which people consult, a wide range of health-care professionals may become involved in aspects of pain management, both in the public and the private sector. In the UK, in this era of 'patient choice' patients have the choice not only of the private or the public sector, as has indeed been the case since the inception of the NHS in 1947, but with the increased range of possible purchasing options available to the GP, there are now a wide range of providers of 'pain management' offering a bewildering array of therapeutic interventions, usually classified as traditional, complementary or alternative medicine. These are found both in clinical and occupational settings.

General versus specialised roles

In an endeavour to clarify what appears to be a confusing situation, it may be helpful to identify a general role for health-care professionals from an additional more targeted role for physical therapists such as physiotherapists, osteopaths and chiropractors.

The key ingredients for a general role for health-care professionals, such as specialist nurses, occupational therapists and physical therapists are shown in Box 9.16. It can be seen that there is overlap with some aspects of the role of the general practitioner. Much of the advice will be fairly general in nature and not dependent on physical examination findings, since the patient will usually already have seen a GP.

For most patients with subacute or recurrent musculoskeletal problems such as back pain, this will entail

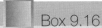

Box 9.16

Key components in a general role for HCPs

- Yellow flag screening
- Reassurance about the recurrent nature of back/ neck pain, and its essentially 'benign' nature
- Provision of simple advice, supplemented by appropriate evidence-based educational and self-help material
- Encouraging re-engagement in normal daily activity
- Patient advocacy in terms of access to other resources.

an individual assessment by a musculoskeletal specialist such as a physiotherapist, chiropractor or osteopath, and the general approach, in common with the other health-care professionals will have to be supplemented by a more specialised evaluation of pain-associated limitations, particularly in function. Occupational therapists may also have a role in the evaluation of specific functional associated limitations.

Although they may differ in their specific biomedical and biomechanical approaches, all consultations will involve discussion of patients' beliefs and expectations, although in 'traditional' biomedical and biomechanical approaches this may not be given a major or systematic focus.

During the past two or three decades, however, there has been increasing recognition of the importance of cognitive factors and this has been reflected in the design of a range of research studies, particularly in the treatment of low-back pain, which have included a focus to a greater or lesser extent on the modification of beliefs and behaviour, in the context of early intervention. The 'psychological' component has ranged from simple educational approaches to specific attempts identify and tackle psychosocial risk factors for chronicity (yellow and blue flags) the primary focus of the intervention.

Format of interventions

While the majority of patients are seen on an individual basis, there has also been a tradition of offering treatment to patients together in a group. Clearly in terms of the simple provision of information there would seem to be an obvious advantage in terms of efficiency of seeing patients in a class. Health-care costs within a financially constrained system such as the NHS, particularly when several different professionals may be involved, may be an important consideration. The original back school as described by Koes et al (1994) with its *primary* emphasis on education was delivered in a group format and has been popular within secondary care (although probably as much on the grounds of efficiency than on any conviction of specific therapeutic benefit as such). Many secondary-care facilities such as hospital physiotherapy departments attempt to systematise health care on a condition-specific basis and thus set up varieties of back pain programmes, some run by individual professionals, others with input from a variety of professionals. The use of therapeutic groups has been a major feature of psychiatric care and staff are required to have appropriate training and supervision. In tertiary-care programmes (Ch. 11) the specific therapeutic advantages of working with groups of patients has been more clearly recognised, but outwith the mental health sector, staff usually do not have specific training in and experience of group therapies, and there is no attempt to use group processes systematically to enable or enhance therapeutic benefit.

There are a number of therapeutic trials of early intervention in low-back pain and they have included a range of treatments, some of which may be delivered to more than one patient at a time, and there appears to be no clearly focused research on the specific therapeutic benefit of treating patients in groups as opposed to individually. (Indeed the term 'group' is frequently used to refer to data which has been aggregated rather than delivered specifically within a group format.) For the rest of this chapter, therefore, psychosocial interventions will be addressed primarily from the standpoint of individual interaction between patients and their therapists. (The specific therapeutic benefit of group treatment per se is discussed in Ch. 11.)

Research studies into psychosocial approaches to early intervention

During the last 20 years, since the beginning of systematic interventions of the effectiveness of physiotherapy, there has been an increasing interest in the nature of such interventions. Common themes have been the need to remobilise the patient, based on a biomechanical appraisal of their pain-associated limitations and provision of recommendations for reactivation, incorporating a range of therapeutic modalities, sometimes with the provision of specific anatomical and physiological education. There is a plethora of studies on the value for musculoskeletal problems of specific therapeutic modalities such as types of manipulation and mobilisation, many of which are to be found in the Cochrane Library (Cochrane Back Group 2006) and they will not be reviewed here. There has not as yet been a synthesis of the results of the trials on early intervention.

In an attempt to synthesise the results of recent research studies, the studies have been classified as Wave 1, Wave 2 or Wave 3 studies, the criteria for which are outlined in Box 9.17.

A comparison of some of these trials will now be presented.

First-wave studies (primary focus on the educational component)

For the purpose of this chapter, educational approaches are viewed as a precursor of the later more clearly focused psychosocial interventions. Many of the early educational approaches seemed to be based on assumption of a 'knowledge deficit' for which provision of

> ### Box 9.17
>
> **Stages in the development of the cognitive–behavioural approach**
>
> **Wave 1 (W1)**
> - Educational approaches (e.g. back schools)
> - Assumption of a knowledge deficit
> - Generic approach
> - No assessment of competency in CB approach.
>
> **Wave 2 (W2)**
> - Specific cognitive and behavioural content
> - Generic approach
> - No specific training in yellow flag elicitation.
>
> **Wave 3 (W3)**
> - Specific yellow flag training
> - Competencies assumed
> - Individualised approach.
>
> **Suggestions for a way forward: Wave 4 (W4)**
> - Screening of patients
> - Subgrouping according to 'modifiable risk profile'
> - Designing tailored interventions
> - Establishing and demonstrating therapeutic competencies
> - Controlled evaluation of outcome.

adequate education was required. The psychosocial intervention in the 'first-wave' studies included a fairly didactic educational approach.

Thus in an early study, Klaber-Moffett et al (1986), in a comparison of back school with an exercise intervention for patients with chronic back pain, demonstrated that that both approaches led to clinical improvement at 6-weeks follow-up. The back school patients, however, continued to improve thereafter. The reasons were not fully explored.

Education per se thus may be of value. Indeed in recent controlled study Frost et al (2004) found that a simple discussion with a physiotherapist concerning the causes of back pain and advice on how to remain active was as successful in the long term as routine physiotherapy treatment, but the level of disability was low and although both groups improved, the improvements were modest, suggesting that the improvements may have been suboptimal.

In a later study Frost et al (1998) demonstrated added value of a fitness programme over and above specific exercises and back school, although the initial levels of self-reported disability were relatively low (mean initial Oswestry score of 23–24).

Second-wave studies (a more developed psychosocial 'CBT' component)

Klaber-Moffett et al (1999), in a randomised controlled trial of low-back pain patients recruited through general practices, compared a progressive exercise programme with usual primary-care management. According to the authors a 'cognitive–behavioural approach' was used. In many ways this study is typical of the 'second-wave' of psychosocial interventions content (Box 9.18) in that cognitive and behavioural factors are located within a framework of reactivation and as such are best viewed primarily as physiotherapeutic rather than a psychotherapeutic approach.

Thus in this study, the intervention consisted of a physiotherapist-led exercise class including strengthening exercises, stretching exercises, relaxation and 'brief education on back care'. The sessions were held in the community, close to the patient. The results demonstrated that, at 6 and 12 months follow-up, the changes in the intervention group were significantly lower than in the control group (and at no greater cost), despite the fact that their intervention was surprisingly brief – only eight 1-hour sessions over 4 weeks. However, the changes in disability even in the intervention group were small and arguably of marginal clinical significance, perhaps a consequence in part of the low initial levels of self-reported disability (mean of 5.5–6.6 out of 24 on the Roland and Morris Disability Questionnaire), suggesting an element of selection on the part of the GPs who referred to the study, with the implication of a possible 'floor effect' in terms of the degree of improvement which was possible. However, the package has proved to be popular and has gained wide acceptance amongst physiotherapists. Development of a manual has helped to standardise the intervention.

In a secondary analysis of the data the same group (Klaber-Moffett et al 2004) demonstrated that those participants who scored more highly on fear-avoidance beliefs were more likely to benefit from the programme. It is not known whether such factors were in fact identified and targeted as such in the intervention group, and the physiotherapists involved seem to have been given only minimal training in cognitive–behavioural techniques and the level of therapist competence is not stated, so the intervention is perhaps better described as 'brief pain management' rather than full-blown CBT. Nonetheless the study is one of the first explicitly to recognise the possible influence of cognitive factors on early community-based interventions for LBP and offers some encouragement for the adoption of an approach as a way of challenging at least one of the obstacles to recovery.

Box 9.18

Typical content of 'second-wave' psychosocial interventions

- Advice and reassurance
- Challenging distorted cognitions about pain and activity and unhelpful attributions
- Practising feared activities
- Targeted increases in habitual physical activity – resumption of ceased activities
- Graded increase in general exercise.

In a recent study, a brief neck pain intervention has been demonstrated to be no better and slightly inferior to routine physiotherapy (Klaber-Moffett et al 2005) but the 'CBT' intervention, described as a 'brief physiotherapy intervention using cognitive-behaviour principles' was limited to one to three sessions, and since the physiotherapists received only 1 day of training, it seems unlikely that specific therapeutic competencies were established.

George et al (2003) compared a simple intervention for patients with acute low-back pain, designed to challenge fear-avoidance beliefs and promote early activation, with standard care. Although the intervention is described as 'Fear-Avoidance Physical Therapy' and therefore a prime candidate for psychologically enhanced physiotherapy, the intervention seems to have consisted essentially of an initial orientation with the *Back Book* (Roland et al 2002), followed by a Fordycian quota-exercise approach, as evaluated by Lindstrom et al (1992), reinforced by completion of treatment logs, which were monitored. As might be expected, participants in the treatment group and the control group improved significantly but those in the treatment group demonstrated greater changes in fear-avoidance beliefs and, although the number of participants was very low, those who were initially higher on fear avoidance appeared to demonstrate greater improvements than similar participants in the control group. In fact it appears unlikely that there was any sort of systematic attempt to address cognitions, over and above the educational material, and although it is stated that the physical therapists 'demonstrated competency in the study protocol by passing a written test' it appears that they had only one training session. We must also keep in mind that fear-avoidance beliefs, although important, are not the only obstacles to recovery in physiotherapy practice (Woby et al 2004).

The UK BEAM Trial (UK BEAM Trial Team 2004) has extended the concept of management using exercise within a cognitive–behavioural framework. The programme developed by Klaber-Moffett was compared to manipulation and GP best care along with groups of combined back class and manipulation. The authors state that the exercise programme comprised 'initial individual assessment followed by group classes incorporating cognitive behavioural principles' and classes ran in local community facilities. In fact all groups benefited from treatment, and the intervention groups did slightly better than best care, but although the differences reached statistical significance there were no clinically significant differences. This is perhaps disappointing since the groups were more disabled that those reported in the earlier studies by Klaber-Moffett et al (1999) and had a slightly longer duration, and therefore the study was presumably less vulnerable to 'floor effects'. A direct comparison of exercise (CBT) vs manipulation vs manipulation followed by exercise (CBT), indicates change in back beliefs in all three conditions at 3 months follow-up, with sustained but reduced change by 12 months. Fear-avoidance beliefs improved only in the two groups which included the exercise (CBT) and the changes in fear-avoidance beliefs were sustained, although significantly reduced at 12 months only in the group which received both treatments. Considered overall, however, the changes were small, and the change in back beliefs were of comparable magnitude in the exercise (CBT) and manipulation groups, suggesting lack of specificity in effect. Furthermore, since all groups initially were oriented to the evidence-based CBT philosophy, this reduced the chance of finding a difference between exercise (CBT) and manipulation. The trial therefore cannot be said to offer a robust evaluation of the specific value either of manipulative techniques or of exercise (CBT).

Third-wave studies (clinicians trained to deliver psychosocial CBT interventions)

Hay et al (2005) compared manual therapy with a simple, individualised CBT pain management approach provided by physiotherapists for patients presenting to their GP with low-back pain of less than 12 weeks. In fact the vast majority had pain for less than 4 weeks, representing a subacute group; most of the group were employed and most of these had lost work due to the pain. However, the level of self-reported disability was much higher than in the previous studies. Physiotherapists were trained in a psychosocial interview strategy, based on a 'stem-and-leaf' approach (Main & Watson 2002) and simple CBT techniques over 3 days with follow-up study days and mentoring. In the final analysis there was some evidence of 'health-economic' differences but both interventions were beneficial and there was little difference clinically between the two groups at 1-year follow-up.

As part of the research audit, using blinded video analysis of sample interventions from each arm, Mullis et al (2006) demonstrated that the therapeutic approaches in the two treatment arms were clearly distinguishable, and indeed seemed to represent a 'hands-on' and a 'hands-off' (pain management) approach as had been intended. Why then was no difference in outcome evident? In an effort to clarify this puzzle, Main et al (2006) undertook further interrogation of the data set by comparing the recorded activity of the treating physiotherapists with psychometric questionnaires completed independently by the participants in the study. These data were compared with details of treatments delivered in the intervention sessions. It was found that only in two-thirds of the patients was the treatment protocol strictly adhered to, and even restricting the analysis to those patients, there was a high level of use of non-specific treatments, thus blurring the differentiation between the two treatment approaches. Fuller details are reported elsewhere (Main et al 2006).

In a recently concluded trial, Johnson et al (2007) compared an active treatment intervention consisting of a 6-week community-based group intervention programme based on active exercise and education using a CBT approach with a control arm comprising usual GP care supplemented with educational material. The active intervention comprised eight 2-hour sessions over a period of 6 weeks delivered by two physiotherapists to a group of between four and ten patients. Each of the intervention sessions started with group discussion and ended with exercise, with the duration spent on exercise increasing throughout the course.

The authors state that the team of therapists were trained to competencies designed to be applicable to the needs of non-psychologists managing musculoskeletal pain conditions in primary- and secondary-care settings. Success of the training in terms of provision of 'evidence of a CBT approach' was evaluated by external examiners using audiotapes of a sample of group sessions and documenting the number of times the various concepts were mentioned during the sessions.

In fact the active intervention had, at most, a small additional benefit in the reduction of LBP and disability. However, there was only modest compliance to the intervention (with only 63% of the subjects attending at least 50% of the eight sessions), the patients in the trial had relatively mild LBP at baseline and the authors wondered whether the brief training for the therapists had been sufficient, noting: 'At times however, it was evident that the therapists found it difficult to adopt the communication style characteristic of a CBT approach and some methods, including challenging patients' beliefs and fears were limited.'

However, the study showed a beneficial influence of patient preference and recommended the targeting of interventions at subgroups.

Conclusions from studies on early psychosocial intervention

It can be seen that even with relevant training and a defined intervention protocol, it cannot be assumed that the intervention has been carried out on the population identified or in the manner intended. It seems clear that in intervention trials of the type recently undertaken a clear picture in terms of treatment outcome cannot be obtained without careful attention to factors such as treatment adherence and protocol violation as major potential confounders. The recent research studies have not been powered to elucidate, or control for, such confounders. Unfortunately in 'real-life' clinical trials there is a perpetual difficulty in deciding how much cost in terms of clinical service delivery and generalisability of findings is acceptable to ensure tighter experimental control.

The principal lessons learned from the recent research studies into psychosocial interventions are shown in Box 9.19.

Box 9.19

Lessons learned from recent randomised controlled trials

Current state of knowledge

- There is high level of consensus about the nature of psychosocial obstacles to recovery in patients with subacute LBP
- A range of methods for the early identification of patients burdened by psychosocial obstacles to recovery are now available
- We can distinguish potentially modifiable from unmodifiable risk factors
- Studies in secondary- and tertiary-care settings have demonstrated that addressing such factors reduces the extent and impact of pain-associated incapacity
- A next logical step is to 'move upstream' and develop a clearer focus on secondary prevention in primary-care settings.

What we have learned from the recent early intervention trials

- Patients at risk of chronicity can be identified in primary care

(Continued)

What we have learned from the recent early intervention trials (Continued)

- A biopsychosocial approach to management appears to be acceptable to such patients and to be beneficial (although to a different extent in different studies)
- To date, biopsychosocial approaches have not been shown to be superior either to usual care (whether delivered by GPs or by physiotherapists) or to other specific physiotherapeutic approaches. There are a number of possible reasons for this, but the strongest contenders appear to be:
  - insufficient training to guarantee competent assessment and intervention
  - protocol violation in terms of delivery of intervention and similarities outweighing the differences in the content of interventions
  - lack of information about the treatment *process*
  - insensitive or inappropriate outcome measures
  - lack of comparability in treatment cohorts across trials.

Conclusion and recommendations

- We still do not know whether, how or for whom psychosocial interventions are effective
- We need to clearly define the competencies we require for the outcomes we desire
- We need to develop and validate the training required to establish the necessary competencies, in association with the 'dose–response curves' required for various levels of risk reduction
- We may be advised to explore possibilities of linking screening, targeting and customising interventions accordingly
- In order to develop more effective interventions we have still a lot to learn about the influence of psychosocial factors on change across time and on the development of chronicity, but at least the nature of the task is becoming clearer.

The issue of competency in delivery of early intervention programmes: using physiotherapy as an example

Much biomedical management is, appropriately, specific to accredited professionals. The situation with regard to psychosocial interventions (or perhaps more accurately to the psychosocial component of biopsychosocial interventions) is somewhat more complex. As previously discussed, in a trivial sense there is a psychosocial component in all therapeutic encounters involving face-to-face relationships. In the first part of this chapter GP-led interventions were discussed and in the previous section physiotherapy-led interventions have been reviewed in detail. In many clinics, nurses, occupational therapists and pharmacists play an important role, the issues of communication and self-disclosure are of relevance, and therefore the general issue of competency arises.

It might be argued that competency in patient interaction ultimately is a question of professional accreditation and the responsibility therefore of statutory professional bodies. Nevertheless, there are a number of general issues specific to biopsychosocial management which need to be addressed. Given that the preponderance of relevant research has been on physiotherapy-led intervention, this will be used as an illustrative example.

What should constitute evidence for competence in physiotherapy-led CBT? Most of the published studies have either not stated the level of training given to the physiotherapist who delivered the programmes or, where stated, the level of training has been remarkably low. In addition, in Wave 1 and Wave 2 studies there is usually no indication of the standard of practice of competence of those performing the intervention and there is no assessment of how the treatment interventions were monitored to ensure that the therapists were indeed delivering what was intended. There was an attempt in the Wave 3 physiotherapy studies (Hay et al 2005, Jellema et al 2005b) to systematise the sort of competencies for which the training was designed. Some suggestions for minimum competency are shown in Box 9.20; however, it must be emphasised that we are talking of skills *in addition to* established clinical musculoskeletal assessment and treatment skills.

Box 9.20

Minimum competencies for a CB approach in physiotherapy

1 Psychosocial assessment and management
- Demonstrates an understanding of the role of psychological factors in the management of chronic pain
- Is able to conduct a simple psychosocial assessment

(Continued)

---

1 Psychosocial assessment and management (*Continued*)
- Is able to identify the key psychosocial obstacles to recovery from incapacity in a variety of patients
- Uses elements of CBT to improve patient understanding of their condition and to enhance treatment outcome
- Can explain physiological and medical information in terms appropriate to the patient's level of understanding
- Integrates physical assessment, interview and questionnaire information into a management plan.

2 Patient-centred treatment
- Leaves responsibility for rehabilitation with the patient – non-directional
- Is able to help the patient define clear, measurable and achievable rehabilitation goals
- Helps the patient to identify potential risks and barriers
- Integrates the patient's social circumstances into the management plan
- Helps the patient make an informed decision about participation in treatment.

3 Patient motivation
- Helps the patient identify obstacles to recovery
- Reflects inconsistencies between patient's aims and behaviour
- Helps the patient see an alternative scenario to incapacity – future orientated
- Reinforces positive behaviours and goal achievement
- Facilitates acceptance of chronic pain.

Conclusions

Can a CB approach be recommended?

The apparent failure of the general biomedical/biomechanical approach to prevent chronicity in a significant subgroup of patients, combined with the evidence of a strong influence of psychosocial factors, perhaps explains the popularity of the CB approach in physiotherapy in recent years. Can we give this shift in focus full-hearted support? Should this approach be seen as a panacea for the future? The results of the low-key CB approach implemented in the Hay et al (2005) trial, despite the acknowledged limitations of the study, suggest that a CB approach to patients is efficacious and is acceptable to patients. It may be that a Wave 4 CB approach (involving screening, subgroup and tailoring interventions) may provide a clearer picture of the specific worth of a CB approach to early intervention. Time will tell its worth.

However, the CB approach should not be uncritically adopted. 'Low-intensity approaches' to the chronically incapacitated do not work (Marhold et al 2001) so it is unlikely that these types of programme will be successful with very incapacitated or distressed patients or those who have been absent from work for a long time (more than 6 months). These patients will always be managed better in a full pain management programme.

Reiteration and recommendation

At this time the implementation of a CB approach should be considered for patients who have only a relatively short history of pain or who, despite having chronic or recurrent pain, remain functional (low disability and distress) and working. If not working, they should show evidence in general of a reasonable level of participation in their domestic or social environment, in activity or work. Many of these problems will be relatively 'low key' and the intervention is likely to centre mainly around issues of mistaken beliefs about pain, injury and activity, unhelpful coping behaviours and difficulty in managing activity, especially work and housework.

This calls for methods for identifying those at risk of not recovering, possibly including the development and refinement of screening tools (Ch. 5) to identify patients with modifiable risk factors and informing the design and implementation of low-cost interventions. Private practitioners, whether physiotherapists, osteopaths or chiropractors, are certainly in a position to deliver effective biopsychosocial interventions, but there is a need also to optimise appropriate use of NHS resources. There is an important role for the GP in this process, although at the time of writing, with the structural turbulence in the NHS, the possibilities for the integration of various health professions across the primary-/secondary-care interface is unclear and the development of simple clear patient pathways is a major challenge.

On balance, however, it would appear that for successful early intervention, the blending of biomechanical skills within a CB approach appears the 'best bet' for delivery of an optimal approach within the biopsychosocial framework, and physiotherapists are in 'pole position' to do this. Many physiotherapists, however, are strongly wedded to manual therapy approaches of various sorts, but a CB approach requires identifying not only goals for intervention but also obstacles to recovery, and the physiotherapist treating the patient must have a level of competence to design and instigate such an approach.

There is an urgent need, therefore to specify and define the level of competence required to implement successful early interventions, without the requirement of the level of skill required for tertiary pain management (Ch. 11) for those with higher levels of pain-associated limitations and significant levels of distress. A refocusing of attention from the cure of pain and 'normalising' biomechanical abnormalities to patient-centred pain management requires a fundamental reconsideration of the nature of early intervention, with development of the role of treating clinician into that of a 'coach' assisting the patient not only in managing the present episode but also preventing future recurrences from triggering a downward spiral into distress and unnecessary health-care consulting.

Key points

- **Education needs to be focused and systematic rather than haphazard**
- **Understanding the nature and process of communication is fundamental**
- **There are a number of key strategies in the assessment and management of pain-associated distress and dysfunctions**
- **The cognitive–behavioural (CB) approach is a helpful framework for the conceptualisation, design and delivery of early interventions**
- **It is important to appreciate both the communalities and the differences between primary-care and secondary-/tertiary-care contexts of health-care delivery**
- **Training to competency is an important precursor of optimal health-care delivery**
- **Competencies are as yet insufficiently understood**
- **Recent research trials into the outcome of an early CB approach are encouraging but suggest the need to develop more clearly targeted interventions at modifiable risk factors.**

References

Burton A K, Waddell G 2002 Educational and informational approaches. In: Linton S J (ed) New avenues for the prevention of chronic musculoskeletal pain and disability: pain research and clinical management, vol 12. Elsevier, Amsterdam, ch 16, pp 245–258

Burton A K, McClune T D, Clarke R D et al 2004 Long-term follow-up of patients with low back pain attending for manipulative care: outcomes and predictors. Manual Therapy 9:30–35

Burton A K, Waddell G, Main C J 2006 Beliefs and obstacles to recovery. In: Halligan P, Aylward M (eds) The power of belief. Oxford University Press, Oxford (in press)

Cochrane Back Group 2006 Issue 2. Cochrane Library

Department of Health 2002 Implementing a scheme for general practitioners with special interests. www.doh.gov.uk/pricare/gp-specialinterests

Deyo R 1998 Low back pain. Scientific American 279:53

Ernst E 2000a Prevalence of use of complementary/alternative medicine: a systematic review. Bulletin of the World Health Organization 78:252–257

Ernst E 2000b The role of complementary and alternative medicine. British Medical Journal 321:1133–1135

Ernst E, Cantor E 2006 A systematic review of systematic reviews of spinal manipulation. Journal of the Royal Society of Medicine 99:189–193

Ernst E, Eisenberg D, Pittler M H et al 2001 The desktop guide to complementary and alternative medicine: an evidence-based approach. C V Mosby, St Louis

Flor H, Fydrich T, Turk D C 1992 Efficacy of multidisciplinary pain treatment centers: a meta-analytic review. Pain 49:221–230

Fordyce W E 1976 Behavioral methods for chronic pain and illness. C V Mosby, St Louis

Frost H, Lamb S E, Klaber-Moffett J A et al 1998 A fitness programme for patients with chronic low back pain: 2-year follow-up of a randomised controlled trial. Pain 75:273–279

Frost H, Lamb S E, Doll H A et al 2004 Randomised controlled trial of physiotherapy compared with advice for low back pain. British Medical Journal 329:708

Gask L, Usherwood T 2003 The consultation. In: Mayou R, Sharpe M, Carson A (eds) ABC of psychological medicine. BMJ Books, London, ch 1, pp 1–3

George Z S, Fritz M J, Bialosky J et al 2003 The effect of a fear avoidance based physical therapy intervention for patients with acute low back pain: a randomised controlled trial. Spine 28:2551–2560

Hay E M 2005 Personal communication

Hay E M, Adebajo A 2005 Editorial: Musculoskeletal general practitioners with special interests: where are we up to? Rheumatology 44:1210–1211

Hay E, Mullis R, Lewis M et al 2005 Comparison of physical treatments versus a brief pain management programme for back pain in primary care: a randomised clinical trial in physiotherapy practice. Lancet 365:2024–2029

Jellema P, Van Der Windt D A W M et al 2005a Why is treatment aimed at psychosocial factors not effective in patients with (sub) acute low back pain? Pain 118:350–359

Jellema P, Van Der Windt D A W M et al 2005b Should treatment of (sub)acute low back pain be aimed at psychosocial prognostic factors? Cluster randomised trial in general practice. British Medical Journal 331 (online): Doi=10.1136/Bmj.38495.686736.Eo

Johnson R E, Jones G T, Wilies N J et al 2007 Randomised controlled trial of active exercise, education and cognitive behavioural therapy for persisting disabling low back pain. Spine (in press)

Kendall N A S, Linton S J, Main C J 1997 Guide to assessing psychosocial yellow flags in acute low back pain: risk factors for long term disability and work loss. Accident Rehabilitation and Compensation Insurance Corporation of New Zealand and The National Health Committee. Wellington, NZ

Klaber-Moffett J A, Chase S M, Portek I et al 1986 A controlled, prospective study to evaluate the effectiveness of a back school in the relief of chronic low back pain. Spine 11:120–122

Klaber-Moffett J, Torgerson D, Bell-Sayer S et al 1999 Exercise for low back pain: clinical outcomes, costs and preferences. British Medical Journal 319:279–283

Klaber-Moffett J A, Carr J, Howarth E 2004 High fear-avoiders of physical activity benefit from an exercise program for patients with back pain. Spine 29:1167–1173

Klaber-Moffett J A, Jackson D A, Richmond S et al 2005 Randomised trial of a brief physiotherapy intervention compared with usual physiotherapy for neck pain patients: outcomes and patients' preference. British Medical Journal 330:75

Koes B W, van Tulder M W, van der Windt D W M et al 1994 The efficacy of back schools: a review of randomised controlled trials. Journal of Clinical Epidemiology 47:851–862

Lindstrom I, Ohlund C, Eek C et al 1992 The effect of graded activity on patients with subacute low back pain: a randomised prospective clinical study with an operant-conditioning behavioral approach. Physical Therapy 72:279–290

Maguire P, Pitceathly C 2002 Key communication skills and how to acquire them. British Medical Journal. 325:697–700

Main C J 2005 Commentary: early psychosocial interventions for low back pain in primary care. British Medical Journal 331 (online):Bmj,Doi:10.1136/Bmj.38498.4950000.E0

Main C J, Watson P J 2002 The distressed and angry low back pain (LBP) patient. In: Gifford L (ed) Topical issues in pain, vol 3. CNS Press, Falmouth, pp 175–200

Main C J, Williams A C De C 2002 ABC of psychological medicine: musculoskeletal pain. British Medical Journal 325:534–537

Main C J, Mullis R, Lewis M, Hay E M 2006 To treat or not to treat. (Submitted)

Marhold C, Linton S J, Lennart M 2001 A cognitive-behavioural return-to-work program: effects on pain patients with a history of long-term versus short-term sick leave. Pain, 91:155–163

Morley S J, Eccleston C, Williams A 1999 Systematic review and meta-analysis of randomised controlled trials of cognitive behavioural therapy and behaviour therapy for chronic pain in adults. Pain 80:1–13

Mullis R, Dziedzic K S, Lewis L et al 2006 Validation of complex interventions in a low back pain trial: selective video analysis cross-referenced to clinical case notes. Contemporary Clinical Trials (in press)

NHS Modernisation Agency 2003 Practitioners with special interests: a step by step guide to setting up a general practitioner with a special interest (Gpwsi) service. www.natpact.nhs.uk/specialinterests

Price J, Leaver L 2002 Beginning treatment. British Medical Journal 325:33–35

Roland M, Waddell G, Klaber-Moffett J et al 2002 The back book, 2nd edn. The Stationary Office, Norwich

Rosen R, Stevens R, Jones R 2003 General practitioners with special clinical interests. British Medical Journal 327:460–462

Secretary of State for Health 2000 The NHS Plan: a plan for investment a plan for reform. Stationary Office, London

Staal J B, Hlobil H, Van Tulder M W et al 2003 Occupational Health guidelines for the management of low back pain: an international comparison. Occupational and Environmental Medicine 60:618–626

Turk D C, Okifuji A 2003 A cognitive-behavioral approach to pain management. In: Melzack R, Wall P D (eds) Handbook of pain management: a clinical companion to Wall and Melzack's textbook of pain, ch 36. Churchill Livingstone, Edinburgh, pp 533–541

Turk D C, Meichenbaum D H, Genest M 1983 Pain and behavioral medicine: a cognitive-behavioral perspective. The Guilford Press, New York

UK BEAM Trial Team 2004 United Kingdom back pain exercise and manipulation (UK BEAM) randomised trial: effectiveness of physical treatments for back pain in primary care. British Medical Journal 329:1377

Vlaeyen J W S, Morley S J 2005 Cognitive-behavioral treatments for chronic pain: what works for whom? Clinical Journal of Pain 21:1–8

Von Korff M, Moore J 2001 Stepped care approach for back pain: activating approaches for primary care. Annals of Internal Medicine 134:911–917

Waddell G, Watson P 2004 Rehabilitation. In: Waddell G (ed) The back pain revolution, 2nd edn. Churchill Livingstone, Edinburgh, pp 371–399

Woby S R, Watson P J, Roach N K et al 2004 Are changes in fear-avoidance beliefs, catastrophizing, and appraisals of control, predictive of changes in chronic low back pain and disability? European Journal of Pain 8:201–210

Chapter Ten

10

Intervention models and techniques

CHAPTER CONTENTS

Introduction

Biopsychosocial conceptualisations of pain and disability emerged as the limits of strict physiological or medical conceptualisations became more apparent. As research accumulated supporting biopsychosocial conceptualisations of pain and disability, there emerged an increasing awareness that psychosocial interventions would be required in order to more effectively treat pain-related conditions.

Over the past three decades, the field has witnessed varying approaches to managing psychosocial factors associated with pain and disability. The different approaches have been loosely tied to different theoretical positions. Table 10.1 illustrates the evolution of different perspectives on the psychology of pain over the past century.

Evolution of psychological approaches to the treatment of pain conditions

The role of subconscious conflicts: the contributions of Breuer and Freud

Psychoanalytic conceptualisations dominated early ways of understanding the psychology of pain. In the absence of discernable organic pathology, chronic pain was viewed as the consequence of unresolved unconscious conflicts. Proponents of this view considered

Table 10.1 Most influential psychological models in the treatment of pain

Proponent(s)	Model	Description
Breuer & Freud (1893)	Studies on hysteria	Model suggested that unresolved psychological conflicts could give rise to the experience of pain. The goal of intervention is to uncover the psychological conflicts giving rise to pain symptoms.
Beecher (1956)	Injury without pain	Model suggested that the manner in which pain symptoms were 'interpreted' would influence the experience and expression of pain. Contributed to elaboration of cognitive strategies for reducing pain and distress.
Engel (1959)	The pain-prone personality	Model suggested that certain personality features could predispose the development of a chronic pain condition. The goal of the intervention is to increase awareness of maladaptive aspects of personality contributing to pain and disability.
Fordyce (1976)	Pain as a learned response	Model suggested that pain expression was determined to a large extent by reinforcement contingencies. Goal of the intervention is to manipulate reinforcement contingencies in order to reduce expression of pain behaviour.
Blumer and Heilbronn (1982)	Chronic pain as the expression of psychic pain	Model suggested that chronic pain could be construed as a variant of a depressive disorder. Goal of the intervention is to treat underlying depression in order to alleviate symptoms of pain.
Turk et al (1983)	Cognitive–behavioural foundations of pain	Model suggested that cognitive appraisal processes and coping strategies influenced the manner in which pain was experienced and expressed. Goal of the intervention is to invoke a variety of cognitive and behavioural techniques aimed at reducing the negative impact of pain on emotional well-being and function.

psychoanalytic techniques to be the treatment of choice for chronic pain conditions. Although psychoanalytic perspectives on chronic pain are still discussed today, they have been embraced by only a minority of clinicians practising in this domain.

The role of cognition: the contributions of Beecher

Beecher's (1956) naturalistic observations of war casualties sparked considerable interest in the psychology of pain. Beecher provided vivid descriptions of soldiers who had sustained severe wounds in combat yet did not request narcotics to alleviate their pain. He suggested that for many soldiers, the wounds may have represented their 'ticket to safety' and thus their pain experience may have been lessened by its positive

reinterpretation. Beecher's ideas would eventually lay the foundation of cognitive–behavioural models of pain that emphasised the importance of cognitive factors such as expectancies, appraisals and attributions of the experience of pain.

The role of personality: the contributions of Engel

In 1959, Engel published his controversial paper, 'Psychogenic pain and the pain-prone patient' (Engel 1959). The notion put forth in the paper was that certain personality features could predispose individuals to the development of pain symptoms. Psychogenic pain later appeared in the DSM-III (APA 1980) as a condition of 'severe, prolonged pain unrelated to organic disease in which psychological factors were etiologically

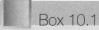

involved'. There followed several reports describing an association between pain and personality.

The role of behaviour: the contributions of Fordyce

Behavioural therapy initially emerged from empirical research on the determinants of learning (Skinner 1953). In the 1960s and 1970s, Wilbert Fordyce and his colleagues applied the concepts of learning theory to the problem of chronic pain (Fordyce 1976, Fordyce et al 1968). Fordyce's approach to treatment focused not on reducing the experience of pain, but on reducing the overt display of pain. The targets selected for treatment were pain behaviours such as distress vocalisations, facial grimacing, limping, guarding, medication intake, activity withdrawal and activity avoidance.

The role of depression: the contributions of Blumer and Heilbronn

Blumer & Heilbronn (1982) expanded on the notion of pain-proneness by arguing that persistent pain could emerge as a variant of a depressive disorder. They described the typical pain-prone individual as female, approximately 39 years of age, and showing evidence of excessive work performance and overactivity prior to the onset of pain. In the words of Blumer & Heilbronn (1982), 'chronic pain is the somatic expression of psychic pain'. They argued that antidepressant medication was the treatment of choice for chronic pain sufferers who showed evidence of pain-prone personality.

Cognitive–behavioural approaches to the management of pain and disability: the contributions of Turk

Cognitive–behavioural approaches have dominated recent intervention research on psychological influences on pain and disability. Current cognitive–behavioural interventions have emerged from the seminal work of Turk and his colleagues (Turk et al 1983). Cognitive–behavioural perspectives proceed from the view that an individual's interpretation, evaluation and beliefs about their health condition, and their coping repertoire with respect to pain and disability, will influence the degree of emotional and physical disability that will be associated with their pain condition (Turk & Okifuji 2002, Vlaeyen & Linton 2000).

Box 10.1

Major types of specific interventions

- Education/information (back schools)
- Behavioural interventions
- Cognitive–behavioural programmes
- Stress management programmes
- Risk-factor targeted interventions.

Specific intervention approaches for chronic pain and disability

The major types of specific intervention for chronic pain and disability are shown in Box 10.1.

Education/information (back schools)

Although back schools were first developed in the late 1960s, the first published reports of the benefits of back schools only appeared in the literature in the early 1980s (Zachrisson-Forsell 1980, 1981). The structure and content of back schools reflected the prevailing view of the time that information could be a powerful tool to effect change in behaviour (e.g. pain-related disability).

Back schools vary widely in terms of content, duration and the intervention disciplines used to administer their programmes. The duration of back school interventions has ranged from a single information session to a 2-month inpatient programme (van Tulder et al 2002). Back school interventions have tended to use group formats with didactic structures in which participants might be exposed to information about biomechanics, posture, ergonomics, exercise, nutrition, weight loss, attitudes, beliefs and coping. As a function of the type of information being provided, the interventionist might be a physician, physiotherapist, occupational therapist, nurse or psychologist.

The marked differences across back schools in terms of content, structure and duration have presented significant challenges to the systematic assessment of their efficacy. A recent review of randomised clinical trials of back school programmes concluded that back schools yielded a greater benefit than treatment-as-usual interventions, that the treatment effect size was small, and that back school programmes implemented within occupational settings appeared to yield the most positive outcomes (Heymans et al 2004).

Behavioural interventions

The first behavioural approaches to the management of pain and disability were conducted within inpatient settings that permitted the systematic observation of pain behaviours, as well as control over the environmental contingencies influencing pain behaviour (Fordyce 1976). Staff were trained to monitor pain behaviour, and to selectively reinforce 'well behaviours' and selectively ignore 'pain behaviours'. The results of several studies revealed that the manipulation of reinforcement contingencies could exert a powerful influence on the frequency of display of pain behaviours (Fordyce et al 1985). The manipulation of reinforcement contingencies was also applied to other domains of pain-related behaviour and shown to be effective in reducing medication intake, reducing downtime, and maximising participation in goal-directed activity.

A number of clinical trials on the efficacy of behavioural treatments for the reduction of pain and disability have yielded positive findings (Sanders 1996). However, given the significant resources required to implement contingency management interventions, issues concerning the cost-efficacy of behavioural therapy for pain and disability have been raised. There has also been concern over the maintenance of treatment gains since reinforcement contingencies outside the clinic setting could not readily be controlled. In order to increase access and reduce costs, behavioural treatments were modified to permit their administration on an outpatient basis. This change in delivery format compromised to some degree the control over environmental contingencies, and required greater reliance on self-monitoring and self-report measures (Sanders 1996).

With its focus on reducing pain behaviour as opposed to ameliorating the pain condition, the early work of Fordyce and his colleagues was at once novel and contentious. Critics voiced their concern that behavioural treatments might only be effective in training stoicism, and were not dealing with the underlying problem. In response to critics, Fordyce pointed to literature indicating that the magnitude of the relationship between pain and disability was modest at best, and that treatments aimed at reducing pain often had no appreciable effect on level of disability (Fordyce et al 1985). According to Fordyce, to effectively treat disability, disability had to be targeted directly.

There has been a recent resurgence of interest in the application of behavioural interventions for the management of pain-related disability. Emerging programmes differ from traditional approaches with greater emphasis on increasing activity involvement and reducing avoidance and escape behaviours (Vlaeyen & Linton 2000). Recent programmes have also tended to adopt a client's return to work as the primary goal of the intervention (Sullivan & Stanish 2003).

Cognitive–behavioural programmes

Programmes of cognitive–behavioural therapy (CBT) for the management of pain and pain-related disability began to appear in the 1980s. Many CBT programmes incorporated concepts drawn from earlier behavioural approaches as well as the information-based approaches used in back schools. The objective of many CBT programmes was to equip individuals with the psychological 'tools' necessary to adequately meet the challenges of persistent pain (Linton et al 1989, Turk et al 1983).

Administered individually or in groups, cognitive–behavioural interventions are currently considered the psychological treatment of choice for individuals coping with pain-related disability (McCracken & Turk 2002, Turk 1996). A number of clinical trials have demonstrated that these types of interventions can assist individuals in learning to manage or control their symptoms, and can lead to clinically significant decreases in emotional distress (Linton & Andersson 2000, Morley et al 1999). There is evidence to suggest that cognitive–behavioural interventions can also impact return-to-work rates, but observed effects have been modest and inconsistent (Morley et al 1999).

It is important to note that the term cognitive–behavioural does not refer to a specific intervention but, rather, to a class of intervention strategies. The strategies included under the heading of cognitive–behavioural interventions vary widely and may include self-instruction (e.g. motivational self-talk), relaxation or biofeedback, developing coping strategies (e.g. distraction, imagery), increasing assertiveness, minimising negative or self-defeating thoughts, changing maladaptive beliefs about pain, and goal setting (Turk et al 1983, Linton & Andersson 2000). A patient referred for cognitive–behavioural intervention may be exposed to varying selections of these strategies. The goals of CBT programmes might also differ across settings and may include pain reduction, distress reduction, increased activity involvement or return to work.

The lack of standardisation of the content of CBT intervention within pain management programmes has likely weakened the demonstrated impact of these interventions. The essentially 'palliative' nature of many intervention techniques subsumed by CBT interventions might also compromise their impact on return-to-work outcomes. An examination of the content of many CBT interventions for pain-related disability also reveals an emphasis on techniques designed to reduce physical (e.g., relaxation) or emotional (e.g., reinterpretation) distress. While emotional distress and pain no doubt contribute to disability, the reduction of emotional distress and pain may not be sufficient to contribute in a meaningful manner to return-to-work potential (Sullivan & Stanish 2003, Sullivan et al 2005).

Stress management programmes

Stress management programmes represent a special kind of cognitive–behavioural intervention. These programmes proceed from the view that, unless properly managed, chronic stresses can lead to the depletion of an individual's physical and psychological resources, thereby increasing the individual's susceptibility to physical or psychological dysfunction (Lazarus & Folkman 1984). Stress management approaches are considered separately from cognitive–behavioural pain management programmes since stress management programmes do not necessarily focus on managing pain symptoms or disability. Furthermore, while CBT programmes are typically used for individuals who are work-disabled, stress management programmes can potentially be used as preventive interventions for individuals who are still working. Stress management interventions might primarily focus on stresses within the workplace (Feuerstein et al 2000, Pransky et al 2002) or on an individual's personal stresses (Pelletier & Cagney 1991). There is considerable variability in the duration of stress management programmes, which can range from two sessions to 8-week programmes (Pransky et al 2002).

Problem-solving therapy is a variant of stress management programmes that has recently been applied to work-disabled individuals (D'Zurilla 1990, Van den Hout et al 2003). Problem-solving therapy proceeds from the view that life stresses can be minimised if an individual is able to use appropriate problem-solving strategies to deal with difficult situations that might be encountered at the workplace or in daily life (D'Zurilla & Goldfried 1971, Nezu & Perri 1989). Problem-solving intervention programmes will typically span 8–10 weeks and might involve didactic lectures, group discussion, and homework assignments. The limited research that has addressed the efficacy of this form of intervention indicates that the addition of problem-solving therapy to the usual forms of treatment might improve return-to-work outcomes (Van den Hout et al 2003).

Risk-factor-targeted interventions

Recent research on risk factors for prolonged pain and disability has prompted the development of risk-factor-targeted intervention programmes. These programmes differ from traditional CBT programmes in that their focus is on a limited set of risk factors, such as fear of pain, pain catastrophising or depression. Graded activity and exposure interventions aimed at reducing fear of movement have been shown to be effective in facilitating return to work and reducing absenteeism (Van den Hout et al 2003, Lindstrom et al 1992, George et al 2003). The premise underlying graded activity or exposure interventions is that disability can be construed as a type of phobic orientation toward activity (Vlaeyen et al 1995). In this model, the reduction of fear of movement is viewed as a critical component of the successful rehabilitation of work disability (Vlaeyen & Linton 2000).

Intervention programmes, such as the Pain-Disability Prevention (PDP) Program, have also been developed to specifically target psychosocial risk factors (Sullivan & Stanish 2003). The PDP Program is a standardised 10-week intervention that uses structured activity scheduling strategies and graded activity involvement to target risk factors such as fear of movements/reinjury and perceived disability. Thought-monitoring and cognitive-restructuring strategies are used to target catastrophic thinking and depression. A recent study showed that treatment-related reductions in pain catastrophising significantly predicted return to work in a sample of injured workers (Sullivan et al 2005).

A programme similar to the PDP Program has been developed for front-line rehabilitation professionals such as physiotherapists and occupational therapists (Sullivan et al 2006). The Progressive Goal Attainment Program (PGAP) is a standardised community-based intervention that aims to reduce risk factors for prolonged work disability, such as pain catastrophising, fear of movement or reinjury, and perceived disability. The rationale behind the development of the programme was that increasing front-line rehabilitation professionals' ability to detect psychosocial risk factors and to intervene accordingly would facilitate the early implementation of risk-factor-targeted interventions. In a recent clinical trial with a sample of individuals who had been work-disabled due to whiplash symptoms for approximately 6 months, 75% of individuals in the PGAP group returned to work compared to 50% who followed usual treatment (Sullivan et al 2006). The later study raises the possibility that psychosocial interventions might be effectively administered by interventionists who are not mental health professionals.

Specific intervention techniques used in pain management

A summary of the major intervention techniques used in pain management is shown in Box 10.2.

Disclosure

Some of the key aspects of disclosure are shown in Box 10.3.

The benefits of disclosure

The key to success in almost any type of intervention is the establishment of a good working relationship. The disclosure of personally relevant or emotionally significant information is one way in which working relationships are built. Communication theory suggests that connections between people occur through the telling of life stories. Stories are the vehicles through which experiences are shared. Our perception that a listener is interested in hearing about our experiences, and in learning about who we are provides the basic foundation of the development of a working relationship.

Box 10.2

Specific intervention techniques used in pain management

- Disclosure
- Cognitive restructuring
- Activity scheduling
- Relaxation and biofeedback
- Hypnosis
- Exposure interventions.

Box 10.3

Key aspects of disclosure

- The benefits of disclosure
- The development of disclosure
- Strategies for the facilitation of disclosure
- Placing boundaries on disclosure.

Research suggests that emotional disclosure following exposure to aversive situations may have beneficial effects on physical and emotional well-being (Pennebaker 1995, Pennebaker & O'Heeron 1984, Pennebaker & Susman 1988). Although emotional disclosure can temporarily heighten distress, many individuals report a lessening of distress after disclosure. The disclosure of emotionally upsetting information has also been shown to have a positive impact on indices of immune function, health status, and health-care utilisation (Esterling et al 1990, Pennebaker et al 1988). The results of one investigation showed that emotional disclosure in patients with rheumatoid arthritis led to significant reductions in affective disturbance and physical symptoms (Kelley et al 1997).

When clients feel better after an interview in which they have disclosed the difficulties associated with their pain condition, they are likely to attribute their increased feelings of well-being to the clinician. This attribution will likely increase the clients' sense that the clinician will be able to help them. In turn, the client's confidence in the clinician's abilities will likely impact positively on the former's adherence to recommended treatments.

By setting the stage for the development of an emotional connection between the patient and the clinician, the clinician builds an additional motivational 'tool' for the rehabilitation process. The patient may not always be ready to participate in arduous rehabilitation treatments on his or her own accord, but might pursue them in order to avoid disappointing the clinician. The stronger the working relationship that has been established between the patient and the clinician, the less likely that the patient will behave in a manner that he or she believes will disappoint the clinician.

The development of disclosure

Patient disclosure should be encouraged early in the first meeting in order to prevent the development of an excessively didactic relationship. Given that the rehabilitation treatment environment is novel to many clients, they will be using early experiences to develop a model of their role in treatment. Interviews that are too specific, or interview styles that are too directive, will entrain a more respondent than participatory role for the client. Interviews that are characterised by checklisting an inventory of signs and symptoms will impede the development of a positive working relationship. Clients are likely to feel that their situation is being compartmentalised, their experience objectified, and their suffering trivialised.

Strategies for the facilitation of disclosure

Patient disclosure can be facilitated by using a broad, open-ended interview style. The clinician must appear genuinely interested in understanding the client's pain experience and how pain has affected his or her day-to-day life. Behind the objective details of the client's descriptions, the clinician should probe for emotional reactions, issues related to the family's adaptation to the client's pain condition, and the client's view of the future.

For the injured client, disclosure can be facilitated with questions such as:

'The letter from your doctor indicates that you were injured on June 4 2005. Can you tell me what happened on that day?'

The clinician should follow a line of questioning that will facilitate disclosure of details concerning the injury or difficulties that have ensued since the injury. This line of questioning should also target the client's understanding of his or her condition.

'So after you injured yourself, what happened next?'
'What did they do at the hospital (or your physician's office)?'
'Did the physician give you a diagnosis or explain what had happened?'

Since the patient is likely to be quite fluent in the details of the injury and his or her treatment-related experiences, the line of questioning described above, in combination with expressions of interest and concern, should facilitate the development of a positive working relationship.

The clinician may then wish to increase the level of intimacy of disclosure by addressing some of the social and emotional aspects of work injury.

'How did your spouse react to your injury?'
'What has it been like being away from work?'
'Of all that you've gone through over the past few weeks, what has been the toughest thing to deal with?'
'Many people who experience symptoms of persistent pain say that they have become more easily frustrated, or more irritable, or more upset. Have you noticed these kinds of changes in yourself? What has been most noticeable?'

By increasing the level of intimacy in the interaction, from injury details to the life impact of injury, the clinician will be fostering the development of an emotional connection with the client. Emotional connections develop as interactions move from lower to higher levels of intimacy and continue to be characterised by a sense of openness, interest and authenticity.

Empathic reflections can be useful when communicating. An empathic reflection is a statement that provides a summary of the emotional themes that were communicated by the client. To a patient who has been disclosing about the impact of pain in his or her life, empathic reflections might take the following forms:

'So this accident has really turned your world upside down.'
'I guess you started to get worried when you saw that you weren't getting better.'
'I guess you never dreamed you would be going through something like this at this point in your life.'
'The whole situation sounds like a nightmare.'

Statements such as these will ring true for the majority of clients with persistent pain. When a patient hears words that capture the essence of what he or she has been communicating, the patient will likely feel that the clinician is listening, is interested and understands.

Placing boundaries on disclosure

The type of working relationship that the clinician will need to build with the patient is similar but not identical to the working relationship that a psychologist might build with a psychotherapy client. Psychologists will use techniques similar to those described above, but will encourage disclosure across several domains of experience. In the treatment of the patient in pain rehabilitation, disclosure will be contained to domains relevant to pain. By restricting the territory of disclosure, the clinician will place implicit boundaries on the material that a patient will feel comfortable disclosing. Restricting the domains of disclosure to pain-relevant information will minimise the probability that the patient will begin to share information about relational conflicts, parental issues or sexual problems. These are all important domains of life, but delving into these issues might detract from rehabilitation goals.

Psychosocial issues should not become the focus of discussion in the first session. The client, however, should be encouraged to view the impact of injury and the process of recovery as one that comprises physical, social and psychological factors.

Cognitive restructuring

Key aspects of cognitive restructuring are shown in Box 10.4.

Theoretical basis

As noted earlier, cognitive–behavioural models of pain and disability proceed from the view that the manner in which individuals think about their situation can influence how they will feel and behave. Cognition is the term used by cognitive–behavioural theorists (and practitioners) to refer to different forms of 'thinking' that might impact on emotion and behaviour.

Cognitive–behavioural theories emerged from cybernetic models of human functioning. In other words, within cognitive–behavioural frameworks, a computer analogue is used to understand how psychological processes operate. This computer analogue is the reason why so much of the language of cognitive–behavioural theory is common to the world of computers. Concepts like input functions, output functions, accessibility, processing, retrieval and storage were essentially transported from cybernetics to psychology.

Lazarus & Folkman's transactional model of stress and Beck's cognitive theory of depression may be considered exemplars of the application of cybernetic models of psychological functioning. Lazarus & Folkman's (1984) transactional model of stress draws a conceptual distinction among the concepts of appraisals, beliefs and coping. Primary appraisals (judgements about whether a potential stressor is irrelevant, benign-positive or stressful) interact with secondary appraisals (beliefs about coping options and their possible effectiveness) and influence whether, and which, coping responses will be attempted.

The nature of cognitive processes

Beck et al (1979) propose that 'depressive schema' may become activated following the occurrence of negative life events. Once activated, depressive schema are said to give rise to a variety of cognitive distortions, including catastrophising, overgeneralisation, personalisation and selective abstraction. In this model, cognitive errors are expected to bias information processing in such a manner as to increase the likelihood of the development of depressive symptoms. Schema activation is said to increase the accessibility of information that is thematically relevant to the event that initiated the schema activation.

Although many of the processes discussed within appraisal or schema models are considered to be automatic, proponents of these models argue that a certain degree of conscious control can be exerted. It is through these conscious control mechanisms that opportunities for intervention arise. In the sections below, intervention strategies used to target different components of pain-related 'cognition' are briefly described. Clinical judgement plays a major role in determining which strategies would be most appropriate in the treatment of a particular patient.

Appraisals are considered to be a significant determinant of emotional and behavioural responses to a stressful situation. Appraisals can be construed as one of the initial steps of perception during which the individual interprets or evaluates the threat value of a particular situation. Any situation can be interpreted in different ways, and different interpretations can lead to different emotional and behavioural outcomes. The patient who interprets an increase in back pain as muscle soreness will feel and behave differently than the one who interprets the same pain experience as a spinal tumour. Individuals who consistently interpret their pain symptoms as indicative of a significant health threat will likely experience heightened emotional distress and heightened disability. Cognitive–behavioural intervention techniques can help patients change maladaptive ways of interpreting pain-related stresses.

Moving from education to active engagement

Education about pain systems is frequently included as an integral component of cognitive–behavioural interventions. The rationale for including education as part of treatment is that providing accurate information about the patient's health condition will reduce the probability that the patient will develop erroneous interpretations of his or her health condition. However,

---

Box 10.4

Key aspects of cognitive restructuring

- Theoretical basis
- The nature of cognitive processes
- The role of monitoring
- Identifying the links between thoughts, emotional responses and pain behaviour
- Modifying negative thoughts
- Developing strategies for behaviour change
- Establishing the links: further therapeutic strategies.

as discussed in the previous chapter, education per se is a relatively weak method of intervention, particularly in patients with chronic pain problems, and education alone will typically not be sufficient to exert a significant impact on mood or functioning.

A major step in assisting a patient to control appraisals of pain-related stresses is to bring the patient to recognise that his or her approach to interpreting pain-related stresses might be disadvantageous. Clinicians will frequently provide patients with examples of how one's interpretation of a situation will influence outcomes.

'If I lost my job tomorrow, and I reacted to this situation by thinking that I will surely lose everything, I will likely feel anxious and fearful. If I reacted to this situation by thinking that now I have an opportunity to find the kind of job that I really want, I will probably feel less anxious or fearful. It's the same thing with pain. We can react to our pain in ways that will make us feel even worse, or we can react to our pain in ways that won't make the situation worse than it is.'

The Pain Catastrophising Scale contains several items reflecting pessimistic or alarmist interpretations of pain symptoms. A patient's responses to this scale can be used as a platform for introducing the patient to the relation between appraisals and negative pain-related outcomes.

'On this questionnaire you noted that you often react to your pain by thinking "It's terrible and I think it's never going to get better". When you think like that, how does it make you feel?'

In response to this question, it is likely that the patient will indicate that he or she felt worse or discouraged. The clinician can then point to another item that was endorsed by the patient, proceeding with a similar question. Again, the patient is likely to indicate that the catastrophic thought resulted in a lowering of mood. The clinician can then summarise the patients' responses and point to the need to change how he or she is reacting to pain symptoms.

'So it seems that sometimes you will react to your pain in ways that make you feel more anxious, fearful or discouraged. I think that this is something we need to work on. If we can change how you are reacting to your pain, we might be able to help you feel better.'

Once a patient recognises the link between pessimistic or alarmist thinking and negative pain-related outcomes,

the next step is to help the patient to modify his or her thinking. The terms 'thought monitoring' and 'reappraisal' are used to describe strategies that can be used to modify previously automatic and maladaptive ways of responding to pain. For thought monitoring, the patient will be asked to keep a log of difficult pain-related situations and to record the thoughts he or she entertained during that situation. For reappraisal, the patient will be invited to consider alternate ways of reacting to difficult pain-related situations.

The role of monitoring

A number of different forms have been developed to assist the patient in monitoring reactions to stressful life situations. Some of these are pain-specific (e.g. Turk et al 1983), while others address broader categories of stressful life situations (e.g. Beck et al 1979).

A number of cognitive theorists have suggested that the beneficial effects of thought monitoring emerge from the 'distancing' required in order to monitor one's thoughts. For example, in order to act as an observer of one's thinking, the individual must be cognitively distanced from the source of the thoughts that are being monitored. Part of the emotional impact of negative thoughts derives from the truth value that is ascribed to the thought and the unitary experience of thought. As such, when the patient thinks 'This will never get any better', the patient also believes this statement and experiences it as a true reflection of reality. But a different emotional experience will ensue from a patient who is monitoring pain-related thoughts and thinks instead, 'There I go again, I was thinking that my condition was not going to get better'. The act of monitoring will decrease the frequency of occurrence of the targets of monitoring and will reduce the emotional impact of the monitored thoughts when they do occur.

An important element of cognitive–behavioural interventions is 'collaborative discovery' (Turk et al 1983). Prescriptive approaches where the patient is informed about the maladaptive nature of his or her cognitions will not be as effective as those in which the patient becomes aware of the maladaptive nature of certain ways of thinking through collaborative exploration with the clinician.

An example of a pain-specific thought-monitoring form is reproduced in Box 10.5. The thought-monitoring form can serve several useful purposes in facilitating treatment progress. It encourages the patient to become an observer of his or her cognitive and behavioural responses to painful or stressful situations. As the patient learns more about the inter-relations among his or her pain-related thoughts and behaviours, the stage

Box 10.5

Example of pain-specific thought-monitoring form

Pain Reaction Record

Date/time	Pain situation	Negative thoughts	What you did	What could you have done differently?
	(Describe situations where your pain was, very intense or a situation where you stopped an activity because of your pain)	(Describe the thoughts that were going through your mind)	(Describe how you reacted to the situation)	(Describe how you could have handled the situation better)

is set to take greater control over the negative impact of painful or stressful situations. By using a thought-monitoring form, the patient can develop skills in reappraisal, cognitive restructuring, self-instruction and anticipatory coping.

The clinician should be prepared for the possibility that the patient will require some degree of coaching before he or she is able to use a thought-monitoring form in the most appropriate fashion.

In the example provided below, the patient describes a situation in which he or she discontinued mowing the lawn due to an increase in pain. The patient entertained pessimistic thoughts about the lack of improvement in his or her condition and then went to bed. In the second example, the patient avoided an activity due to pain, reacted with very negative thoughts about himself, and then took medication and watched television.

Identifying the links between thoughts, emotional responses and pain behaviour

The clinician should proceed in a step-by-step fashion, retracing the sequence of events, reactions and thoughts that led to the discontinuation of an activity. As the clinician 'recreates' the problem situations described in the thought-monitoring form, he or she should use the opportunity to model the correct method of recording if it appears that the patient proceeded with some confusion.

By reviewing each of the problem situations, the hope is that the patient will learn that painful situations can trigger a sequence of cognitive and behavioural 'events' that ultimately culminate in lowered mood and activity termination. The patient is then in a better position to appreciate how modifying cognitions triggered by pain can be beneficial.

Identifying the nature and function of maladaptive thoughts

The maladaptive consequences of negative thoughts can best be illustrated for the patient by asking him or her about emotional responses to the negative thoughts. Although the clinician may wish to appeal to the relation between negative thoughts and activity discontinuation, the patient may not readily grasp this relation as maladaptive. To the patient, discontinuing an activity due to pain will likely seem totally reasonable.

The maladaptive effects of negative thoughts will most easily be grasped in relation to their effects on emotional well-being. The clinician can explore the client's emotional reactions in the following manner:

'Here you indicate that you were mowing the lawn and then you stopped because it was hurting too much. And the thought that went through your head was that you would never get better. How did you feel at that moment? How were you feeling when you thought that you were never going to get any better?'

Since emotional reactions are also automatic responses to negative thoughts, it is likely that the patient will reflect that he or she felt down, or depressed, or sad, or hopeless. The clinician can then further explore how long the patient felt that way, and whether the patient shared his or her feelings with anyone. Finally, the clinician can highlight that the client's reaction to feeling down was to go to bed:

'So it seems that your pain went up, you thought that you were never going to get better, that made you feel down, and then you went to bed.'

If the clinician hopes to engage the patient in monitoring and modifying negative thoughts associated with pain, he or she will need to repeatedly demonstrate the causal chain that is triggered by the pain situation. A similar causal chain can be traced in the second situation that the patient described:

'In this situation, it appears that you avoided an activity due to your pain, you then thought of yourself as useless, which made you feel really down, and then you took medication and watched TV.'

After a number of examples have been covered in this manner, the patient will become more fluent with regard to the relationship between pain situations, negative thoughts, negative emotions and further activity reduction. The clinician's next task is to highlight the maladaptive nature of these cognitive and emotional reactions:

'I guess what we're seeing in these different situations is that when you stop or avoid an activity due to pain, you are very likely to think in rather negative ways. This negative thinking then causes you to feel very badly, either down, or depressed or frustrated. And then, feeling like that

just makes you want to lie down or take medication. That doesn't sound like a very pleasant way to live. I'm starting to see a pattern. It's like this chain of events that is triggered by the situation; then the negative thoughts and negative emotions kick in, and then everything seems hopeless. It's like everything starts spiralling down.'

Once the clinician has reviewed the problem situations recorded in the thought-monitoring form, the patient should be encouraged to consider alternate ways of responding to increases in pain.

Modifying negative thoughts

In order to develop the ability to modify the negative thoughts that accompany problematic pain situations, the patient must first learn to generate alternate ways of responding to pain 'after the fact'. The sequence of cognitive and behavioural events that are triggered by a problematic pain situation is so rapid that these events are experienced as instantaneous. The more that the patient engages in thought monitoring, the more the sequence is slowed. One effect of becoming an observer of one's thoughts is to slow down the sequence of internal reactions to specific situations. Then, as the patient explores alternate ways of reacting, the sequence of internal events is slowed even further, and ultimately the sequence can be interrupted.

'Let's look at this last column of the example of the thought-monitoring form. This is where we want to see how we could have responded differently to each problem situation. Sometimes we overestimate what we are able to do. We get into trouble when halfway through the activity we realise it's too much for us. A way to prevent this is to slow down just a bit. One might be able to complete 10 minutes of cleaning in the garage, but 25 minutes causes too much pain. If we cut back to 10 minutes, we may find that we are able to meet the goal we set for ourselves, and be less likely to think negatively about the situation.

Our negative thinking gets us into trouble. Telling ourselves that we are getting worse will lead to discouragement and a sense of giving up. We can try to prevent our discouragement by telling ourselves that increases in pain are normal, and that they are temporary.

As usual, we need to stay positive and remain confident that we will make progress and that we will recover.'

Developing strategies for behaviour change

After examining the entries in the thought-monitoring form, the clinician should engage the patient in a discussion of what could have constituted alternate responses to the problematic pain situations.

'Here you noted that you went to bed when your pain got worse after mowing. What could you have done differently?'

The patient who is making progress will be able to reflect that he or she could have planned to mow for a shorter period of time or could have engaged in a lighter form of activity until the pain subsided. The patient should also be encouraged to maintain a positive attitude even when situations are difficult. In order to progress, the patient must become a 'mental coach' to him- or herself, so as to maintain the drive to persist through difficult situations.

Establishing the links: further therapeutic strategies

In order to effect meaningful change in the frequency and impact of negative pain-related cognitions, thought-monitoring exercises might need to be used for several weeks. In the example provided above, the patient was initially not asked to complete the section addressing how he or she might have reacted differently. Our experience has been that it is easier to engage the patient in reappraisal of difficult pain-related situations once he or she has developed a clear understanding of the impact of thoughts on emotions and behaviour. In the second week of treatment involving thought monitoring, the clinician can invite the patient to consider alternate ways of reacting to difficult pain-related situations. An example of a week 2 form is shown in Figure 10.1.

Like the first time that the thought-monitoring form was used, the clinician should take a step-by-step approach to retracing the sequence of events that unfolded in the problematic pain situation. The goal is to reinforce the notion that the apparently 'instant-aneous' experience of the external and internal components of the problem situation is actually an ordered sequence of thoughts, emotions and behaviours.

'Let's start with the first situation: you say that you were going to take your son to the hockey game but decided not to do so because the pain was too bad?'

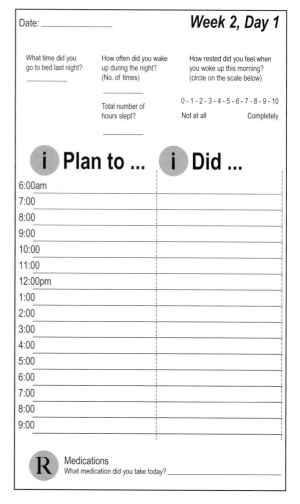

Figure 10.1 • Example of a week 2 form.

Patients with pain will often avoid going to places where they must remain essentially immobile for a long period of time, particularly if the setting is one associated with cold temperatures. The patient may not be in intense pain when making the decision, but chooses to avoid the situation in light of his or her expectation that the situation will lead to intense pain. Patients will inevitably feel bad as they reflect on a decision where they let someone down:

'When you thought that you let your son down, how did you feel?'

Once again, the clinician is assisting the client in drawing a link between a negative thought and a negative feeling. This situation is a challenging one because the solution lies not only in changing the negative thoughts. The solution involves not giving in to the temptation to avoid potentially painful situations. The patient has thus placed the avoidance of potential pain over the emotional needs of the son. The patient might not be entirely aware of the dynamic, but regardless of the level of awareness, the patient will feel the sting of the emotional consequence of the decision. In this case, the patient realises that the situation would have had a better outcome if only he had tried to go, even for a short time.

In this example, the patient is able, upon reflection, to invoke strategies learned in relation to changing activity and pacing so as to manage an increase in pain. The thought-monitoring form can be a powerful tool, and requires minimal active intervention from the clinician in order to yield positive outcomes. The tool functions as a cognitive mirror held up to the self, and much change occurs as a direct result of this self-observation.

Since individuals typically do not like to feel bad, most will be motivated to alter their way of thinking or their way of behaving in a manner that will reduce the negative impact of pain on their emotional well-being. With guidance, the client can also be helped to realise that most negative thoughts associated with pain lead to a further reduction in activity:

'I have been glancing over the first thought-monitoring form you completed and I'm noticing an interesting pattern. Whenever you had negative thoughts in reaction to a problematic pain situation, your activity level went down. The more negative thoughts you had, the less active you became. It seems to me that one advantage of learning to control these negative thoughts will be that you will feel better emotionally. Another advantage is that you will probably be able to remain more active. And as we have discussed at various points in the programme, activity is going to be the key to positive results.'

Using activity scheduling as a pain management intervention

The key aspects of activity scheduling are shown in Box 10.6.

The critical importance of re-establishing activity

Activity mobilisation or activity participation have been central themes in many chronic pain treatment

Box 10.6

Key aspects of activity scheduling

- The critical importance of re-establishing activity
- The use of structured activity schedules
- Applications of structured activity scheduling.

programmes. Whether promoted through information pamphlets, communication with primary-care physicians, or the direct intervention of physical therapists, pain patients have been urged to resume their regular activities as soon as possible.

Although the literature supports activity mobilisation as an effective means of minimising disability associated with pain, the magnitude of treatment effects has frequently been disappointing. The treatment effects associated with information provision, back education, or exercise have been sufficiently modest to lead many clinical investigators to question whether such programmes can be cost-effective (Waddell 1998).

Information-based intervention programmes such as medical advice or pamphlets often proceed from an overly simplistic view of the necessary conditions of behaviour change, and, consequently, their impact on behaviour change is often negligible. Physical therapy interventions circumvent some of the limitations of information-based interventions by providing direct guidance in activity involvement. These interventions, however, proceed from the assumption that the performance of the physical manoeuvres constituting a therapeutic exercise regimen will contribute to increased involvement in social, recreational or occupational activities. There are indications, however, that such transfer effects do not occur automatically. In order to promote activity participation, structured activity scheduling techniques must be used. The clinical use of structured activity scheduling techniques is described in detail elsewhere (Sullivan & Stanish 2003, Sullivan et al 2006) and will be only briefly addressed in this chapter.

The use of structured activity schedules

It is clear that activity participation interventions are important with respect to their effects on improving physical function. Recent research suggests that structured activity scheduling can lead to meaningful decreases in psychosocial risk factors such as catastrophic thinking, fear of pain, disability beliefs and depression (Sullivan et al 2005).

Applications of structured activity scheduling

An example of a structured activity scheduling form is shown in Figure 10.1. In intervention programmes such as the Progressive Goal Attainment Program (PGAP) or the Pain Disability Prevention (PDP) Program, clinicians guide patients as to ways of increasing their involvement in activity domains that defined various life roles (e.g., parent, spouse, worker) prior to the development of a debilitating pain condition. By increasing participation in life role activities, pain-related disability can be reduced.

If an individual has been avoiding activities due to fears that activity will increase pain or be harmful, structured activity scheduling can be used as a type of exposure technique. In orchestrating the patient's involvement in various activities, the clinician must be mindful of the distinction between graded activity and exposure. Graded activity simply refers to steadily increasing the client's involvement in different tasks. An error that is sometimes made by patients is to participate in an activity until their pain symptoms increase in severity. Although a patient can make progress with this type of approach, more often than not, the approach will have limited success. If the patient uses pain severity as the gauge to determine when to discontinue an activity, the patient is still allowing pain to control his or her activity. The ultimate lesson learned is 'when it hurts, I stop'.

A better strategy is to decide on a specific amount of time that a task will be performed, or a specific subcomponent of the task that will be performed. The patient aims only to complete the agreed upon time or task units, and discontinues once the goal has been attained, regardless of his or her current level of pain. If the goals are chosen appropriately, it will be rare that a patient will need to discontinue the activity due to intolerable pain. When, for instance, the patient attains the goal of washing the dishes for 15 minutes, or of vacuuming one bedroom, he or she terminates the task assignment with a sense of mastery and accomplishment. These feelings will be important in determining the patient's motivation to pursue more difficult task challenges. In contrast, when a patient persists until he or she is no longer able to tolerate the pain, each task assignment is experienced as a failure.

Structured activity scheduling can also be useful in reducing the frequency of catastrophic thinking. For individuals who experience a high frequency of catastrophic thoughts, these thoughts will be more likely to be accessible to consciousness when no other stimulus is competing for attention. Sedentary activities such as resting have minimal attention demands, and consequently, the high-frequency pain catastrophiser experiences a state of consciousness characterised by the presence of catastrophic, alarmist and pessimistic thoughts. By engaging in an attention-demanding task, the attentional requirements of the task will partially consume the attentional resources of consciousness, reducing the degree to which the individual will be able to engage in catastrophic thinking. Reducing the frequency of catastrophic thinking has also been shown to yield reductions in depressive symptoms (Sullivan et al 2006).

For the patient experiencing depressive symptoms, the clinician should encourage the patient to incorporate as many enjoyable activities in his or her weekly schedule as possible. In home-based activity programmes, there is often a tendency to overemphasise participation in household chores. Household chores (e.g. cooking, cleaning) are ideal activities from which to build an activity routine because the tools or equipment necessary for their execution are readily available, and it is likely that the client possesses the required skills. Household chores can also be easily incorporated into a structured schedule of activity and the patient has considerable control over determining the intensity and duration of activity involvement. For patients with depressive symptoms, however, it will be important to ensure that the patient's activity schedule contains activities that are considered by the patient to be pleasurable and meaningful. Depression impacts negatively on an individual's level of engagement and interest in their environment. Re-engagement in life role activities will be maximised when activity involvement is associated with pleasure, achievement and a positive sense of self-worth.

Finally, structured activity scheduling can be used to change disability beliefs. Participation in setting activity goals is important because it engages the client in a process in which he or she must envisage a future that is different from the present. Implied in disability beliefs is the idea that the future will not differ from today. The process of setting activity goals and then making plans to work toward those goals will challenge and weaken such disability beliefs.

Relaxation and biofeedback

The key approaches to relaxation are shown in Box 10.7.

Muscle relaxation training

Relaxation, as a treatment method, refers to techniques aimed at reducing tension. A number of

Box 10.7

Key approaches to relaxation

- Muscle relaxation training
- Meditation and autogenic training
- Biofeedback.

different approaches to inducing a relaxed state have been described in the literature (Benson 1975). Progressive muscle relaxation emphasises the relaxation of voluntary skeletal muscles (Jacobson 1948). The underlying theory is that stress-related conditions (including pain) can be caused or exacerbated by sustained muscle contraction (Blanchard et al 1990). In a typical relaxation protocol, the patient is taught to alternate contraction and relaxation of different muscle groups. For example, the clinician might ask the patient to contract specific muscles, to focus for a few seconds on the feelings of tension associated with contraction, and then ask the patient to relax the muscles. The clinician proceeds in this manner until all major muscle groups of the body are relaxed.

In order to reduce tension in the shoulders, the clinician might proceed as follows:

'I'd like you now to turn your attention to the muscles of your shoulders. I would like you to pull your shoulders up and back, and to tighten these muscles as much as you can. Notice the feelings of tension and tightness in these muscles. Keep focusing on these feelings of tension, and … now … relax. Let your shoulders fall back to their normal position, let them go completely. Let your shoulders hang loose, let them become completely relaxed. Feel the warm sense of relaxation flow through these muscles, making you feel calm, rested and completely relaxed.'

The intent of relaxation training is to assist the patient in developing relaxation skills. It has been suggested that 7–10 sessions of treatment might be required in order to develop the skills required to use relaxation techniques effectively (Arena & Blanchard 1996). The duration of the sessions can be reduced over time, as the patient's increasing proficiency permits contraction and relaxation of larger groupings of muscles. Once the patient has developed relaxation skills with the assistance of a clinician, the patient can continue to self-manage his or her tension through home-based programmes. Home-based exercises can be supplemented by the use of audiotaped

relaxation instructions. Relaxation audiotapes are commercially available through bookstores or health-needs outlets. Clinicians frequently provide the patient with an audiotape of a previous session. A detailed description of a progressive relaxation procedure for pain patients is provided by Arena & Blanchard (1996).

Meditation and autogenic training

Other forms of relaxation training include meditation and autogenic training (Lichstein 1988, Luthe 1969, Kabat-Zinn 1982). Meditation and autogenic training combine techniques for muscle tension reduction and strategies intended to facilitate the attainment of cognitive or spiritual relaxation. With these approaches, the patient might be provided with a word or a phrase that is repeated quietly. In autogenic training, the patient might be asked to repeat phrases such as 'I am feeling relaxed', 'My legs are heavy and warm', or 'My whole body feels comfortable'. Meditation will often involve certain postures such as the lotus position (e,g., sitting cross-legged). In addition, students of certain forms of meditation will be prescribed a 'mantra'. The mantra is repeated mentally to rid the mind of tension-related thoughts and induce a spiritual calm (Kabat-Zinn 1982, 1985). It is likely that over time, the autogenic phrase or mantra will become associated with the relaxed state, and repeating the word or phrase might be sufficient to induce relaxation.

Biofeedback

Biofeedback can be viewed as a form of targeted relaxation. In biofeedback, electrodes are attached to the surface of the skin over the painful muscle region. The electrical output of the muscles is amplified and converted into an auditory (e.g. tone) or visual (e.g. dial) signal. The amplitude of the tone or deviation of the dial varies with the electrical output of the muscle. Since muscle tension is associated with greater electrical output of the muscle tissue, the amplitude of the tone or deviation of the dial will increase and decrease in response to increasing and decreasing tension. In essence, the patient receives 'feedback' about the level of tension in the muscle region. The patient is taught to use cognitive or visualisation strategies to reduce the amplitude of the biofeedback signal.

Relaxation techniques, autogenic training or meditation are typically used to induce total body relaxation. With biofeedback, the objective is to achieve relaxation in a specific muscle region. A drawback to the use of biofeedback is the specialised equipment required for treatment. There is research to suggest that treatment effects with progressive relaxation are comparable to those obtained with biofeedback (Arena et al 1995). As such, there might be advantages to considering a trial of relaxation treatment before considering the use of biofeedback.

Biofeedback and relaxation have been used extensively in the treatment of headache, sometimes as the sole or primary treatment (e.g., Arena & Blanchard 1996). Biofeedback and relaxation have also been used in the treatment of low-back pain (and other musculoskeletal conditions), but rarely as the sole treatment. For chronic low-back pain, relaxation and biofeedback are more likely to be included as a component of a multipronged interdisciplinary approach to pain management (Ostelo et al 2006).

The results of clinical trials suggest that relaxation, biofeedback and meditation can be effective techniques for reducing emotional distress, subjective tension and pain intensity (Blanchard et al 1990, Ostelo et al 2006). It is not clear that these techniques (in isolation) have a meaningful impact on function, disability or return to work.

Hypnosis

The key aspects of hypnosis are shown in Box 10.8.

The origins of hypnosis

The use of hypnosis in the control of pain has its origins in the work of Anton Mesmer. As discussed in Chapter 2, Mesmer believed that the infusion of 'magnetic fluid' into the body could effect cures of a variety of health conditions, including pain. In the mid-1800s, Mesmer's techniques were adopted by English and Scottish surgeons as a means of inducing a 'painless sleep' during surgical procedures (Hall 1986). Today, hypnosis is rarely used as a substitute for pharmacological methods of anaesthesia, but hypnosis is often included as a component of pain management programmes (Evans 1990, Hawkins 1988, Syrjala & Abrams 2002).

Although the mechanisms by which hypnosis influences pain perception are not entirely understood,

research supports the view that hypnosis can have a meaningful impact on pain experience. Factors related to distraction, relaxation, dissociation, suggestibility and absorption have all been discussed as mechanisms of hypnosis (Hawkins 1988, Watkins & Watkins 1990). Hypnosis has been shown to increase cutaneous pain threshold (Hajek et al 1991) and reduce pain associated with aversive medical procedures (Weinstein & Au 1991), childbirth (Weishaar 1986) and headache (VanDyck et al 1991).

Patient selection

Hypnosis describes both an experiential phenomenon and a collection of intervention techniques. The clinician intending to use hypnosis for pain control might consider using a test of hypnotisability, trance induction techniques and analgesic suggestions. Since patients vary in their level of hypnotic susceptibility, some clinicians may only consider using hypnotic pain control techniques on patients who demonstrate an adequate level of hypnotisability.

If a patient passes the hand levitation test (reflecting a moderate level of hypnotisability), he or she probably possesses the necessary level of hypnotisability to benefit from hypnotic pain control techniques. For this test, the patient would be asked to sit with eyes closed, both arms resting on the armrests of a chair. Gently touching the wrist of the patient, the clinician might proceed as follows:

> 'I am now tying a piece of string around your wrist. This string is holding two red helium balloons that are hovering in the air, just above your head. With the string tied around your wrist, you can feel the balloons tugging at the string. As you focus on the feeling of the balloons tugging at the string around your wrist, you notice that your hand is becoming lighter and lighter. Your hand feels lighter and lighter, and you know that if you let them, the balloons will lift your hand off the armrest. Now just let the balloons slowly lift your hand off the armrest.'

For patients who are hypnotisable, the hand will begin to rise off the armrest. Patients who respond to this suggestion will likely be able to respond positively to analgesic suggestions.

Hypnotic techniques

A variety of techniques can be used for trance induction. Many clinicians will use a combination of guided

---

Box 10.8

Key issues in hypnosis

- The origins of hypnosis
- Patient selection
- Hypnotic techniques
- Utility in pain management.

---

imagery and a relaxation protocol to induce a hypnotic trance. The reader is referred to Hawkins (1988) for a detailed description of trance induction techniques. It is important to note that many clinicians do not consider it critical that the patient enter a trance in order to benefit from analgesic suggestions.

Analgesic suggestions are essentially sensory-based metaphors that capture the theme of pain reduction. If the patient has previously indicated to the clinician that ice applied to the painful region yields some degree of pain reduction, imagining ice being applied to the painful region might be used as an analgesic suggestion. Patients can also be asked to imagine a pain thermometer where the mercury rises with increasing pain. Patients might be asked to imagine that the thermometer reading is decreasing, and in turn, decreasing their pain experience. Dissociative suggestions might also be used. In this case, patients are asked to 'separate' themselves from the source of pain; their pain might still persist, but they are less affected by it.

Utility in pain management

Hypnotic pain control strategies have been used to manage procedural pain in both children and adults (Syrjala et al 1992, 1995). Hypnotic pain control strategies are typically taught/used prior to exposure to a painful procedure, and patients might then be coached through the procedure by a clinician (Liossi & Hatira 1999, 2003, Montgomery et al 2002). Albeit its utility for acute procedural pain, hypnosis may have limited applicability for persistent pain. The high attentional resource demands of hypnosis might interfere with a person's ability to engage in any other activity while utilising the strategy. The attentional resource demands of hypnosis also places limits on the duration of time that it can be invoked to deal with a pain episode.

Exposure interventions

Some important issues in the use of exposure interventions are shown in Box 10.9.

Box 10.9

Key issues in the use of exposure interventions

- The relationship between fear, avoidance and disability
- Patient selection
- Utility of exposure techniques in pain management.

The relationship between fear, avoidance and disability

There is growing recognition that, for many patients, fears of pain or of movements that might cause pain, are a significant contributing factor to disability. For some, pain-related fears might be more important determinants of disability than pain itself (Crombez et al 1999, Vlaeyen et al 1995). Vlaeyen and his colleagues have suggested that interventions that have yielded positive outcomes in the reduction of phobias might also be useful in the treatment of chronic pain (Vlaeyen & Linton 2000).

Exposure is considered the treatment of choice for the reduction of fear and avoidance associated with phobias. Most intervention programmes used to treat phobias involve a graded exposure approach. In such programmes, the clinician works with the patient to build a fear hierarchy. Fear-arousing stimuli are ranked in terms of the level of fear they generate. Treatment then proceeds by exposing the patient to stimuli that are associated with mild levels of fear, then slowly moving up the hierarchy. Individuals who have intense fears of certain situations, animals or objects anticipate that contact will be associated with negative or catastrophic outcomes. Exposure can be useful in that it demonstrates that the anticipated negative outcomes do not occur. This same approach can be used to reduce pain-related fears.

Although randomised clinical trials of the use of exposure for chronic pain have yet to be reported, a number of published case studies suggest that this type of intervention might be beneficial, at least for some chronic pain patients (Boersma et al 2004, Vlaeyen et al 2002). It has been suggested that exposure to feared movements/activities may yield clinically significant reductions in fear, and improvements in function.

Exposure treatment for pain-related fear is primarily considered for patients who obtain high scores on measures of pain-related fear. In other words, not all chronic pain patients are considered candidates for this type of intervention. Intervention duration ranges from 6 to 10 weeks, with two or three sessions per week, with each session lasting approximately 90 minutes (Boersma et al 2004).

Patient selection

Scores on the Tampa Scale for Kinesiophobia (TSK) are often used as the basis for selection. Patients are considered potential candidates if they obtain a score which is greater than 35 on the TSK. In the studies reported to date, patients have been asked to rank, in order of intensity of fear, photographs depicting various activities of daily living. The Photograph Series of Daily Activities (PHODA) is the instrument that has typically been used to develop an activity–fear hierarchy (Kugler et al 1999). The interventionists who have used exposure interventions have included physiotherapists, kinesiologists and psychologists, alone or in treatment teams. During treatment sessions, patients are repeatedly exposed to movements involved in different activities. Activities are also prescribed in-between sessions in order to assist the patient to play a greater role in the self-management of his or her fears. Over time, patients learn that their fears of catastrophic outcomes are largely unfounded and their level of fear decreases.

Utility of exposure techniques in pain management

An advantage of exposure treatment for chronic pain is that it is very behavioural and concrete, and might thus be applicable even in cases where the client is not sufficiently literate to participate in other forms of psychological intervention. A disadvantage is that not all patients might be willing to participate in an intervention that will expose them to activities that they fear will make their condition worse.

Conclusions

The aim of this chapter was to provide brief descriptions of non-pharmacological interventions for the management of chronic pain. These interventions might be useful as stand-alone interventions, as combinations of interventions, or as part of comprehensive interdisciplinary treatment programmes. In clinical decision making concerning the type of interventions to be used, the clinician must first decide what will constitute the main target of intervention. Is the goal to reduce pain, to reduce suffering, or to reduce disability? It is important to consider that interventions used to reduce pain and suffering will not necessarily have an impact on disability.

The process of combining intervention techniques must also consider the conceptual consistency of the specific intervention techniques. It might be difficult for a patient to understand that he must remain as active as possible, avoid sedentary activities, yet practice relaxation exercises. It is beyond the scope of this chapter to address all combinations of intervention techniques, but the clinician should consider the issue of conceptual compatibility when tailoring intervention techniques to specific client needs.

Key points

- There is a range of possible interventions from education to systematic cognitive–behavioural interventions
- Mental health psychology has provided the basis for the development of many such interventions
- Although the specific focus of intervention in the context of pain management may be different, they are derived from the same cognitive and behavioural substrate
- Specialised professional training is required in using what can be powerful therapeutic techniques
- Such techniques are more commonly offered to patients with severe or persistent pain problems
- They are often used as the primary pain management intervention, whether as a precursor to or instead of a multidisciplinary pain programme, but may also be built in as part of a comprehensive pain management programme
- As a precursor to assessment with a view to intervention, specific attention should to paid to facilitation of self-disclosure
- Most of the techniques can be subsumed under the headings of cognitive restructuring, activity scheduling, stress/relaxation approaches, hypnosis or exposure paradigms.

References

APA (American Psychiatric Association) 1980 Diagnostic and Statistical Manual of Mental Disorders, 3rd edn. American Psychiatric Association, Washington, DC

Arena J G, Blanchard E B 1996 Biofeedback and relaxation therapy for chronic pain disorders. In: Gatchel R, Turk D C (eds) Psychological approaches to pain management. Guilford Press, New York, 159–186

Arena J G, Bruno G M, Hannah S L et al 1995 A comparison of frontal electromyographic biofeedback training, trapezius electromyographic biofeedback training, and progressive muscle relaxation therapy in the treatment of tension headache. Headache 35(7):411–419

Beck A T, Rush A J, Shaw B F et al 1979 Cognitive therapy for depression. Guilford Press, New York

Beecher H K 1956 Relationship of significance of wound to pain experienced. Journal of the American Medical Association 161:1609–1613

Benson H 1975 The relaxation response. Morrow, New York

Blanchard E B, Appelbaum K A, Radnitz C L et al 1990 Placebo-controlled evaluation of abbreviated progressive muscle relaxation and of relaxation combined with cognitive therapy in the treatment of tension headache. Journal of Consultation and Clinical Psychology 58(2):210–215

Blumer D, Heilbronn M 1982 Chronic pain as a variant of depressive disease: the pain-prone disorder. Journal of Nervous and Mental Disease 170:381–406

Boersma K, Lintona S J, Overmeer T et al 2004 Lowering fear-avoidance and enhancing function through exposure in vivo: a multiple baseline study across six patients with back pain. Pain 108:8–16

Breuer J, Freud S 1893 Studies on hysteria. Republished 1957, Basic Books, New York

Crombez G, Vlaeyen J W, Heuts P H 1999 Pain-related fear is more disabling than pain itself: evidence on the role of pain-related fear in chronic back pain disability. Pain 80(1–2):329–339

D'Zurilla T J 1990 Problem-solving training for effective stress management and prevention. Journal of Cognitive Psychotherapy: An International Quarterly 4:327–355

D'Zurilla T J, Goldfried M R 1971 Problem solving and behavior modification. Journal of Abnormal Psychology 78:107–126

Engel G 1959 'Psychogenic' pain and the pain-prone patient. American Journal of Medicine 26:899–918

Esterling B A, Antoni M H, Kumar M et al 1990 Emotional repression, stress disclosure responses, and Epstein-Barr viral capsid antigen titers. Psychosomatic Medicine 52:397–410

Evans F J 1990 Hypnosis and pain control. Australian Journal of Clinical and Experimental Hypnosis 33(1):1–10

Feuerstein M, Huang G D, Shaheen M et al 2000 Ergo-stress management for your health: managing job stress and reducing ergonomic risks. Monograph, Washington, DC

Fordyce W E 1976 Behavioral methods in chronic pain and illness. C V Mosby, St Louis

Fordyce W E, Fowler R S, Lehmann J F et al 1968 Some implications of learning in problems of chronic pain. Journal of Chronic Disease 21:179–190

Fordyce W E, Roberts A H, Sternbach R A 1985 The behavioral management of chronic pain: a response to critics. Pain 22:113–125

George S Z, Fritz J M, Bialosky J E et al 2003 The effect of a fear-avoidance-based physical therapy intervention for acute low back pain: Results of a randomized control trial. Spine 28:2551–2560

Hajek P, Radil T, Jakoubek B 1991 Hypnotic skin analgesy in healthy individuals and patients with atopic eczema. Homeostasis in Health and Disease 33(3):156–157

Hall H 1986 Suggestion and illness. International Journal of Psychosomatics 33:24–27.

Hawkins R 1988 The role of hypnotherapy in the pain clinic. Australian Journal of Clinical and Experimental Hypnosis 16(1): 23–30

Heymans M W, van Tulder M W, Esmail R et al 2004 Back schools for non-specific low-back pain. The Cochrane Database of Systematic Reviews, issue 4

Jacobson E 1948 Progressive relaxation: a physiological and clinical investigation of muscular states and their significance in psychology and medical practice. University of Chicago Press, Chicago

Kabat-Zinn J 1982 An outpatient program in behavioural medicine for chronic pain patients based on the practice of mindfulness meditation: theoretical considerations and preliminary results. General Hospital Psychiatry 4(1):33–47

Kabat-Zinn J, Lipworth L, Burney R 1985 The clinical use of mindfulness meditation for the self-regulation of chronic pain. Journal of Behavioral Medicine 8(2):163–190

Kelley J E, Lumley M A, Leisen J C C 1997 Health effects of emotional disclosure in rheumatoid arthritis patients. Health Psychology 16:331–340

Kugler K, Wijn J, Geilen M et al 1999 The photograph series of daily activities (PHODA). Heerlen, The Netherlands

Lazarus R, Folkman S 1984 Stress, appraisal and coping. Springer, New York

Lichstein K L 1988 Clinical relaxation strategies. Wiley, New York

Lindstrom I, Ohlund C, Eek C et al 1992 The effect of graded activity on patients with subacute low back pain: a randomized prospective clinical study with an operant-conditioning behavioral approach. Physical Therapy 72:279–290

Linton S J, Andersson T 2000 Can chronic disability be prevented? A randomized trial of a cognitive-behavioural intervention and two forms of information for patients with spinal pain. Spine 25:2825–2831

Linton S J, Bradley L A, Jensen I et al 1989 The secondary prevention of low back pain: a controlled study with follow-up. Pain 35(2):197–207

Liossi C, Hatira P 1999 Clinical hypnosis versus cognitive behavioural training for pain management with pediatric cancer patients undergoing bone marrow aspirations. International Journal of Clinical and Experimental Hypnosis 47:104–116

Liossi C, Hatira P 2003 Clinical hypnosis in the alleviation of procedure-related pain in pediatric oncology patients. International Journal of Clinical and Experimental Hypnosis 47:4–28

Luthe W 1969 Autogenic therapy. Grune & Stratton, New York

McCracken L M, Turk D C 2002 Behavioral and cognitive-behavioral treatment for chronic pain. Spine 27:2564–2573

Montgomery G H, Weltz C R, Seltz M et al 2002 Brief presurgery hypnosis reduces distress and pain in excisional breast biopsy patients. International Journal of Clinical and Experimental Hypnosis 50:17–32

Morley S, Eccleston C, Williams A 1999 Systematic review and meta-analysis of randomized controlled trials of cognitive behavior therapy and behavior therapy for chronic pain in adults, excluding headache. Pain 80:1–13

Nezu A M, Perri M G 1989 Social problem-solving therapy for unipolar depression: an initial dismantling investigation. Journal of Consulting and Clinical Psychology 57:408–413

Ostelo R W J G, van Tulder M W, Vlaeyen J W S et al 2006 Behavioural treatment for chronic low-back pain. The Cochrane Database of Systematic Reviews, issue 1, art no: CD002014. DOI: 10.1002/14651858.CD002014

Pelletier K R, Cagney T 1991 Building skills for stress management. The Stay Well Company, San Bruno, CA

Pennebaker J W 1995 Emotion, disclosure, and health: an overview. In: Pennebaker J C (ed) Emotion, disclosure, and health. American Psychological Association, Washington, DC, pp 255–270

Pennebaker J W, O'Heeron R C 1984 Confiding in others and illness rates among spouses of spouses of suicide and accidental death victims. Journal of Abnormal Psychology 93:473–476

Pennebaker J W, Susman J R 1988 Disclosure of traumas and psychosomatic processes. Social Science and Medicine 26:327–332

Pennebaker J W, Kiecolt-Glaser J K, Glaser R 1988 Disclosure of traumas and immune function: health implications for psychotherapy. Journal of Consulting and Clinical Psychology 56:238–245

Pransky G, Robertson M M, Moon S D 2002 Stress and work-related upper-extremity disorders: implications for prevention and management. American Journal of Industrial Medicine 41:443–455

Sanders S H 1996 Operant conditioning with chronic pain: back to basics. In: Gatchel R J, Turk D C (eds) Psychological approaches to pain management: a practitioner's handbook. Guilford Press, New York, pp 112–130

Skinner B F 1953 Science and human behavior. Macmillan, New York

Sullivan M J L, Stanish W D 2003 Psychologically based occupational rehabilitation: the Pain-Disability Prevention Program. Clinical Journal of Pain 19:97–104

Sullivan M J L, Ward L C, Tripp D et al 2005 Secondary prevention of work disability: community-based psychosocial intervention for musculoskeletal disorders. Journal of Occupational Rehabilitation 15:377–392

Sullivan M J L, Adams H, Rhodenizer T et al 2006 A psychosocial risk factor targeted intervention for the prevention of chronic pain and disability following whiplash injury. Physical Therapy 86:8–18

Syrjala K L, Abrams J R 2002 Hypnosis and imagery in the treatment of pain. In: Gatchel R, Turk D C (eds) Psychological approaches to pain management. Guilford Press, New York, ch 9, pp 187–209

Syrjala K L, Cummings C, Donaldson G W 1992 Hypnosis or cognitive behavioural training for the reduction of pain and nausea during cancer treatment: a controlled clinical trial. Pain 48:137–146

Syrjala K L, Donaldson G W, Davis M W et al 1995 Relaxation and imagery and cognitive-behavioural training reduce pain during cancer treatment: a controlled clinical trial. Pain 63(2):189–198

Turk D C 1996 Biopsychosocial perspective on chronic pain. In: Gatchel R J, Turk D C (eds) Psychological approaches to pain management. Guilford Press, New York

Turk D, Okifuji A 2002 Psychological factors in chronic pain: evolution and revolution. Journal of Consulting and Clinical Psychology 70:678–690

Turk D C, Meichenbaum D, Genest M 1983 Pain and behavioral medicine: a cognitive-behavioral perspective. Guilford, New York

Van den Hout J H C, Vlaeyen J W S, Heuts P H T G et al 2003 Secondary prevention of work-related disability in non-specific low back pain: does problem-solving therapy help? A randomized clinical trial. Clinical Journal of Pain 19:87–96

VanDyck R, Zitman F G, Linssen A C et al 1991 Autogenic training and future oriented hypnotic imagery in the treatment of tension headaches. International Journal of Clinical and Experimental Hypnosis 39(1):6–23

van Tulder M W, Esmail R, Bombardier C et al 2002 Back schools for non-specific low back pain. The Cochrane Library, issue 3, Oxford

Vlaeyen J W, Linton S J 2000 Fear-avoidance and its consequences in chronic musculoskeletal pain: a state of the art. Pain 85(3):317–332

Vlaeyen J W, Kole-Snijders A M, Boeren R G et al 1995 Fear of movement/(re)injury in chronic low back pain and its relation to behavioral performance. Pain 62(3):363–372

Vlaeyen J W, de Jong J R, Onghena P et al 2002 Can pain-related fear be reduced? The application of cognitive-behavioural exposure in vivo. Pain Research and Management 7(3):144–153

Waddell G 1998 The back pain revolution. Churchill Livingstone, London

Watkins J G, Watkins H H 1990 Dissociation and displacement: where goes the ouch? American Journal of Clinical Hypnosis 33(1):1–10

Weinstein E J, Au P K 1991 Use of hypnosis during angioplasty. American Journal of Clinical Hypnosis 34(1):29–37

Weishaar B B 1986 A comparison of Lamaze and hypnosis in the management of labor. American Journal of Clinical Hypnosis 28(4):214–217

Zachrisson-Forsell M 1980 The Swedish back school. Physiotherapy 66:12–114

Zachrisson-Forsell M 1981 The back school. Spine 6:104–106

Section **Four**

Tertiary pain management programmes

SECTION CONTENTS

Chapter 11 focuses on the content of tertiary pain management programmes, considered from both individual professional and interdisciplinary perspectives with discussion of both individualised and group approaches to intervention. The chapter includes a summary of the British Pain Society's key criteria for pain management programmes and related pain treatment services.

Chapter Eleven

11

Tertiary pain management programmes

Part 1 Introduction

While the majority of patients do not become significantly incapacitated with pain, and while a further proportion will benefit from appropriate early intervention, some patients develop a level of pain-associated incapacity that requires intensive rehabilitation in the form of multi- or interdisciplinary pain management. Depending on the health-care setting they may be offered a variety of products from functional restoration programmes (FRPs), occupational rehabilitation such as that offered in the Workmen's Compensational Board (WCB) or pain management programmes (PMPs) of varying lengths, complexity and duration, offered both in the public and private sector. There are many variants of these programmes, but little in the way of controlled comparisons, and sometimes the labelling on the package bears little resemblance to its contents.

The specific focus on pain reduction for chronic pain patients can be seen as a logical extension of skills developed by anaesthetists in the management of postoperative pain. Unfortunately, such pharmacological and modality treatments proved less successful in treatment of complex or long-standing pain problems than had been hoped. Agencies such as the WCB found themselves carrying increasing costs of chronic incapacity in injured workers unable to return to work. The shift in emphasis led to the identification of a wider set of objectives for treatment than pain reduction. This chapter will focus primarily on the sort of tertiary-care programmes offered in the NHS. Traditionally, these have been primarily clinically rather than occupationally focused, although there have been recent examples of occupationally focused pain management (Watson et al 2004) and it seems likely that there will be further development of this kind of approach.

The origin and development of modern pain management

In his textbook of pain, Bonica (1990) outlines the origins and development of multidisciplinary and interdisciplinary pain programmes. Bonica reports that his experience as a military anaesthetist led him to appreciate the difficulty in managing some of the more complicated pain problems. He developed the view that such patients could be best managed by a multidisciplinary/interdisciplinary team, each contributing his or her own specialised knowledge. Shortly after the Second World War, the first such clinic was established in Tacoma General Hospital in Washington State and ran for 13 years. The problems encountered at that time seem strikingly familiar:

> They included (a) the resistance by many physicians to accept the team approach and their reluctance to refer patients to the group, especially if the physician was in the same speciality as one of the members of the group; (b) difficulty in co-ordinating the time of conferences so that all of the key persons and the referring physician could attend; (c) difficulty in discussing the problem frankly, especially failure(s) of the referring physician and other specialists to make a correct diagnosis or to carry out effective therapy; (d) the cost of the comprehensive evaluation which was then considered too high (Bonica 1990, p. 198).

The majority of the early clinics were anaesthetically led, either modality oriented or syndrome oriented; and about two-thirds of the clinics were in the USA.

Seattle model

The approach of the University of Washington Pain Center in Seattle, often referred to as the 'Seattle model', has become world-renowned. It has pioneered multidimensional treatment, research, education and interdisciplinary working. Their conceptualisation of pain as consisting of nociception, suffering and pain behaviour represented a radical departure from the traditional medical model (Ch. 2). The Seattle model was not only an example of a practical implementation of a biopsychosocial model of pain, but also an illustration of the mutual interdependence of clinical practice, teaching, training and research. In an almost immeasurable sense, the Seattle model has served as an inspiration to the rest of the world.

Although most pain management programmes now would define themselves as cognitive–behavioural in their orientation, the power and incisiveness of the behavioural component (Fordyce 1976) in the original Seattle model was fundamental to the development of modern interdisciplinary pain management.

The cognitive–behavioural perspective

As discussed particularly in Chapters 2 and 9, during the last 20 years there has been increasing interest in cognitive aspects of pain. The arrival of a major textbook on cognitive–behavioural approaches to pain (Turk et al 1983) represented another significant phase of conceptual development. It had been observed that there were similarities between chronic pain patients and depressed patients both behaviourally and cognitively. Aspects of the treatment of cognitive distortion and learned helplessness in patients with depression were blended with training in cognitive coping strategies for pain derived essentially from the hypnosis literature. These cognitive approaches were combined with some of the behavioural methods outlined by Fordyce into a comprehensive approach to pain management known as cognitive–behavioural therapy, or CBT (perhaps termed more appropriately the cognitive–behavioural approach, or CBA). This has become the framework from which most current pain management programmes are derived. Simply put, the behavioural model focuses primarily (and some would say exclusively) on what patients are doing. Cognitions, if deemed relevant at all, are seen as being of secondary importance. In contrast to the radical behavioural approach, the CBA aims to change the way patients think, challenge their beliefs about their pain and therefore influence how they behave.

The challenge of interdisciplinary pain management

As stated in Chapter 1, models of illness have considered the influences on pain and disability at various stages of chronicity. Once a chronic pain syndrome is clearly established, there may be a large number of interacting factors influencing the content and manner of the patient's clinical presentation. Main & Spanswick (2000) offered a way of conceptualising chronic disability in a model comprising a number of stages, summarised in Box 11.1.1 and depicted in Figures 11.1.1 to 11.1.7.

We have found that breaking down the model into components such as these can be used as the basis for case discussion to facilitate understanding and communication across the team.

Case Study 11.1.1 (p. 247) illustrates the stages in development.

Major ingredients of a PMP

PMPs contain many ingredients (Loeser 1990) but there are, however, a number of common themes and key elements, and the development of the modern interdisciplinary PMP has to be seen against the backdrop of

Box 11.1.1

Elements of the Salford Model

Stage 1. The development of deconditioning and disuse
Stage 2. The influence of fear and avoidance
Stage 3. The influence of depression
Stage 4. The influence of anger and frustration
Stage 5. The influence of iatrogenics
Stage 6. The influence of the family
Stage 7. The influence of socio-economic and occupational factors.

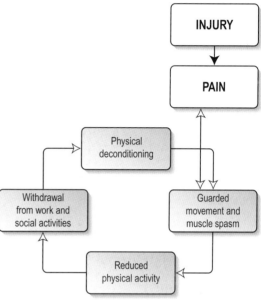

Figure 11.1.1 • The development of deconditioning and disuse.

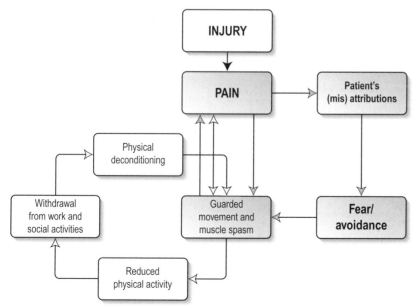

Figure 11.1.2 • The influence of fear and avoidance.

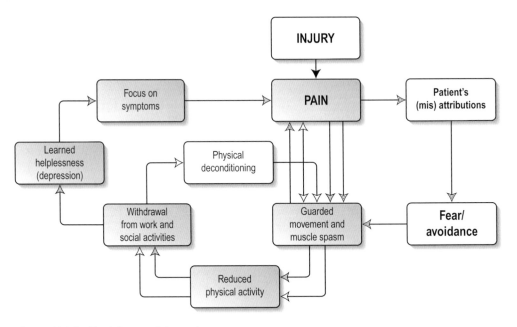

Figure 11.1.3 • The influence of depression.

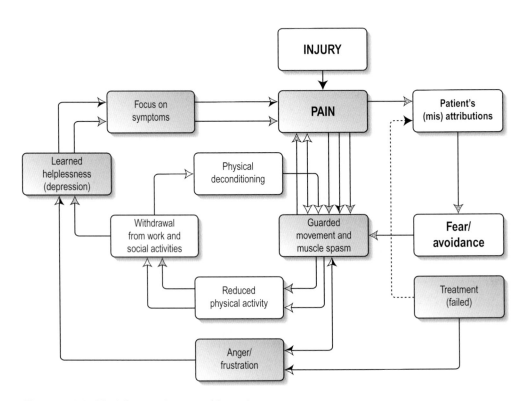

Figure 11.1.4 • The influence of anger and frustration.

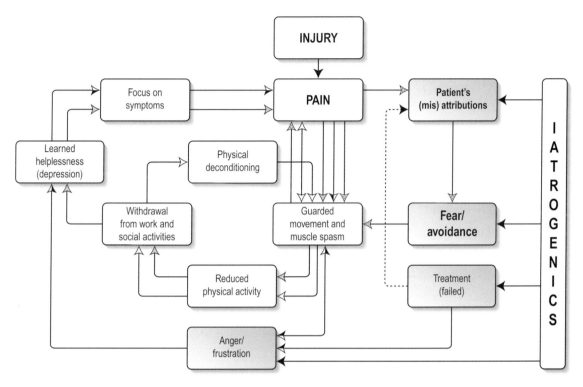

Figure 11.1.5 • The influence of iatrogenics.

these earlier programmes. Every PMP contains a number of discrete elements blended into a package of care. Each of these elements has its own pedigree as an approach to treatment, and each element has its origins in a particular perspective on the nature of pain. The major features of modern PMPs are shown in Box 11.1.2 (p. 248).

Major therapeutic objectives of PMPs

In practical terms there are five major therapeutic foci under which most other therapeutic ingredients can be subsumed. Some of the major therapeutic objectives are outlined in Box 11.1.3 (p. 248).

Treatment of stiffness and immobility through reactivation

Treatment of stiffness and immobility are cornerstones of individualised approaches to manipulation and mobilisation, as offered by many physiotherapists, osteopaths and chiropractors. Recent systematic reviews have found some evidence of effectiveness at very acute stages of

incapacity, but there is no evidence for their effectiveness for chronic pain. Furthermore, as essentially passive techniques, they do not encourage patients to help themselves. More appropriate self-directed physiotherapeutic approaches are discussed in Part 4 of this chapter.

Increasing fitness/strength and reversal of the 'disuse syndrome'

Loss of strength and fitness are key features of many chronic pain patients. Sophisticated functional restoration programmes, or FRPs (Mayer & Gatchel 1988) place considerable emphasis on restoration of muscle power and fitness as a way of achieving increased functional capacity. The 'sports medicine' approach has often been attempted by the time patients arrive on PMPs. In most PMPs there is insufficient time to achieve significant changes in strength or aerobic fitness by the end of a programme. A large proportion of therapeutic effort is directed at educational and psychological obstacles to change. It is not usually possible to schedule as rigorous a programme of activity as is found on most FRPs. It is expected nonetheless than some progress in restoration of strength and fitness will

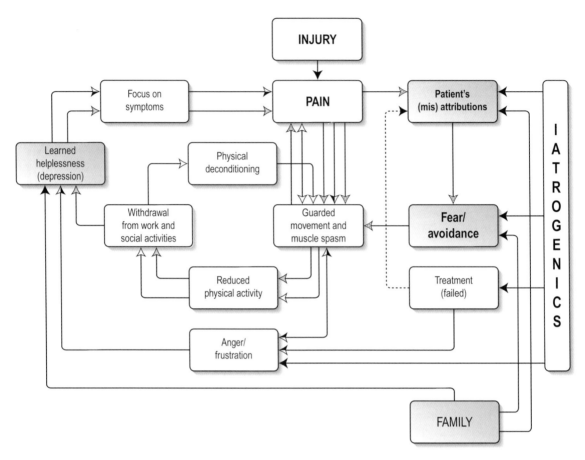

Figure 11.1.6 • The influence of the family.

be achieved and this will serve as the basis from which further change will develop.

Minimising the psychological impact of chronic pain

The treatment of distress or depression is an important ingredient of PMPs, although treatment on an individual basis will not always be indicated. Many PMPs contain sessions of individual psychological therapy, using the sort of techniques described in Chapter 10. As aforementioned, the cognitive–behavioural approach is the treatment modality of choice for cognitive dysfunction or maladaptive coping strategies. The more recent focus on the role of fear and avoidance behaviour can be seen as a further development of this integrated perspective (Vlaeyen et al 1995) but will also include general counselling focused on psychological obstacles to

participating fully in the rest of the PMP. In PMPs such problems are tackled primarily within groups since, to the extent that distress is based on loss of confidence and misunderstanding about the nature of their pain, being part of a group may alleviate the problem to a considerable extent. Most depression is reactive to (or secondary to) the pain-associated incapacity (Ch. 3) and restoration of function with associated increase in quality of life may go a long way to 'treat' the depression.

Modifying unhelpful pain behaviour

A focus specifically on pain behaviour is critical. Patients must be encouraged to 'walk the walk' rather than just 'talk the talk'. Modification of pain behaviour can take many forms. In many of the early clinics, biofeedback was routinely used to try to reduce physiological arousal in general and muscle tension in particular. Stress reduction programmes are now part of every competent PMP, although their specific effects are unclear. The psychological

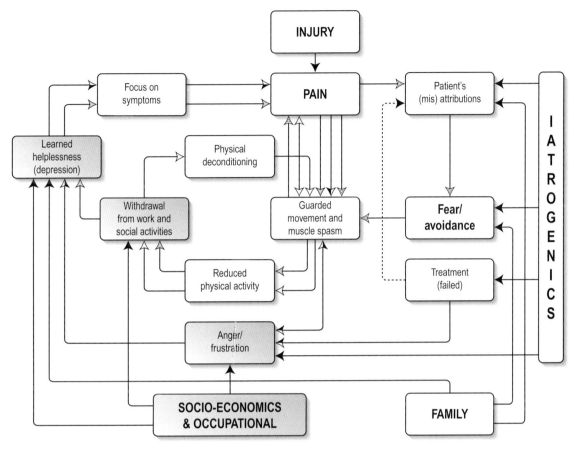

Figure 11.1.7 • The influence of socio-economic and occupational factors.

Case study 11.1.1

Stage 1. The development of deconditioning and disuse

Mr S. was a very fit building labourer aged 30. He sustained a back injury at work when he fell off a plank, which had not been secured properly. He experienced immediate pain in his back. He had to leave work early and was taken home by a friend. By the next day he was in severe pain and was very stiff.

He was advised by his GP to rest up and was given analgesics and anti-inflammatory drugs. He was also given a sick note for 2 weeks. Mr S. did not notice any change in his pain. He felt unable to exercise (he was previously very active in sports).

Stage 2. The influence of fear and avoidance

By the end of the second week Mr S. was concerned that he had seriously injured his back. His pain was still severe and he had become progressively more and more stiff. Any attempt on his part to become more active produced excruciating pain and stiffness, which did not settle for several hours. Following further advice from his GP he continued to rest and avoid activity. He was convinced that if he tried to do too much before his back 'healed' he would damage himself further.

Stage 3. The influence of depression

As the weeks went by Mr S. became more demoralised. Not only was he not able to go to work, but he was unable to get out of the house. He could not go to the gym and he had lost contact with his workmates. Slowly his mood drifted down and he began to focus on his pain, which was preventing him from doing almost anything.

Stage 4. The influence of anger and frustration

Mr S. tried on a number of occasions to 'get moving' as he was becoming very frustrated at his lack of fitness

continued ...

and reliance on others, including his wife, for trivial things. However, each time he tried to do something it simply caused a lot of pain and he would have to rest in bed for days. His GP had sent him to physiotherapy. The physiotherapist tried some mobilisations but Mr S. had got very much worse afterwards. The physiotherapist was worried about Mr S.'s condition and had suggested a referral to a specialist. Mr S. was now convinced there was something seriously wrong. He avoided anything that would aggravate the pain until he saw the specialist.

Stage 5. The influence of iatrogenics

Mr S. was eventually seen by a specialist. Some X-rays were taken and the specialist told Mr S. that he had arthritis of the spine. He suggested some injections and more physiotherapy. Unfortunately neither of these helped. In fact they seemed to make his pain worse. The specialist said there was no more he could do and that Mr S. would have to learn to live with it. If his pain got any worse he should come back. Mr S.'s worst fears had come true. He knew he had a progressive disease, 'arthritis'. He wondered how he would be when he was 60. He became very angry with his GP and his employer who he felt were not helpful. He was soon made redundant. He could not understand why more could not be done for him.

Stage 6. The influence of the family

By now Mr S.'s wife had gone back to full-time work and had to do everything around the house. She left him meals ready each day so that he would not have to do too much. She would not let him do anything for fear of yet more pain. She went to her GP to insist on another specialist appointment. She felt there was perhaps something else wrong. She was worried her husband would end up in a wheelchair.

Stage 7. The influence of socio-economic and occupational factors

Mr S. had been called for a medical for his disability benefit. The examining doctor hurt him during the assessment. Mr S. later learned that the doctor felt there was nothing wrong with him and his benefits were withdrawn. Meanwhile Mr S.'s trade union was seeking compensation on his behalf. Mr S. therefore had to undergo a number of medical examinations from doctors instructed by his union's solicitors and those of his previous employers. Mr S. felt insulted when he read some of the reports, which seemed to imply he was putting it all on and malingering. He became very angry and depressed. His wife and family, meanwhile, had to adjust their lifestyle as the family's income had effectively halved.

Box 11.1.2

Defining characteristics of PMPs

- Behavioural rather than a disease perspective
- Focus on pain management rather than cure
- Blend of ingredients
- Interdisciplinary skill-mix
- Incorporation of group therapy
- Emphasis on active rather than passive approaches to treatment
- Promulgation of self-help and patient responsibility.

Box 11.1.3

Major therapeutic objectives

- Treatment of stiffness and immobility through reactivation
- Increasing fitness/strength and reversal of the 'disuse syndrome'
- Minimising the psychological impact of chronic pain
- Modifying unhelpful pain behaviour
- Restoration of function including occupationally oriented rehabilitation.

boost in re-establishing some control over their incapacity may be as important as specific counter-conditioning of the pain response. Operantly maintained pain is hard to assess and even harder to 'treat' since the focus of attention may be the family or environmental context. Although it may be extremely difficult to effect change in such parameters within the context of a PMP, clarification of their nature may enable patients to make more informed choices.

Considerable change can be effected within PMPs, particularly on inpatient programmes, but unless changes are made also in the patient's own environment, the PMP will only lead to short-term changes. Assessment of such factors are extremely important in clinical decision making (Ch. 5) and may be best viewed as potential obstacles to change rather than patient goals which are likely to be achievable.

Restoration of function including occupationally oriented rehabilitation

Finally, sources of funding and specification of outcome in terms of occupational parameters have led to a number of programmes which are particularly occupationally focused (Chs 14 and 15). Some PMPs incorporate ergonomic assessment of the workplace and simulate specific work tasks. As such they resemble some of the FRPs. In some countries there are strong interfaces between health and education which have allowed the development of shared initiatives, including both clinical management and ergonomic redesign. PMPs differ in the extent to which such arrangements are possible, perhaps because specific competencies in biomechanics and ergonomics are necessary. Increasing emphasis on reduction in sickness absence as an outcome criterion, however, is likely to lead to the development of this aspect of pain management.

Conclusion

Behavioural analyses of the circumstances in which pain occurred shifted focus to individuals' responses to their pain and the determinants of pain-associated incapacity. The broader perspective required a broader range of skills packaged into treatment programmes which including a variety of components delivered by several health-care professionals. The modern interdisciplinary PMP for the chronic pain patient represents the latest development in a process which began four decades ago with the recognition of the limitations of traditional 'nociceptive' models in the conceptualisation of chronic pain and pain-associated incapacity.

The powerful influence of iatrogenic distress and dysfunction as a consequence of excessive and inappropriate treatment has been recognised. The lessons learned in PMPs about the characteristics of chronic pain have highlighted therapeutic possibilities for early intervention. It seems likely that during the next decade there will be an increasing shift from primary prevention to secondary prevention and from chronic care to subchronic care. Nonetheless, there will always be a need for intensive rehabilitation for the chronically and significantly incapacitated patient.

It is not possible to overstress the importance of the behavioural perspective as an alternative to the disease/pathology model in offering a new and alternative understanding of pain. It has led to the focus on pain management as an alternative to cure, which is not available for many pain conditions.

Whatever the blend of therapeutic ingredients, an interdisciplinary skill-mix is required and the group milieu is essential. Arguably, patients learn as much from each other as from staff. It should be remembered, however, that there is more to group therapy than sitting in a circle. Specific competence in the therapeutic use of groups is exceedingly important (see Part 6 of this chapter).

Finally, perhaps most important of all as a defining characteristic of PMPs is the promulgation of self-help and personal responsibility. This is evident particularly in the emphasis on active rather than passive approaches to treatment. In the rest of this chapter a more detailed presentation of the key ingredients of modern PMPs is offered.

An extract from the revised edition of the 'Recommended Guidelines for Pain Management Programmes for Adults', produced by the British Pain Society (2007) is presented in Appendix 11.1.1.

Key points

- **Tertiary PMPs incorporate a blend of professional skills and perspectives**
- **Modern interdisciplinary pain management is now of age**
- **It is not possible to overstress the importance of the shift from the biomedical to biopsychosocial perspective of illness**
- **Chronic pain is better understood as an illness than a disease in optimal adjustment to which active engagement and involvement of the patient is critical, and the role of the health-care professional is more that of a coach than a therapist.**

References

Bonica J J 1990 Multidisciplinary/interdisciplinary pain programs. In: Bonica J J (ed) The management of pain, 2nd edn. Lea & Febiger, Philadelphia, ch 9, pp 197–208

British Pain Society 2007 Recommended guidelines for pain management programmes for adults. British Pain Society, London

Fordyce W E 1976 Behavioral methods for chronic pain and illness. C V Mosby, St Louis, MS

Loeser J D 1990 Interdisciplinary, multimodal management of chronic pain. In: Bonica J J (ed) The management of pain, 2nd edn. Lea & Febiger, Philadelphia, ch 100, pp 2107–2120

Main C J, Spanswick C C (eds) 2000 Pain management: an interdisciplinary approach. Churchill Livingstone, Edinburgh

Mayer T G, Gatchel R J 1988 Functional restoration for spinal disorders: the sports medicine approach. Lea & Febiger, Philadelphia

Turk D C, Meichenbaum D H, Genest M 1983 Pain and behavioural medicine: a cognitive-behavioural perspective. The Guilford Press, New York

Vlaeyen J, Kole-Snijders A M J, Boeren R G B et al 1995 Fear of movement/(re)injury in chronic low back

pain and its relation to behavioral performance. Pain 62:363–372

Watson P, Booker C K, Moores L et al 2004 Returning the chronically unemployed with low back pain to employment. European Journal of Pain 8(4):359–367

APPENDIX 11.1.1

Key criteria for pain management programmes (PMPs) and related pain treatment services

Adapted from Recommended Guidelines for Pain Management Programmes for Adults, British Pain Society (2007, www.britishpainsociety.org.uk).

Aim of a pain management programme

Its aim is rehabilitation and long-term self-management for people whose lives are adversely affected by persistent pain. This is achieved by the application of cognitive and behavioural principles to problems of pain, disability and emotion, and by the application of physical rehabilitation principles to the problems of pain and disability, delivered by a multidisciplinary team in either an inpatient or outpatient setting.

Content and delivery of pain management programmes

A PMP aims to improve the physical, psychological, emotional and social dimensions of quality of life of people with persistent pain, using a multidisciplinary team working according to behavioural and cognitive principles. The problems of people with persistent pain are formulated in terms of the effects of persistent pain on the individual's physical and psychological wellbeing, rather than as disease or damage in biomedical terms, or as deficits in the individual's personality or mental health.

PMP participants apply the programme content to goals important to them, where pain has had significant negative impact. They aim to improve their quality of life, working towards their optimal level of function and self-reliance in managing their persistent pain. Pain relief is not a primary goal, although improvements in pain have been reported. Return to work or improved function at work is an important goal for many, but not for all.

A PMP consists of education and guided practice.

Education

Education is provided by all members of the multidisciplinary team, according to their expertise, using an interactive style to enable patients to raise and resolve difficulties in understanding material or in applying it to their particular situations or problems.

Some of the information refers to pain mechanisms, to associated pathologies, and to healthy function and normal processes:

- Anatomy and physiology of pain and pain pathways; differences between acute and persistent pain
- Psychology and pain; fear and avoidance; stress, distress and depression
- Safety and risk in relation to increased activity
- Exercise for better health and improved function
- Advantages and disadvantages of using aids, treatments and medication
- Self-management of flare-ups and setbacks
- Other information introduces treatment principles and rationales
- Mutual influence of beliefs and ways of thinking, emotions and behaviour
- Using cognitive strategies to deal with the psychological effects of persistent pain and stress
- Principles of goal setting
- Scheduling and regulating goal-directed activity, using pacing
- Using cues and reinforcement to help change habits; generalisation and maintenance of changes
- Strategies to improve sleep.

Guided practice

An opportunity is given for guided practice in use of the methods outlined above to abolish unhelpful habits and build helpful habits of activity and of thinking. Guided practice also enables patients to use help from staff to apply these changes to their individual goals, starting from their current level of performance and increasing at a manageable rate. Patients are instructed to practise in their home and other environments, monitoring what they do and reviewing progress with staff regularly, adjusting goals and methods as necessary.

The core components are:

- Exercise to improve fitness and mobility, to improve confidence in movement and activity, and to enable increases in goal-related activity. People with persistent pain who are fearful of activity-related pain or injury are less likely to transfer exercise gains to improvements in general function
- Gradual return to goal-defined activities, from self-care to work, social activities and sports. This consists both of analysis of barriers and areas requiring specific change, and synthesis of the various movements, positions and tolerances into the integrated activity
- Pacing activity by quota: this is simplest with repetitive exercise which can be counted or timed and increased at a steady rate. Goals involving reduction of medication and use of aids can be achieved using the same method
- Identification, elaboration and challenging of appraisals, beliefs and processing biases related to pain and activity, using cognitive therapeutic methods
- Relaxation skills to enhance breaks, rest and sleep, and as foundation for attention control methods
- Graded increase in safe but feared activities, increasing according to resolution of anxiety
- Improvement of communication skills with family, friends and others, such as work colleagues, or health care professionals.

The inclusion of additional components will depend on available resources but should always be properly evaluated. Sacrificing core components for other content for which evidence is poor or lacking is to be discouraged.

Outcomes

There is no single primary outcome, since multiple problems imply multiple outcomes, and goals are to a large extent determined by patients themselves. However, outcomes can generally be subsumed under the following domains, which were agreed at a National Consensus meeting in 2000 of staff from UK PMPs:

- Reduced distress/emotional impact
- Normalising of beliefs and information processing (fears, catastrophic thinking, self-efficacy)
- Increase in range and level of activity/physical performance (observed, self-rated)
- Reduced pain experience

- Reduced healthcare use (e.g. medication, consultations)
- Improved work status where relevant.

Outcome evaluation should be standard practice so that pain management staff can describe to patients, referrers and purchasers the range of patients with whom they work and the range of changes which the PMP brings about, in both the short and longer term.

Delivery

The dimensions in which programmes may vary in terms of clinical input to patients are intensity, length, size of group, individualisation of clinical input, and competence and training of staff.

Intensity and range

Historically, these programmes have been delivered as outpatient programmes, for days or part-days over weeks, or as more intensive, usually residential, programmes.

Outpatient programmes of at least 25–30 hours have produced evidence of efficacy, but more intensive programmes achieve greater improvement.

Group format

PMPs are delivered to groups because this format normalises the experience of pain and maximises opportunities to draw on the experiences of group members. It is also cost effective.

Group size varies but most groups aim to have between 8 and 12 participants. Aspects of the group dynamic are weakened with smaller numbers.

Individualisation of clinical input may be patient-led (as it is largely in goal selection), or may be guided by patient characteristics according to standardised measures.

Staff skills

Staff training is addressed in Section 5; there are no data specifically from PMPs on staff skills in relation to outcome.

Patient referral and selection

This treatment should be offered when indicated by persistent pain causing distress, disability, and a negative impact on quality of life.

Pain management components should be offered alongside the treatments intended to abolish or reduce the pain.

The optimal timing of a PMP in relation to other treatment will vary in individual patients but will always entail careful discussion between patient and therapist(s).

Although most people attending PMPs have musculoskeletal pain, the methods are applicable to visceral, neuropathic, phantom and central pain, and to pain from identified disease such as osteoarthritis and rheumatoid arthritis.

Assessment for inclusion in a PMP should include appropriate medical screening to exclude treatable disease, to discuss treatment options or the lack of them, and to introduce the concepts of persistent pain and pain management.

Assessment for a PMP is made by one or more members of the clinical staff, possibly the whole team, in relation to inclusion and exclusion criteria, to arrive at a clinical judgement about the extent to which the PMP can address the patient's needs, and to agree the proposed plan with the patient.

It is helpful to give potential attenders written information about the nature and scope of the proposed treatment.

Resources

PMPs should be properly resourced with time, personnel and facilities. Efficacy has been demonstrated for the entire package, rather than for specific components, so reduction of any of these may adversely affect outcome. Behavioural interventions, like drugs, can be diluted until they are no longer effective.

Time

Shortening a programme may reduce its efficacy or render it ineffective.

A crucial principle of pain management programmes is interdisciplinary work, close teamwork between diverse professionals who together have the necessary skills and competencies to provide the assessment and programme content. In this context, the combined competencies of the team are as important as individual qualifications.

Personnel

Competencies can be described as core and specific:

- Core competencies relate to the knowledge and skills required to be part of a multidisciplinary team and to deliver cognitive behavioural therapy in a group environment. These are transferable,

in that all members of the team should be able to provide these effectively
- Specific competencies are the knowledge base and specific skills with which specialist training equips the individual. These are not transferable.

Key staff

- Medically qualified person with a special interest in pain management. This will normally be a consultant with sessions in a pain clinic, but the role can be filled by any medical specialist, such as GP, neurologist, or rheumatologist, with appropriate training
- Chartered clinical psychologist or British Association for Behavioural and Cognitive Psychotherapies (BABCP)-registered cognitive behavioural therapist with appropriate training and supervision
- Physiotherapist (State Registered). Standards of practice for work in pain management programmes are described on *www.ppaonline.co.uk/standards.html*.

Other clinical staff

A number of other health professionals have skills which are extremely useful for the delivery of PMPs:

- Occupational therapist, whose training includes many relevant aspects, and whose role covers group work, goal setting, planning and pacing a return to activities, retraining and return to work. Training requirements are described on *www.notpa.org.uk*
- Nurse, whose role may include medication review, rationalisation and reduction when agreed; health advice and information; and liaison with the patient's family and other agencies, such as primary care practitioner, pharmacist, etc. Recommendations for nursing practice in pain services, including in pain management, are described within *www.britishpainsociety.org/pdf/nurse_doc.pdf*
- Pharmacist, whose role includes education and planning of medication reduction
- Assistant psychologists can have an important role in data collection and analysis, and in implementing graded exposure programmes.

Non-clinical staff

- Administrative/secretarial staff. A pain management programme needs secretarial and administrative support appropriate to its organisational needs

- Graduate patient (ex-patient), whose role includes patient education and serving as a role model for patients.

Leadership

Leadership within local management structures and in the daily running of the team and programme is crucial. The discipline or title of the leader(s) is less important than their identification and recognition of these roles. Consideration should be given to professional and clinical support and supervision for the post-holder(s).

True interdisciplinary teams require cross-discipline management structures.

Team working

Working together as a team requires time to meet and arrive at shared understandings of patients' needs and staff provision. Team members also need to appreciate one another's areas of unique and shared expertise. All staff can benefit from discussion with the clinical psychologist or equivalent on the application of cognitive and behavioural principles to their area of work.

Training

There is currently no recognised pain management training. Staff bring generic and specific skills from professional training, and learn from peers in the pain management field and from published accounts. It is a mistake to think that generic single discipline training is sufficient for transfer to the needs of an effective cognitive behavioural intervention.

Continuing professional development

All staff working as part of an interdisciplinary PMP should have adequate access to continued within-discipline education and development specific to the area of pain, as well as to their own broader areas of professional interest.

Facilities

A PMP requires designated space suitable for its activities and where any necessary equipment can be accommodated, including:

- A disabled-friendly venue
- Access to public transport
- A room large enough for the group
- Adequate floor space for exercise and relaxation practice
- Availability of private area(s) for individual discussion
- Easily accessible toilet facilities
- Refreshment facilities
- Office space.

PMPs are often delivered within hospitals or health centres, but alternative venues such as gyms or community centres are suitable, and may be optimal.

Part 2 Setting the scene: Introduction to the PMP

PART CONTENTS

Although it is recognised that clinics may vary considerably in programme delivery, content and staffing, a number of common features characterise pain management. The successful programme blends specific uni-professional skills into an integrated package that is consistent in terms of its overall philosophy of care and balance of emphasis. In a mature programme, there will have developed a degree of commonality across the professionals involved. *What* is delivered is more important than *who* delivers it. Most of the programmes would align themselves with a cognitive–behavioural approach (CBA), although other psychotherapeutic perspectives may be incorporated. The primary focus, however, is on improvement of function rather than cure of pain and the development of personal responsibility and self-help skills appear to be fundamental to success.

> ### Box 11.2.1
>
> **Aims of interdisciplinary pain management programmes**
>
> - To improve patients' management of their pain and related problems
> - To help patients improve their level of physical functioning
> - To help patients reduce their use of medication
> - To help patients become less dependent upon the health-care system
> - To reduce patients' use of the health-care system
> - To reduce patients' level of depressive/anxiety symptoms
> - To improve patients' level of self-confidence and self-efficacy
> - To address patients' fear and avoidance of activity that may be painful
> - To help patients return to useful and gainful activities.

> ### Box 11.2.2
>
> **Techniques of pain management**
>
> - Didactic teaching (e.g. pain pathways, anatomy)
> - Interactive teaching (e.g. drugs, problem solving)
> - Skill training (e.g. stretches, exercises, relaxation, pacing)
> - Practice (e.g. problem solving, exercises)
> - Evaluation and check on progress.

Until relatively recently, the specific importance of addressing maintenance of change and the management of 'flare-ups' has perhaps been insufficiently recognised.

General aims

The aims of pain management programmes (Box 11.2.1) are well known and have been documented in other texts (Main & Parker 1989). How these aims are addressed and delivered will vary between programmes. This may be dependent more upon local resources, rather than philosophy. Nevertheless, there is a minimum amount of input that is required to produce change. Most, if not all, programmes should include three main components of delivery. These include education, skill acquisition and practice/implementation. All of the professionals involved in the running of the programme will include elements of the above.

Usually the specific medical input will be primarily educational, although the teaching should be as interactive as possible and not restricted to a didactic approach. The professionals involved in the psychological and physical activity sessions may use the range of techniques listed in Box 11.2.2.

Programme structure

Most PMPs are offered either on a sessional basis over a number of weeks or as a much more intensive 16–20

day programme offered 4 or 5 days per week over 3 or 4 weeks. Clinics differ in the extent to which a complete evaluation will have been possible at the time of initial acceptance for a PMP, so all patients should be given a detailed pre-programme evaluation. This will allow for the evaluation of any important clinical change since the time of initial referral, but will also permit the fine-tuning of specific objectives for participation in the PMP. These must be agreed with the patient. Typically this initial evaluation might include psychometric evaluation, assessment of pain, physical function, and exercise tolerance, medication use and determination of specific objectives for participation in the PMP. Parts of this baseline assessment can be used for comparative purposes with assessment at outcome (usually at the end of treatment and at 3-, 6- or 12-month follow-ups). These follow-up assessments should be regarded as an integral part of the programme and not as an 'optional extra', since follow-up evaluations permit some 'fine-tuning' in terms of goal-setting and the opportunity to discuss the management of 'flare-ups'.

Wherever possible a partner or significant other should be invited to attend both initial assessment and follow-up assessments.

Establishing the interdisciplinary ethos

As discussed below, effective pain management requires an interdisciplinary approach in which a consistent approach is offered to the patient. (This contrasts with the sessional multidisciplinary approach in which different professions work consecutively with the patient and a degree of inconsistency may creep in.)

Ideally there will be a small number of sessions at which all of the team members will be present. The first session is the most important. Most sessions, however, will be led by one of the team and a number of topics may be covered by more than one professional (e.g. pacing of activity and management of flare-ups). Although the topic may be the same, individual professionals will cover that topic from their own stand-point at the same time as pointing out the links with other team members' sessions. This will provide a consistent message from the different team members and add weight to its importance.

Preparation for the programme

Before the programme commences, the team involved in the delivery of the programme should meet to discuss the timetabling and the content of the programme. Adequate time for this must be set aside. All team members must be aware of their responsibilities. The team should discuss each of the patients on the programme specifically to identify individual barriers to progress. It is worth reviewing the assessment data again at this stage. The team members may not have been involved in the assessment of every patient so it is important that they become familiar with the details of each patient prior to starting the programme. This will enable the team to plan the specific content of the programme more efficiently. It should allow the team to anticipate problems rather than simply reacting to events on the programme. In addition the team will be able to agree a common strategy with any of the anticipated problems that may arise on the programme, thereby presenting a common message to the patients.

The group programme by its nature will address general issues that may or may not be relevant to any particular patient. In practice, most of the issues covered will apply to most of the participants but the programme must allow for some individualisation in order to address any specific problems that individual patients may have. Some time must therefore be allocated to individual sessions. The remaining patients can quite reasonably be set other tasks that they can be doing during such sessions.

The initial session(s) of the programme

The first session of the first day is probably the most important session (Keefe et al 1996). It is desirable for all team members to be present. If possible, the patients should attend with their partners or 'significant others'. The fundamental purpose of this session is to explain again (this should have already been done before the patients were listed for a programme) the reasons why the patients have been invited to attend the programme. The patients and their partners will need reassurance

that the patients' pain is real and is taken seriously by the team. The patients should have been convinced that no further treatment or investigation is indicated and agree that a primary focus on activity rather than pain is the best way forward. The patients' partners must be helped to share this understanding. (It should be recognised of course that full 'sign-up' to the PMP objectives in terms of actual behaviour change may only develop during the PMP, but initial agreement to the plan is essential.)

The session should outline the details of the programme and the expectations of outcome. It is helpful to establish 'house rules' regarding behaviour, attendance and the disclosure of sensitive information. These may differ in different clinics. Patients (and partners) who are not comfortable with continuing on the programme following this session must either be persuaded to 'sign-up' or be removed from the programme. It is important that every effort is made to elucidate the patients' and partners' feelings about starting on a rehabilitation programme. Only then can any specific worries or fears be tackled. These may be addressed either in the group setting or on an individual basis. It cannot be emphasised enough that major barriers to progress must be addressed early on in the programme and preferably before the end of the first session.

The patients and partners will need some time to get to know each other. Time should be made for patients and partners to introduce themselves and express their expectations of the programme. In addition to general issues and making introductions it is worth ensuring that there are short presentations from each of the team members. This gives an opportunity for team members to introduce themselves and to explain their role in the programme. This should cover reassuring patients' fears about activity and 'psychology' and giving them realistic expectations of outcome.

Both patients and partners are often confused and faced with a large amount of information on the first day. Therefore try not to overload them with too much information. The prime aim is to sell the programme to them and identify specific barriers that will need addressing as early as possible. Box 11.2.3 lists general points to be covered in the initial session.

The medical introduction

One of the functions of the physician in pain management programmes is to give credence to the programme and techniques used. Unfortunately patients do still take more notice of what doctors say than other professionals. For this reason it is worth letting the physician

Box 11.2.3

Important features of the initial session

- Check patient's (and partner's) understanding of the purpose of the programme
- Explain again the purpose and specific aims of the programme
- Reassure the patient (and partner) of the reality of the pain
- Allow the patient (and partner) to raise questions concerning treatment and investigations
- Outline and explain the reasons for 'house rules'
- Each team member gives a short introduction outlining the future sessions
- Sell the programme
- Allow time for patients to get to know each other
- Try not to overload the patient (and partner).

Box 11.2.4

Medical points in the introduction

- Limitations of the medical model
- Accepting iatrogenic distress and confusion
- Acknowledging the reality of the patients' pain
- Illustrating the complexity of the pain system:
  - chronic pain is different from acute pain
  - lack of relationship between pain and injury.
- Reasons for investigations and the value of diagnostic tests
- Pain management as 'the end of the road'
- It is 'safe' to participate in a rehabilitation programme
- Hurt does not mean harm
- Brief overview of structure of the rest of the PMP.

start the introductory session. The introduction should be pitched at a very simple level and a number of points emphasised that will be repeated by colleagues in the team later (Box 11.2.4).

Limitations of the medical model

Over-reliance on the narrow biomedical model in the management of chronic pain has been a theme running through this textbook. Such a model has use in the management of acute pain problems and diseases of an identified pathology. Until the commencement

of their current chronic problem, patients may have been successfully treated by the medical model for different problems and have always held out hope that it would triumph in the end. To this end they may have subjected themselves to many interventions, most of which will have failed totally and some of which may have offered only temporary relief. The ability to produce temporary relief may well have reinforced their view that cure may be ultimately possible. This belief has to be challenged.

Accepting iatrogenic distress and confusion

Being told that one's pain is unlikely to go away, that the actual cause (such as in musculoskeletal pain) may not be clearly identifiable and that the results of scans and X-rays are not helpful in explaining the current situation is very upsetting for the patient (van Tulder et al 1997). This in turn may lead to a degree of hostility or anger. Doctors must be prepared to be the 'Aunt Sally' and accept that patients' anger with their previous medical and other advisors may be directed at them. It is not helpful simply to blame other doctors or health-care professionals for the patient's predicament (Loeser & Sullivan 1995).

Acknowledging the reality of the patients' pain

Great care must be taken to emphasise that the absence of obvious or treatable pathology does not imply the pain is imaginary or 'psychological' (i.e. psychogenic). It is helpful to explain the complexity of the pain system in a lay-person's terms. This should reinforce the reality of the pain experience in the absence of ongoing tissue injury or damage. A number of models may be used. Most patients have heard of amputees feeling pain in an absent limb and understand that sports players may not experience pain from an injury until the game is finished.

Illustrating the complexity of the pain system

The complexity of pain transmission, and the multiple factors that affect pain perception, is one of the early topics of education because it is fundamental to establishing the belief in patients that they can gain control over the intrusive nature of the pain. Most patients have rudimentary understanding of pain via nerve conduction and that the pain is 'felt' in their brain. Unfortunately most are likely to have had reinforced the misconception that persistent pain can be explained only by persistent nociception. In addition they also believe, again erroneously, that the intensity of pain is determined solely by the severity of the tissue injury or damage. They need to be helped to understand the difference between acute and chronic pain.

It is best to use examples of (acute) painful experiences that the patients may have had in the past to explain the variable pain experience from any given injury. Individual experiences can be recalled to suggest the important role of attention, anticipation, fatigue, stress and emotion in the perception of pain. This will allow the introduction of the 'gating mechanism'. It is important that the participants are made aware of the difference between increased perception of pain and increased nociceptive transmission. The role of descending inhibitory influences on 'shutting the gate' or modulating the pain gate can then be used as a reason for the teaching of pain-modulating techniques such as relaxation, distraction and mobilisation.

Reasons for investigations and the value of diagnostic tests

Many patients, like many clinicians, have a 'fixation' about identifying a structural component or cause of their pain problem. They require a cause that can be clearly identified. Introducing them to the concept that pain may result from changes in the sensitivity of nerves and the 'mistransmission' of previously non-painful stimuli can be very useful in offering an alternative explanation of their pain that does not require identification of a 'source' by scans, blood tests or other investigations. This, of course, is the basis of much current thinking on the role of neuroplastic change in the generation and maintenance of chronic pain (Ch. 1).

Pain management as 'the end of the road'

Patients have been 'selected' for pain management because there are no other options. This may be true, but that does not mean that they are unlikely to benefit. It should be emphasised that patients are selected on the basis of their likelihood of therapeutic benefit and not simply because there are no other options. In this respect pain management should be considered comparable to surgery.

It is 'safe' to participate in a rehabilitation programme

Doctors should emphasise that the patients have been carefully assessed and every effort has been made to check that there is no ongoing tissue injury or damage. They should explain this in a way that will allow any patients to challenge this if they feel that they have *not* been investigated adequately. This may then need to be dealt with on an individual basis if necessary. Often an explanation about the interpretation of investigations is enough to defuse such a problem. Despite careful assessment and counselling prior to listing a patient for a programme there will still be occasions when patients raise questions for the first time on the programme.

Hurt does not mean harm

Given that both patients and partners will be faced with an enormous amount of new information the doctor must finish with only one important message. This should be that 'hurt does not mean harm' in the case of chronic pain and it is 'safe' for the patients to exercise in spite of their pain. It should be emphasised that on the basis of the patient's initial assessment, the team is confident that it is safe for the patient to participate in the PMP, that the agreed objectives are appropriate.

Brief overview of structure of the rest of the PMP

The session should include a brief overview to the rest of the PMP with emphasis on the importance of addressing all facets of pain management. Box 11.2.5 gives an additional summary of the major educational points to be covered in the medical introduction.

Physiological effects of pain and inactivity

It is appropriate for this topic to be addressed by a physiotherapist. Almost all patients on PMPs will have had 'physiotherapy' and possibly 'exercises' to no avail. It is safe to assume that they will view this part of the programme with some scepticism, suspicion and even fear. The physiotherapist must therefore gain the patients' confidence and explain how this programme will differ from their past experiences.

It is important to explain the differences between conventional physiotherapy, which the patient is likely to have had, and the physiotherapy on the PMP. Commonly the physiotherapist will outline the sorts of conventional treatment that the patient may have had (Box 11.2.6) and then encourage the patients to comment.

Most of the comments from the patients regarding previous physiotherapy are negative. At this point

Box 11.2.5

Summary of the major educational points of the medical introduction

Simple explanation of the pain system

- Injury does not *always* produce pain (e.g. sports injury)
- Pain can occur in the absence of injury (e.g. post-amputation)
- Other factors influence pain perception.

Reasons for investigations

- Limitations of investigations
- Interpreting the results
- Why doctors give differing answers.

Conclusions

- The patients have been carefully assessed to look for continuing damage
- It is safe for the patients to exercise in the presence of their chronic pain
- Hurt does not equal harm
- The programme aims to help patients improve physical functioning in spite of pain
- The programme is designed to help the patients learn skills to manage their pain more successfully.

Box 11.2.6

Traditional physiotherapy treatments

Types of treatment

- Symptomatic pain relief (e.g. electrotherapy)
- Manipulation/mobilisation
- Other 'hands on' treatments
- Education/advice.

Aims of traditional physiotherapy

- To seek cause for painful symptoms
- Directed towards alleviating and curing symptoms.

Note: The physiotherapist is generally 'in charge' of the treatment and the patient is the 'passive recipient' of the treatment.

For chronic pain, physiotherapy is likely to be of short-term benefit only.

Box 11.2.7

The adverse effects of repeated or prolonged episodes of physiotherapy for chronic pain

- Reliance on the physiotherapist for treatment
- The physiotherapist takes control of managing the pain problem
- The physiotherapist may actively discourage patients' attempts to manage their own problem
- Conflicting diagnoses/opinions
- Demoralisation as a result of repeated failed treatments.

the physiotherapist should outline the problems with repeated or prolonged physiotherapy (Box 11.2.7).

However, some patients may have had relief from some passive forms of therapy; in these cases it is important to get the patient to identify the difference between short-term symptomatic relief and the gradual downward spiral of loss of function. From this the patient should be helped to discriminate between therapies that have short-term benefit but have not addressed the problem of increased incapacity.

Most patients identify with the problems outlined in Box 11.2.7. This allows for discussion and reassurance from the physiotherapist that past experiences will not be repeated on the programme.

Most patients are very aware of the effects of inactivity (Bortz 1984). Through group discussion, the physiotherapist can get the patients to identify the changes that they have experienced since they have had chronic pain. Most will relate reduced strength and fitness, increased fatigue, weight gain and depressed mood.

Having explained the effects of inactivity the physiotherapist should now outline the major benefits of exercise. The beneficial effects of exercise in the management of pain need to be understood early on in the programme if compliance with exercise is to be achieved (these are discussed later). Box 11.2.8 lists the goals of physiotherapy in pain management.

It is important to warn patients that they may expect discomfort and an increase in their pain following exercise. It should be explained that this is a normal concomitant of exercising muscles and joints that have not been used for some time. This is also critical if compliance with exercise is to be achieved.

A frequent charge made by patients is that the discomfort they feel following exercise in the muscles and

Box 11.2.8

The goals of the physiotherapy component of the pain management programme

- To learn about the effects of inactivity
- To learn about the importance and benefits of exercise
- To increase flexibility, strength, cardiovascular and respiratory fitness, i.e. to recondition the body
- To increase levels of general activity and function despite the pain
- To manage daily activities more effectively (managing the over-/underactivity cycle)
- To learn about the benefits of goal setting and pacing
- To learn about posture and biomechanics and apply these skills in everyday activities
- To learn how best to manage acute flare-ups.

Box 11.2.9

Responsibilities of physiotherapist and patient

- Skills are combined with other team members
- Aims to help the patient improve function and quality of life despite the pain
- Pain/symptoms are not the focus of attention
- Therapists are responsible for teaching pain management skills
- The patient is responsible for applying the skills.

The psychological effects of chronic pain

Almost all patients with chronic pain are suspicious of psychological issues and psychologists. They usually interpret any attempt to look at psychological issues as meaning that their pain is, in effect, imaginary. Past experience with health-care professionals has sensitised many against considering any of the psychological influences or consequences of pain. Many have had previous consultations in which the patient's pain has either implicitly or occasionally explicitly been said to be psychological. Psychologists in teams therefore have a difficult task ahead of them before they even speak. Many of these potential barriers will have been addressed at the assessment, but that may have been several weeks or months ago. Patients (and their partners) will require further reassurance that their pain is taken seriously.

joints away from the 'injured' area is not of the same quality or intensity of that coming from the 'injured' area. In this situation it may be useful to reinforce the points made by the doctor about the increased sensitivity of the pain system (neuroplastic changes). It is important to explain in understandable lay-person's terms that non-painful stimuli (e.g. stretch) may be misrouted up the pain system in patients with chronic pain. Using the metaphor of an 'oversensitive burglar alarm system' may be helpful in conveying this difficult concept.

Finally the physiotherapist should outline briefly the approach to be taken in subsequent sessions, and the responsibilities of each party (Box 11.2.9).

It should be explained that the focus will be on activity not pain, and emphasised that the physiotherapist is not being unkind. The reality of patients' pain is not in question. There is little that can be done to change patients' pain in itself and there is therefore little point in the therapist responding to complaints of pain or pain behaviour. The physiotherapist should reinforce that the purpose of the programme is to help the patients manage their pain more successfully. Choosing simply to ignore the patient when they demonstrate pain behaviour without explanation can result in some people becoming angry (both patients and spouses). This is why it is essential to give this explanation of the staff action, or lack of it, right at the start of the programme.

Perhaps the best way to begin to gain the patients' confidence is to outline simply the normal consequences of chronic pain (Gatchel 1996). Presenting the details of a number of traps (Peck & Love 1986) that patients find themselves falling into demonstrates that there are a number of profound and serious consequences to chronic pain. Individual patients will realise that they are no different from many other patients treated on the programme. The psychologist can then explain that not only is the pain a problem, but there are now a number of new other problems. These may well have occurred as a consequence of the pain, but nevertheless will need addressing.

Figure 11.2.1 shows how patients can slip almost insidiously into decreasing levels of activity following well-meaning advice to 'take it easy'. This ultimately can lead to withdrawal from all rewarding activities, a slide into depression and a subsequent focusing on and decreasing tolerance of pain. The pain alone is perceived

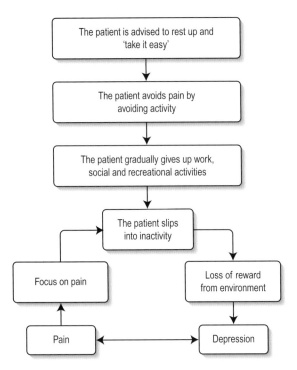

Figure 11.2.1 • The 'take it easy' trap. Adapted from Peck & Love (1986).

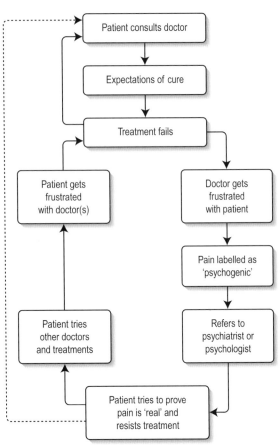

Figure 11.2.2 • The chronic treatment trap. Adapted from Peck & Love (1986).

as the barrier to any activity, when in fact many other barriers now exist. The use of such a simple model to outline the natural consequences of chronic pain and decreased activity enables patients to identify with it. They can begin to understand how they have become so disabled without blame being implied. By avoiding blame the patients are more likely to address the issues rather than become angry or resistant.

Figure 11.2.2 demonstrates the chronic treatment trap into which many patients fall. In the beginning both patient and doctor expect a resolution of the problem. In the case of the patient with chronic pain, treatment fails to provide a cure. Other treatments will be tried and they too fail. The doctor becomes progressively frustrated with the patient. The failure to respond to treatment must be because the pain is not 'organic' and the patient is then sent for 'psychological' treatment. The patient, who knows the pain is real, resents such inferences and tries to prove the pain is real by not participating in psychological treatment and searching for more physical treatments. Unfortunately this only proves unsuccessful and leads to more and more failed treatment, which confirms to the doctor that the pain is mainly psychological or has a major psychological component.

Patients identify well with this model. They often feel they have been 'labelled' and treated dismissively. Giving an understanding of the very different nature of chronic pain enables them to understand why treatment has failed and why doctors (and other health-care professionals) are frustrated as well. No blame should be aimed at either the doctors or patients. The purpose of demonstrating these models is to explain that what has happened to the patient is common and that the consequences of chronic pain are profound.

Figure 11.2.3 outlines the chronic medication trap. This is perhaps the commonest trap that ensnares patients. This occurs largely out of the helplessness of the doctor as well as the patient. The figure charts the development of tolerance leading to the patient asking for something stronger. Invariably psychological dependence occurs and in some cases physical dependence as well. Patients' reliance upon tablets makes them feel bad about their predicament and others will often point

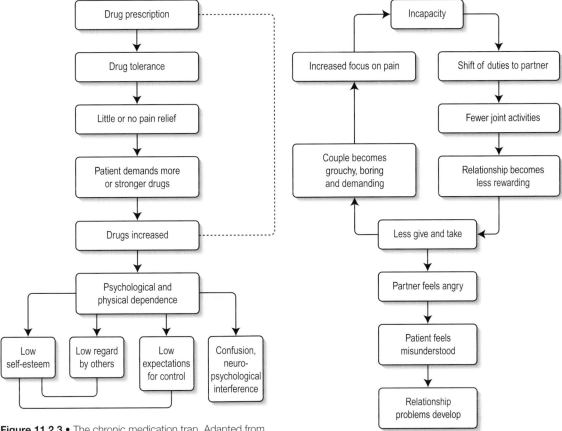

Figure 11.2.3 • The chronic medication trap. Adapted from Peck & Love (1986).

Figure 11.2.4 • The chronic resentment trap. Adapted from Peck & Love (1986).

out they are becoming addicted, which only makes them feel worse. Patients do indeed become reliant on tablets as the only way to control or manage their pain and therefore do not attempt any other strategies. A number of patients suffer subtle neuropsychological changes as a consequence of either toxic doses of medicines or drug interactions. Most patients are not aware of this effect until they eventually withdraw from medication.

Some patients may have stopped analgesic medication because it does not help. Most patients, however, continue to take analgesics even when these are not helpful. All patients identify with the 'medication trap'. Many do not understand why this has occurred. The psychologist should not blame the doctor or the patient, but simply point out that this is simply what happens, that it is not helpful and will need to be addressed.

Figure 11.2.4 shows the effects of chronic pain upon relationships. Very few relationships emerge unscathed from the effects of the chronic pain and the associated

incapacity. As can be seen from the figure the consequent incapacity leads to changes in the ability of the couple to enjoy activities together. This in turn leads to a less rewarding relationship and commonly to problems with communication. Ultimately the couple focus on the pain as the cause of all of their problems and its cure as the only solution. This topic is often the most important theme to emerge during the partner session later in the programme.

Some patients may be in the middle of one of the traps, or have been through some of the problems outlined. Most patients identify with most if not all of the traps described above. No blame is attributed. The traps are simply a description of what happens to people. On the basis of these 'ripples' from the pain and associated incapacity, the psychological issues can be addressed more openly and with little resistance or hostility from most patients. Such an explanation allows the psychologist to lay the ground for subsequent sessions and allay the fears of the patients.

The psychologist now moves on to begin to link mind and body in very simple terms. It should be explained that pain will have an effect emotionally as well as physically and these in turn can affect each other. Patients will, therefore, have to address all of the effects of and the issues surrounding the pain if they are to take control and master it.

The psychologist will give a very brief outline of the sorts of things that the group will be doing during the sessions later in the programme. Finally questions are invited from patients and partners.

Conclusion

The whole process of the first day is carried out with as little didactic and as much interactive teaching as possible. The patients and partners are encouraged to interrupt if they do not understand anything. The patients are encouraged to stand up if sitting for any length

becomes uncomfortable. This is the beginning of the patients taking more responsibility for their own conditions.

Key points

At the end of the first day the patients should have an understanding of the following:

- **Their pain is real and taken seriously**
- **They have been assessed to ensure that it is safe to exercise in the face of pain (hurt does not equal harm)**
- **The consequences of their chronic pain (physical and psychological) are common and can be regarded as normal**
- **The programme is designed to help them learn to improve their quality of life despite their pain**
- **The philosophy of the programme is 'self-help' and they are responsible for their own management.**

References

Bortz W M 1984 The disuse syndrome. Western Journal of Medicine 141:691–694

Gatchel J G 1996 Psychological disorders and chronic pain: cause-and-effect relationships. In: Gatchel R J, Turk D C (eds) Psychological approaches to pain management: a practitioner's handbook. Guilford Press, New York, ch 2

Keefe J K, Beapre P M, Gill K M 1996 Group therapy for patients with chronic pain. In: Gatchel R J, Turk D C (eds) Psychological approaches to pain management: a practitioner's handbook. Guilford Press, New York, ch 10

Loeser J D, Sullivan M 1995 Disability in the chronic low back pain patient may be iatrogenic. Pain Forum 4:114–121

Main C J, Parker H 1989 The evaluation and outcome of pain management programmes for chronic low back pain. In: Roland M, Jenner J R (eds) Back pain: new approaches to rehabilitation and education. Manchester University Press, Manchester, pp 129–156

Peck C, Love A 1986 Chronic pain. In: King N J, Remenyi A (eds) Healthcare: a behavioural approach. Grune & Stratton, Sydney, ch 14

van Tulder M W, Assendelft W J J, Koes B W et al 1997 Spinal radiographic findings and non-specific low back pain. Spine 22:427–434

Part 3 **Medical component**

PART CONTENTS

Pain pathways

The patient's model of pain will often have been challenged at the introductory session or in the first day of the programme. It is important to expand on this later to give the patient a better understanding of the pain system and the reasons behind the variability in pain experience following injury. The patient should understand that the complexity of the pain system has only recently been understood and indeed we still have much to discover. It is important that emphasis is laid on the fact that our knowledge of the pain system is based on good scientific evidence and is not simply theory or pseudoscientific ramblings. It is important also for them to appreciate that some health-care practitioners may be unaware of the new research and might still describe and consider pain in an outdated medical model. Figure 11.3.1 is a simple model of the pain pathway.

It is not necessary to go into immense detail, but it is important to explain enough to give the patient an understanding of the reasons behind the various treatments that are used and why some treatments do not work (e.g. cutting nerves). The doctor should not be tempted to use only a didactic lecturing style. Because of the complexity of the pain system and the difficulty that

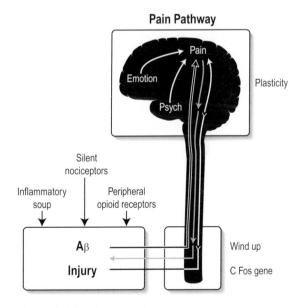

Figure 11.3.1 • The pain pathway.

we as professionals have in understanding it, the doctor should constantly check patients' understanding. It is best to use models and examples that patients may have experienced or know about already. For example, simply asking the patients about their experience of twisting an ankle in detail will bring out the detail of first and second pain. This then enables the doctor to show the patients that a single event (the injury to the ankle) produces two entirely different pains. The system therefore must be more complicated than a simple stimulus–response system.

Getting the patient to understand increased nerve sensitisation can be misunderstood if the patient perceives that you are inferring that the pain is not real or they are exaggerating the report of pain, or worse that they are weak and therefore report more pain than others. A simple experiment which often challenges this is to demonstrate that the amount of pressure required to produce pain in one area (their back for example) does not cause pain in a pain-free area and is insufficient to cause damage. Then ask the patient to explain why pressure which cannot cause damage causes pain. The conclusion is that there is something sensitive about the painful area which is not telling them about damage (the pressure exerted could not cause damage). They can then start to understand that the problem is better explained by transmission of 'false' information rather than by injury.

It is often useful to explain that the nervous system modulates all incoming information from the peripheral nerves and will filter out unimportant information almost to the extent that the person may not be aware of it, for example, the selective deafness of children called to meal times, or the sensation of the wristwatch, which does not normally enter consciousness. Similarly the nervous system will enhance and pay much more attention to information that is deemed important, threatening or annoying, for example, the squeak in the car, the whimper of a newborn baby or the sound of footsteps behind one when walking in the dark. Pain has been for all their life a way of telling them about danger and damage, the pain they have now is no longer informing about damage but the response is the same and it takes a lot to try and ignore it.

Most patients can identify with examples of this. It should be explained that pain signals are treated in much the same way. They are, of course, regarded as important signals and may well be enhanced, especially if the patient is fearful of their meaning (Box 11.3.1).

At the end of the session(s) on pain pathways, patients should be confident that their usual chronic pain does not signify further damage or harm and when it increases it does not signify a new injury. They should

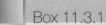

Box 11.3.1

What the patient should understand after the session on pain pathways

- There is not a simple one-to-one relationship between the degree of injury and the amount of pain experienced
- There are good 'physical' or 'physiological' explanations for injury without pain and pain without injury
- The patients' pain is not 'imaginary' pain, all in the head or 'psychological'
- Pain signals are modulated by local and central factors
- Chronic pain is not the same as acute pain
- The chronic pain the patient feels is not a sign of ongoing damage
- Chronic pain usually cannot just be switched off
- Non-pain stimuli (e.g. stretching or pressure) may send pain signals in patients with chronic pain
- An increase in the patients' usual pain with or without exercise does *not* signify a new injury
- Acute pain (new) is a useful signal but must be differentiated from the old pain.

also understand that a new pain in an area they have not had pain in before *may* indicate damage and it may require attention. Similarly a new sensation of pain which is very different from their usual pain which they have not experienced previously should be reported and checked out. Patients should therefore become more confident of increasing activities in spite of their pain and become less fearful of movement. Unless patients understand the model of pain and are able to be confident that they will not deteriorate physically as a consequence of increasing their physical activities they will not participate in the programme or make any progress.

Diagnoses and investigations

This session has the potential to stir up a significant amount of anger that patients may have with the medical and other professions. The doctor entrusted with this session must be prepared to take the brunt of patients' anger with the medical profession in general. Patients' experiences are very variable. Most patients have had a

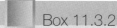

lot of previous investigations and (unsuccessful) treatment. They often feel they have been passed from pillar to post with little explanation of their condition. They may have been given to understand that they have 'spinal arthritis' or a 'degenerative spine' when the X-rays simply show age-related changes. It may have even been implied they are imagining their pain or it is not real pain. Patients can be helped to understand that we age on the inside as well as the outside and wrinkles and baldness do not mean you cannot function; such changes are part of ageing and are normal but some people get them sooner than others.

There is considerable distress and dismay when imaging does not provide the explanation a patient was looking for. We have all spoken to the patient who has had an MRI scan which has proved normal only to state that they were 'devastated' with the result. It is worth spending some time explaining that scans are essentially pictures and tell us nothing of the function of the back in normal use and certainly tell us nothing about everyday muscle function or whether nerves are sensitive or not. Scans tell us about the structure, not about whether the thing works properly. An analogy would be asking them if they would buy a car from a photograph or a series of photographs (of the engine, the interior, the exterior); most will say no. Asked why, they will reply that it will not tell you if it works. Likewise a few scratches on the paintwork and the occasional dent does not mean that it is not a fully working car; it may not look perfect but it can be reliable.

It is sometimes helpful to invite a specialist from outside the team (e.g. a spinal surgeon). Care should be taken in choosing whom to invite. The relevant person should have a good understanding of pain management programmes and the specific reason for their session. They should be warned that patients on such programmes can often become very angry during this session. Patients often feel that investigation, tests and diagnoses have not been explained fully (Box 11.3.2). They frequently feel they have been treated dismissively. As a consequence they may become quite hostile to the doctor in this session. It is worth ensuring that another regular team member is at this session not only to provide some support for the doctor but also to gain first-hand knowledge of what was said.

Limitations in diagnostic tests and in the potential value of surgery may be addressed most convincingly by a surgeon who will be able to put surgery into context and explain why certain investigations are performed and how they should be interpreted. The surgeon invited to participate must fully understand, however, the purpose of the session and be able to deal with fairly frank exchanges without becoming defensive or

Box 11.3.2

The points patients should understand after the session on investigations, tests and diagnoses

- The reasons why certain investigations are performed
- The limitations of particular types of investigations
- The interpretation of the results of investigations
- What do people without pain show on investigations?
- What are the known causes of chronic pain?
- What treatments are available?
- Just how effective are the treatments?
- Why can't pain be stopped?
- What is the future likely to be for a patient with chronic pain?

hostile. Patients have often invested a lot of hope in an orthopaedic appointment only to find that they were not offered an operation. This often leave the patient feeling they are inoperable or have been 'fobbed-off'. The good reasons why operations are not offered can be explained. Finally they may be able to give the patients an understanding that as yet some problems do not have a medical solution.

At the end of this session any residual fears regarding further investigations should have been addressed. This may require time to be spent with individuals to either reassure particular patients or institute further investigations in order to reassure them. It must be said that investigating such patients further at this late stage should be very rare and will probably exclude them from the programme until the issues have been clarified. Most issues, however, can be more than adequately addressed in the group setting. The team should feel able to draw a line under these issues and feel comfortable that no further discussions should be held unless an entirely new problem occurs.

Medicines: how to get the best out of them

A lot of information is available about medicines, their use and potential problems associated with them (Box 11.3.3). It is best to tackle these at two sittings, avoid didactic teaching (remember how boring pharmacology lectures were!) and get the patients to do most of the work.

A significant proportion of patients with chronic pain problems persist in using medication of various types despite little in the way of prolonged or sustained benefit. Many have been prescribed medication, which is normally designed to help with short-term problems during the initial phase of the pain. There is evidence in the literature that the level of medication usage, and in particular misuse, correlates with the level of psychological distress (Spanswick & Main 1989). In other words the more distressed patients are the more likely it is that they will use analgesics and/or tranquillisers and also the more likely that they will use them in doses above the recommended maximum. It is for this reason that some education regarding medication usage is important. It cannot be assumed that medication usage will automatically change following a pain management programme unless it is specifically addressed.

Patients should be warned in one of the first sessions by the doctor that they may well experience more pain in the first few days or weeks of the programme. This is usually because they are using muscles they have not used for some time. They should be asked specifically *not* to increase their medication usage, but to begin to take it on a time-contingent (by the clock) basis rather than an as-needed or pain-contingent basis (Fordyce 1976). It may be helpful to ask them to complete a drug usage form to indicate what medicine they are taking and when, and to fill this in each day, recording *all* pain-related and psychotropic medication they use. This will enable the team to establish the patient's baseline use of medication.

Introduction to use of medicines

Many patients have no understanding of the medicines they are taking or the rationale for their prescription. The medications are often taken in a haphazard way. Frequently patients gain little benefit despite high doses.

It is important, therefore, to offer some education addressing the points above. It is useful to allow patients to do much of the work in finding out about the various types of drugs and to get them to report back the detail of what they have learned. However, it is important to give a basic structure into which they can hang the detail.

The patients should, therefore, have been set 'homework' in one of the sessions prior to this first session on medicines. They may be given copies of drugs information leaflets, a pharmacists' formulary or even the BNF (British National Formulary 2006) and asked to look up a number of drugs including the medicines they are likely to either be taking or have taken in the past. The patient group can be asked then to divide themselves into subgroups and to allocate to each subgroup a specific type of medicine to look up. At this session each subgroup is asked to tell the rest of the group what they have learned about the various medicines they were asked to investigate. In order to help the patients make sense of the information they will discover they should be directed to searching out the benefits, the side-effects and the major problems with each type of medication they look up.

The patients may be quite daunted by this task and will need some guidance. The doctor's task is to act as interpreter, as drug information is often not designed for the lay-person. The doctor should guide the patients through the meaning of the medical terms and translate the information in terms that the patients can understand. Patients may be frightened by the description of side-effects and complications. The doctor should take care to reassure patients about the safety of the medicines they have read about and put the side-effects into context.

At the end of the presentations and the subsequent discussions within the whole group and with the doctor, the patients should have an understanding of the various types of medication outlined in Box 11.3.4. They should understand the basic modes of action of NSAIDs, opioids, tranquillisers and night sedatives. They should understand why such medications are prescribed. It is important to reiterate what has been said in the introductory session. No blame of either the patient or their doctor should be implied. The patients may become angry at realising they have been prescribed medication that has not been helpful and may have caused significant

Box 11.3.4

Medication

- Non-steroidal anti-inflammatory drugs (NSAIDs)
- Opioids and opioid-containing medicines including co-compounds
- Paracetamol
- Tranquillisers (benzodiazepines)
- Antidepressants (tricyclic antidepressants, newer antidepressants, selective serotonin reuptake inhibitors (SSRIs))
- Anticonvulsants
- Others.

Box 11.3.6

Opioids

- Related to morphine
- Work at morphine receptors
- Key-and-lock mechanism
- Physical dependence
- Psychological dependence
- Development of tolerance
- Withdrawal effects
- Long-term-use effects (possibly enhancing pain)
- Interaction with benzodiazepines (central effect)
- Why use them?
- The body's own morphine.

Box 11.3.5

NSAIDs: main teaching points

- Act by inhibiting enzymes that normally enhance pain
- A peripherally acting painkiller
- Not addictive
- Some potential problems with gastric side-effects
- Some central side-effects.

problems. The doctor must emphasise that most of the medications discussed are very useful in the early phase of a pain problem or during the acute episode.

The opportunity should also be taken to answer any questions, doubts or worries about any other medication that the patients may be taking.

NSAIDs

Box 11.3.5 shows a simple outline of the important points to be made with regard to NSAIDs. Explaining how the NSAIDs came to be discovered and used originally and why they have been so successful is important. The message should not be entirely negative about drugs, but rather putting their use into the context of other conditions and diseases (e.g. osteoarthritis). The emphasis should be made, as with all medication, that often patients do not necessarily find them helpful if taken all of the time, although they may be helpful during acute episodes of pain (McQuay & Moore 1998a).

Opioids

Many patients are horrified to discover that they are taking medication that includes an opioid, a drug related to morphine (Box 11.3.6). Some become quite angry, especially if they have become physically dependent on them. It is therefore important to explain the rationale for using opioids in acute pain and exactly how effective they can be. Their use in chronic pain, however, is not associated with quite so much success (Jamison 1996, Molloy et al 1997). Of course all episodes of chronic pain began with an acute episode and therefore it is quite reasonable to use opioids in the acute phase (McQuay & Moore 1998b). It is important to reinforce that no blame should be attached to either the prescriber or the patient. The British Pain Society produce an excellent leaflet for patients which explains the reasons for the use of opioids in persistent pain (www.britishpain society.org).

Paracetamol

It is surprising how many patients do not know that compounds like co-codamol contain paracetamol. It is, fortunately, becoming less common, but considering the potential danger of inadvertent overdose of paracetamol it is very important. Indeed it is the paracetamol rather than the opioid content that is dangerous in the taking of such compounds in excessive doses. There are records of patients consuming as many as 28 co-codamol per day!

Emphasis should be made that in therapeutic doses paracetamol is safe and sometimes helpful even for chronic pain. More importantly it is not addictive

Box 11.3.7

Tranquillisers

- Sedatives
- May help sleep in short term
- Originally thought not to be addictive
- Now known to produce 'physical' dependence within 3 weeks
- Psychomotor effects
- Enhanced effect on cognition with concurrent opioid
- Withdrawal effects
- Psychological dependence, 'habit'.

Box 11.3.8

Antidepressants

- Tricyclic antidepressants often prescribed as analgesics
- Analgesic effect separate from antidepressant effect
- Well-documented dose–response curve
- Useful non-addictive night sedation
- Significant side-effects can limit use
- More recent SSRIs less sedating; no known analgesic effect.

and relatively free from side-effects such as gastric irritation.

Tranquillisers and night sedatives

Most patients with chronic unrelieved pain develop sleep problems if they did not have them before. In addition some patients become increasingly anxious and worried about their pain and increasing disability. A significant number are prescribed night sedatives, which usually means a benzodiazepine. Fortunately there is a trend for fewer patients to be prescribed diazepam for pain even if some muscle spasm is associated with it. Such treatment almost invariably does not help the pain and simply sedates the patient, who subsequently finds it more difficult to cope. Some pointers about tranquillisers are given in Box 11.3.7.

Having already explained the mechanisms of the actions of opioids, it is a simple matter to use that basis for the teaching of the effects of benzodiazepines. It is worth putting benzodiazepines into context. It should not be implied that the drugs themselves are bad, but rather that they need to be used appropriately in appropriate circumstances to reap the best benefit. The patients should have noted from their reading of the BNF that they are not recommended for more than 6 weeks.

Antidepressants

Depression as a part of the clinical picture with chronic pain is neither uncommon nor unsurprising. A number of patients end up taking antidepressants of one type or another. Many, if they have already been to a pain clinic, will have been prescribed a tricyclic antidepressant

for the analgesic effect rather than the antidepressant effect (Box 11.3.8).

It is important to emphasise that the analgesic effect seems to be entirely separate from the antidepressant effect. Patients often need some reassurance that antidepressants are not tranquillisers or addictive. They are frequently not aware of the reason for their prescription. It is therefore important to spend some time explaining their use. Mention should be made of the SSRI (selective serotonin reuptake inhibitor) antidepressants. Some patients may have been prescribed these. Although their effectiveness in depression is not challenged, they do not appear to have a specific analgesic effect.

Anticonvulsants and other membrane stabilisers

A small number of patients will have been prescribed anticonvulsants (or other membrane stabilisers) for their pain problem (Bull et al 1969, Loeser 1994, Monks 1994). There is some evidence in the literature that they can be helpful, particularly in neurogenic pain of a shooting nature. Patients, pharmacists and some doctors become confused as to the rationale for their prescription. It is not possible to educate the whole of the medical and pharmacy staff. Therefore, educating patients is the most efficient way of ensuring these drugs are used in the appropriate way by them.

It is important that patients understand why they have been prescribed, how they work and how they should take them (Box 11.3.9). Many patients will take them 'as required', which is probably the least effective way of using them.

Box 11.3.9

Anticonvulsants and other membrane stabilisers

- Useful in pain of a 'shooting' or paroxysmal nature
- Often used in pain of a neurogenic origin
- Need to be taken regularly 'by the clock'
- May cause sedation, tremor, gastric irritation and other side-effects
- Long-term use requires blood monitoring
- Not addictive.

Box 11.3.10

Definitions in patients' language

Tolerance

- The ability of the body to 'get used to' a medicine
- Often leads to a decreasing effect from the drug and the need either to increase the dose or to move on to a 'stronger' medicine
- Does not happen with all medicines
- Most common with opioids, tranquillisers and night sedatives
- Can happen in a short time (less than 6 weeks).

Psychological dependence

- A habit
- Commonly results from repeated actions in association with a trigger
- Inability to perform the habit makes people feel anxious and focus on the original symptoms
- Easily reinforced.

Physical dependence

- Involves the development of tolerance
- 'Physical symptoms', usually unpleasant, develop following sudden cessation of medication
- The physical symptoms may include some that are similar to those for which the medicine was taken
- All withdrawal symptoms stop eventually, even without treatment
- Withdrawal symptom profile varies according to the medicine and between individuals.

Other medication

During the medication education part of the programme it is often a good time for patients to ask the questions they always wanted to ask about their other medicines. This should be actively encouraged, although it is obviously not the main thrust of the education. It is important to emphasise to patients that although they will be encouraged to make less use of analgesics and tranquillisers they should continue on all their other medicines that they take for other purposes (e.g. blood pressure tablets).

Patients should be set a homework task at the end of this session. It is worth indicating the topics to be covered in the next session and ask the patients to prepare some questions they may wish to ask and to put some thoughts down on paper. Given that the next session will be on addiction and tolerance, the group should be asked to prepare any questions they have and write down their thoughts about addiction and getting used to medicines.

Tolerance, addiction and how to get the best out of medicines

Although this second session on medication could be given in entirely a didactic way, it is best to use techniques that involve as much activity from the patients as possible. The doctor should check that patients understood the content of the previous session on medicines and that there are no further outstanding worries or questions. It may be worth reassuring the audience by explaining that many patients find these sessions difficult and often raise questions about tablets and medicines.

It is best to use the term 'dependence' rather than 'addiction'. The word addiction is often used in a judgemental way and is best avoided. The discussion should identify the difference between physical dependence and psychological dependence.

The doctor should then ask the group members to give their own understanding of dependence and tolerance. At the end of the discussion with the group it should be possible to write down definitions of physical and psychological dependence and tolerance (O'Brien 1996, Reisine & Pasternak 1996). The discussion can then move on to what the patient can do to avoid these problems. Box 11.3.10 outlines the main teaching points of this part of the session.

No blame should be attached to either patients or their prescribing doctor. This session should emphasise

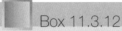

Box 11.3.11

Reasons for reducing and withdrawing from medication

- Significant improvement in cognitive functioning (especially with opioid/benzodiazepine combination)
- Loss of potentially significant side-effects (e.g. constipation, gastric problems)
- Feel more 'in control'
- Improvement in self-esteem
- Analgesics often make little or no change to long-term pain anyway
- Return of positive short-term response for acute episodes (see tolerance above).

Box 11.3.12

Common reasons for failing to stop medicines

- Abrupt withdrawal leads to a much greater chance of profound withdrawal symptoms
- Stretching out the time interval between tablets produces withdrawal symptoms
- An increase in pain is a common withdrawal symptom, reinforcing the 'need' for tablets
- The patient has no other strategies to manage the pain to replace the tablets
- General practitioner may inadvertently reinforce regular medication.

that this is simply what happens. It does not happen to everyone, nor does it represent a problem in everyone, even though they may have noticed some of the physical effects. The ultimate aim of this session is to point out that continuous use of some pain medicines is often not helpful and can be counterproductive.

Patients must be given some positive reasons for medication reduction and withdrawal (Box 11.3.11). These should be outlined before going on to techniques of how to withdraw from tablets.

Some patients become overenthusiastic and will wish to stop everything immediately. Some may become quite angry at any implication they are to blame as they have tried to stop medicines but have been unsuccessful because the pain becomes intolerable. Time should be taken to address these feelings and explain why many patients are unsuccessful in their attempts to stop tablets (Box 11.3.12). For example, simply stopping tablets or stretching out the time in between tablets is more likely to provoke withdrawal symptoms. This, however, is the commonest strategy that patients adopt.

At this point the principles of drug withdrawal should be outlined and the patients then set the task of working out for themselves precisely how they propose to come off all or some of their medication. However, before any attempt is made to withdraw, patients should learn to change their habit of taking medicines. Patients must start to take their medicines on a 'time-contingent' basis or 'by the clock' rather than contingent upon their pain. This will help break the 'pain–pill' habit and must be in place before any attempt at withdrawal is made.

At this point, if not before, the patients are asked to keep a drug diary to help them monitor their own medication usage. This will give them an insight as to

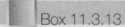

Box 11.3.13

Principles of drug withdrawal

- Choose to reduce or withdraw from one drug at a time
- Choose the easiest one first (probably the opioid)
- Start by stabilising level of medication usage
- Change from pain-contingent to time-contingent medication
- Keep timing of medication the same (do not extend time between medications)
- Reduce the amount taken by a small amount (half a tablet) at a time
- Reward success.

how much they actually are taking and may well change their behaviour just by the fact that they are monitoring the situation. Having established baseline, patients should follow the guidelines outlined in Box 11.3.13 while continuing to monitor their tablet consumption.

The patient plan should first establish taking medicine on a time-contingent basis and not only as response to pain. Having established regular medication, patients should concentrate on reducing the amount of drug/medication by a small amount every few days or weeks. This should be done with the aim of coming off the chosen medication within a specific period of time. This will vary according to which type of medication is being withdrawn. In general, opioids may be withdrawn much

Case study 11.3.1

Chronic back pain

Mrs J. has had a chronic back pain problem for some 8 years. She has tried most medications but has found them not helpful and has become desperate to find something that works. Over a prolonged period she has ultimately ended up taking a significant number of different medicines. These include anti-inflammatory drugs (diclofenac), an opioid (dihydrocodeine), up to 16 tablets a day, a night sedative (temazepam) and an antidepressant (amitriptyline).

Despite the use of all of this medication her pain is still severe. It appears to get much worse if she tries to stop any of the tablets. She doesn't like taking all of this medication and tries to stretch out the time in between her ordinary painkillers (dihydrocodeine). This simply seems to make her pain much worse and reinforces her feeling that she needs to continue taking the tablets in spite of the fact they do not help very much. Mrs J.'s use of painkillers had become very

haphazard and on occasions she would take four or five at a time to try to get on top of the pain.

Towards the end of the pain programme Mrs J. had managed to organise her medication use so that she was taking her tablets on a regular time-contingent basis (even though still at a higher dose than the recommended maximum). She picked one medication (dihydrocodeine) and decided to reduce this slowly by reducing her consumption from four tablets every 6 hours to three and a half every 6 hours. When she had got used to the new level (after several days) she reduced this further to three tablets every 6 hours. She continued with this technique for several weeks until she was not taking any dihydrocodeine. She noticed by reducing her medication this way that there was very little change in her pain. She then planned to tackle her use of other tablets one at a time until she was on a minimal level of medication.

quicker than benzodiazepines, which might take several months (Hobbs et al 1996). It may be necessary to change the patient's medication in order to facilitate withdrawal. For example, some compound analgesics that contain an opioid and paracetamol are best prescribed separately so that the opioid component can be withdrawn separately from the paracetamol or more slowly if necessary.

It is important to stress that if the patients do get any withdrawal symptoms these will eventually disappear. The negative aspects of withdrawal should not be over-emphasised; many patients get none at all. Patients should be encouraged to plan the withdrawal and use the medication-monitoring forms to assess their progress and identify any problems. This allows patients to monitor their reduction of tablets and enables the staff to reinforce the changes the patient has achieved. Some patients may have difficulty in completing such forms so it is important to go through it with them individually if necessary. Patients should be encouraged to ask questions about their medication if they are not sure, and to check with the doctor on the programme that they are managing their medication correctly. Be sure to keep the patient's GP informed.

The patients must understand that medication reduction and withdrawal is a long-term plan and should not be instituted in haste. They should not be expected to make major changes in a few weeks, particularly if they are increasing their level of exercise at the same time.

Much of the teaching about medication will have necessarily dwelt on the negative effects of continuous use. It is important to point out that medicines can be

of significant help, particularly during acute episodes of pain. It is worth revisiting the 'mission statement'. This emphasises that continuous use of medicines for reducing pain is usually not helpful in the long term. Analgesic use for short periods during acute episodes has been shown to be helpful (McQuay & Moore 1998a–c). If patients are able to reduce their medication to the lowest level possible (preferably zero) then they are likely to gain some help during acute flare-ups without having to exceed the maximum recommended dose. In addition, patients will have been taught other techniques to help them manage acute episodes more effectively. This prepares the way for the last session with the doctor. An example is given in Case Study 11.3.1.

The management of flare-ups

During the last week there is a session with the doctor that is entitled 'the emergency card'. An important part of this session is devoted to the 'sensible use' of medication. During the course of the programme the patients will have learned to use a range of skills in managing their pain. They are taught to recognise the difference between their usual pain, which may simply be increased in intensity, perhaps as a response to unpaced exercise, and a new pain, which they have never had before. Patients are encouraged to pay little attention to their 'old' pain, and in particular not to continue to seek further curative treatment or to manage it solely with medication. With a new pain they are encouraged to seek appropriate advice if it does not settle in due course.

Box 11.3.14

Major points for the emergency card

- Don't panic; this will get better
- Assess 'is this a new pain or my old pain?'
- Physical and mental relaxation
- Possibly stretching exercise
- May need to rest up (max. 2 days bed rest)
- Keep active; potter if possible
- Cut back on exercises
- Begin to pace exercises up slowly again
- May need some painkillers to help restore function
- Visit general practitioner only for prescription for painkillers
- Retain control; don't allow oneself to be referred again
- Work out why this happened (lack of pacing, etc.)
- Congratulate self for managing it well.

Box 11.3.15

Guidelines for the use of medicines during acute episodes of your usual pain

- Keep on the lowest level of painkillers (preferably none) when not in the midst of a flare-up
- Use all of the other techniques you have learned to 'manage' this episode
- Medicines can be useful as a tool to help you institute the other techniques
- NSAIDs (if they do not give you significant side-effects) can be used on a regular basis for a short time (4 weeks maximum) if helpful
- Combination analgesics (e.g. co-codamol) may be added or used alone. These should be taken 'by the clock' (not on a pain-contingent basis) for a maximum of 3 or 4 weeks. The dose should then be reduced and stopped
- The medicines should be used as a 'tool' to help in restoring activity.

The session centres around the patients making their own plans for what they are going to do when they get an acute flare-up of their pain. The doctor poses the questions and the patients as a group have to come up with the answers. Thus the patients have an investment in the resulting plans. It is often useful to give an explanation of the 'emergency card' system that exists in many hospitals to make sure the hospital's response to a 'red alert' is not chaotic but well ordered and thought out. It should be pointed out that hospitals often 'practise' and then make changes in the light of experience. The patients should be encouraged to produce their own 'emergency card', and practise what they will do and make changes in the light of experience.

The group members should be taken through, step by step, exactly how they will feel when they have an acute flare-up and what they have learned that will help them to manage it more successfully than they have in the past. They should understand that they will need to plan what they are going to do during an acute episode as they are unlikely to think rationally at the time. The doctor's role in this session is simply to guide the discussion and make sure all the relevant points are made. Box 11.3.14 shows the points that should have been made by the group by the end of the session.

In the past, tablets were the first and in some cases the only way many patients had of trying to cope with and manage their old pain and flare-ups of their old pain,

even if it did not help much. The patients are encouraged to continue to use *all* the skills they have learned and not to resort to medication in the first instance.

The doctor should give specific recommendations for what types of medicines may be used and how they should be used during acute episodes. These guidelines are outlined in Box 11.3.15. They are not absolute, but should give an indication of how to get the best out of medicines. The doctor should inform the patients that these guidelines will also be sent to their GP, so that medicines are not inappropriately withheld during acute episodes and that the patients are supported in their efforts to keep medication to a minimum at other times.

The doctor should not, however, concentrate on medicines at this stage but rather encourage the group to come up with the solutions on the basis of what has been learned on the programme. It is often best to use a case example to focus the discussions. The patients should be set homework to make their own 'emergency card', which should detail what they are going to do when they have an acute flare-up. They should be encouraged to get the help of their partners (if appropriate) to help in the plan of action. This will give the partner a specific supportive role rather than over-protective role in helping patients to manage their own pain.

Finally the patients must be directed to practising their emergency system. Just as novices practise the routine *before* making a parachute jump, so the patients must practise their emergency plan when they are in a good phase so that their response to an acute episode becomes almost a habit.

A patient's guide to how to survive the health-care system

It has been said that the health-care system itself should have a health warning! Many of the patients on pain programmes have been on a circuitous route before ending up on a pain management programme. They have little understanding as to why they have apparently been passed from pillar to post with no answers or helpful treatment (Loeser & Sullivan 1995).

Basing this session on the experiences of the patients in the group will make it more relevant to them. This is best done by briefly going through the referral pathway of one or two of the patients. Rather than simply giving answers as to why, for example, referral between a number of specialists occurred, the doctor should encourage the group to come up with some of the potential reasons. This should promote discussion on a number of topics ranging from 'why did I see a different doctor in the same clinic each visit?' to 'why didn't I get an MRI scan at my first visit?' Of course it is not possible to know the precise reasons in any given case, but the doctor should give the patients an idea of the thoughts that may have been going through the treating doctor's mind and a better understanding of how the health-care system works.

Patients have no understanding of differential diagnoses, what diseases different specialists see or the specificity and sensitivity of various tests. They do not usually have an understanding that test results are not necessarily absolute and that ultimately a judgement has to be made with regard to diagnosis and treatment.

One of the most important points to be made is the fact that doctors, be they GPs or specialists, are no less human than the patients they see and are subject to bias and other human frailties. If the doctor is pressurised by the patient to 'do something' at any cost, the patient should understand that the doctor may respond emotionally rather than intellectually. In other words, upon seeing a very distressed patient pleading for help, the doctor may be tempted to offer treatment to the patient even though the likelihood of major help is very small. This may be offered to help doctors cope with their sense of helplessness rather than being based on their knowledge and experience. The doctor and the

Box 11.3.16

Learning points for surviving the health-care system

- When consulting your general practitioner or specialist be explicit about what you want (e.g. 'I only need some painkillers for a short time')
- Put the doctor at ease
- Explain you are taking responsibility for managing your old pain
- Do *not* get angry or aggressive
- Do *not* pressurise the doctor if there is nothing that can cure your problem
- If you have a new pain, explain it is not your usual pain but a new one you have not had before
- If you are anxious take someone with you. The other person will remember what is said better than you
- Write down the questions you want to ask, so you don't forget anything
- If you are to undergo investigations ask what is being sought
- If you are offered treatment, ask what is the expected outcome and the risks
- Avoid being reinvestigated or treated for your old pain.

patient usually regret this decision later. Patients frequently do not have an understanding of the effect of the pressures that they put upon their doctors. They tend to feel they are being denied treatment when the doctor is appropriately resistant to the patient's imploring that something must be done.

The group should be invited to come up with solutions as to how to get the best out of consultations with their doctors. This may be approached by asking the group to come up with ideas of how to make life as difficult as possible for the doctor. Having identified these behaviours the group could then be asked how they could modify their behaviour to put the doctor at ease and thus get the most out of the consultation.

It is impossible to anticipate all of the points that may be covered in this session. There are, however, a number of important learning points. These include the importance of the patients' behaviour in determining how the doctor reacts. The specific learning points are outlined in Box 11.3.16.

Conclusion

It is important not to overmedicalise the PMP. The doctor's role in the programme should be supportive of the other members of the team. There are a small number of sessions in which the doctor may participate with other team members present. These include the initial session (see above) and the session with the partners. The reason for both is essentially the same: to reinforce the 'hurt does not equal harm' message and act as a resource to answer any remaining medical questions that may arise.

Finally the doctor may be required at any time during the programme to evaluate any new problems that may arise. It is always likely that a new episode of pain may be due to another pathological event, for example another disc prolapse, and one must always keep an open mind and examine and reassure the patient and refer if required.

Key points

- **The medical component of the programme should integrate with and facilitate the sessions led by other team members**
- **The following topics should be covered:**
  - **pain pathways**
  - **special tests, investigations and diagnosis**
  - **medication use and misuse**
  - **tolerance, physical and psychological dependence**
  - **the management of flare-ups**
  - **how to make the best of the health-care system.**
- **Time should be set aside to answer patients' specific queries.**

References

British National Formulary 2006 British Medical Association, London and Royal Pharmaceutical Society of Great Britain, London (www.bnf.org)

Bull J, Quinbrera R, Gonzalz-Millan H et al 1969 Symptomatic treatment of peripheral diabetic neuropathy with carbamazepine: double-blind crossover study. Diabetologia 5:215–220

Fordyce W E 1976 Behavioural methods for chronic pain and illness. C V Mosby, St Louis

Hobbs W R, Rall T W, Verdoon T A 1996 Hypnotics and sedatives. In: Hardman J G, Gilman A G, Limbird L E (eds) Goodman and Gillman's the pharmacological basis of therapeutics, 9th edn. McGraw-Hill, New York, ch 17, pp 362–373

Jamison R N 1996 Comprehensive pretreatment and outcome assessment for chronic opioid therapy in nonmalignant pain. Journal of Pain and Symptom Management 11(4):231–241

Loeser J D 1994 Tic douloureux and atypical facial pain. In: Wall P D, Melzack R (eds) Textbook of pain. Churchill Livingstone, New York, pp 699–710

Loeser J D, Sullivan M 1995 Disability in the chronic low back pain patient may be iatrogenic. Pain Forum 4:114–121

McQuay H J, Moore R A 1998a Oral ibuprofen and diclofenac in post operative pain. In: An evidence based resource for pain relief. Oxford University Press, Oxford, ch 10, pp 78–83

McQuay H J, Moore R A 1998b Injected morphine in post operative pain. In: An evidence based resource for pain relief. Oxford University Press, Oxford, ch 13, pp 118–126

McQuay H J, Moore R A 1998c Paracetamol with and without codeine in acute pain. In: An evidence based resource for pain relief. Oxford University Press, Oxford, ch 19, pp 58–63

Molloy A R, Nicholas M K, Cousins M J 1997 Role of opioids in chronic non-cancer pain (editorial). Medical Journal of Australia 167:9–10

Monks R 1994 Psychotropic drugs. In: Wall P D, Melzack R (eds) Textbook of pain. Churchill Livingstone, New York, pp 963–989

O'Brien C P 1996 Drug addiction and drug abuse. In: Hardman J G, Gilman A G, Limbird L E (eds) Goodman and Gillman's the pharmacological basis of therapeutics, 9th edn. McGraw-Hill, New York, ch 24, pp 557–577

Reisine T, Pasternak G 1996 Opioid analgesics and antagonists. In: Hardman J G, Gilman A G, Limbird L E (eds) Goodman and Gillman's the pharmacological basis of therapeutics, 9th edn. McGraw-Hill, New York, ch 23, pp 521–555

Spanswick C C, Main C J 1989 The role of the anaesthetist in the management of chronic low back pain in back pain. In: Roland M, Jenner J R (eds) New approaches to rehabilitation and education. Manchester University Press, Manchester, pp 108–128

Part 4 Physiotherapy component

Introduction

Physical activity is perhaps the most powerful component in pain management programmes. Increasing fitness is important not only in reversing the problems associated with prolonged restricted activity, but in giving a powerful signal to patients that they are beginning to regain a degree of control over their musculoskeletal system. It is extremely rare for a patient not to improve on at least one physical performance score and even simple improvements can be used to motivate the patient. Patients can see and record their progress and see progress in the members of the group. It is therefore extremely important from both the physical and the psychological point of view.

Effect of chronic pain on activity

Over time chronic pain patients will have reduced their levels of physical activity. Although there is some controversy over the role of physical decline and reduced physical activity in chronic pain, those who attend pain management usually represent the least physically active of people whom we might describe as chronic pain patients. People can be classed as having chronic pain when the symptoms have only been of 3 months' duration. But many people who have persistent symptoms are likely to be working and relatively active and compare relatively favourably with the pain-free population, which is increasingly sedentary. By the time people reach pain management (at least in the UK) they have become increasingly physically inactive and have often lost their job. The physiological effects of this are a gradual physical deconditioning of the patient (through the avoidance of activity) characterised by reduced strength and flexibility and reduced aerobic capacity (Bengtsson et al 1994, Bennett et al 1989, Jacobsen et al 1991). Because of the reduced level of activity, chronic pain patients are also more likely to be overweight than the normal population.

Effects of increase in physical activity level

Influence on mood

Increases in physical activity levels have been associated with an improvement in mood evidenced by reduction in depressive symptoms and anxiety. This does not, however, necessarily imply a cause–effect relationship. People who are depressed tend to be less active than those who are not depressed. Improvement in mood may be a result of improved self-efficacy or achievement and engagement in group activity rather than a direct result of the physical conditioning. Many of the studies that have identified a relationship between improvement in mood following exercise have been conducted on depressed or anxious populations rather than people with chronic pain (North et al 1990). Despite these reservations most research into the area does seem to indicate that exercise does improve mood.

Evidence of an analgesic effect

Data on an analgesic effect of exercise has been equivocal. Observations of endurance runners led some to infer that increased fitness was related to increased pain tolerance. Initial research into the area suggested that beta endorphins were produced during physical exercise and that this may occur at low levels of exercise intensity. However, the work of Gurevich et al (1994) and Donovan & Andrew (1987) suggests that it occurs only at high levels of exercise intensity. To confuse the issue further, Droste et al (1991) found that the *perceived* level of intensity was related to the biggest changes in pain thresholds and that this was independent of endorphin levels. Changes in pain report associated with participation in exercise has been widely reported (see below), although the mechanism still remains unclear.

Initial effect of increased exercise

Once patients attempt to restart exercise they will experience an increase in pain or post-exertional soreness, which most of us feel after unaccustomed exercise. This may reinforce their perception that they have reinjured themselves. Increased pain engendered by post-exertional pain in an unfit individual with chronic pain can also serve to increase excitation of pain receptors in an already sensitive pain system, presumably through secondary central sensitisation (Corderre et al 1993, Henriksson & Mense 1994, Mense 1994).

Physical capacity as an outcome measure

Some authors have suggested that an increase in physical capacity leads to an improved outcome as measured by reduced disability and reduced pain report, a reduction of recurrence of symptoms and reduced work absence. These studies usually refer to programmes that rely on physical and psychological interventions. There is a wide

variation in the improvements on each of the different physical measures within subjects (e.g. muscle strength, cardiovascular fitness and range of motion). It is extremely difficult to establish the influence of specific improvements on disability, recurrence and maintenance of change. Physical exercise sessions are a valuable tool to desensitise fearful patients by allowing them to approach physical exercise in a carefully regulated and safe way, thus overcoming their fear of activity. In this respect the increases in physical capacity observed are more likely to be linked with an increased willingness of subjects to engage in tests of capacity and this translates into other daily activities, which is reflected in observed increases in activity and on self-report assessments.

Techniques for increasing physical activity

The key aims of the physical activity component of the programme are summarised in Box 11.4.1.

Goal setting and pacing

Limited physical capacity and lowered pain tolerance restrict function in chronic pain patients. As has been mentioned above, engaging in activity may exacerbate the pain immediately or some time after the activity has finished. Although patients are educated to remain active despite the pain it is essential that they do not precipitate the pain to such an extent that they have

Box 11.4.1

Aims of physical activity component

- Overcome the effects of physical deconditioning
- Challenge and reduce patients' fears of engaging in physical activity
- Reduce physical impairment and capitalise on recoverable function
- Provide a safe and graded approach to the re-engagement in physical activity
- Help patients accept responsibility for increasing their functional capacity
- Promote a positive view of physical activity and health
- Introduce physically challenging, functional activities to rehabilitation.

to limit their activity. Conversely, some patients avoid activity to such an extent that they do not progress and do not achieve improvement.

Pacing exercise has been described by Gil et al (1988) as moderate activity–rest cycling. It is a strategy to enable patients to control exacerbations of pain by learning to regulate activity and, once a regimen of paced activity is established, gradually to increase their activity level. The converse of this is the 'overactivity–pain–rest' cycle, illustrated in Figure 11.4.1.

Chronic pain patients often report levels of activity that fluctuate dramatically over time. On questioning at initial assessment they report that they frequently persist at activities until they are prevented from carrying on by the ensuing level of pain. This leads them to rest until the pain subsides or until frustration moves them to action, whereupon they then try again until defeated once again by the increase in pain. Over time the periods of activity become shorter and those of rest lengthen. Achievements become smaller and disability increases, as the individual becomes more anxious and fearful of activity and progressively demoralised. A typical pattern of activity can be seen in Figure 11.4.2.

Through engaging gradually in exercise and not precipitating a flare-up, patients can be given a measure of control over their condition. This can be reinforced with a measured increase in activity with respect to distance walked or repetitions of an exercise to enhance the patients' self-efficacy.

The purpose of pacing and goal setting is to regulate daily activities and to structure an increase in activity through the gradual pacing up of activity. Activity is paced up by timing activity or by the introduction of quotas of exercise interspersed by periods of rest or change in activity (Fordyce 1976, Gil et al 1988, Keefe et al 1996). Pacing activity requires the patients to break down activities into both activity and rest periods and to subdivide tasks into sections that enable rests to be taken. The patients must learn also to identify activities that they find stressful and pain provoking (often, but not always, the most strenuous). These activities are assigned longer rest periods and shorter activity periods. Gradually the length of the activity times can be increased and the rest periods reduced. Some patients find it very difficult to pace activities, these usually are people who have rather fixed timetables for performing tasks. These are often self-imposed, 'Once I start the ironing I have to finish it' or 'There is no point in cleaning only half the house'. They may report that certain activities hurt them, for example 'Vacuuming the house is painful' only to find out that the patient always does the whole house in one go. It is important to distinguish between the work tasks (the things the patient has to do/wants to do) from the work style (how they go about doing them). It is often not the task but the way in which it is done with reference to intensity, duration and posture that is the main problem. These need to be addressed.

In summary, although patients are encouraged to remain active despite the pain, it is necessary not to precipitate pain to such an extent that they feel they have to limit their activity. The important principle is that they remain active rather than descend into periods of prolonged rest. What may appear to be a relatively easy task in fact often requires a lot of discipline on the

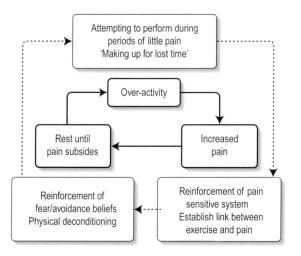

Figure 11.4.1 • The over/under-activity cycle. From Keefe et al (1996). Reproduced with permission of the Guilford Press, New York, USA.

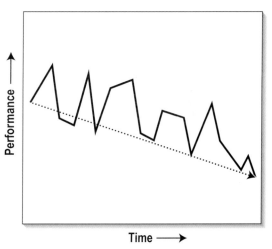

Figure 11.4.2 • A graphic representation of poor pacing leading to a gradual reduction in performance.

part of the patient. Once engaged in a task it is often easier to continue until it is completed rather than take time out to rest. Some individuals find the use of clocks or kitchen timers useful to remind them to change between activity and rest periods.

Goal setting

Goals should be set in three separate domains:

1 *physical*, which relates to the exercise programme the patient follows and sets the number of exercises to be performed or the duration of the exercise and the level of difficulty
2 *functional/task*, which relates to the achievement of functional tasks of everyday living such as housework or hobbies and tasks learned on the programme
3 *social*, where the patient is encouraged to set goals relating to the performance of activities in the wider social environment. It is important that goals are personally relevant, interesting, measurable and achievable.

The influence of psychological factors on performance

It is important to distinguish physical *capacity* from physical *performance*. Physical capacity is determined by physiological constraints. Thus, no matter how hard I try, I cannot touch the ceiling if my arm is not long enough. Physical performance on the other hand is influenced by many different psychological factors. Among the most important of the psychological factors is self-efficacy (or belief that one can actually carry out the task in question). In setting goals therefore it is important to consider the patient's expectations.

Self-efficacy

The concept of setting goals in pain management is supported by two influential pieces of psychological theory. Locke (1967) suggested that increased task performance is facilitated by the setting of specific but challenging and attainable goals. Demotivation and a sense of failure occur if the goals set are unattainable. According to Bandura (1977) two forms of expectation may lead to increased performance (Ch. 2). These are *efficacy expectations* (or the belief that one has the personal ability to perform actions that will lead to specific outcomes) and *outcome expectations* (or the belief that specific outcomes can be achieved as the result of specific

---

Box 11.4.2

Methods of increasing self-efficacy

- By information from others including professionals
- Vicarious learning from others
- Personal experience and practice
- Generating physiological arousal and 'psyching' oneself up to do things.

From Bandura (1977)

---

behaviours). Of these, efficacy expectations may be the most potent determinants of change in pain management. Previous research has demonstrated a close link between increased self-efficacy and good outcome from rehabilitation and pain management with respect to increased activity, increased positive coping and reduced pain behaviour (Bucklew et al 1994, Burkhardt et al 1994).

In the initial stages of the rehabilitation programme patients may suffer from low self-efficacy. Failure to perform a task (total inability to perform an exercise) or incompetent performance of the task (failure to reach the required level of performance, e.g. required number of repetitions) leads to a fall in perceived self-efficacy. Continued goal attainment will reinforce self-efficacy and lead to a perception of mastery over the task or problem (managing to exercise despite the pain). Increases in self-efficacy can be brought about in a number of ways or strategies (Box 11.4.2).

In pain management programmes, many patients demonstrate lack of self-confidence. Being part of a group is often particularly helpful in facilitating progress. It is most important therefore that goals are set that encourage successes but are sufficiently challenging to ensure progress.

The establishment of appropriate goals

The setting of goals should be a matter of negotiation between the patient and the therapist. The use of goal-setting charts is an essential platform on which to build. Examples of such charts are shown in Appendix 11.4.1.

Patients set a target for activities each week and record their achievements on the charts. Through this process they not only monitor their progress but also become more accurate in setting attainable goals. Goal-setting can also be used as a problem-solving exercise. Patients are asked to set specific goals (e.g. travelling to visit relatives). They then have to identify the physical goals (e.g. increase sitting tolerance) that will help them to be successful. The specific barriers to achieving those goals are also identified (e.g. increased stiffness/discomfort on a long journey). Strategies are developed to overcome these (e.g. taking breaks, performing stretches). It is also useful for patients to discuss the consequences of the goal, both positive (visiting friends, re-establishing contacts) and negative (possible increased pain the next day). They should plan how they are going to deal with the negative consequences (alteration in medication, stretching exercises and change in activity levels).

Involvement of relatives and family

It is usually desirable, and sometimes essential, to involve family members in the rehabilitation process. Introducing pacing may have a significant effect on the routines of the rest of the family. Patients may have to develop strategies that assist them in overcoming barriers presented by relatives and friends in a non-confrontational way. Care should be taken to explain the concepts of pacing and goal setting clearly to them also. They too can often be a barrier to the achievement of goals through their desire to protect the patient from injury. They should be advised not take upon themselves any task during the patients' rest period or complete tasks for them because patients are taking a long time to complete it. The way in which everyday work within the house is performed may need addressing. It may be usual for patients or their families to complete work around the house during the day and leave the evening for 'relaxing'. This usually results in a drive to complete tasks quickly rather than spread them throughout the day. It is sometimes difficult to facilitate such changes in family patterns of behaviour. Suggestions of change to family members may meet with resistance. Group tasks during pain management programmes often identify social skill deficiencies in managing interpersonal relationships. Appropriate assertiveness can be perceived as aggressiveness. A particular advantage of group, as opposed to individual, treatment is that it provides a non-threatening context for training in various aspects of communication skills.

The importance of regular review

Goal setting is an integral part of pain management, and while the patients are in contact with the pain management team, goals should be constantly set and reviewed. The patients should set themselves both short- and long-term goals at the end of the programme. This helps the patients to focus on future attainment and assists the maintenance of change once the formal pain management interventions have been completed. It should be emphasised to the patients that pain management is a process and that they must continue by themselves, rather than rely only on future attendances at a pain management centre. Furthermore, the pain problem is likely to remain with them to a variable degree for life, so management of goals has to become a life skill.

Approaches to reactivation: aerobic conditioning

Most patients attending pain management programmes have been physically inactive for a long period of time. Reduced physical activity leads to a reduction in cardiovascular fitness and a feeling of fatigue on the resumption of physical activity. Many patients are discouraged from performing physical activities not only because of the effect it may have on their level of pain but also because of the effects of fatigue on a deconditioned system. Chronic pain is frequently associated with heightened awareness of somatic symptoms, and sufferers may become acutely aware of their bodily sensations. Some patients, particularly those with fibromyalgia, report very high levels of fatigue on the resumption of activity. Although there is some evidence for abnormalities in muscle energy availability in fibromyalgia, increasing levels of physical activity have been demonstrated to reduce the subjective feeling of fatigue if the patient is encouraged to adhere to a regimen where activity is increased gradually. Activities aimed at increasing the range of motion of joints and muscle strength may not address the effect of reduced cardiovascular function. It is therefore essential that an increase in general aerobic physical fitness is incorporated in a pain management programme. Regular performance of some sort of aerobic exercise is also important for future health management and to foster a positive attitude to health. Reductions in pain report and increases in physical function on objective testing have been reported for rehabilitation programmes utilising aerobic exercise alone (Burkhardt et al 1994, Martin et al 1996, Wigers et al 1996).

Types of aerobic conditioning

Paced walking, swimming, stationary exercise cycle, stair walking, use of a stair climber and non-impact aerobic classes have all been suggested as ways of increasing physical fitness in chronic pain patients (Bennett 1996, Bennett et al 1996, Burkhardt et al 1994, Haldorsen et al 1998, McCain et al 1988, Martin et al 1996). The exercises should be performed at least three times each week for best effect. Where possible, patients should exercise to 60–70% of aerobic capacity or should pace themselves up to achieve this level of intensity if maximum advantage is to be gained. It is essential that the exercise can also be continued at home; paced walking and stair walking are obvious examples.

The planning of exercise

Endurance exercises need not involve expensive equipment. Stair walking or paced walking around a circuit (either indoors or out of doors) is an excellent form of aerobic conditioning in the early stages of rehabilitation and something that the patient can continue at home. The patient is encouraged to set initial targets and advance these gradually. Although it is preferable if patients set goals based on the attainment of heart rate targets using pulse meters, many will be unable or unwilling to do so because of the restriction imposed by pain or fear of exacerbating their condition. It therefore might be more advisable to set goals based on time, speed or resistance of the conditioning exercises chosen.

Strategies for enhancing compliance

Compliance with exercise is more likely if the individual finds it interesting and rewarding. Exercising in a gym may not be suitable for all. Some people may not have access to such facilities outside of the programme; others may not be motivated by this form of exercise, indeed gym exercise is performed by only a very small minority of pain-free people so can be considered relatively abnormal. Developing activities that are patient and family orientated and can be integrated into the normal daily routine will help to improve adherence. Exercise should become part of life, not an intrusion into it.

Approaches to reactivation: stretching

Deconditioning from inactivity or restricting joint range to a limited range of motion leads to reduction in the length of soft-tissue structures. This will limit the ranges of available motion in joints and distort the normal body biomechanics. Such distortions can in

themselves contribute to nociception or even the risk of further injury.

The influence of injury

Many of the patients on pain management programmes have an initial injury as the precipitating event in their pain history. Scar tissue that develops following injury responds to stresses and mobility by orientating along the lines of stress. Scar tissue formed under the influences of graduated stress and motion is stronger and more pliable than that formed in the absence of movement. This applies also to other non-contractile connective tissue. This makes movement and particularly stretching an essential component of the rehabilitation of deconditioned subjects.

The importance of careful initial assessment

It is not possible to go into detail of the types of problems that may be encountered in specific conditions. Most chronic pain patients have widespread symptoms and often have been particularly avoidant of exercise; hence the problems will affect not only a localised area and generalised stretching exercises will be indicated. The importance of a thorough physical examination must be stressed here. Limited ranges of motion should already have been identified and the problems and areas for improvement discussed with the patient. Although the patients are treated in a group setting the emphasis on treatment targets must be individualised to maximise improvement. Not all patients will be able to achieve the desired starting position for stretching exercises and modification of the positions will be required for some. The therapist should progress the starting position to facilitate improved stretching as increased range is achieved.

Types of stretching

There are at least two main schools of stretching technique. The first favours sustained stretching, where the tissue is taken to its limit and the stretch is maintained for a recommended period of at least 5–6 seconds. Most authorities (Magnusson 1998) suggest longer (greater than 15 seconds) if it can be tolerated. The second is ballistic stretching where dynamic rhythmic, bouncing exercises are performed from the resting length of the muscle to the limit of the range in repetitive movements.

Exaggerated guarding and increased myotatic stretch reflexes have been identified in those with painful muscles (Corderre et al 1993, Mense 1994). Additionally, psychological factors have been demonstrated to be closely associated with abnormal guarding patterns of muscle activity (Watson et al 1997). (As discussed in previous chapters, the interaction between psychological factors and guarding may be a key factor in the development of chronic disability.) Such abnormalities of movement could potentially lead to ineffective stretching and at worst injury to the muscle; therefore the ballistic stretching technique is inadvisable.

Sustained stretching, where the force is gradually applied, results in less stiffness in the muscle tendon unit for the same amount of elongation, and slow stretches are less likely to trigger a myotatic stretch reflex (Garrett 1996). In addition, there is some evidence that the sustained stretch of 6 seconds allows for inhibition of muscle activity in the stretched muscle to occur. This has been attributed to the stimulation of the Golgi tendon organ, which leads to reflexive inhibition of muscle activity (so-called autogenic inhibition) (Hutton & Atwater 1992).

Theoretical basis for 'prescription' of exercise

There has been much controversy over the type of stretching exercise that is most suitable to gain an increase in the extensibility of soft tissue. In addition to this there is a further discussion on the need for a 'warm-up' period prior to stretching. Most of the research on the benefits of different types of stretching and the relative benefits of warm-up has been conducted on normal subjects or athletes of varying levels of performance ability. There is still little conclusive evidence to demonstrate that warm-up exercises improve the extensibility of the muscle tendon unit unless the level of exercise is quite vigorous and sustained, something which is not achievable in the group under consideration here. Passive warming with hot packs similarly has little evidence for its efficacy. Some patients may benefit from hot packs prior to exercise but it must be emphasised that this is a means to an end and must not be seen a passive form of therapy by the patient.

Practice

It is important to be systematic about advice given concerning practice. Stretching exercises should be performed according to quota (number of stretches to be performed) and endurance targets (the length of time for which the stretch is to be held). An example of a stretching regimen is given in Appendix 11.4.1.

The initial emphasis is on increasing the length of time the stretch is maintained until the patient can achieve at least a 6-second hold. The number of repetitions as well as length of hold can then be increased gradually. Stretching exercises should be performed at the beginning and at the end of exercise sessions. Introducing regular stretching into daily work and home routines, especially between different activities and after periods of static work (e.g. reading, typing) is essential. The patient should also identify other times when stretching is beneficial, for instance to break up prolonged static postures, as in the goal-setting example given above. Combining the muscle relaxation skills and distraction techniques learned on the programme with stretching will increase the effectiveness of the stretch.

Effect of joint range activities

Motion through complete joint range is required to assist in the nutrition of the cartilage of synovial joints as well as in the maintenance of the length and strength of the soft tissue of the joint, such as the joint capsule and ligaments. Repeated motion through a restricted range results in limitation of joint range through the shortening of such structures and an impoverishment of joint nutrition.

Low-impact full-range free exercises are an elementary component of a warm-up and warm-down programme in most exercise regimens and this is so in pain management programmes. They should be combined with stretching exercises to capitalise on increased range of motion.

Approaches to reactivation: strengthening and endurance exercises

Theoretical basis

Loss of muscle strength and endurance has been identified in many types of chronic pain patient, and it has been suggested that a reduction in the strength and endurance of the muscles, particularly those involved in posture and lifting activities, contributes to the persistence of chronic pain. The evidence for this is still rather tenuous as increases in strength, although related to a reduction in pain, explain less improvement than psychological factors. However, exercises aimed at increasing the strength and endurance of muscle groups is an established component of pain management. Monitoring an increase in strength in particular can be motivating for some patients.

Like most physical-training modalities there are many differing ideas on what is the best way to increase muscle strength. A general rule of thumb is that strength training occurs when the muscles are exercised at an intensity of greater than 40% of maximal force with a relatively low number of repetitions; any lower force than this and a higher number of repetitions would tend to increase endurance. Exercise at greater intensity than this tends to increase muscle bulk and strength. Very high percentages of maximal force (greater than 60%) with low repetitions give the greatest increases in maximal force as an effect of training (Olsen & Svendsen 1992).

Practice

Strengthening exercises can be in the form of free exercises where the starting position is adjusted to increase the load on the muscle groups or can incorporate free weights and weight-resistance equipment. Strengthening exercises should be introduced with caution as discomfort associated with post-exertional muscle soreness and stiffness is inevitable. This is especially true for those suffering from musculoskeletal pain (e.g. back pain, fibromyalgia). Movements should be smooth and fluid. Exercises at highest resistance values or which emphasise the eccentric component of exercise have been demonstrated to be associated with a greater incidence of muscle damage and increased post-exertional soreness, so these are to be avoided.

Like the stretching exercises, strength training will need to be specific to the patient's own problem and generalised to combat the effects of deconditioning. A simple generalised strengthening regimen is shown in Appendix 11.4.1.

Muscle coordination

There is good evidence that all forms of muscle pattern coordination deteriorate with reduced physical activity, and improvement in hand–eye coordination and other similar outcomes has been demonstrated following rehabilitation. Other researchers would go further and suggest that poor muscle coordination is a cause of ongoing pain. Examples of this include the transversus abdominis and multifidus implicated in persistent back

pain. Indeed, differences in muscle function between healthy individuals and those with chronic pain have been demonstrated. However, research comparing general exercise versus specific exercise therapy, including spinal stabilisation designed to correct the imbalance between muscles acting around the lower abdomen and spine, have failed to demonstrate that specific exercises are superior to general exercise. Furthermore, compliance with exercises is poor but compliance with physical activities, especially if enjoyable, is likely to be better, so one would favour encouraging increases in enjoyable physical activity over highly specific exercises. The evidence for exercise regimes appears to favour generalised exercise over specific exercises.

Reducing pain behaviour

The subject of pain behaviour and its modification has been addressed specifically in Chapters 2 and 10, but it is relevant to revisit the topic briefly in the context of specific physiotherapeutic reactivation.

Pain behaviours are 'all outputs of the individual that a reasonable observer would characterise as suggesting pain' (Loeser & Fordyce 1983). Most commonly these are verbal complaints, altered posture and movements, and deviation from normal behaviour (lying down and/or resting for long periods). Patients are relatively unaware of their demonstration of such behaviour and the effects that it has on other people. Pain behaviours are closely associated, not only to pain intensity, but also to fear of pain accompanying activity, low self-efficacy and psychological distress (Keefe & Block 1982, Waddell et al 1993, Bucklew et al 1994, Watson & Poulter 1997).

The most florid pain behaviour is often demonstrated during exercise sessions. Operant behavioural theories suggest that the physiotherapist should ignore all pain behaviours and recognise only well behaviours and improved function (Fordyce 1976). This may not be as productive as is often claimed. Well behaviours and achievements should be acknowledged, but simply ignoring pain behaviour without explanation can be counter-productive. An explanation by the clinician to the individual or the group that all are attending for a significant pain problem is helpful. The clinician can then acknowledge their difficulties with this chronic pain, but that the focus will be on what is attempted *despite* the pain, rather than responding to demonstrations of pain. The clinician needs to make sure the patient understands that they believe the reality of their pain but, although they might ask them to do things that are uncomfortable, they will never ask the patient to do things that could result in injury.

As mentioned above, family and partners often respond to pain behaviours in a solicitous manner and in doing so unwittingly reinforce the behaviour. This is rarely overt manipulation by patients. Asking patients and partners to identify the behaviours and their responses to them, is a useful way of demonstrating the interaction between the expectation of pain, beliefs about pain and their own reactions. Video-recording patients during standardised tasks is an established method of recording pain behaviours (Keefe & Block 1982, Watson & Poulter 1997). Patients are often unaware of their pain behaviour, so video-recording, especially when they are performing tasks and interacting with others, is a useful way of providing feedback on their pain behaviour. From this discussion we can identify how the behaviour might be counterproductive and how it might be changed.

Ergonomics, lifting and handling exercises

Theoretical basis

The principles of good posture and more importantly, recognition of risk factors for poor working environments and working practices can be taught in general terms of advice that all should follow (including the healthy) with specific advice for the particular patient group (e.g. low-back pain or headache patients). Grossly stressful activities such as bending and twisting of the lumbar spine when the upper body is carrying a load, prolonged task performance or static postures without a break and prolonged exposure to vibration of the lumbar spine have all been demonstrated to increase the risk of developing musculoskeletal pathology.

In teaching good lifting, handling and posture the therapist should avoid leaving the impression with patients that a moderately poor posture or inefficient working practices will irreparably damage their musculoskeletal system. There is no convincing evidence to date that it does. Many people work in less than ideal working situations without ever becoming incapacitated or losing significant time from work owing to musculoskeletal pain. In those subjects who already have a significant level of pain such postures and inefficient working positions will lead to an increase in pain in an already sensitised pain system with a consequent risk that they may be unable to perform their work sufficiently well to remain employed. The performance of some tasks is likely to initially increase the patient's level of pain and discomfort. Although the patient

should be warned of this, care must be taken. If over-emphasised it is possible to reinforce fear-avoidance behaviour inappropriately through the provision of artificially strict rules on posture and task performance.

Persistent static postures are not a good idea for anyone, let alone a person with a chronic pain problem. The longer a person sits or stands in one position the more likely they are to experience symptoms and feel pain and stiffness once they do change posture. Patients must adopt a healthy attitude to their posture and be aware that regular changes of posture are required. Although they will be encouraged to increase their sitting tolerance or standing tolerance to a level which makes it possible to perform everyday tasks such as cooking a meal or going out to visit friends, remaining in one posture for a long time should be avoided. Simple strategies to ensure this might mean the use of timers to remind them to change posture. The changes in posture can be incorporated with a brisk walk, stretching exercises or a 'mini-relaxation' session. Some people are self-conscious about this but explanation to people that they will need to get up and move around, in a meeting for example, can help overcome this.

Practice

Patients should become skilled in the appraisal of risk, but the concept of risk needs to be considered carefully. Most movement is not harmful and it is important to reassure patients about this. Patients are given information on good working and lifting postures and the correct execution of movements. They are then asked to consider a variety of practical situations in which they have to identify risk in lifting and handling situations. These are everyday activities such as ironing, carrying shopping, cleaning cupboards, or dismantling large items (e.g. a table) and transporting them. The patients are asked to analyse the tasks to identify good and poor postures and make adjustments to the working environment to make the task less stressful. They must not get the impression that daily movements or activities are inherently dangerous or will lead to irreparable harm. Through participation in a practical task these principles can be linked to pacing activities. It seems logical that the way one improves or returns to an activity is to do it and practise until the required performance is achieved. Many 'rehabilitation' approaches do not seem to have understood this, have forgotten it or have been seduced by new 'fix-all' exercise prescriptions. It seems a vague hope that improved function can be brought about by sole adherence to a series of abstract exercises.

Few people get pleasure out of exercise for its own sake. Waddell (1998) reminds us that active exercise is not the same as active rehabilitation. Specific exercises that are remote from the activities the patient needs to do in daily life are likely to be less effective than specific management. Patients must practice the type of activities they find difficult and particularly those that they are afraid to do.

Finally, the interesting interplay between psychological factors and performance has been investigated in a series of single case experiments (Vlaeyen et al 2001) that have demonstrated that a graded exposure technique where subjects repeatedly practise feared movements can be successful in improving the outcome of treatment over and above the effects of graded non-specific exercise. Subjects were required to identify and grade exercises they were worried about or that they feared would increase their pain or cause damage. These exercises were then practised starting with the least feared and progressing onto the most feared. Feedback on performance was given with positive reinforcement to challenge fears. However, it is not clear if reducing fear of one specific activity generalises to other feared activities (Goubert et al 2002, Crombez et al 2002). Neither has the research demonstrated that patients will adhere to or become adept at practising feared movements without close supervision. Despite these concerns, on the evidence currently available it would appear advisable to include the identification and performance of feared movements/activities as part of an overall rehabilitation strategy.

Practice and practical work

A pain management programme offers an important opportunity to instigate meaningful changes and the importance of practical implementation with practice and corrective feedback cannot be overestimated.

From Figure 11.4.3 the cycle of education shows that those receiving education must have the opportunity to practise the new information to test its validity and to enhance retention of the knowledge. This is particularly important in the performance of activities such as specific exercises and pacing. Written examples (or 'paper case studies') can be used to help the patient identify problems with pacing and barriers to goal achievement in a non-threatening way. However, intellectual understanding does not always lead to a practical solution. It is very important that patients practise the skills taught in a way to make meaningful changes in their own personal life.

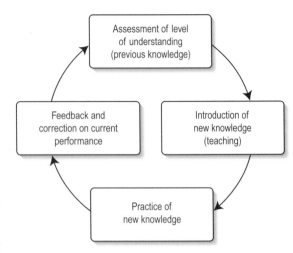

Figure 11.4.3 • The cycle of education.

Practical tasks can be developed during the pain management programme. The groups are given assignments to complete and it is often helpful to videotape sections of these tasks for discussion with the group later. These tasks must be practical and require individuals to pace their activities. Examples of such tasks include emptying a cupboard of equipment and weights and transferring it to another cupboard, or planting up large patio planters with bulbs and plants. The number of tasks depends on the inventiveness of the staff and the group! These practical tasks allow patients to identify tasks within their capability, which they can plan. Examples are shown in Case Studies 11.4.1–11.4.3.

The use of a systematic goal-setting approach to the instigation of a reactivation and strengthening exercise programme for 'Mr B.' is shown in Appendix 11.4.1.

Conclusion

Re-engaging patients in physical activity and physical exercise is an essential part of all approaches to pain management. With long-established 'disuse syndromes' a careful analysis of the pain-associated incapacities is essential. Increase in tolerance for exercise and re-establishment of activities require a planned and systematic approach. Although each rehabilitation protocol must be individualised, the general principles outlined should be the key features of all physical activity modules within pain management programmes.

Case study 11.4.1

'Mrs D.'

Mrs D. has suffered from fibromyalgia for 7 years and her husband has gradually taken over domestic activities such as cooking and cleaning. Mrs D. has set preparation of the meals as one of her goals. Her husband is concerned that she will be overdoing things and will suffer a setback if she takes this upon herself and is unwilling to relinquish the task.

They come to an agreement that Mrs D. will prepare the evening meal every other evening and will start with simple meals that are relatively quick and easy to prepare, based on some convenience foods. Initially the meal preparation will not require the use of heavy pans. Her pacing strategy includes laying the table for the evening meal in the mid-afternoon, preparing any vegetables required throughout the day and keeping the length of time she is actively engaged in cooking (frying, stirring food) to under 20 minutes. Part of the agreement is that her husband washes up on her cooking days and vice versa. One of the potential barriers identified was the oversolicitous behaviour of the husband. Both agreed that he should be out of the kitchen during the preparation of the meal.

Case study 11.4.2

'Mr A.'

Mr A. is 63 and retired; he has chronic low-back pain. He presents as mildly disabled, highly motivated but tense and frustrated at his lack of progress despite previous treatments. Like many back pain sufferers his pain is very variable and he reports days when the pain is relatively mild. He tries to capitalise on these good days by performing many of the tasks he is unable to do on the days when his pain limits his activity. This leads to an increase in pain to which he responds by increasing his pain-relief medication and restricting his activity until the pain subsides. Once the pain subsides he resumes his activities, once again doing as much as he can on good days and resting and restricting his activity when the pain increases.

Prior to commencing pain management he is asked to keep a pain and activity diary. These demonstrate days of intense physical activity (gardening, washing the car) followed by days of reduced activity (lying in bed, watching television) with an increase in medication consumption. Over time Mr A. has gradually reduced his activities. (A graphic representation of his physical performance is similar to that given in Fig. 11.4.2, p. 277)

He was asked to write down a list of tasks he wanted to achieve. As a keen gardener many of these were related to the return to this hobby. He then assigned levels of difficulty to each of a series of gardening-related tasks according to the degree to which they might be expected to increase his pain. All were perceived as pain-provoking to a different degree. The tasks ranged from planting seed/thinning plants in trays at a bench (low risk); weeding and hoeing (moderate risk) to digging (high risk).

He then assigned times, including rest periods, to each of the tasks that he thought he could comfortably perform. Low-risk activities were allowed 15 minutes of activity followed by a series of stretching exercises then 5 minutes of relaxing in a chair. Moderate-risk activities were assigned 10 minutes with stretching and 10 minutes of resting. Since he has a tendency to become engrossed in his hobby (and not notice the passage of time) he planned to use a kitchen timer to help regulate rest and activity periods. He also limited the length of time he would engage in gardening (initially for an hour) before he took a prolonged break or went for a gentle walk. The high-risk activities were not initially included in the plan but were to be introduced as he gained control of pacing his activity and improved his physical endurance.

Case study 11.4.3

'Mr B.'

Mr B. has chronic low back pain. He reports a considerable degree of disability and has recently taken to using a wheelchair when travelling out of the house. He has become unemployed because he felt his job as a delivery van driver and lifting boxes of cleaning fluids was injuring his back (since he always had increased pain at the end of a day at work). Gradually he found it difficult to perform his hobbies of playing darts and pool so he stopped and thus restricted his social activities. As his usual physical activities have become increasingly difficult (because they increase his pain), he has reduced his overall activity level and now spends more time reclining in bed or on the settee to reduce the exercise-associated pain. His wife helps him to dress each morning. He is now very fearful that any activity will increase his pain and is extremely reluctant to perform physical activities and uses a wheelchair if he needs to walk more than 50 metres.

Although Mr B. is now very physically disabled, he is not yet suitable for a comprehensive pain management

continued ...

programme since he requires help in dressing and spends long periods reclining. Following negotiation with the physiotherapist he has identified a programme to be performed at home with targets to be reached. These can be seen in his plan (Appendix 11.4.1).

His targets were reviewed weekly with the physiotherapist and new goals set. In addition to the exercise plan he aims to reduce the amount of time he spends reclining each day. Currently he spends most of the day reclining on a settee or on the bed. He has agreed to stop reclining on his bed, to restrict each period of reclining on the settee to 30 minutes maximum with immediate effect and gradually to increase his sitting tolerance. He will intersperse the planned restriction of 'downtime' with 'pottering' around the house, and eventually increase his walking distance in his garden. His aim is to eliminate reclining within 2 months and increase sitting tolerance to 1 hour within the same time frame.

In a plan developed in discussion with his wife, he aims eventually to dress himself every day, beginning with having help dressing his lower body only, progressing to having help only with his shoes and socks within 1 month, and be fully independent within 2 months. If he achieves these goals within the agreed time frame he will then be reviewed for possible inclusion on a full pain management programme.

Long-term goals

1 To become independent with dressing – to dress self every day within 2 months
2 To increase sitting tolerance to 1 hour within 2 months
3 To increase walking tolerance
4 To eliminate reclining within 2 months
5 To carry out a regular exercise programme to increase fitness in preparation to attend a PMP.

Present difficulties

1 Poor fitness/flexibility
2 Reliant upon wife for help
3 Poor fitness and tolerance for sitting
4 Poor fitness and tolerance for walking
5 Poor sitting/walking tolerance/reduced fitness.

Key points

- **Systematic assessment**
- **Re-education where necessary**
- **Problem analysis**
- **Phased re-introduction of increased level and range of function**
- **Positive reinforcement of progress**
- **Inclusion where possible of significant others.**

References

Bandura A 1977 Self-efficacy: towards a unifying theory of behavioral change. Psychological Review 84:191–215

Bengtsson A, Backman E, Lindblom B et al 1994 Long term follow-up of fibromyalgia patients: clinical symptoms, muscular function, laboratory tests: an eight year comparison study. Journal of Musculoskeletal Pain 2:67–80

Bennett R M 1996 Multidisciplinary group treatment programmes to treat fibromyalgia patients. Rheumatic Diseases Clinics of North America 22(2):351–367

Bennett R M, Clarke S R, Goldberg L et al 1989 Aerobic fitness in patients with fibrositis. A controlled study of respiratory gas exchange and ^{133}xenon clearance from exercising muscle. Arthritis and Rheumatism 32(10):1113–1116

Bennett R M, Burkhardt C S, Clarke S R et al 1996 Group treatment of fibromyalgia: a 6 month outpatient programme. Journal of Rheumatology 23:521–528

Bucklew S P, Parker J C, Keefe F J et al 1994 Self efficacy and pain behavior among subjects with fibromyalgia. Pain 59:377–384

Burkhardt C S, Mannerkorpi K, Hedenberg L et al 1994 A randomised, controlled trial of education and physical training for women with fibromyalgia. Journal of Rheumatology 21:714–720

Corderre J T, Katz J, Vaccarino A I et al 1993 Contribution of central neuroplasticity to pathological pain: review of clinical and experimental evidence. Pain 52:259–285

Crombez G, Eccleston C, Vlaeyen J et al 2002 Exposure to physical movements in low back pain patients: restricted effects of generalisation. Health Psychology 21:573–578

Donovan M R, Andrew G 1987 Plasma beta endorphin immunoreaction during graded cycle ergometry. Sports Medicine 17:358–362

Droste C, Greenlee M, Schreck M et al 1991 Experiments in pain thresholds and plasma beta endorphin levels during exercise. Medical Science and Sports Exercise 23:334–345

Fordyce W E 1976 Behavioural methods for chronic pain and illness. C V Mosby, St Louis

Garrett W E Jr 1996 Muscle strain injuries. American Journal of Sports Medicine 24(suppl):S2–S8

Gil K M, Ross S L, Keefe F J 1988 Behavioural treatment of chronic pain: four pain management protocols. In: France R D, Krishnan K R R (eds) Chronic pain. American Psychiatric Press, Washington, DC, pp 317–413

Goubert L, Francken G, Crombez G et al 2002 Exposure to physical movement in chronic back pain patients: no evidence for generalisation across different movements. Behav. Res. And Ther. 40:415–429

Gurevich M, Kohn P, Davies C 1994 Exercise induced analgesia and the role of reactivity in pain sensitivity. Journal of Sports Medicine 12:549–552

Haldorsen E M H, Kronholm K, Skounen J S et al 1998 Multimodal cognitive behavioural treatment of patients sicklisted for musculoskeletal pain: a randomised controlled study. Scandinavian Journal of Rheumatology 27:16–25

Henriksson K G, Mense S 1994 Pain and nociception in fibromyalgia. Pain Reviews 1(4):245–260

Hutton R S, Atwater S W 1992 Acute and chronic adaptations of muscle proprioceptors in response to increased use. Sports Medicine 14(6):406–421

Jacobsen S, Wildshiodtz G, Danneskiold-Samsoe B 1991 Isokinetic and isometric muscle strength Rheumatology 18(9):1390–1393

Keefe F, Block A 1982 Development of an observational method for assessing pain behavior in chronic pain patients. Behavioral Therapy 13:363–375

Keefe F J, Beaupre P M, Gil K M 1996 Group therapy for patients with chronic pain. In: Gatchel R J, Turk D C (eds) Psychological approaches to pain management. Guilford, New York, pp 259–282

Locke E A 1967 Towards a theory of task motivation incentives. Organisational Behavior and Human Performance 3:157–189

Loeser J D, Fordyce W E 1983 Chronic pain. In: Carr J E, Dengerink H A (eds) Behavioral science in the practice of medicine. Elsevier, New York, pp 341–346

McCain G A, Bell D A, Mai F M et al 1988 A controlled study of the effects of a supervised cardiovascular fitness training program on the manifestations of primary fibromyalgia. Arthritis and Rheumatism 31:1535–1542

Magnusson S P 1998 Passive properties of human skeletal muscle during stretch maneuvers. A review. Scandanavian Journal of Medicine and Science in Sports 8(2):65–77

Martin L, Nutting A, Macintosh B R et al 1996 An exercise program in the treatment of fibromyalgia. Journal of Rheumatology 23(6):1050–1053

Mense S 1994 Referral of muscle pain: new aspects. American Pain Society Journal 3(1):1–9

North T C, McCullagh P, Tran Z V 1990 Effect of exercise on depression. Exercise and Sports Science Review 18:379–383

Olsen J, Svendsen B 1992 Medical exercise therapy: an adjunct to orthopaedic manual therapy. Orthopaedic Practitioner 4:7–11

Vlaeyen J W, de Jong J, Geilen M et al 2001 Graded exposure in vivo in the treatment of pain-related fear: a replicated single-case experimental design in four patients with chronic low back pain. Behavior Research and Therapy 39:151–166

Waddell G 1998 The back pain revolution. Churchill Livingstone, Edinburgh

Waddell G, Newton M, Henderson I et al 1993 Fear-Avoidance Beliefs Questionnaire (FABQ) and the role of fear-avoidance beliefs in chronic low back pain and disability. Pain 52:157–168

Watson P J, Poulter M E 1997 The development of a functional task-oriented measure of pain behaviour in low back pain. Journal of Back and Musculoskeletal Rehabilitation 9:57–59

Watson P J, Booker C K, Main C J 1997 Evidence for the role of psychological factors in abnormal paraspinal activity in patients with chronic low back pain. Journal of Musculoskeletal Pain 5(4):41–55

Wigers S H, Stiles T C, Vogel P A 1996 Effects of aerobic exercise versus stress management treatment in fibromyalgia: a 4.5 year prospective study. Scandinavian Journal of Rheumatology 25:77–86

APPENDIX 11.4.1

Goal-setting charts and exercise programme for Mr B. (Case Study 11.4.3)

Goal setting
Goal 1
Long-term goal

To dress independently within 2 months.

Short-term goal

To begin having help with dressing of lower half only. To progress to having help with shoes and socks only within 1 month.

Plan

Key:
L = help with lower half only
S = help with shoes and socks only
S_1 = help with shoes and socks, one foot only
I = fully independent with dressing

Week one

Mon.	Tue.	Wed.	Thurs.	Fri.	Sat.	Sun.
L	(full help)	L	L	(full help)	L	L

Week two

Mon.	Tue.	Wed.	Thurs.	Fri.	Sat.	Sun.
L	(full help)	L	L	(full help)	L	S

Week three

Mon.	Tue.	Wed.	Thurs.	Fri.	Sat.	Sun.
L	S	L	S	S	L	S

Week four

Mon.	Tue.	Wed.	Thurs.	Fri.	Sat.	Sun.
L	S	L	S	S	S	S

Week five

Mon.	Tue.	Wed.	Thurs.	Fri.	Sat.	Sun.
S_1	S	S_1	S_1	S	S_1	S_1

Week six

Mon.	Tue.	Wed.	Thurs.	Fri.	Sat.	Sun.
S_1	S	S_1	S_1	S_1	S_1	S_1

Week seven

Mon.	Tue.	Wed.	Thurs.	Fri.	Sat.	Sun.
I	S_1	I	I	S_1	I	I

Week eight

Mon.	Tue.	Wed.	Thurs.	Fri.	Sat.	Sun.
I	S_1	I	I	I	I	I

Goal 2

Long-term goal

To increase sitting tolerance to 1 hour within 2 months.

- Mr B. must work out his present *baseline* for sitting—that is, how long he can sit for at the moment without overdoing it. Some patients work this out by taking their average ability of the specific activity over several days.
- He must then decide upon the *pacing interval*— that is, exactly how he intends to increase his sitting tolerance in order that sitting can be built up gradually in a paced manner. Making a written plan and recording progress in a chart is helpful

(see below). He should set daily targets for 1 week at a time, recording this in the 'G' column, and make a note of his achievement in the 'A' column.

- At the end of each week he should evaluate his progress. If there is difficulty reaching the set daily targets, the pacing interval may need to be reduced. If daily targets are easily achieved the rate of pacing may be increased.

Goal: to increase sitting tolerance

G = the daily target (min)
A = a record of what is actually achieved (min)

Week one

Goal	Baseline (min)	Pacing interval	Mon.		Tues.		Wed.		Thurs.		Fri.		Sat.		Sun.	
			G	A	G	A	G	A	G	A	G	A	G	A	G	A
Increase sitting tolerance	7	1 min each day	7		8		9		10		11		12		13	

Week two

Mon.		Tues.		Wed.		Thurs.		Fri.		Sat.		Sun.	
G	A	G	A	G	A	G	A	G	A	G	A	G	A
14		15		16		17		18		19		20	

Week three

Mon.		Tues.		Wed.		Thurs.		Fri.		Sat.		Sun.	
G	A	G	A	G	A	G	A	G	A	G	A	G	A
21		22		23		24		25		26		27	

Week four

Mon.		Tues.		Wed.		Thurs.		Fri.		Sat.		Sun.	
G	A	G	A	G	A	G	A	G	A	G	A	G	A
28		29		30		31		32		33		34	

Week five

Mon.		Tues.		Wed.		Thurs.		Fri.		Sat.		Sun.	
G	A	G	A	G	A	G	A	G	A	G	A	G	A
35		36		37		38		39		40		41	

Week six

Mon.		Tues.		Wed.		Thurs.		Fri.		Sat.		Sun.	
G	A	G	A	G	A	G	A	G	A	G	A	G	A
42		43		44		45		46		47		48	

Week seven

Mon.		Tues.		Wed.		Thurs.		Fri.		Sat.		Sun.	
G	A	G	A	G	A	G	A	G	A	G	A	G	A
49		50		51		52		53		54		55	

Week eight

Mon.		Tues.		Wed.		Thurs.		Fri.		Sat.		Sun.	
G	A	G	A	G	A	G	A	G	A	G	A	G	A
56		57		58		59		60		61		62	

Goal 3

Long-term goal

To increase walking tolerance.

As for goal 2, Mr B. must establish his *baseline* for walking tolerance, decide upon the *pacing interval* and gradually increase his walking tolerance in a paced manner. (Week one only is illustrated.)

G = the daily target (min)
A = a record of what is actually achieved (min)

Week one

Goal	Baseline (min)	Pacing interval	Mon.		Tues.		Wed.		Thurs.		Fri.		Sat.		Sun.	
			G	A	G	A	G	A	G	A	G	A	G	A	G	A
Increase walking tolerance	4	1 min every other day	4		4		5		5		6		6		7	

Goal 4

Long-term goal

To eliminate reclining within 2 months.

Short-term goal

To restrict each period of reclining on the settee to 30 min interspersed with walking and sitting.

Mr B. may set himself a plan to gradually reduce the amount of time he spends reclining. He may record his plan in a chart; an example of such a chart is illustrated below. Each time he reclines during the day he should not do so for longer than his planned time limit for that day. (Weeks one and two only are illustrated; G and A as before.)

Week one

Goal	Baseline (min)	Pacing interval	Mon.		Tues.		Wed.		Thurs.		Fri.		Sat.		Sun.	
			G	A	G	A	G	A	G	A	G	A	G	A	G	A
To eliminate reclining	30	Reduce by 1 min each day	30		29		28		27		26		25		24	

Week two

Mon.		Tues.		Wed.		Thurs.		Fri.		Sat.		Sun.	
G	A	G	A	G	A	G	A	G	A	G	A	G	A
23		22		21		20		19		18		17	

Exercise programme

To improve flexibility and fitness slowly, increase confidence with feared movements and ultimately help in the achievement of specific activity-related goals, a structured exercise programme is followed.

Daily stretching exercise programme

Patients are taught a stretching programme and given written instructions in order that they may continue the exercises at home. Patients must take responsibility for carrying out and progressing their own exercises at home. Their progress is reviewed by the physiotherapist, usually at weekly intervals.

Instructions

Think of three 'Ss' when carrying out the stretching exercises: *Slow, Sustained* and *Steady.*

- Move slowly into the stretching position.
- Sustain (hold) the stretch beginning with a slow count of 5 seconds.
- Steadily release the stretch and return to the start position.
- Repeat each stretch twice only.
- Progress by gradually increasing the length of hold for each stretch up to a maximum of 20 seconds.
- Set your targets at the beginning of each week for the length of hold and record your achievements each day. An example of a record chart is shown below.
- Carry out a gentle warm-up before the stretches as already shown.

Daily stretching exercise schedule

In this example Mr. B. has decided to increase the length of hold by 1 second every other day. A selection of exercises is chosen in consultation with the physiotherapist. Full instructions for each exercise can be found in the stretching exercise patient booklet that is provided. (Week one only is illustrated.)

G = daily target for the stretching programme; this refers to the length of time in seconds each stretch is held

A = record of achievements

Week One

Exercise	Mon.		Tues.		Wed.		Thurs.		Fri.		Sat.		Sun.	
	G	A	G	A	G	A	G	A	G	A	G	A	G	A
Side bend	5		5		6		6		7		7		8	
Arching	5		5		6		6		7		7		8	
Rotation	5		5		6		6		7		7		8	
Knee to chest	5		5		6		6		7		7		8	
Hamstrings	5		5		6		6		7		7		8	
The cat	5		5		6		6		7		7		8	
Knee rolling	5		5		6		6		7		7		8	
Thigh stretch	5		5		6		6		7		7		8	

Strengthening exercise programme

Strengthening exercise may be incorporated into Mr B.'s rehabilitation programme. This may be best introduced at around the third week. At this stage Mr B. will be familiar with the stretching programme and his confidence with exercise may have started to increase. A strengthening exercise programme is selected in joint consultation between Mr B. and the physiotherapist.

- Set your initial exercise baseline (i.e. the number of repetitions you feel you can achieve without overdoing it). It is important to set your initial quota at an easily achievable level to help you gain confidence and reduce fear of injury. Five repetitions is usually a reasonable starting point for most people. Initially set your daily target each day before beginning your strengthening programme. Then after the first week set your daily targets for the week ahead. It is important to follow your exercise programme according to your set plan and not according to pain levels.
- For some exercises it is beneficial to hold for a count of 5 seconds. This is indicated as (H) in the

exercise chart. For these exercises it is not necessary to increase the length of hold.

- Progress by increasing the number of repetitions you do up to a maximum of 15 repetitions. You may choose to progress the various exercises at different rates depending upon the fitness of specific areas of your body.

Strengthening exercise schedule

G = daily target for the strengthening exercises; this refers to the planned number of repetitions

A = record of achievements

H = hold this exercise for 5 seconds only

Exercise	Mon.		Tues.		Wed.		Thurs.		Fri.		Sat.		Sun.	
Name	G	A	G	A	G	A	G	A	G	A	G	A	G	A
Pelvic tilt (lying) (H)	5													
Head arms by side, lift (H)	5													
Diagonals	5													
Leg straightening	5													
Wall slide	5													
Leg lifting (lying)	5													
Opposites all fours	5													

Part 5 **Psychological component**

PART CONTENTS

Introduction

The importance of specific psychological interventions as facets of pain management has been addressed specifically in Chapter 10 where a detailed appraisal of commonly used psychological techniques was presented. Such techniques are often delivered on a one-to-one basis. However, psychological issues form a major part of interdisciplinary pain management programmes. In this chapter a number of additional issues are relevant in the delivery of tertiary pain management programmes. These are shown in Box 11.5.1.

Without doubt the psychological input is a key component of the PMP. In addition to clarifying the patients' understanding of the psychology of pain and coaching in the development of positive, adaptive pain coping strategies, there needs to be a major focus also on tackling psychological obstacles to reactivation and improved function. Even the simplest of exercise programmes for chronic pain patients can meet with resistance, which necessitates addressing the patient's concerns.

Although a number of such concerns will have become apparent at the time of initial assessment and negotiation of treatment objectives, it is not uncommon

Box 11.5.1

Focus of psychological intervention

Enhancing overall participation in programme
- Contextualising emotion and reintroducing the biopsychosocial context of pain and disabilty
- Understanding the stress–pain interface.

Teaching basic management of emotions, cognition and pain behaviour
- Defusing anger, hostility and resentment using cognitive reappraisal
- Training in stress reduction techniques
- Cognitive restructuring
- Changing behaviour using problem-solving techniques.

Tackling interpersonal relationships
- Assertiveness and communication
- The use of role-play as a vehicle for learning about interpersonal behaviour
- Engaging partners.

for the extent of such concerns to become apparent only when the patient is actually confronted with the necessity of behavioural change.

Enhancing overall participation in programme

It can be difficult initially to engage some patients in a PMP. It is important to recognise obstacles to engagement and attempt to deal with them as soon as possible.

Defusing anger, hostility and resentment using cognitive reappraisal

It is not uncommon for patients to express anger during the assessment process. The assessment team will have begun the task of addressing the issues that have given rise to such emotions. However, it is unlikely that all of the issues will have been addressed by the time the patient enters the programme. Keefe et al (1996) identify dealing with anger and high levels of emotional distress as one of the most common and important problems encountered when running a group programme. Often much of patients' anger is directed either at their previous treatment (and clinical advisors) or at the benefit or legal system. Such emotions can be extremely destructive, functioning as a sort of 'red mist' hindering patients' emotional adjustment and preventing a clear focus on the rehabilitation process.

It is important, therefore, to hold a session specifically aimed at defusing these destructive emotions early in the PMP, and thus help to reduce the chance of their re-emergence later on. The doctor will have attempted to provide an explanation to the patients. However, psychologists will need (in their session) to allow patients to discuss any feelings of anger, hostility or resentment about previous consultations and previous treatments and their general experience within the health-care system. These emotions may also be directed towards the legal system, benefits agencies, employers and relatives.

It is sometimes helpful to begin with depiction of some of the more common causes of anger, hostility and resentment, as shown in Table 11.5.1. This allows the patients an opportunity to begin to identify their own emotions and the cognitions which may underlie them. This process may generate a significant emotional response from the group. Group skills in handling these emotions are essential, and the inability to provide

straightforward answers should be acknowledged rather than covered up. Patients often cope better with 'don't knows'. It is essential that the team members communicate well. Truthful and *consistent* answers must be given by each team member. In addition, specific questions may be raised in this session that will need to be addressed by doctors at their next session, or if necessary before the start of the next session. (The issue of competence in group therapy is addressed in Part 6 of this chapter.)

Despite early clarification and attempted 'defusing' it is not uncommon for these issues to resurface from time to time later in the programme. However, repeated focusing on the anger surrounding previous treatments or assessments can be destructive for both the individual and the group. Regular meetings of the team will enable a consistent stance to be taken. Expression of strong doubts in response to answers to medical queries may in some cases be indicative of resentment of the overall management approach and may only be solved by individual sessions.

Table 11.5.1 Common causes of anger, hostility and resentment in chronic pain patients

Agent (object of anger)	Action (reason for anger)
Causal agent of injury/illness	Chronic pain
Medical health-care providers	Diagnostic ambiguity; treatment failure
Mental health professionals	Implications of psychogenicity or psychopathology
Attorneys and legal system	Adversarial dispute, scrutiny and arbitration
Insurance companies; social security system	Inadequate monetary coverage or compensation
Employer	Cessation of employment; job transfer; job retraining
Significant others	Lack of interpersonal support
God	'Predetermined' injury and consequences; ill fate
Self	Disablement; disfigurement
The whole world	Alienation

From Fernandez & Turk (1995), reproduced with permission

Using emotion to reintroduce the biopsychosocial context of pain and disability

At the beginning of the PMP most if not all patients will still subscribe implicitly, if not explicitly, to the medical model of assessment and treatment of their pain problem. Despite careful counselling by the assessment team they may believe that their pain is a symptom of underlying injury or disease that needs to be diagnosed and then treated by doctors. It is important to move the patient away from this model. The patients must be presented with an alternative model of pain, which acknowledges their suffering and explains continuing pain without ongoing disease or damage. The *usual* consequences of chronic pain should be outlined and the patients helped to understand the biopsychosocial model of chronic pain. It is also important that from the start of a programme patients feel that the team understands their problems. It is worth revisiting and discussing the patient traps presented in the opening session as a way to begin to gain patients' confidence; in addition it can help to form common bonds between group members and also provides a useful introduction to a biopsychosocial model of pain.

Describing the development of chronic pain and the biopsychosocial model

The development of chronic pain and disability should be described, with the focus on it being a developing process in which different factors play a significant role at different points in time (as discussed above in Ch. 9). The patients should come to understand that, whether pain onset is insidious or traumatic, a sequence of events is set up that can lead to unhelpful treatment, job loss, immobility, negative emotions and the inability to cope. Patients should realise that some of these factors, such as failed surgery, may not be within their control but that others, such as family relationships, may very well be.

As patients recognise their own history in the description of the development of chronic pain and disability the clinician can then challenge their causal attribution of single, identifiable and treatable somatic factors for their pain. Patients must come to understand that there is no simple treatment which will 'cure' their pain. Understanding of the multiple factors involved in the development of pain and disability should then lead the patient on to the understanding that treatment also has to involve multiple factors.

Developing an understanding of the stress–pain interface

The ability to cope with chronic pain in daily life can be reframed as the ability to cope with stress. Pain and the problems it can lead to (e.g. work loss leading to financial difficulties) are major stressors. Many patients will also have other non-pain-related stressors in their lives. In order to develop effective stress management techniques the patient first needs a basic understanding of the psychophysiological stress reaction and its influence on cognitive, emotional and behavioural functioning.

The use of stress 'experiments'

To demonstrate psychophysiological arousal and its consequences, patients can be put through a stressful event that provokes physical, mental and behavioural reactions strong enough for them to be able to describe their experience. Development of simple role-plays or presentation of video clips of mild–moderate stressful situations from everyday life can be used. Alternatively, this can be developed in the group by introducing a relaxation exercise with a built-in anticipated stressor such as a performance task. This task, introduced in such a fashion during the initial stages of pain management, is enough in some cases to provoke quite a strong stress reaction. For illustrative purposes it may be advisable initially to select non-pain situations in order to demonstrate the nature of stress responses.

It is, however, extremely important that the psychologist leading such 'experiments' should be familiar with such methods and be prepared to deal with the possibility of having to debrief some patients and rebuild constructive group participation. These potentially powerful experiential techniques can stimulate in-depth discussion of stress responses, which are usually very familiar to the patient but so far have often been unexplained.

Explaining the stress response – the 'fight or flight' reaction

One very useful method to explain the stress response is by describing it in terms of the 'fight or flight' response. This includes giving the patient a basic understanding of sympathetic and parasympathetic nervous systems and the roles that they play in this response. Individual differences in reactions will need to be explained carefully along with the effect that stress can have on coping mechanisms. Knowledge and understanding will in itself alleviate some of the patients' worries and enable them to put symptoms within a more appropriate context. It will also increase their awareness of their own personal responses to perceived stressors. Using this approach, patients are given the opportunity to understand their symptomatology fully with regard not only to the physical but also the mental and behavioural consequences.

The ABC of stress

Knowledge and understanding of stress are the basis of being able to implement changes and progress to more appropriate coping styles. A major goal of pain management lies in the ability to change unhelpful or negative thinking (cognitive restructuring). In order to achieve this patients are best helped by making use of the ABC of stress (Antecedents, Beliefs, Consequences; these may be emotional or behavioural). This simplified model of understanding the role of unhelpful cognitions and the effect they can have on emotions and behaviour gives patients a first insight into the effects of stress and allows them to start self-monitoring. Distorted or negative thinking patterns are then open to appraisal and change.

Ellis's (1962) simplified therapeutic technique has several advantages. It matches patients' daily experience and is easy to understand. It provides a tangible skill to change a patient's appraisal of a stressful event and consequently the emotional and behavioural responses. An example of the technique is shown in Box 11.5.2.

The dangers are that the complexity of the problem is often underestimated and implementation into daily life often takes persistent application and the ability not to be demoralised by making mistakes.

Once patients have developed the ability to identify the ABCs they can then move on to the final stage, which is disputing or challenging their beliefs.

Box 11.5.2

Example illustrating the ABC of stress

A Patient doing some gardening experiences an increase in pain

B Patient believes that the back has been harmed, thinks 'I can't cope with this pain, I'm useless, I'll never be able to get back to doing the things I used to do'

C Patient rests, takes painkillers, feels depressed.

Training in stress reduction techniques

Relaxation has been demonstrated to be a valuable technique in pain management. It gives patients a skill that in many cases can quickly lead to significant benefits and also gives them an immediate sense of control. The importance of the latter cannot be stressed too strongly as frequently those attending such groups will, at the outset, feel that they have no techniques at all with which to manage their pain problem effectively. However, it is important to recognise that it is only one of a number of techniques and forms only part of the treatment approach to chronic pain.

There are a number of different relaxation techniques available (Bernstein & Borkovec 1973, Jacobson 1974) and some patients may have previous experience with some of these. It is therefore important to start with a careful assessment of patients' previous experience and any problems that they may have encountered. Any worries, misconceptions or unrealistic expectations need to be addressed. (Details of the specific relaxation techniques follow.) The deep relaxation methods, relaxed imagery, autogenic relaxation and progressive muscular relaxation are usually done during a period of time set aside for relaxation. The brief methods (diaphragmatic breathing and modified progressive muscle relaxation) are often done during the day when patients feel themselves becoming tense. To be truly successful, relaxation should be a skill the patient can call upon during everyday activities and not simply something that is done in a darkened room.

Ideally, relaxation is best taught from start to finish by the same clinician to allow careful monitoring of progress and for the personal preferences of patients to be integrated as far as is possible.

The impact of relaxation should not be underestimated. It has been shown that unresolved psychological traumas may surface during relaxation. Such problems need to be dealt with efficiently and speedily by the psychologist.

Diaphragmatic breathing

One relaxation technique that can be easily demonstrated, learned and applied in almost all daily life situations is diaphragmatic breathing. This method may be the technique of choice for some patients and it is advisable to start relaxation sessions with this technique. Commonly, most patients will have some initial difficulties but with repeated practice they can develop the skill quite quickly.

Box 11.5.3

General guidelines for teaching relaxation exercises

- Address posture and find a comfortable position
- Begin with abdominal breathing
- Wear loose comfortable clothing
- Importance of scheduling, space and time (aim to be undisturbed for 30 min)
- Anticipate 'unsuccessful' sessions and don't lose confidence or become disheartened
- Develop a relaxed *approach* rather then simply applying a technique.

Often the realisation that they have been using chest or shoulder breathing can be an eye-opener for patients and the majority of patients are often unaware of the relationship between poor breathing and psychophysiological arousal.

Progressive muscle relaxation

The overall goal of progressive muscular relaxation (PMR) is to enable patients to become aware of muscle tension and to have the ability to produce muscle relaxation in different muscle groups in daily life. In PMR, tensing and relaxing of the muscles are used to achieve an increase in muscle relaxation. All muscle groups in the body that are amenable to voluntary relaxation are systematically relaxed. The general rule is that the first step consists of tensing a muscle for approximately 5 to 7 seconds, and the second step of trying to relax the same muscle for at least 25 seconds. There is evidence that relaxation can be effective in managing pain in those individuals who can master the technique (NIHTA 1996) although some have pointed out that relaxation is rarely used in isolation from other cognitive techniques, so it is difficult to evaluate the effect (Arena & Blanchard 2002).

Concentration on tensing and relaxing is important because it will both enhance the effect and at the same time help to decrease unwanted intrusive thoughts and images. It is not necessary to tense muscles completely. Two-thirds of the possible muscle tension is sufficient. The purpose of getting patients to first tense their muscles is to raise awareness of the difference between a tense and a relaxed muscle. General guidelines for teaching relaxation exercises are shown in Box 11.5.3.

Although relaxation training is best done lying down it is also possible to carry out the exercises in a sitting position if lying down proves too difficult. Patients may use a towel or a pillow under their head, lower back and knees if desired. Ideally start off with a few minutes of abdominal breathing. Loose comfortable clothing should be worn. When practising at home patients should schedule relaxation into their daily routine. They will need to find time and physical space where they are able to be undisturbed for approximately 30 minutes. If difficulties are experienced with learning to relax it is important to encourage the patient to continue, as most difficulties are of a short-term nature. Patients should also be made aware that relaxation may not work every day and that forcing it through may have detrimental effects on motivation and self-efficacy. It is important to develop a relaxed approach rather than simply applying a technique.

Initially the patient should start off with full PMR. Once this has been sufficiently mastered the patient should progress to combining muscle groups. One of the advantages of this is that relaxation can be applied in a shorter period of time with the same effect. Following this, patients can then progress to the use of relaxation without tensing.

As much time as individuals need should be allowed for them to reach this position, although with regular practice 4–6 weeks should be sufficient. At this stage the patient omits tensing muscle groups and instead simply concentrates on the different muscle groups without tensing and simply concentrating on the feeling of relaxation.

Use of imagery techniques

Once patients have mastered diaphragmatic breathing and PMR, and have shown good insight into the application of these techniques within pain management, it is possible to enhance the effect of relaxation by introducing techniques such as guided imagery and visualisation. Such techniques take the process of relaxation a step further by introducing elements of hypnotherapeutic interventions, which can be used effectively in pain management. These can improve the quality of the relaxation experience, increasing perceived self-control and self-efficacy. Such methods can be introduced by explaining that they are techniques aimed at enhancing mental relaxation. It is advisable that such techniques are initially practised on their own and then combined with the physical relaxation methods.

Applying relaxation in daily life

It is important that patients get into the habit of using relaxation as part of their everyday routine. Patients

Box 11.5.4

Ways of implementing relaxation skills

- *Normal relaxation.* This is just practising relaxation for 15 to 30 minutes, at least once a day. As far as possible this should be kept up despite difficulties although if other stressors make this very difficult then a short break is acceptable
- *Brief relaxation.* This means a relaxation of about 5 to 10 minutes during the day when activities are deliberately stopped. This can be done in almost any position, sitting or standing, and it should be done several times a day in real life
- *Mini relaxation.* This is relaxing for anything from a few seconds to a few minutes and should be done as often as possible. It will help to make relaxation a habitual skill in almost any situation. Patients should be encouraged to identify particular 'trouble spots' for muscular tension and to focus particularly on these areas.

N.B. Such techniques should be used only when it is safe to do so.

Box 11.5.5

Common difficulties in mastering relaxation

- Initial self-consciousness
- Experience of pain when tensing a muscle
- Lack of initial response
- Complaint of lack of time in which to practise relaxation
- Unrealistic expectations of therapeutic benefit
- Confusion between deep relaxation and sleep
- Problems with imagery techniques.

can be advised to practice in the following ways. Some alternative strategies are outlined in Box 11.5.4.

Common difficulties encountered in mastering relaxation skills

Some problems which may be encountered with teaching relaxation are shown in Box 11.5.5.

Initial self-consciousness

Initially patients may feel self-conscious or embarrassed when practising exercises as a group. This should be acknowledged before the start of teaching and a certain amount of embarrassed 'giggling' expected.

Experience of pain when tensing a muscle

When practising PMR some patients may experience pain when tensing a muscle. When this occurs it may be because too much tension is being applied or the muscle is already on a high level of tension and any slight increase will cause pain or muscle spasm. As relaxation skills improve, these problems should subside. If,

however, pain persists then focusing on the tensing without actually tensing the muscle may be used.

Lack of initial response

A frequent complaint of patients is that after practising for two or three sessions they declare that 'the exercises don't work'. The importance of regular practice should be stressed; it can be useful here to use the analogy of learning to drive. Just as you don't expect to be able to go out and drive on a motorway in the rush hour after two or three driving lessons so you cannot expect to master relaxation after a short period of time.

Complaint of lack of time in which to practise relaxation

Patients may complain of lack of time in which to practise relaxation; such problems need to be discussed in detail and often a problem-solving approach to time management is helpful. However, there are instances where personal difficulties and family issues may need to be addressed. Lack of assertiveness may also be responsible. Generally speaking, patients will need to address the issue of practising skills as part of the overall changes they are making to their lifestyle if they want to manage their pain successfully.

Unrealistic expectations of therapeutic benefit

Some patients may have the unrealistic expectation that religiously practising relaxation will automatically lead to success (i.e. pain relief and control of pain-related problems). Such beliefs need to be tackled at the outset, and relaxation should be presented as one part of a series of techniques which will be used by them to manage their chronic pain problem.

Confusion between deep relaxation and sleep

There may be confusion between deep relaxation and sleep, and the difference between the two states should be explained. Those patients who find that they consistently fall asleep during relaxation (a problem that tends to occur when relaxation is practised at the end of the day) should be encouraged to practise at a time of day when they are less tired.

Problems with imagery techniques

Some patients can have problems with imagery techniques, particularly in the generation of images. One useful strategy is to ask them to spend a few minutes looking at a painting or picture and then shutting their eyes and trying to describe it to themselves.

Cognitive restructuring and chronic pain

A major goal of pain management is to teach patients to change unhelpful or negative thinking (cognitive restructuring). Patients need to learn to recognise that their thoughts about their pain and themselves can affect not only their levels of stress and mood state but also their behaviour.

Typical cognitive errors within chronic pain

Clinicians working with depressive or anxious patients have identified a number of typical cognitive errors such as 'all-or-nothing thinking' or 'expecting the worst to happen'. With regard to chronic pain patients there are a number of distorted and/or negative cognitions that need to be addressed.

The tendency of chronic pain patients to 'catastrophise' and the negative effect that this has on psychological functioning (particularly in its contribution to depressed mood) has been demonstrated by numerous studies. If this is pointed out, patients readily accept and acknowledge this difficulty. There may be erroneous expectations of decline, increased disability and insurmountable pain at some future time. Past medical treatment failures may well have enhanced such thoughts.

'All-or-nothing thinking' may be equally frequent as it represents patients' expectations within a medical model approach. Common thoughts include: 'Unless the pain can be cured nothing will be of any help' and 'Unless I can return to how I used to be or how I should be then nothing will be of benefit'.

Patients may hold a number of erroneous beliefs about their pain that affect their behaviour. For example the belief that 'hurt equals harm' is very commonly held by patients with chronic pain and can lead to reduction and avoidance of activities.

Identifying cognitive errors and incorporating them within stress and pain management

The ability to identify cognitive errors and the effect that these have on both the patients' emotional and behavioural responses should enable patients to be able to change dysfunctional cognitive coping styles in general. Based on other elements of the programme such as education about chronic pain, patients may be in a position to adopt a management approach on the basis of the biopsychosocial model rather than remaining on the treatment approach based on a medical model. This is particularly important for patients who perceive pain management as a further 'treatment' that is simply enhanced by a few helpful skills such as exercise and relaxation.

Patients may well vary in their initial abilities to identify their own cognitive errors. When teaching patients how to identify such errors it can be of value to start with case examples. Once patients have the ability to recognise the major types of errors made then they can proceed to identify their own errors in thinking and the effects that these have on both their emotional functioning and behaviour. Techniques that can be of value here are diary keeping, where patients record their activities, thoughts and mood, and asking patients to recall the types of thoughts that they have when having a flare-up or dealing with stressors.

Changing behaviour using problem-solving techniques

Use of 'paper patients', case studies or video material

Problem solving has been identified in many studies as a valuable approach and is a major treatment component in many pain management programmes. The aim of problem solving is to enable the patient to use effective coping strategies to deal with the problems identified.

Box 11.5.6

Stages in problem solving

1 Decide which problem to tackle
2 Describe and break down the problem into small parts
3 Pick one part to work on
4 Think of as many ways as possible of dealing with part identified
5 Evaluate how realistic each way is; look at both the positive and negative consequences for each way
6 Pick the method that you decide is the best
7 Plan how you are going to put this into action
8 Carry it out
9 Evaluate how successful you were.

Patients are best made familiar with the technique by presenting them with a 'case study' that demonstrates the most common problems that chronic pain patients develop. The advantage of using a hypothetical case study is that this is not perceived as threatening by the patients. It is often easier to 'solve' someone else's problems than one's own.

When working on such a case study, patients should work together in small groups. This adds another important dimension to the course. It builds mutual trust and enables patients to realise that discussing even personal issues within a group setting may prove to be beneficial.

Principles of problem solving

Having identified problems using a case study, patients should then be introduced to the stages of problem solving, as outlined in Box 11.5.6.

Application of problem solving

The first stages of problem solving (steps one to seven) should initially be practised using case examples as this will be less threatening to the patients. Patients may initially need considerable help with this, particularly in breaking problems down and in generating solutions. Hawton & Kirk (1989) suggest that one way to aid a patient to generate solutions is to use 'brainstorming', as many potential solutions as possible, no matter how unlikely they seem, are generated; the authors also suggest that if the therapist proposes solutions that are obviously inappropriate this can help to facilitate patients' involvement. Once patients feel comfortable with the method they can then generate their own problem lists and start working on their own solutions.

Tackling interpersonal relationships

From a passive or aggressive to an assertive style

Pain management skills are skills that patients need to apply in daily life both within their family and their working environment. In order to be successful, assertiveness and good communication are essential. Most patients will describe difficulties in these areas, as they have become passive and withdrawn or angry and disaffected. Feelings of guilt with regard to those close to them may also impair good communication.

It is important that patients learn to recognise the difference between expressing what we feel and think to others in an aggressive way, a passive way and an assertive way. Assertiveness should be stressed as one way in which patients can feel that they are more in control of situations and less helpless.

Sessions relating to these topics should be placed towards the end of a course. The group will need to develop a degree of trust between the members if these sessions are to be of value. The topic is best introduced as a further skill that will help to put pain management into practice, rather than as a personal deficit. Describing different styles such as the aggressive or passive communication style may give patients a good opportunity to discuss and assess their own difficulties in these areas.

Use of role-play as a vehicle for learning about interpersonal behaviour

Simple exercises such as 'repeated refusal' or 'repeated request' will provide a simple understandable start for role-plays. Initially patients may feel inhibited about participating in such role-plays. To overcome these initial difficulties only volunteers should be used and the clinician may need to function as a role model and to participate in the majority of role-plays. One way of practising role-play techniques is shown in Box 11.5.7.

Box 11.5.7

Use of role-playing techniques

- Explain each role and the situation in very concrete terms
- Split the group up and give the members observational tasks such as the non-verbal communication of participants
- Participants are allowed to feed back their experience first with particular emphasis on how they felt during the role play. Audience and clinician should then feed back after this
- Make sure that all difficulties that may have occurred are resolved.

Box 11.5.8

Key facets of sleep hygiene

- Avoid stimulants such as caffeine, smoking, alcohol and proprietary painkilling or cold remedies which contain stimulants, particularly late in the day
- Avoid excessive intake of liquid for some hours before sleep
- Timetable analgesic medication appropriately
- Stay in bed only when asleep and restrict the time in bed if not sleeping
- Get up and go to another room and read or perform routine tasks until feeling sleepy then return to bed
- Only use the bed for sleep (or physical intimacy).

Role-play should be aimed at giving the patient the opportunity to try out new or different behaviours in a supportive situation. Every role-play should conclude with a general discussion emphasising the points learned.

As the group increases in confidence the participants should be invited to contribute any particular situations that they would wish to role-play. Assertiveness practice can be usefully combined with problem-solving sessions as many solutions to problems will require assertiveness to put them into practice.

Sleep management

Poor sleep is a very common feature of chronic pain and is implicated in the development and maintenance of muscle tenderness (Moldofsky 2001, Wolfe 1996). Medication may help but is rarely sufficient as poor sleep is a consequence of a combination of factors. The field of sleep and sleep management is a sophisticated and developing field of research, a major review of which is beyond this textbook, but given the clinical impact of pain on sleep the subject will be addressed briefly.

Advice on sleep management and good sleep hygiene is important. In the context of pain management it can be seen as a specific application of a combination of relaxation techniques and specific behavioural intervention with the ultimate objective of facilitating normal physiological function. It seems reasonable therefore to discuss it in this section of the chapter.

The success of a sleep programme can be evaluated by the use of sleep diaries or standardised questionnaires (e.g. Pittsburgh Sleep Quality Index (Buysee et al 1989)).

Specific management of insomnia secondary to chronic pain using CBT alone has had some success

(Currie et al 2002, Currie et al 2000) although the improvements that have been reported have been criticised for not being clinically important (NIHTA 1996). However, those who improve their sleep demonstrate decreases in distress and pain-associated disability (Currie et al 2002). Sleep hygiene management involves making the patients aware of the habits they have which are not conducive to successful sleep and trying to change them (Buysee & Perlis 1996, Perlis et al 2001). The main techniques are summarised in Box 11.5.8.

Sleep hygiene and relaxation are combined for best effect, but patients must also be taught how to refrain from reacting to intrusive negative or worrying thoughts. In one experiment negative thoughts and rumination about pain and disability were associated with difficulty in getting to sleep (Smith et al 2001), whereas pain report was negatively correlated with the length of time from falling a sleep to reawakening.

In conclusion, although there have been no systematic evaluations of the contribution of a sleep hygiene programme as part of a comprehensive PMP, it would seem advisable to include sleep hygiene as part of the PMP.

Working with partners (or significant others)

The partner session

Partners' and family members' behaviour can exert a powerful influence on chronic pain patients' coping behaviour. Solicitous behaviour will reinforce maladaptive coping strategies as much as neglect or withdrawal by disaffected spouses (Chs 2 and 4). Partners and family members are not to blame as they are reacting in a way not dissimilar to patients; their often unhelpful responses are in most cases well meant and may be based on a poor understanding of the process of chronic pain. For example, spouses who believe that 'hurt equals harm' are likely to tell partners to avoid those activities that provoke pain and to advise them to adopt coping strategies such as increasing medication and resting.

Partners should ideally be present at the initial assessment. During the feedback given at the end of the assessment it needs to be made explicit that if a place is offered on a programme then partners are expected to become involved and, if the programme requires it, to attend for certain sessions. Only if patients and partners become aware of the seriousness of this part of the programme will they make an effort to participate.

For pain management to be applied successfully in daily life both partners and family members need to have an understanding of the approach. In addition, flare-ups and setbacks may be dealt with more efficiently and without resorting to use of health-care resources if this support is available from the partner. A partner session is therefore an important element in a comprehensive PMP.

Structure of partners' session

Ideally 2–3 hours should be set aside for this session. Partners are best seen by the team by themselves for up to 1 hour. This should preferably take place in the same setting as the main programme.

The time should be devoted to individual questions from the partners, who will by this time have formed some impressions of how the programme has affected their spouse. This part of the session also gives the team the opportunity to observe partners' understanding and commitment to pain management and to identify any potential problems with particular couples.

As a next step partners and patients should meet informally during a break and then meet with the whole team. A final discussion, facilitated by the team, should aim to start the process of making the expectations and the understanding of both patients and partners explicit and correcting any misconceptions.

How to get partners involved

One of the great challenges of the partners' session is how to get partners involved. In order to avoid passive reception (i.e. expecting an informative lecture from the clinicians) techniques that have been shown to be successful in other group work or group settings should be used.

One such technique may be to let partners answer a simple questionnaire regarding their expectations after the patient has participated in a pain management programme. This questionnaire must be filled in anonymously and should be returned to the clinical psychologist who will prepare and lead the session. In most cases questions will reveal unrealistic expectations and poor knowledge about the rationale of pain management. The answers may then be summarised and presented on a flip chart to both patients and partners. Patients will then be given an opportunity to comment on the expectations and hopefully correct the obvious errors. In most instances this will stimulate a discussion amongst patients and partners, although careful facilitation will be necessary.

Conclusion

The psychological component is a vital part of the PMP. It is not possible to run a cognitive–behavioural rehabilitation programme for chronic pain patients without focused psychological sessions. Many of the obstacles to progress that might initially appear to be physical or practical in nature may be underpinned in fact by significant psychological factors. By working in close collaboration with the physician and in particular the physiotherapist such obstacles may be more readily identified and addressed. There are specific psychological skills that patients will need to acquire if they are to be successful in maintaining their progress and continuing to improve when they have completed the programme. Finally, in addressing bruised or dysfunctional relationships, and in optimising therapeutic benefit from groups, specific psychological expertise is required.

Key points

- **Psychological input aims to educate, to teach positive skills for coping with pain and to address barriers to progress**
- **Issues of anger, hostility and resentment need to be addressed**
- **Relaxation techniques, identifying cognitive-thinking errors, problem solving and assertiveness training are all valuable techniques that**

(Continued)

need to be incorporated within the group programme
- **Involvement of partners can be of particular therapeutic benefit**

- **Specific psychological expertise is needed in order to maximise therapeutic benefit from groups.**

References

Arena J G, Blanchard E B 2002 Biofeedback and relaxation therapy for chronic pain disorders. In: Gatchel R, Turk D C (eds) Psychological approaches to pain management. Guilford Press, New York, pp 159–185

Bernstein D A, Borkovec T D 1973 Progressive relaxation training: a manual for the helping professions. Research Press, Champaign, IL

Buysee D J, Perlis M L 1996 The evaluation and treatment of insomnia. Journal of Psychology and Behavioural Health March:80–93

Buysee D, Reynolds C, Monk T et al 1989 The Pittsburgh Sleep Quality Index: a new instrument for psychiatric practice and research. Psychiatry Research 28:193–213

Currie S R, Wilson K G, Pontefract A J et al 2000 Cognitive-behavioral treatment of insomnia secondary to chronic pain. Journal of Consulting and Clinical Psychology 68:407–416

Currie S R, Wilson K G, Curran D 2002 Clinical significance and predictors of treatment response to cognitive-behavior therapy for insomnia secondary to chronic pain. Journal of Behavioral Medicine 25:135–153

Ellis A 1962 Reason and emotion in psychotherapy. Lyle Stuart, New York

Fernandez E, Turk D C 1995 The scope and significance of anger in the experience of chronic pain. Pain 61:65–175

Hawton K, Kirk J 1989 Problem solving. In: Hawton K, Salkovskis P M, Kirk J et al (eds) Cognitive behavioural therapy for psychiatric problems. Oxford Medical, Oxford, pp 406–426

Jacobson E 1974 Progressive relaxation. Midway reprint. University of Chicago Press, Chicago, IL

Keefe F J, Beaupre P M, Gil K M 1996 Group therapy for patients with chronic pain. In: Gatchell R J, Turk D C (eds) Psychological approaches to pain management. Guilford Press, New York, pp 259–282

Moldofsky H 2001 Sleep and pain. Sleep Medicine Reviews 5:387–398

NIHTA (NIH Technology Assessment) 1996 Integration of behavioral and relaxation approaches into the treatment of chronic pain and insomnia. NIH Technology Assessment Panel on Integration of Behavioral and Relaxation Approaches into the Treatment of Chronic Pain and Insomnia. Journal of the American Medical Association 276:313–318

Perlis M L, Sharpe M, Smith M T et al 2001 Behavioural treatment of insomnia: Treatment outcome and the relevance of medical and psychiatric morbidity. Journal of Behavioral Medicine 24:281–296

Smith M T, Perlis M L, Carmody T P et al 2001 Presleep cognitions in patients with insomnia secondary to chronic pain. Journal of Behavioral Medicine 24:93–114

Wolfe F 1996 The fibromyalgia syndrome: a consensus report on fibromyalgia and disability. Journal of Rheumatology 23:534–539

Part 6 The nature of therapeutic groups

Introduction

In many clinics patients will have been assessed individually, but aspects of treatment are often delivered to more than one patient at a time, and patients thus may find themselves as part of a group. Traditionally, health education has often been delivered to groups of patients, and this fairly didactic approach is often a feature of back schools or educational classes. In terms strictly of information transmission, an educational class has obvious benefits in terms of organisation and efficiency. Chronic pain patients, however, clearly

Box 11.6.1

The nature of therapeutic groups

- Advantages and disadvantages of groups
- Preparing for group participation
- Enhancing participation in groups.

Box 11.6.2

Advantages of group-based treatment

- Efficiency and consistency of information transmission
- Educational benefit from being part of a group
- Additional therapeutic benefits from being part of a group.

require more than 'education' in the traditional sense. Their understanding of their condition may be suffused with emotion and misunderstandings. Emotional and cognitive obstacles to recovery of function can become vehicles for recovery, but treating such patients in groups requires understanding of the nature of group processes. The key elements in the management of therapeutic groups are outlined in Box 11.6.1.

Advantages and disadvantages of groups

The main advantages of group-based as opposed to individually based treatment are shown in Box 11.6.2.

Efficiency and consistency of information transmission

Often the use of treatment in groups is advocated on the grounds of efficiency, and in a financially constrained health-care system it is hard to justify the delivery of a full pain management package to an individual patient. Almost every patient who has 'earned' a place on a pain management programme, in any event, probably will already have had courses of individualised treatment possibly from a range of health-care personnel. PMPs differ widely in content and organisation; they may also differ in therapeutic style ranging from the traditional didactic

educational approach having its origin in the early 'back schools' to more modern problem-based approaches which are much more experiential in style. Nonetheless, since iatrogenic distress and confusion is characteristic of many chronic pain patients, it is necessary to begin with the transmission of the fundamentals of pain management to orientate patients towards the biopsychosocial approach. Thus the move from the Cartesian model to the Gate Control Theory cannot be addressed without provision of a number of 'building blocks' of basic information to the entire group of patients, since it cannot be assumed that they are all 'starting from the same place'. Preparation of visual materials to assist the educational process offers the opportunity to establish a consistent foundation to the therapeutic group. There are therefore clear advantages in terms of efficiency in delivering teaching in a group format.

Educational benefit from being part of a group

There is, however, also a considerable educational advantage in groups. Patients have the opportunity to listen to and observe each other in their interactions with the staff in matters of clarification and reorientation. They have the opportunity also to discuss 'paper patients' and participate in role-play, both powerful learning modalities.

Additional therapeutic benefits from being part of a group

Arguably the most powerful reason for establishing a group format, however, is the potential therapeutic benefit from sharing experiences within the group. A frequently underestimated feature of chronic pain is the gradually increasing sense of alienation which can happen with the failure of treatment, disappointing encounters and displays of helplessness or irritation by family members. The group can offer a safe environment in which to identify, address and explore the wider impact of pain on function, relationships and well-being.

Preparing for group participation

Nonetheless, most patients profess initial reluctance to participate in groups. They may be anxious at the thought of disclosing their difficulties in front of strangers. Such anxieties of course may also be a feature of

Box 11.6.3

Some reasons for anxiety about participation in groups

- Fears of having to disclose sensitive or embarrassing information
- Anxieties about not understanding the teaching
- Becoming upset in front of others.

Box 11.6.4

Strategies for enhancing group participation

- Role of the group leader
- Establishing the therapeutic climate
- Repeating the 'rules of engagement'
- Facilitating self-disclosure
- Reinforcing 'success'
- Managing group dynamics
- Removing group members.

individual encounters with health-care professionals, but being confronted by a group of strangers can be viewed with alarm. There may be a number of alternative reasons for such anxieties. A number of these are shown in Box 11.6.3.

It is important therefore at the time of assessment to elicit patients' concerns and attempt to allay their fears. In so doing it is helpful to describe not only the content of the group programme, but the level and type of participation which will be expected from the patient and the 'rules of engagement' in matters of self-disclosure. It should be stressed that individual patients will not be pressurised to disclose sensitive information, and absolute guarantees need to be given by the staff that information that they may have about individual patients will under no circumstances be disclosed to other patients without the patient's explicit permission. Clinics vary in the extent to which they enter into formal contractual arrangements with patients and while there is much to be said for requiring a specific undertaking from a patient that they will participate in the full programme, there can be a danger of bruising the therapeutic relationship if negotiation of participation is seen as overly unsympathetic.

Enhancing participation in groups

While the majority of patients who agree to participate in groups complete the programme and appear to derive at least some therapeutic benefit from it, a number of patients drop out or appear to derive little benefit from being part of a group. It is important to recognise that there are a number of ways of participating in groups and even passive participants are nonetheless part of the group. It is not uncommon for a patient who shown little evidence initially of active participation to suddenly 'emerge' at later stages. Patients differ in their social skills and verbal fluency. The group

can have powerful influences on thought and feelings as well as behaviour. A number of strategies for enhancing participation are outlined in Box 11.6.4.

Role of the group leader

The role of the group leaders is of paramount importance. They should have had experience and training in the running of therapeutic groups. Groups can develop powerful emotional temperatures and patients can become significantly distressed. It should be stated that the role of the group at all times is to support its members and not 'sit in judgement' about them. It is therefore important at the time of selection for the group to appraise not only the patient's likelihood to benefit from the group, but also the probability of them helping others as opposed to damaging them.

Establishing the therapeutic climate

As aforementioned, an initial level of anxiety is to be expected in any encounter with strangers. General reassurance about the nature of the group followed by simple introductions can be helpful.

Repeating the 'rules of engagement'

Prior to participation in the group, all patients will have been 'worked up' in terms of their preparation by a member of staff. However, they may have been assessed by different individuals. It is important therefore at the start of the group to restate the 'rules of engagement' so that any misunderstandings can be addressed and important reassurances given. Each PMP needs to establish its own way of operating but at the very least the rules should include the right of the staff to exclude a patient, either in the patient's own interest, or for the sake of others; exclusion if under the influence of alcohol or recreational drugs; and prohibition of inappropriate intimacy between patients during the lifetime of the group.

Facilitating self-disclosure

The group programme should begin with simple group participation exercises as a way of 'desensitising' the patient to being part of a group. Challenging or potentially threatening topics initially should be avoided. Thus the most important single object of the initial session should be to persuade the patients to continue to the second session! Initially there should be absolutely no pressure on patients to disclose details of their individual circumstances, but frequently a less-inhibited patient will decide to do so. However, discussion of pain-associated problems can often be facilitated by illustrative examples provided by the staff, either verbally or in the form of a 'paper patient' which can be used as the basis for discussion.

Reinforcing 'success'

It is important to try to ensure that patients' self-confidence becomes re-established or developed. Any positive contributions to the group in terms of helpful observations or adaptive changes to their own circumstances should be recognised and positively supported, although tempered if necessary with a degree of caution about the importance of pacing.

Managing group dynamics

It is often observed that groups can 'have a life of their own' and indeed every group comprises not only different individuals but has its own emotional climate and rate of development. At times distress and anger may emerge during the group. Often such emotions will be directed at people outside the group (such as healthcare professionals, employers or family members) but at times strong emotions can become generated within the group towards particular individuals, whether staff or fellow patients. It is important wherever possible to address such issues prior to the end of the session, or at the beginning of the following one. The staff must take responsibility for the emotional health of the patients in their care and it is therefore advisable for the staff to conduct a brief appraisal at the end of each group to identify emotional issues or misunderstandings which threaten to impair the therapeutic value of the group.

Removing group members

Occasionally a patient will be so destructive or unhelpful that he/she will have to be asked to leave the group. If such a circumstance is more than an extremely rare occurrence the issue of patient selection will have to be addressed. However, it is never possible to predict absolutely how a patient will behave when in a group. As aforementioned, staff must have the right to exclude a patient.

Concluding observations

The therapeutic value of groups is well recognised as part of the treatment of mental health conditions. Unfortunately it is extremely difficult to evaluate, since measures are needed not only of individual patient participation but also their interactions with others. Despite the widespread use of groups in pain management programmes, there has been virtually no research directed either at the specific therapeutic value of being part of a group, or of the additional value of group participation over and above individual therapy.

Anecdotally, despite initial apprehension it would appear that a significant number of chronic pain patients do seem to feel that the group support and opportunity to compare their own situation with that of other patients is therapeutic in its own right. It is certainly true that groups can 'take on a life of their own' and therefore if the group moves beyond the transmission of information or shared problem-solving to focus specifically on the emotional impact of pain and pain-associated limitations on patients and their relationships, then the group should be led by a member of staff with appropriate professional competence and experience of running therapeutic groups.

The interdisciplinary team should as a matter of course discuss the impact of the group and establish systems of recording the occurrence of meaningful interactions within the group.

Part 7 **Maintenance and management of flare-ups**

Introduction

In patients who have responded positively to pain management, it is important to address the issue of maintenance of treatment gains. Marlatt & Gordon (1995) identified four steps in relapse prevention. The essence of their recommendations is shown in Box 11.7.1. They include such techniques in an 'emergency-card', which patients have developed at the end of the treatment programme.

Bradley (1996) addresses the issues of high-risk situations and relapse prevention, and notes that nearly all CBT interventions in patients with rheumatoid arthritis (RA) include some element of relapse prevention training (Bradley et al 1987). He cites Keefe & van Horn (1993) who suggest: 'relapse tends to occur when patients' symptoms increase in intensity, their perceived abilities to control symptoms are compromised, and their psychological distress is magnified'. If patients stop their effort at coping in response to setbacks they are likely to experience a major decline in pain control, functional ability or psychological status. It is suggested that there are critical components designed to help patients cope with a relapse. They identify four phases of treatment, shown in Box 11.7.2.

There is a substantial emphasis on relapse prevention in the Salford programme. At the conclusion of the pain management programme the patients will have been required to identify their own specific goals for the immediate and long-term future. These will have addressed specific areas including medication use, management of acute flare-ups, use of the health-care system, targets for exercise and relaxation, return to social and family activities, the potential for the return to gainful activities (return to work) and other areas

Box 11.7.1

Steps in relapse prevention

- Stopping and paying attention to cues that a setback is occurring
- Keeping calm and using relaxation to prevent an overemotional response
- Reviewing the circumstances leading up to the setback
- Implementing appropriate coping strategies.

specific to that patient (e.g. improving communication with partner).

It is important to prepare the patients on the pain management programme for their return home. Most patients comment upon the loss of immediate support upon return home, even if the programme has been a largely outpatient-based programme with attendance only once or twice per week. The patients gain a great deal from the mutual support and camaraderie on the course from their fellows as well as the obvious support and encouragement they gain from the staff. By the end of the programme the patients have usually become good personal friends and provide each other with significant moral support, particularly when difficulties are encountered. Patients often describe that they leave a programme on a 'high'. This may be to the extent that they have not adequately addressed how they are going to manage on their own at home.

Others do become more anxious about their ability to manage on their own at home, but fail to plan for this. The mutual support of the group may even distract them from focusing their attention on the necessary plans for the future. It is vital, therefore, to help the patients on the programme to plan how they will manage their return to their home (and possibly work) environment.

In addition to the issues of relapse prevention contained within the actual teaching programme, there are a number of other key features which should be addressed during the postprogramme period. They are shown in Box 11.7.3.

Advice to the patient and family

The programme will have helped patients to focus on their own specific problems. Patients will have been set the task of identifying the problems they anticipate and how they propose to manage or solve them. They will have set specific targets that they expect to achieve and the time-scale in which they propose to do this. Patients should be helped to develop explicit written plans that they have agreed. It is important that the patients are the main instigators of this and that the staff do not coerce or dictate the agenda.

In many PMPs at least one session of the programme will have been devoted to the partner (significant other). The prime objective is to educate the partner, improve communications between the partner and the patient and enable the couple (patient and family) to plan how they will manage at home without the immediate support of the group. It is vital that the partner understands the need for the patient to retain control and not to take over managing the patient's pain and other related problems. Written instructions for the partner may be helpful but it is more important that the patient and partner work on the ground rules themselves. A failure to educate partners in how they should behave may lead to patients losing control and returning to unhelpful strategies, including seeking further cures for their pain.

How things can go wrong

Case Study 11.7.1 illustrates the type of problem which may develop if patients have not planned their progress at home carefully and in some detail. It also illustrates the importance of educating the patient's partner.

Neither the patient nor the partner had plans for how to manage acute flare-ups. They both therefore resorted to previous behaviour (calling the GP for more help) in the panic and stress of the acute situation.

Box 11.7.2

Four phases of treatment

- Practice in identifying high-risk situations that are likely to tax patients' coping resources
- Practice in identifying early signs of relapse such as increases in pain or depression
- Rehearsal of cognitive and behavioural skills for responding to these early relapse signs
- Training in self-reinforcement for effective displays of coping with possible relapse.

Box 11.7.3

Key features needing to be addressed after the programme

- Advice to the patient and family
- Advice to the referring agent and GP
- To follow up or not?
  - the purpose of follow-ups
  - frequency and timing of follow-ups
  - content and organisation of follow-up sessions.
- Management of 'cries for help'
- Post-programme support groups
- Accessing return to work
  - barriers to return to work
  - preparation for return to work.

Case study 11.7.1

A problem after the programme

Mrs G. is a 48-year-old housewife with a 7-year history of low-back pain. She had seen a large number of specialists in a search for an explanation of her ongoing pain and a cure. Scans had not revealed any structural cause and she felt reassured by the team's explanation of her ongoing pain. She attended all of the sessions of the pain management programme and made substantial progress both physically and emotionally. She felt that she had gained a great deal from the programme but was fearful of how she would manage at home. Her husband was often away from home for extended periods of time and she had few friends locally.

Mrs G.'s husband had noticed a major improvement, but was fearful of her 'overdoing it'. He was unable to attend the partner session. He tended to be overprotective when at home, insisting on doing everything (although he felt quite resentful).

Mrs G. had made only vague plans by the end of the programme. For example, she expressed a wish to walk more without specifying any detail or how she was going to achieve this and monitor it. She had not discussed any of her plans with her husband.

When at home Mrs G. suffered an acute flare-up. Her husband had to return home and he arranged with her GP for her to be admitted to the local hospital.

Box 11.7.4

Advice to patients

- Have written plans for managing acute flare-ups
- Practise these regularly
- Make sure that you have discussed this with your partner (family)
- Explain exactly how your partner/family can help
- Have plans (time and space) for your exercises and relaxation
- Have specific short-term targets (e.g. increase walking tolerance to 15 minutes by 1 month's time)
- Plan for moral support (e.g. involve friends, family or keep telephone contact with group)
- Visit your GP and explain what you are doing
- Ask for GP's support and help (not more medicines or referrals)
- Translate gains into something pleasurable/useful (e.g. going out for coffee)
- Plan to do something to keep the mood and morale up (e.g. go to cinema, visit friends).

A summary of advice that may be given to patients is shown in Box 11.7.4.

Advice to the referring agent and general practitioner

In addition to the discharge letter at the end of the programme both the referring agent and in particular the patient's GP should be sent specific guidelines to help with the further management of the patient after the programme (Box 11.7.5). The guidelines should include the philosophy, aims and objectives of the programme. Such guidelines simply outline the purpose of the programme and the general principles of management in the community after the programme. Any specific detail that relates to a particular patient should be included in the discharge letter (e.g. detail of the gradual withdrawal of medication).

Sending such detail to referring agents is important, to indicate to them not only how the patient has done but also how the patient should manage the future and avoid unnecessary further evaluations and treatments. Communication with the patient's GP is, however, vital. It is the GP to whom the patient is likely to turn in the event of an acute flare-up. Therefore GPs must be given the rationale and details of the long-term plan if they are to be actively involved in the patient's management. It is vital that the patient does not get 'mixed messages'. GPs must have details of what the team members have told patients and what is expected of them.

GPs must also be given an understanding of what the long-term plans are and precisely what their roles in these are. The outline of the general principles of pain management will be useful as well as specific instructions relating only to their patient. For example, GPs must be involved in managing any changes in medication. They must be informed as to what changes are to be made, how they are to be made and the rationale behind this. Only then is their cooperation likely to be achieved.

Despite communicating with GPs problems can still occur. If GPs are not convinced that pain management is appropriate or, for example, that reduction

Box 11.7.5

Advice to GPs on how they can support their chronic pain patients in management of their pain

Management of flare-ups

1 Short period of rest is acceptable for a maximum of 48 hours
2 Check pacing
3 Look for other stressors
4 Accept that explanations may not always be possible
5 Prevent the patient relapsing into models of pathology as causes of pain
6 Encourage gradual increase in activity
7 Medication may be increased on a time contingent basis for short periods to enable restoration to normal levels of activity as soon as possible.

General advice

1 Reinforce that what has been learned at the pain centre should be exploited for an *unlimited* length of time
2 Avoid return to medical model:
   - emphasise no structural or pathological cause for the pain
   - emphasise no specific medical intervention will cure pain
   - emphasise hurt does not indicate harm.
3 Encourage continued activity and pacing of activity; use exercise programme taught at pain centre and avoid prolonged rest
4 Actively encourage continuing use of stress reduction and relaxation training techniques
5 Encourage continued medication reduction:
   - avoid opioids (alone or in combination) for long-term use
   - avoid hypnotics and benzodiazepines.
6 Avoid artificial aids to mobility (e.g. walking sticks, corsets, etc.)
7 We would not anticipate putting the patient through a further full programme but occasional top-ups may be available according to clinical indications at the time.

of medication is sensible in the face of chronic pain then they are likely to unintentionally undermine the patient's progress. This is far more likely to occur if they have not been given specific guidelines and reasons for pursuing this line of management.

It should be remembered that the care of the patient rests with the GP. They may be under considerable pressure (from the patient or the family) to do something in the event of an acute flare-up. It is very difficult to resist in the heat of the moment unless the team has given explicit (written) support. All patients should therefore be given a copy of the guidelines that are to be sent to their GPs. This ensures that there are no misunderstandings and gives explicit permission to the GP to remain firm in neither prescribing inappropriately nor referring the patient for further specialist appointments or treatments that are not clinically indicated.

The guidelines will also give the GP the confidence to refer the patient to a specialist if 'new' pain problems arise that are clearly different from the 'chronic' and long-standing problems. The clinical decision rules, therefore, become explicit. The pain management team, the patient and the GP will share an agreed understanding of the specific reasons for further investigation or the appropriate refusal of this if indicated.

Finally it should be recalled that in an effort to prevent miscommunications following the PMP, certain clinics previously were accustomed to give copies of discharge letters to patients. There is now in the UK a requirement, with only a small number of specific clinical exceptions under the Data Protection Act, to allow patients full access to their records.

To follow up or not?

Most pain management programmes include some form of follow-up sessions as an integrated part of their programme. It is essential to have some assessment of longer-term progress of patients if the purchasers are to be persuaded that pain management programmes are a worthwhile investment. In addition the team cannot audit either outcome or the content of the programme without some evaluation of the patients' progress other than that demonstrable at the end of the programme.

The purpose of follow-up

Monitoring patients' progress

The patients will have set themselves specific goals and targets at the end of the programme with the help of the team members. The prime purpose of at least the first follow-up session should be to monitor the patients' progress in achieving their goals, identifying any problems and helping the patients to plan how to overcome these and set their targets for the future.

Despite warning patients that they will come across problems when they are at home, setbacks often come as a shock and can be very demoralising. Many patients leave the programme on a 'high', often buoyed up by the support of the group, thinking that they have got on top of their problems. They expect to make continuous improvement and do not anticipate any setbacks. Setbacks should be regarded as normal, however. The patients must be encouraged to learn from their experience, identify specifically what went wrong and why. They should then plan how they will manage such problems in the future and anticipate what other problems may occur.

Troubleshooting

'Troubleshooting' is often done in a group setting. This enables other members of the group to offer a different perspective on problems identified. It will demonstrate that setbacks are common and group members may well come up with the solution to the problem. This is an essential part of the programme and can be done only after the patients have had a chance to practise their skills on their own at home. It is the only way of assessing how much patients have learnt and is an integral part of the learning process on the programme.

An opportunity for evaluating outcome

Follow-up sessions present an opportunity to measure outcome. This may be done formally by asking patients to fill out questionnaires that they will have completed prior to starting the programme. Patients may be asked to keep medication diaries for the week prior to follow-up sessions and comparisons may be made with pre-programme measures and with the patients' declared goals. Finally, physical measures may be performed (e.g. timed walk) to indicate performance of specific tasks. Such data are vital to audit not only the performance of individual patients but also the efficacy of the programme as a whole. Changes in outcome may then be investigated to determine whether there have been changes in case mix, programme content, programme delivery or clinical decision making.

Auditing the programme

Whereas auditing outcome is vital to maintaining standards the content and style of delivery should also be audited. Patients should be encouraged to give constructive criticisms of both some time after the programme. This may be done anonymously by questionnaire.

The team may also identify specific problems arising after programmes at the follow-up sessions that can alert them to specific weaknesses in either content or delivery. Thus follow-up sessions should include time for team debriefing in order to audit the session and the programme. Changes can then be made and the effect monitored in successive programmes.

Frequency and timing of follow-ups

There is no absolute rule. Clearly it is not possible nor desirable to follow up groups indefinitely. It would seem to be counter to the ethos of the programme of teaching patients to become less dependent upon others to manage their pain and other associated problems.

Ideally some sort of short-term follow-up should be organised 4–6 weeks after conclusion of the PMP. This is when problems are likely to emerge, and leaving these for too long can be counterproductive. It allows the patients enough time to test out their skills, identify problems and weaknesses and get help within a reasonable time. There are no scientific data to support this view, but our experience has shown that leaving the first follow-up for too long can lead to patients failing and becoming demoralised or catastrophising. It is then much harder to help them regain control.

The nature and frequency of follow-ups is resource dependent and sometimes 3-month follow-ups are arranged but in many clinics a substantive follow-up and reassessment is arranged at around 6 months after the PMP. In any event, follow-up sessions should be regarded as an important and integral part of the programme. Patients are asked to commit themselves to coming to all the follow-up sessions at the beginning of the programme.

Attendance at the 1-month follow-up is usually good. The follow-up rate can be expected to decrease in proportion to the length of the follow-up period. For programme evaluation purposes, every effort should be made to follow up at least 80% of the patients.

General organisation of follow-ups

All follow-up session times and dates are given to patients when they accept the invitation to treatment. The patient is asked specifically to agree to come to all the sessions of the programme, the preprogramme assessment and all of the follow-up sessions.

Wherever possible the follow-up sessions should be staffed by the same team members as the programme itself. There are occasions when this is not possible (e.g. sickness or holidays). There must be at least one member of the original team at these sessions. It is not appropriate to have an entirely different set of staff. The group will have developed good rapport with the staff and this cannot be established quickly at a single session. (For research purposes, however, an independent follow-up clearly is desirable.)

Content of 4–6-week follow-up

The first follow-up session (at 4–6 weeks) should follow a similar pattern to sessions on the programme itself. All of the team members should be involved. The purpose will be to monitor progress and to ask for feedback from the patients regarding any specific problems they have had. Ideally the patients will be seen initially by each of the treating clinicians (usually physician, physiotherapist and psychologist and perhaps nurse). It is useful for the whole group to be seen together.

The doctor may have to reassure some of the patients if they have concerns about the cause of any increase in pain or any new symptoms that may have emerged. It is important not to be dismissive but take such problems seriously. On occasions it may be necessary to re-evaluate patients (including re-examination) in order to reassure them and be very positive in reinforcing the notion that in their case hurt does not mean harm. The doctor should review the patients' progress with medication reduction and encourage them to continue towards their goal of drug reduction.

Occasionally patients may have experienced problems with the health-care system. The doctor should reinforce the patients' avoidance of further assessments, treatments and emergency use of the health-care system unless there is clear indication to do so. For example, it is appropriate to consult their GP if a new pain or symptom emerges, but further consultations because they have had an exacerbation of their usual pain not only will not be helpful, but may lead them into further and repeated assessments and unhelpful treatments.

Both the physiotherapist and the psychologist should run very similar sessions. They should assess progress so far (as a group) highlighting the positive and allowing the other members of the group to offer solutions to problems that patients may bring up. Essentially the session is one of reinforcing patients' problem-solving skills, and helping them to set their goals for the next 3 months. In addition the psychologist should revise relaxation skills with the group and the physiotherapist will revisit specific and general exercises. Finally the opportunity should be taken to perform some physical measures of performance, for example the speed walk, to provide some outcome data.

9.00–10.30	Introduction and problem-solving review (physiotherapist + psychologist)
10.30–11.00	Break
11.00–11.30	Problem-solving review/physio review (physiotherapist + psychologist)
11.30–12.30	Relaxation (psychologist)

Figure 11.7.1 • Three-month booster session timetable.

Subsequent follow-ups

The follow-up sessions at 3 and 6 months should allow a gradual change of emphasis. There should be a gradual reduction in the medical input as the programme itself progresses and likewise with the follow-up sessions. Therefore by the 3-month follow-up the sessions should include only the physiotherapist and psychologist. The aim of the sessions at this stage is to facilitate the patient's self-management. Figure 11.7.1 shows the outline of a 3-month booster. As can be seen the time allocated is reduced to half a day and emphasis should be placed on maintenance of change and long-term goals.

The 6-month follow-up should include specific time for patients to complete questionnaires and other tests to allow audit of outcome. By emphasising the importance of outcome data, patients are usually compliant in attendance and cooperation.

Management of 'cries for help'

Cries for help immediately after the programme are not common. They usually indicate that the patient has panicked or catastrophised following a flare-up. Although it is important to encourage patients to take responsibility for their own pain and related problems it is better that they be allowed access to the team rather than risk being lost in the health-care system. Most patients are aware that following the programme they should take control of their pain and associated problems. A small number lack confidence in doing so. Problems that do arise can usually be managed by advice given over the telephone. Rarely the patient may need to attend the centre for a physical check to ensure that a 'new' problem has not arisen.

Most centres will not have resources to allow continuous unlimited follow-up, and in general this is not consistent with a patient-centred self-directed approach.

Case study 11.7.2

A rereferral to a pain centre

Mrs W. had been referred to the pain centre by the department of rheumatology for a lumbar sympathetic block. She had a long history of back pain and continuing sciatica which had not been helped by decompressive surgery some 8 years previously. A diagnosis of neurogenic pain had been made and it was felt that a sympathectomy should be attempted. Rather than simply act as technicians and perform the block without further evaluation the pain centre decided to review the patient.

At interview it became apparent that the leg pain was not of major importance to the patient but that her back pain was the major problem. She had become very disabled and despondent. On further questioning and introduction to the potential for self-management (pain management techniques) Mrs W. revealed she had been on a pain management programme elsewhere and had benefited greatly from it, but now did not have the control she had had.

Following the 'apparent' failure of these techniques her GP had referred her to a number of other specialists who had instituted further investigations and repeated treatments to no effect. In desperation she had been referred to a department of rheumatology at a teaching hospital that was linked informally to a pain management programme.

Only when referred to the pain centre did it emerge that she had attended and made good initial progress on a pain management programme. She explained that she lived in an isolated village and had not managed to remain in contact with other members of her group nor had she been able to motivate herself to keep up with her exercises and relaxation. When it was put to her that she might benefit from returning to the original programme for a booster and to institute workable plans for managing at home she was anxious to take up the offer.

She was duly seen by the original pain management team, included on a booster programme and made good progress.

Allowing such access would eventually flood the centre with follow-up patients and no time could be given to new patients. Patients often do not understand this. The patients must, therefore, learn to manage their problems in the future without continuous reference to the staff at the centre. Limited access should be allowed as the danger of unhelpful treatment or management (as has usually happened in the past) is very likely. Both the patient and the GP should therefore at least seek advice from the centre if there are clear signs that the patient is not managing well.

The commonest reason for problems arising is the failure of patients to maintain the skills and techniques they have learned on the programme. This is more likely to be the cause with patients who develop problems some time after the end of the programme (e.g. 1 to 2 years later). Occasionally such patients may return to the centre via other departments to whom they have been referred. An example is given in Case Study 11.7.2. It can be seen from this actual case that the patient ultimately was 'rescued' by good fortune. Patients and their GPs should be encouraged to seek advice from the centre before being referred back into the health-care system. The GPs should be encouraged to check that the patient has been able to continue with all of the advice from the centre before referring elsewhere.

Post-PMP support groups

There is little evidence in the literature to support the efficacy of post-programme support groups in helping patients to maintain progress (Linton et al 1997). Commonly patients who have benefited from the social contact wish to continue after the programme. Patients who have been able to incorporate the skills learned on the programme in their normal life usually do not wish to be involved in such groups. Many self-help groups tend to be attended by those patients who have made the least progress in changing lifestyle. They are at risk of focusing on pain and mutual support in their invalidity and failing to address the need to focus upon return to useful activity.

Not all support groups are unhelpful. Some are well focused on helping their members keep out of the health-care system and are truly focused on maintenance of change. It has to be said that such successful groups are not common. They require a dynamic person with substantial time and energy to lead them. Burnout among the leaders is common as some group members make unrealistic demands upon the leaders.

Any formal arrangements with such groups should be taken on only with considerable care. The groups should be independent. Support in the way of occasional talks to encourage members to keep active and reinforce self-reliance is wise. Any further participation is likely to be counterproductive. A number of self-help groups have arisen in the UK. Most have not lasted very long and only a few seemed to be firmly focused on helpful activities.

Finally, there is a danger that support groups may be used as a 'dumping ground' for patients who have either failed on the programme or are not suitable. This is unreasonable, as the members of the group will potentially be faced with patients who are least likely to benefit from any encouragement to change their lifestyle. Such groups may ultimately become a 'mutual moaning society', of little value to the members or the centre.

Not all support groups are so disastrous. Some provide good emotional and physical support for patients with long-term pain and disability. Support must be given to the leaders of such groups in order to prevent burnout and help maintain a group that is of significant help to the centre.

Accessing return to work post PMP

Return to work as an outcome measure has been suggested by many as the true measure of successful pain management. Despite this there are very few studies that demonstrate that pain management programmes assist people in returning to work. This may be because those attending pain management, in some centres at least, are so disabled and deconditioned that return to work is not an achievable goal. Others may contend that return to work should be the focus of pain management only where patients identify it as one of their own desired goals.

As mentioned in the introduction to this chapter, there are international differences in the configuration and availability of work rehabilitation and in North America the focus of pain management is primarily on functional change in general, and on work capability in particular. In the UK traditionally the primary focus has been on pain, pain-associated limitations and on quality of life rather than work capability as such, although there has been a move recently to develop occupationally focused rehabilitation programmes, and some PMPs are now developing such extensions and interfaces. Sheer practicalities of funding, referral mechanisms and availability have deterred such developments in the NHS, but a number of private sector organisations are now offering work rehabilitation and are certainly worth considering for a proportion of patients on completion of their PMP.

Research evidence is lacking on the specific value of work-focused rehabilitation as an adjunct to or extension of tertiary PMPs, but it certainly cannot be assumed that even significant clinical change will guarantee successful return to work which may require addressing important additional issues.

Preparation for return to work and for work retention are discussed in detail in Chs 14 and 15.

Conclusion

Pain management should be regarded as a process rather than a single event. The patients, their partners and the treating team should be focused on the maintenance of change after the group programme has finished. Patients should be made aware of their commitment to all of the follow-up sessions prior to commencing the group programme. From the very beginning of the programme the patients must commit to planning short-, middle- and long-term goals. They must, with the help of the team, identify the barriers to continued progress and plan in detail how they will address them. Others, including their partners, (potential) employers and GPs, will need to be recruited to assist.

Key points

- **Relapse prevention and management should be addressed both on the pain management programme and at subsequent follow-up sessions**
- **Specific advice with regard to both prevention and management of relapse should be given to patients, their families and their GPs**
- **Advice should include specific details of the planned management of any 'flare-ups'**
- **Follow-up sessions should be regarded as an integral part of the pain management programme**
- **Follow-up sessions should be focused on maintenance of skills and 'troubleshooting', and include audit measures**
- **Adopt specific plans to manage 'cries for help'**
- **Offer support for those who wish to return to work.**

References

Bradley L A 1996 Cognitive-behavioural therapy for chronic pain. In: Gatchel R J, Turk D C (eds) Psychological approaches to pain management: a practitioner's handbook. Guilford Press, New York, ch 6, pp 131–147

Bradley L A, Young L D, Anderson K O et al 1987 Effects of psychological therapy on pain behavior of rheumatoid arthritis patients: treatment outcome and six-month follow-up. Arthritis and Rheumatism 30:1105–1114

Keefe F J, van Horn Y 1993 Cognitive-behavioral treatment of rheumatoid arthritis pain: maintaining treatment gains. Arthritis Care and Research 6:213–222

Linton S J, Hellsing A L, Larson I 1997 Bridging the gap: support groups do not enhance long-term outcome in chronic back pain. Clinical Journal of Pain 13(3): 221–222

Marlatt G A, Gordon J R 1995 (eds) Relapse prevention. Guilford, New York

Part 8 **Conclusions**

PART CONTENTS

Consistency of approach

Although the content of the group programme has been dealt with in different chapters, this has been done for pragmatic reasons. It is important to understand that the running of the programme is very much a team effort. There are many issues and topics that cross the boundaries between the various professions of the team. Consistency of approach is vital and will enable patients to link psychological issues and physical activity.

There must be regular scheduled time for team members to meet to discuss the progress of individuals and the group as a whole. Problems can then be identified and important issues raised can be addressed as soon as possible, if necessary allowing patients' concerns to be addressed individually.

Regular 'handing over' of sessions will contribute to presenting a consistent approach. Adopting a 'Kardex' or written record of the group's and individual's progress is of great help in keeping all members of the team informed and helps in the formulation of the discharge letter at the end of the programme. Each team member should record the content of his or her session with the group and write comments in the individual's record if appropriate.

The advantage of developing explicit 'house rules'

It can be very helpful to have a written set of 'house rules' so that patients understand the explicit responsibilities both of the team and of themselves. They should be developed and agreed by the team before they are presented to patients. These should be given to patients prior to their agreeing to opt into treatment. The rules should be reinforced at the first session of the programme. They should not be thought of as some sort of straightjacket limiting reactivity to fluid and dynamic clinical situations, but they can serve as a useful reminder of what was agreed. Such rules protect the staff and allow for a more objective means of assessment

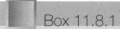

of the patient's behaviour in cases where either non-compliance or disruptive behaviour threatens the group.

Monitoring progress

Throughout the group programme the patients' progress is monitored, both by the team and by the patients themselves. The need to monitor progress is made explicit from the very beginning of the programme. Patients attend the centre just prior to the first session for completion of various questionnaires and assessments of physical function. The need to collect outcome data is stressed to patients and they must agree to participate in this as a condition of attending the programme.

The patients are asked to bring a loose-leaf file with them. This will enable them to keep a written record of their progress including charting their exercises and progress towards their declared goals. They are encouraged to make notes during the teaching sessions and keep the various handouts from team members in their file. Thus they are able to develop their own handbook to which they can refer later.

The importance of individual reviews

Each patient is interviewed at the end of the first week by the team. This may seem a little daunting for the patient, but is done in as relaxed a manner as possible. Patients are invited to give their own assessment of their progress and to identify any specific problems or barriers (Box 11.8.1).

The team members feed back their view of the patient's first week offering support, advice and praise where it is appropriate. Occasionally it is clear that the patient is making no progress or progress is very slow. The team will try to identify the specific barriers with the patient and come to a conclusion as to whether the patient should continue with the group or if there are appropriate alternatives (individual management).

Patients may be given advice as to how to tackle their problem and their progress will be reviewed at the end of the second week. Rarely, patients are destructive to the cohesion of the group or non-compliant and may be invited to leave.

If a patient has to leave the group for any reason, it is important to discuss this with the group after the event to ensure that the group understands the reasons

Box 11.8.1

Potential problems on the programme

- Patient does not understand model
- Patient not convinced of the pain management model
- Patient still considering other treatments
- Difficulty in coping with pain
- Acute flare-up of pain
- Difficulty in concentration
- Patient's anger unresolved
- Socioeconomic factors
- Overprotective partner
- Partner undermining confidence or gains
- Patient failing to observe 'house rules'.

and does not lose its morale. Frequently the group members anticipate patients dropping out, as they are aware that that patient was not engaged.

The setting of task assignments

During the second week of the programme the group is set the task of putting pain management techniques into practice. A session is set aside during the third week. The patients have to decide upon a task, which they will do 'as a group'. It must incorporate activity that demonstrates the need for planning, pacing, physical activity and patients monitoring their own performance. Although some guidance may be given, essentially the group must decide what it wishes to do. Such task assignments have varied from 'American line dancing' to a major gardening project. The purpose of this is to place responsibility firmly with the patients and allow them to put their knowledge into practice in a very practical way.

Group review

At the end of the second week and at the end of the final week the patients' progress is reviewed in a group setting. In particular the issues surrounding the 'task assignment' are discussed and feedback on performance is given. Commonly problems do occur with the task assignment. It is important for the patients to use this as a learning experience upon which they can build.

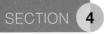

The end of the programme

It is important to impress upon the patients right from the very beginning that the purpose of the programme is for the patients to develop the necessary skills to manage their pain for the rest of their lives. They should not regard their treatment as being completed at the end of the programme. The programme is simply an opportunity to learn and develop lifelong skills. Perhaps the most important period is the first 6 months after the end of the programme when they should be implementing all that they have learned. They will, of course, need to continue with such skills indefinitely.

The patients must have committed themselves to the follow-up sessions at the very beginning of the programme as a prerequisite for inclusion on the programme. It is vital that the later sessions concentrate on getting patients to identify the specific goals they wish to achieve by the time they come for the follow-up session. They should be directed not only to picking realistic goals but also to identifying the difficulties and barriers to reaching their goals. They should have specific plans as to how they are going to address and overcome the barriers that they have identified. Finally the patients must receive feedback on their performance on the programme. This should be honest and include an analysis of the good points and any specific weaknesses or worries the team may have about the patient. Although it is important to boost the patient's confidence, this should be done with a degree of realism. The patient otherwise will leave the programme on something of a 'high' and will not be adequately prepared for the reality of life without the immediate support of the team or the other participants.

By the end of the programme all patients should have explicit goals and targets for the next 4 weeks (Box 11.8.2). They should have plans for managing an acute flare-up of their pain should that occur.

Box 11.8.2

Patient plans

- Targets for exercises and physical activity
- Planning for relaxation and exercise
- Management of tablets and medicines
- Involvement of partner/significant other and family
- Managing acute flare-ups
- Planning middle and long-term goals.

The importance of careful documentation and discharge letters

Adequate documentation of patients' status prior to commencing the programme, and their progress and status at the end of the programme is vital. Time should be allocated for the team to meet after the programme to discuss the content of the discharge letter. Patients' GPs should be given a summary of their progress and any potential problems that may be anticipated. They should also be given details of the aims and objectives of the pain management programme together with the patient's specific goals. This can be recorded in a 'Record of achievement' such as that illustrated in Appendix 11.8.1.

Concluding observations on tertiary interdisciplinary PMPs

Some pain is curable but we are not able to cure all pain and a significant number of patients suffer from recurrent or chronic pain. A proportion of patients are able to manage their pain such that it is neither very distressing nor significantly disabling. A further proportion of patients established on a trajectory of chronicity respond beneficially to early intervention. There are, however, a residue of significantly dysfunctional chronic pain patients who develop psychologically mediated chronic pain syndromes. Such patients need multiprofessional help delivered by a competent team of clinical pain specialists offering an integrated programme designed to address the obstacles to re-engagement in purposeful activity. Not all patients of course respond to this approach, but a significant proportion appear to benefit at least in part, as a consequence in part of the teaching and encouragement they receive from staff but probably also as a consequence of interactions with fellow pain sufferers.

It is to be hoped that in our financially constrained health-care systems it will be possible to retain such programmes as part of the spectrum of care, because, ironically, to the extent that secondary prevention is successful, this may lead to an increasingly challenging case-mix of patients who require the high level of professional skill which characterises effective interdisciplinary PMPs.

Key points

- An integrated approach to the delivery of a pain management programme is essential
- Individual team members' responsibilities must be explicit
- Frequent informal meetings of the team members will ensure early identification of problems both with individual patients and with the group as a whole

(Continued)

- Close team working will produce a consistency in approach and avoid mixed messages
- Clear goal setting with the patients by the end of the programme will prepare the patients for the future and should be the focus of the follow-up sessions
- Detailed discharge letters are vital to helping the patient's GP support the patient in the community and avoid unnecessary use of the health-care system.

APPENDIX 11.8.1

Record of achievements, plans and barriers

Name: _____

My achievements so far:	
My plans for the next 3 months:	
Barriers to achieving my goals:	

Section **Five**

Occupational perspectives

Chapter 12 begins with consideration of the economic impact of pain and disability, from both a societal and an individual perspective, and of the particular influences of compensation and litigation. A review of methods used in the assessment of lying, faking and deception precedes an overview of the personal impact of ongoing litigation and the nature of psychological and psychiatric evaluation of painful personal injury. Finally, the issues of deception, malingering and exaggeration specifically are addressed.

In Chapter 13, the focus is on psychological aspects of work. A review of the literature on work stress leads to a wider consideration of occupational factors associated with poor health and well-being. Risks of work-related illness and injury and long-term disability are then considered. A conceptual framework is offered for the relationship between occupational factors, and recovery from injury. A distinction is made between targets for intervention and obstacles to recovery. Finally, 'blue flags' (perceived obstacles to work) are distinguished from 'black flags' which are *not* a matter of perception, and affect all workers equally.

In Chapter 14, the need for a specific occupational focus within a pain management approach is stressed. The focus is on Type-I interventions or interventions which have the individual worker as the prime focus of intervention. A review of traditional clinical approaches,

back schools, functional restoration programmes, and provision of modified work will conclude with examples of some recent return-to-work initiatives in the UK. Finally, more recent approaches to secondary prevention of work disability, including the specific targeting of risk factors, are presented.

In Chapter 15, Type-II, workplace- (or system-) focused interventions are discussed. Various depictions of the employee–organisational interface are described. The role of 'black flags,' such as working conditions and content-specific aspects of work, as economic and organisational obstacles to return-to-work is discussed. There follows a description of key organisational structures and processes and their influence on work retention and rehabilitation. Different types of workplace interventions are defined. We then review the nature of organisational management of absence, health management policies and their relationship with workplace absence and sub-optimal performance. We stress the importance of the social climate at work, the importance of relationships and the need to develop paths back into sustained employment. We highlight the role of employers and modified work within such policies, including specific targeting of workplace or system-related psychosocial risk factors. Finally we offer a number of recommendations for health and absence management within an organisational context.

Chapter Twelve

Economic and medicolegal influences on pain and disability

CHAPTER CONTENTS

Introduction

In Chapter 4 the social influences on perception of pain, response to pain and the treatment process were considered. In the previous chapters the major emphasis has been on clinical aspects of pain, but in the next four chapters the primary emphasis will be on economic and occupational factors. In this chapter, following a brief overview of economic influences on pain and response to treatment, the influences of medicolegal factors will be addressed. In Chapter 13 an overview of the interface between pain and work will be presented. In Chapter 14, the focus will be occupationally oriented pain management, viewed primarily with reference to the individual worker, while in Chapter 15, pain-associated work limitations, or work disability will be viewed primarily from a workplace or system-based perspective. The primary focus will be on musculoskeletal disorders and on low-back pain, for which the clearest picture is available.

The economic impact of pain and disability

The costs

The clearest data on the costs of pain reference musculoskeletal disorders, and low-back pain in particular. Back pain has been estimated to cost the NHS £1 billion per annum, and cost employers between £5 billion and £11 billion, depending on the method used by Mandiakis & Gray (2000). It has also been estimated that primary-care management of patients with chronic pain accounts for 4.6 million appointments per year in the UK, equivalent to 793 full-time GPs, at a total cost of around £69 million (US$105.6 million) (Belsey 2002).

Musculoskeletal problems are one of the major causes of disability across the world. The impact of pain on economies is enormous, with the cost of back pain alone equivalent to over one-fifth of a country's total health expenditure, and 1.5% of its annual gross domestic product (GDP) (Mandiakis & Gray 2000). In terms of health conditions, it represents three times the total cost of all types of cancer.

Within the UK for example, musculoskeletal problems account for over 23% of recipients of Incapacity Benefit (DWP 2005), a state benefit for long-term inability to work due to sickness.

It has been estimated that in the UK the total cost of back pain amounts to over £12 billion (Mandiakis & Gray 2000), which is equivalent to 22% of UK health-care expenditure; 2.5 million people have back pain every day of the year. Nearly 5 million working days are lost each year due to back problems; 13% of unemployed people give back pain as the reason for not working (Backcare 2005) and 80% of people with back pain on incapacity benefit at 6 months are likely to be on benefit at 5 years (Aylward 2004).

In the UK, the annual cost of absenteeism has been estimated at over 1% of GDP but it is known that health-risk factors and disease also adversely affect worker productivity (Chatterji & Tilley 2002). A US study found that lost productivity due to presenteeism (ill-health when at work) was on average 7.5 times greater than productivity due to absenteeism and for some conditions, including migraine and neck/back/spine pain, the ratio was approaching 30 to 1 (Employers' Health Coalition 2000).

Finally, Waddell (2004), on the basis of 1998 figures, estimated the relative annual costs in terms of NHS costs and private health-care costs to be around £845 m and £301 m respectively, but these were almost insignificant in comparison with an estimate for social security benefits of £3600 m and for sickness absence of £1350 m–£3500 m (depending on how lost production costs are calculated). His total in the £6–8.2 bn range is comparable with the Phillips et al (submitted) estimate. However the figures are drawn up, the impact of back pain is considerable and represents a massive burden to the economy.

The nature of economic factors

As highlighted above, economic costs of pain can be considered at an individual as well as at a societal level.

For a particular individual, the economic effects of pain and pain-associated incapacities can vary from the inconsequential to the catastrophic. The most powerful economic influences can be seen when individuals are compromised in their ability to work, but the economic impact on a particular individual will depend on a number of factors such as those shown in Box 12.1.

In a sense, for a particular individual, the overall economic impact can be most simply understood in terms of the *net costs of sickness*, i.e. with an economic model (Aylward 2003). The real costs may not be perceived by individuals until they actually find themselves in the situation. They may have made inadequate financial provision, or even no provision at all for such an eventuality. In the event of significant injury, pessimism about being able to obtain further employment may be considerable. It is not uncommon to find distress bordering on panic and despair amongst individuals who perceive their job to be at risk because of their sickness record. Response to painful injury is affected not only by the perception of pain and expectation of outcome of treatment, but also by attitudes towards work and perceived entitlements in the event of work-related incapacity (whether temporary or permanent). Cross-culturally, there are major differences in social policy affecting injured workers.

Over the last 30 years, however, there has been a steady increase in the number of people on disability or incapacity benefits, and in the length of time people stay on benefits, *in the absence of any evidence of a corresponding increase in physical disease or impairment*. Furthermore, there has been a huge increase in the number of people being awarded retirement on health grounds, particularly non-specific low-back pain. Improved clinical management has had no apparent beneficial impact on these social security trends. In the UK it has been recognised that significant alleviation of the increasing economic burden of back pain may require fundamental changes in levels of employment, in social policy and in cultural attitudes

Box 12.1

Influences on the economic impact of inability to work

- Current financial commitments
- Length of work loss
- Entitlement to various benefits
- Insurance in the event of sickness
- Alternative sources of income.

and behaviour about sickness. It does appear that sickness and incapacity benefit cannot be considered in isolation. In terms of clinical practical management the potential impact of economic influences on consultation and response to treatment has to be recognised along the length of the continuum from early consultation in primary care (Ch. 10) to tertiary rehabilitation (Ch. 12) and reintegration into work (Chs 14 and 15).

The psychological impact of economic factors will be addressed in the next section.

Psychological impact of economic factors on the individual with pain

Economic hardship resulting from unemployment is well recognised, but an individual's economic situation can also directly influence treatment seeking and response to treatment. It also has to be taken into account as part of the assessment of the patient and in clinical decision making about whether or when to offer pain management. The major spheres of influence are summarised in Box 12.2.

Increase in personal stress

As highlighted in Chapters 2 and 3, pain itself can be considerably stressful, particularly if it is disturbing sleep and affecting activity. The unpleasantness of the pain and demoralising effects of its limiting effects can be enhanced still further if it has a significant financial impact, whether in terms of ability to work, or in terms of quality of life.

Box 12.2

Possible adverse effects of economic factors

- Increase in personal stress
- Increase in family hardship
- Strain on relationships
- Treatment seeking and legitimisation of symptoms
- Acceptance of treatment by the patient
- Acceptance or rejection for treatment by the health-care professional.

Increase in family hardship

The economic impact may be felt not only by individuals, but also by their family. This can further enhance feelings of despair, frustration and sometimes guilt. As aforementioned, the family may or may not have the organisation or opportunity to mitigate the economic impact.

Strain on relationships

Families of chronic pain patients sometimes seem to have made remarkable adjustments to mitigate financial loss without apparent strain on relationships, but even the strongest of relationships can be strained by economic adversity. Even if it is possible to mitigate the hardship, this may be only at the cost of placing a significant strain on relationships. Frequently, partners of the major breadwinner will feel obliged to increase their hours of work or find a new or better paid job to compensate for the shortfall. This may result in increasing tiredness, impaired quality of life and resentment at having to make major changes to the pattern of family life. There may be effects also on relationships with the extended family, if help with childcare becomes necessary in order to obtain further paid work.

Treatment seeking and legitimisation of symptoms

A major factor in consulting doctors is the search for a diagnosis and cure. There are, however, other factors affecting treatment seeking. Sick certification by a medical practitioner may be necessary for entitlement to benefits of various sorts. In the UK, self-certification is permitted for up to 5 days, after which medical ratification is required for entitlement to benefit. Employers vary in the amount of self-certification they will tolerate in an individual period before formal appraisal of health status is initiated (see Ch. 15), but it is certainly the case that legitimisation of the complaint is a major factor in consultation with doctors. In families under strain, particularly with prolonged sickness absences, doubts may have been raised about the 'legitimacy' of the pain, and whether patients are genuinely as incapacitated as they claim. (As discussed below, such doubts may have been raised within medicolegal reports.)

Acceptance of treatment

Many chronic pain patients find themselves in a difficult situation. They may be dependent on the receipt of sickness benefits or some sort of compensation to avoid desperate financial hardship. Improvement as a result of treatment may put incapacity-related benefits at risk. While it could be argued that such a situation requires a 'social policy solution', it can nonetheless represent a real dilemma for pain patients whose medical history may decrease their chance of re-employment, irrespective of re-establishment of their physical capacity and perceived ability to work. Sometimes their pessimism is a function of their lack of confidence, but there may be significant economic anxieties about embarking on rehabilitation without satisfactory guarantees.

Acceptance for treatment and response to treatment

Consideration of economic obstacles to recovery is also important in the context of clinical decision making. It may be that the development of integrated clinical and occupational programmes, both for work retention and for rehabilitation into work, will overcome some of these obstacles to recovery. On a large scale, changes in social policy in terms of sickness benefit and phased return to work may also be required and can be thought of as 'black flags' (Chs 14 and 15). Such matters are beyond the influence of pain clinicians, and a difficult judgement, about whether such influences constitute a relative or an absolute barrier to acceptance for treatment, may have to be made. In the former case, if change in economic circumstances is anticipated, it may be decided to defer treatment. Sometimes, however, the power of the economic obstacles to recovery may be considered to be a contra-indication to pain management.

The special influence of compensation and litigation

Arguably, few issues in clinical medicine generate as much emotion as the nature of pain and pain-associated incapacity in the context of personal injury litigation. Indeed many of the early investigations into chronic pain and its psychological features were addressed from a forensic perspective, in which any apparent mismatch between symptoms and signs and persistence of pain beyond expected healing time was viewed with innate suspicion (Collie 1913). Many chronic pain patients today find themselves embroiled in litigation, at the heart of which is the acceptance or not of chronic pain as a valid

clinical phenomenon and, sometimes, the legitimacy of psychologically mediated chronic pain syndromes. Involvement in personal injury litigation can not only be distressing, but may also adversely affect acceptance for treatment and response to it. A brief appraisal of the influence of litigation on chronic pain and pain-associated incapacity will therefore be undertaken. The line of reasoning presented below has been developed from a number of previous publications (Main 1999, 2003, Main & Spanswick 1995, Main & Waddell 1998).

History of personal injury (PI) litigation

Although it is possible to find award of damages for emotional distress as early as the fourteenth century, a significant increase in PI legislation followed the construction of the railways in the second half of the nineteenth century. Mendelson (1988) offers a fascinating account of the polarisation that developed between those who considered 'railway spine' to be due to an *organic* cause and those who viewed the condition as a type of 'nervous shock'. In a legal context the phrase 'nervous shock' has been used to refer to identifiable psychiatric illness and not simply to emotional states such as anxiety, sadness or grief, which were not considered to be injuries, and were not therefore compensable.

In the evaluation of painful injuries, there are a small number of important overarching questions which will be of relevance in most assessments. These are outlined in Box 12.3.

Terminology

The terms 'compensation' and 'litigation' can be somewhat confusing, since their precise meaning differs across different countries and in differing economic systems. In some contexts, 'compensation' is used in the literature as synonymous with 'financial influence' and in other contexts seems to refer to 'involvement in adversarial litigation'. The term 'litigation' itself will differ in interpretation depending on whether or not there is a 'no-fault' compensation system and on whether the system is essentially adversarial in nature.

The term 'secondary gain' is frequently found in medicolegal reports. The term is actually Freudian in origin. It referred originally to emotional benefits resulting from illness, which were being presented as distressing or unpleasant. In its original sense the term did not

Box 12.3

Key questions in the evaluation of painful injury

- Has the individual been injured?
- What is the nature of the injuries?
  - has the individual suffered a 'psychological injury'?
  - psychiatric disorder
  - post-traumatic stress disorder (PTSD)
- Is there any neuropsychological impairment?
- Is the patient suffering from a chronic pain syndrome?

refer to a perceived benefit sought by the individual. In the medicolegal context, the term frequently has a pejorative or unsavoury connotation and is taken to refer to supposed advantages, whether realised or anticipated, as a consequence of being involved in litigation. Technically, the term is often used to imply that the claimant is at best exaggerating symptoms or incapacity for financial gain, and at worst that the individual is actually fraudulent. In such a context the term may be used in support of an allegation of deliberate exaggeration or even malingering.

In fact, all sorts of adversity may have their compensations. As mentioned in the previous chapter, pain-associated incapacity may lead to changes in family patterns. Sometimes adversity brings couples closer together. Most claimants pursue compensation or litigation with some expectation of outcome. The desired outcome is not always financial, although in high-value claims, particularly in the context of current poverty, it may be the dominant feature. Some litigants want justice of a different sort, such as the righting of a perceived injustice, 'legitimisation' of their continued disability, or even retribution. Pursuit of litigation should not be viewed as inherently suspicious. It may offer the best or only way out of a major predicament.

In fact, impaired quality of life and inability to work often represent such an adverse set of circumstances that it is hard to imagine that such a 'career path' would have been chosen simply in pursuit of anticipated financial gain. Outcome of litigation is uncertain, the pursuit of it can be stressful (see below), and even successful litigation does not always bring significant financial reward.

Compensation, litigation and outcome

The effects of compensation on treatment outcome

According to Mendelson (2003) compensation and litigation have an adverse effect on outcome of both conservative and surgical treatment, but he concludes:

the adverse effect of compensation and/or litigation on the outcome of some injuries sustained in compensable circumstance can be modified by specific intervention and treatment programmes that stress early mobilisation and return to the work-place, appropriate activity and exercise, and avoidance of other factors that may promote learned pain behaviour (p. 223).

Follow-up studies after the conclusion of litigation

Mendelson (2003) takes issue with the 'cure by verdict' implied by earlier writers such as Kennedy (1946) and Miller (1961), a view which has been extremely influential. He considers such views to be 'inaccurate and simplistic', stating 'there are many factors which influence outcome following compensable injury and also the behaviour of disability claimants and a new paradigm is needed' (p. 229).

Factors influencing the outcome of compensable injuries

Mendelson (2003) does, however, list a number of factors which appear to have an influence on outcome of compensable injuries, shown in Box 12.4 (overleaf). The list notes features which most assessors may have noted at times during assessment, but of course they are as much a feature of chronic pain in general as of litigating pain patients, include variables of unknown validity and reliability and no opinion is expressed on their strengths as predictors, whether individually, or in combination.

Concluding observations

The effects of compensation on claims, clinical outcomes and rehabilitation are summarised in Box 12.5 (overleaf). It would appear that compensation claimants have a somewhat poorer prognosis in response to

Box 12.4

Factors influencing outcome of compensable injuries

- Personality
- Demographic factors
- Cultural factors
- Interpersonal dynamics
- Occupational factors
- Psychological reaction
- Physical factors
- Economic factors.

Box 12.5

Effects of compensation on claims, clinical outcomes and rehabilitation

Effect of compensation on claims

- There is no evidence that compensation changes the actual injury rate
- 10% increase in compensation level produces 1–11% increase in claims rate
- 10% increase in compensation level produces 2–11% increase in duration of disability
- This affects 'verifiable' injuries such as fractures as much as more subjective soft-tissue injuries.

Effects of compensation on clinical outcomes

- Compensation patients have poorer clinical outcomes and more disability
- These findings have been criticised:
  - these men often have heavier physical jobs
  - they may have other psychosocial differences
  - they may get different treatment.

Effects of compensation on rehabilitation outcome

- Compensation patients respond less well to pain management and rehabilitation
- These findings have been criticised:
  - there are methodological flaws in many of these studies; they are often small samples of highly selected patients with poor diagnostic criteria; follow-up is poor
  - there is a failure to allow for other factors such as job demands
  - differences are small.
- Despite all of this, more than 75–90% of workers/compensation patients do respond well to health care, recover rapidly and return to their previous work
- Despite this, many compensation patients do benefit.

Waddell (2004, Box 13.4, p. 258), reproduced with permission

treatment, but the magnitude of the effect varies in different studies, and frequently research design does not permit determination of the specific effect of compensation over and above other factors.

Methods used in the assessment of lying, faking and deception

A number of approaches to the detection of lying, faking and deception are shown in Box 12.6.

Self-report measures designed specifically to detect faking

There have been a number of ways in which evaluation of distortion of self-report has been investigated. The most widely used test has been the Minnesota Multiphasic Personality Inventory (MMPI) or its successor the MMPI-2 (Keller & Butcher 1991), which according to Helmes & Reddon (1993) offers no significant improvement over the original. The original MMPI contained 556 items yielding scores on ten clinical and three validity scales. The vast majority of the items on the revised version (MMPI-2) are unchanged, and the same scale names have been retained. Since the original questionnaire was developed, there have been a vast number of scales produced by combining subsets of items. The test has been popular in the investigation of feigned cognitive deficits in the context of neuropsychological evaluation (Frederick 2003), but it has also been used with pain to measure malingering and defensiveness. Greene (1997) documents a plethora of small scales with seductive titles purporting to capture facets

of malingering but no convincing evidence that either these new scales, or the original validity scales, are adequately validated as stand-alone measures, and they seem to be capable at best of raising questions about the style and context of communication, which might merit further investigation.

Arbisi & Butcher (2004), having expressed the view that 'Psychometric instruments such as the MMPI-2 that contain dimensional, empirically derived validity

Box 12.6

Methods employed in the detection of lying, faking and deception

- Self-report measures designed specifically to detect faking
- Elicitation of behavioural responses to examination
- Non-verbal behaviour, speech content and the ability to detect deceit
- Muscle testing
- Diagnostic blocks
- Polygraphy and symptom validity testing
- Use of functional magnetic resonance imaging (fMRI)
- Video surveillance and other types of fraud investigation.

Box 12.7

Principal uses of the MMPI/MMPI2 in detection of malingering in chronic pain

- Psychiatric comorbidity
- 'Objective' confirmation of a claim of psychiatric morbidity following an injury
- Malingering of somatic complaints
- Detection of inconsistent responding
- Detection of exaggeration or feigning
- Detection of defensiveness or impression management.

scales can play a critical role in the detection of feigned or exaggerated pain' (p. 384), review the usefulness of the test in characterising patients with chronic pain, in predicting outcome, and in identifying profiles of litigating patients.

Characterising patients with chronic pain

The use of the MMPI in the identification of distinct personality types for chronic pain patients has not been successful, nor have the early attempts to distinguish 'organic' from 'functional' pain (an enterprise which now seems to be fundamentally flawed). There does appear to be evidence, however, of consistent elevation on certain of the clinical scales across various studies of chronic pain patients. According to Arbisi & Butcher (2004), using clustering techniques, four groups generally emerge: an elevated psychopathology group; a group with elevations on the 'neurotic triad', i.e. Scales 1 ('Hysteria'), 2 ('Depression') and 3 ('Hypochondriasis'); a group with elevations only on Scales 1 and 2; and finally a group with a normal profile.

Predicting outcome

Having reviewed the literature, Arbisi & Butcher (2004) find some association between Scale 1 and occupational outcome, stating that 'there is no clear evidence that elevations on the Hysteria scale per se are associated with a conscious attempt to feign chronic pain or somatic symptoms' (p. 386).

Identifying profiles of litigating patients

They conclude, 'There does not appear to be a particular profile type or scale elevation associated with compensation seeking in chronic pain patients' (p. 386).

Possible applications

In the second part of their review, Arbisi & Butcher (2004) identify six main ways in which the instrument may be used. They are shown in Box 12.7. The reader is referred to the article for a detailed discussion of each of these aspects.

However, having recommended the use of the MMPI for the provision of an 'objective and dimensional perspective', for the assessment and quantification of self-report, and for a relative comparison of symptomatic status and level of distress as compared with other groups, Arbisi & Butcher (2004) conclude, 'The MMPI-2 cannot independently make dichotomous judgements regarding the source of the chronic pain complaint or the absolute accuracy of the self-report' (p. 390).

Helmes & Reddon (1993) offered a trenchant critique of the general structure of the MMPI in terms of overlap in item content not only across clinical scales, but also across clinical and validity scales, the multifactorial nature of many of the scales, and the lack of cross-validation of item selection; they express doubts specifically about the worth of the validity scales and their interpretation.

Conclusion

On the evidence available, self-report measures would appear to be of little value specifically for the detection of deception or malingering in patients with chronic pain.

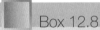

Behavioural responses to examination (Waddell signs or WS)

According to Fishbain et al (2004), there are basically two types of malingering: commissions and omissions, i.e. conscious distortions of problems, events or symptoms and withholding information, respectively.

Waddell et al (1980) produced a set of behaviour signs (originally termed 'non-organic' signs) which could be elicited during a physical examination, and were independent of standard signs of physical impairment. Waddell et al (1980) found, however, that they were associated with psychological distress such as heightened somatic awareness and depressive symptoms (Main et al 1992), and perhaps best understood as a type of pain behaviour. Subsequently these became widely misused and misinterpreted as indicators of hysteria, insincerity of effort or even malingering (a use for which they were never originally validated), prompting Main & Waddell (1998) to attempt to clarify their interpretation. Their interpretation was confirmed by Fishbain et al (2004) who, following an extensive recent review, concluded, 'There is little evidence for an association between WS and secondary gain, and thereby, malingering. The preponderance of the evidence points to the opposite conclusion: no association' (p. 408).

In fact the whole concept of exaggerated pain behaviour has been recently challenged by Sullivan (2004) who has offered a trenchant critique of the use of exaggerated illness behaviour as evidence of malingering, arguing from a philosophical, historical and clinical perspective that we have been misled by pseudoscience into relying on medical tests which are essentially moral and social in nature.

Non-verbal behaviour, speech content and the ability to detect deceit

There has been a long tradition within social psychology of investigation of the nature of communication, and in particular the verbal and non-verbal components of speech. These investigations have extended into the investigation of lying and deceit. However, DePaulo et al (2003), having reviewed more than 110 studies, concluded that typical deceptive speech content and non-verbal pain behaviour does not exist, and according to Vrij & Mann (2003), 'both laypersons and professional lie catchers alike are commonly mistaken when they try to detect deceit' (p. 359). They report a series of studies in experimental or forensic settings in which they have investigated judgements about

> ### Box 12.8
>
> **Critical issues in the use of muscle testing for determination of sincerity of effort**
>
> - The use of force variability is not sufficient to distinguish sincerity of effort
> - The shape of force output curves similarly is not sufficient
> - Reliable and clinically useful methods of differentiating effort levels have not been established
> - Many studies have questionable or at least unknown generalisability to patient samples and actual functional capacity.

deceit and they claim that lie detection skills can be easily improved, expressing optimism about the usefulness of training programmes aimed at enhancing skills in detecting deceit. They offer interesting observations but to date their methods do not seem to have been employed in the evaluation of painful personal injury.

Muscle testing

Determination of sincerity of effort using muscle testing has also been the subject of much study but is beyond the remit of this chapter. Having reviewed the available literature, Robinson & Dannecker (2004) identified a number of critical issues in terms of measurement and validation (Box 12.8). They concluded:

> It is critical that other explanatory variables such as fear of injury, pain, medications, work satisfaction, and other motivational factors be considered. It is our opinion that there is not enough empirical evidence to support the clinical application of muscle testing to determine sincerity of effort (p. 392).

Diagnostic blocks

Bogduk (2004) recommended the use of diagnostic nerve blocks in the investigation of spinal pain for which the cause is not evident, and concluded:

> A positive response to diagnostic blocks demonstrates that the complaint of pain is genuine, and by implication, refutes any contention that the patient is malingering (p. 409).

They noted further, however:

'negative responses do not exclude a genuine complaint of pain, for patients may have a source of pain which is not amenable to testing with diagnostic blocks' (p. 409).

Polygraphy and symptom validity testing

The use of polygraphy or 'lie-detection' is widely used in North America by government agencies. A polygraph records physiological responses, such as galvanic skin response (GSR), respiratory rate and heart rate, to various 'challenges' in which the subject is asked to answer a number of questions. In terms of paradigms, most popular are the Guilty Knowledge Test (GKT) and Control Question Test (CQT), used in forensic settings and the relevant/irrelevant technique (IRT), used in pre-employment screening. (The latter will not be reviewed.)

The GKT (Ben-Shaker & Furedy 1990) is a type of multiple-choice detection procedure in which the subject is asked to choose one of a set of answers to a series of questions, the correct answer to which should not be known to an innocent party.

The CQT (Ben-Shaker & Furedy 1990) is more widely used in forensic settings, and there are large number of procedural variants but in general it is assumed that, when compared with innocent subjects, guilty people will produce enhanced physiological responses to forensically relevant questions in comparison with control questions.

Iacano & Patrick (1997), however, consider that 'the methodological problems with analogue and field studies make it impossible to accurately estimate CQT validity' (p. 260). The most trenchant criticism, however, seems to not to be in the correct detection rate (estimated between 77% and 98% in various studies), but in the percentage of innocents falsely classified (with estimated range from 64% to 77%) (Iacano & Patrick 1997). They restate the cautions expressed in the previous edition of Rogers's textbook (presented in Box 12.9).

Use of functional magnetic resonance imaging

There have been attempts to investigate the cognitive components of deception. In experimental studies (Spence et al 2003), the published data using functional magnetic resonance imaging (fMRI) 'clearly implicate specific regions of the frontal cortex in the functional

Box 12.9

Limitations in the value of videotape evidence

- Offer only samples of behaviour
- Samples may or may not be 'representative' of the claimant's typical behaviour
- Usually are unable to replicate the actual physical demands of work in terms of physical demand or posture
- Do not capture possible after-effects of exertion
- Ratings and interpretation is of unknown reliability, particularly in the assessment of mild levels of pain-associated limitations
- Differences on footage taken at different times may illustrate variability in clinical condition rather than inconsistency in behaviour suggestive of deception.

anatomy of deception' and recommend the further elucidation of deception through novel brain-imaging techniques; but such laboratory investigations are clearly still at an early stage and not as yet developed for, or validated in, forensic settings.

Video surveillance and fraud investigation

Videotape evidence is sometimes adduced by defendants in an attempt to discredit claims of pain-associated incapacity. Typically, covert footage will be obtained of the claimant engaged in a range of activities, and experts will be asked to give a view on whether the behaviour displayed on the videotape is consistent with their own assessment of the claimant. Indeed videotape evidence, if it clearly discredits the claimant, can represent the turning point in a case. This is usually only the case if the video evidence clearly and unambiguously contradicts the claimant's self-report. Usually, however, videotape evidence is less conclusive and indicative of a degree of exaggeration at best. The court then has to decide whether the degree of inconsistency evident between the videotape footage and the claimant's limitations, as stated or evaluated during a clinical examination, is outwith the normal variability in pain-associated limitations, or beyond an acceptable degree of imprecision.

The scientific basis of videotaped evidence, however, has not so far been sufficiently developed to determine when a sample of behaviour obtained on a video can be said to constitute a fair and representative sample of the

Box 12.10

Problems with reliance on polygraph testing

- Inadequate research addressing their validity
- Need for psychologists to rely on polygraphers inadequately trained in psychophysiology and psychometrics
- Dearth of information on clinical populations.

Box 12.11

The personal impact of personal injury litigation

- Need for additional assessments
- Contrasting clinical opinions
- Protracted nature of litigation
- Adverse influence on decision to treat
- Attributions of exaggeration, faking and malingering
- General self-confidence and level of distress
- Need to convince.

behaviour concerned. A number of limitations in the use of videotape evidence are presented in Box 12.10.

Visual evidence nonetheless appears to exert a powerful influence on judges, particularly when confronted with a claimant reporting pain (which the judge cannot see) in circumstances when the two sides offer markedly different medical opinions. Thus videotape evidence may be helpful, and indeed conclusive, in determination of level of pain-associated incapacity, but should be interpreted with caution, and viewed as only part of the evidence in the case.

Kitchen (2004) offers an interesting review of the detection of fraud from the perspective of the UK Department for Work and Pensions (DWP). Five thousand of the Department's 125,000 are directly involved in the investigation of fraud, frequently based on allegations made by members of the public. To establish fraud there has to be evidence of a deceptive act (such as failure to declare income), intended financial advantage, and dishonest intent (either through admission of dishonesty or evident in behaviour).

The personal impact of ongoing litigation

The psychological impact of engagement in adversarial litigation can be considerable, and if sufficiently marked may constitute a psychological obstacle to recovery. Some of the major influences of ongoing litigation are summarised in Box 12.11.

Need for additional assessments

In cases of personal injury, the litigation process almost always requires the claimant to undergo additional examinations specifically for medicolegal purposes. These often include a physical examination, which can be painful. The purpose of the assessment is not always made clear, and not infrequently claimants may believe they are being assessed with the primary purpose of offering treatment. Claimants who are fearful of pain or further injury find the prospects of such an examination extremely alarming. Patients with a history of distressing encounters with health-care professionals also may find the prospects of assessment distressing. A proportion of patients may have been emotionally traumatised by the accident and its sequelae. Even though only a minority of patients will report symptomatology of a nature and severity sufficient to constitute an unequivocal post-traumatic stress disorder, many find it emotionally difficult to recall the details of the accident or injury. Finally, the adversarial nature of litigation does not encourage good doctor–patient rapport during assessments carried out on behalf of defendants.

Contrasting clinical opinions

Contrasting clinical opinions are frequently evident in reports prepared for medicolegal purposes. This can be confusing and distressing for pain patients, and may become part of significant iatrogenic distress, as is evident in a significant proportion of patients attending PMPs (Ch. 11).

Protracted nature of litigation

Completion of the process of litigation may take years. Patients often are bewildered and distressed about this. They cannot understand why this should be so, particularly in cases such as motor vehicle accidents in which liability is frequently accepted and completion of the case hinges only on the extent of damages. Some claimants become extremely angry with their legal advisers, whom they blame for the delay. As time passes by, claimants' coping strategies may become exhausted and they may abandon the claim.

Adverse influence on decision to treat

It is perhaps not always fully acknowledged that clinical decisions are influenced by the fact of ongoing litigation. Although it may in certain circumstances be sensible to defer treatment until the conclusion of litigation, some doctors are unwilling even to see patients with ongoing litigation, far less offer them treatment. Some doctors appear to view claimants with considerable suspicion and the doctor–patient relationship can be adversely affected on both sides. A minority of claimants find themselves in a virtually impossible situation in which their legal advisers recommend further treatment before they are willing to conclude the case, whereas the relevant clinicians are unwilling to undertake such treatment until the conclusion of litigation.

Attributions of exaggeration, faking and malingering

Possibly the most distressing aspect of litigation for chronic pain patients is that they may find themselves subject to attributions of exaggeration, faking or even malingering. Attribution of malingering as such is a matter for the court and not for a medical expert (Mendelson 1988) but medical experts are frequently asked by solicitors to give a view on whether they consider plaintiffs to be exaggerating their symptoms or even faking incapacity. Some clinicians nonetheless seem to consider that judgements do lie within their province as experts and appear to have considerable confidence in their ability to do so. According to Faust (1995), however: 'some malingerers practice deception for a living, and can easily outmatch the physician who lacks the same type of experience, mental set and willingness for exploitation that sometimes characterises the professional con artist'.

Impact of litigation on general self-confidence and level of distress

In potentially high-value claims, it is not uncommon for defendants to engage surveillance operators to undertake covert surveillance of the claimant. Claimants are frequently distressed to see secret videos taken of themselves engaging in a variety of activities, particularly if it casts doubt on their credibility. (They may be even more distressed if they become aware of the surveillance at the time it is being carried out.)

From the aforementioned it is easy to understand how claimants can become highly distressed about the litigation process. They may believe they established good rapport with the assessing clinician and feel that the latter was 'on their side', until they gain sight of the report that has been produced. Usually they will not know that they have been the subject of videotape surveillance. They may find sensitive aspects of their personal history revealed in reports. They may find significance that they do not accept given to aspects of their musculoskeletal history. Finally, they may find themselves the subject of what they perceive as a 'character assassination', with attributions of inconsistency, lack of motivation to get better and even lying. They may come to have doubts themselves about the reality or legitimacy of their pain or associated incapacities.

Need to convince

With genuine claimants such an emotional onslaught as described above can lead to the firm conviction that no one believes them, and they need to convince doctors of their bona fides. Ill-advisedly, they may exaggerate in an attempt to convince. They may not be entirely aware of this. Even when it is clear that a conscious element is present, a distinction should be made between 'exaggeration with the intention to convince' and 'exaggeration with the attempt to deceive'. This distinction, however, can be extremely difficult to establish, and may need a detailed history of the patient's symptom presentation to previous assessors (both clinical and medicolegal). This issue will be addressed in more detail later in this chapter.

Concluding reflections on the impact of litigation

Economic factors can have a profound influence on treatment seeking and response to treatment. Financial difficulties as a result of inability to work and the need for benefits to ensure some sort of limited financial security are frequently the most powerful effects of painful injuries. The distress associated with such difficulties can be magnified considerably in the context of adversarial litigation, such that the litigation process itself can short-circuit recovery. Much of the helplessness is associated with fears about the future course of symptoms and lack of confidence in return to work. The specific influence of occupational factors on work disability will be addressed in Chapters 14 and 15.

Psychological and psychiatric evaluation of painful personal injury

There are many types of expertise called upon in the evaluation of personal injury, but arguably psychological and psychiatric evaluation represents a particular challenge in that it highlights the presence of Cartesian dualism at the heart of the medicolegal system, frequently requires an evaluation of 'mismatches' among signs, symptoms and claimed disability, and inevitably requires evaluation of the veracity of the claimant.

Some issues of terminology

As discussed in Chapters 3 and 8, there are established diagnostic procedures such as DSM-IV (1994) for the determination of psychiatric injury. The term 'chronic pain syndrome' is now increasingly referred to in medicolegal reports, and it now seems that chronic pain in certain circumstances may be considered as compensable in its own right and not simply as a mental illness deemed to have resulted from the accident.

The term 'chronic pain syndrome' (CPS), however, can be somewhat ambiguous. A number of different terms have been used to address painful symptoms that are not considered fully explicable on the basis of physical findings. At the simplest level, CPS can be used to describe the symptoms and effects of chronic pain. In this usage, the term is defined essentially by a time parameter, time course and a range of effects (e.g. on function). There is no particular imputation regarding the nature of the symptoms themselves. Usually, however, in using the term CPS one infers that aspects of the symptoms are psychological in nature, and either have a psychosomatic origin predating the injury in question or are indicative of a type of 'psychological injury' that is attributable to the accident. As has been suggested previously (Main & Spanswick 1995), the term 'functional overlay' is often used simply as a diagnosis of exclusion, since it is assumed ipso facto that if the symptom pattern is not considered fully explicable on the basis of the underlying physical characteristics, then it must be psychologically mediated. Such an assumption is unsafe unless psychological factors have specifically been investigated.

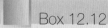

Box 12.12

Purpose of psychological evaluation

- Detection of specific psychological injury (such as a diagnosable psychiatric disorder (e.g. DSM-IV)
- Determination of a psychologically mediated pain syndrome
- Evaluation of the genuineness or veracity of the client.

We recommend that where clear psychological influences have been identified, the term 'psychologically mediated pain syndrome' is preferred to CPS. Where no such influences can be identified, and the persistence of the pain has not been explained, the issue may amount to taking a view about the credibility of the pain complaint, about which a forensic rather than a clinical opinion may be required.

The nature of psychological and psychiatric opinion

In the majority of cases of personal injury, such as road traffic accidents, liability for the original accident may not be in dispute; but the key issue may be one of extended causation, i.e. the extent to which a *chronic* pain syndrome can be considered to be attributable to the accident in question. In such an evaluation, issues both of independent causation and the claimant's credibility may arise. The extent to which a psychologically mediated chronic pain syndrome should be classified as a psychiatric injury or not has been the subject of some debate. In considering such issues, it is important to consider the objectives for a medicolegal assessment. These are shown in Box 12.12.

Difficulties in clinical diagnostics can lead to problems in assessment of 'condition' in medicolegal contexts. Historically, 'psychological injury' was defined in terms of identifiable psychiatric disorder, and although 'pain and suffering' were explicitly identified in terms of grounds for compensation, they were not recognised as an injury as such. The DSM-IV (1994) recommends differentiation of *Somatoform Disorder* from *Pain Disorder*, and states:

An additional diagnosis of Pain Disorder should be considered only if the pain is an independent focus of clinical attention, leads to clinically significant distress or impairment, and is in excess of that usually associated with the other mental disorder (p. 461).

Most personal injury claimants on which an expert psychological opinion is sought would be considered to have a Pain Disorder rather than a non-pain-related mental illness.

According to Shapiro & Teasell (1998); there already exists a diagnosis in DSM-IV which is not considered as a mental disorder but is consistent with a biopsychosocial conceptualisation of chronic pain, i.e. *Psychological Factors affecting a General Medical Condition*, the criteria of which are shown in Box 12.13.

In summary, psychiatric diagnostic criteria are not particularly helpful in elucidating the psychological features associated with chronic pain. However, these problems are of more than academic significance. If chronic pain and pain-associated incapacity cannot be explained in terms of physical signs or structural damage; and if the presenting problem is a chronic pain syndrome rather than a diagnosable mental illness, it could be argued that the claimant has not sustained a recognised injury and therefore is not entitled to be compensated. If on the other hand it is accepted that chronic pain is a genuine medical condition, characterised primarily by psychological and behavioural dysfunction, and frequently with equivocal physical signs, then assessment of injury by a psychologically competent pain specialist becomes the appropriate basis for the medicolegal case.

Arriving at a psychological opinion therefore, is a complex task involving the integration of a number of different clinical dimensions. The major focus may rest less on the origin of the pain (which in the case of specific accidents may be relatively unambiguous), and more on the nature of the injury and the components of the resultant incapacity. In arriving at an overall opinion it is therefore necessary to integrate a range of perspectives. Each component of the psychological opinion should if possible be clearly appraised before any attempt is made to integrate the opinion. Although at times problematic in terms of quantification of 'injury', in a proportion of patients, the litigation process itself can have a significant influence on the manner and content of symptom presentation.

The context of deception and malingering

Halligan et al (2003) offer a range of circumstances (including personal injury litigation) in which health-related deception may occur. They are shown in Box 12.14. The list makes interesting reading in that it can thus be seen that when viewed through a long lens, there are many types of deception, which are probably viewed by the general public with varying degrees of opprobrium. It will be suggested later that malingering can be located on a dimension ranging from inconsistency in behaviour at one end to fraud at the other. Robinson (2003), in reflecting from a sociological perspective upon malingering, particularly in the context of *Paid Sickness Absence (PSE)* and *Pensionable Early Retirement (PER)* has identified a number of societal

Box 12.13

DSM-IV criteria for psychological factors affecting a general medical condition

- A general medical condition is present
- Psychological factors adversely affect the medical condition in one of the following ways:
  - the factors have influenced the course of the general medical condition as shown by a close temporal association between the psychological factors and the development or exacerbation of, or delayed recovery from, the general medical condition
  - the factors interfere with the treatment of the general medical condition
  - the factors constitute additional health risks for the individual
  - stress-related physiological responses precipitate or exacerbate symptoms of the general medical condition.

Reproduced from Shapiro & Teasell (1998, p. 26)

Box 12.14

Examples of health-related deception

- Health insurance fraud
- Prescription fraud
- Medical competency
- Personal injury compensation
- Medical collusion and attorney coaching
- Sickness absence
- Early retirement due to ill-health.

> ### Box 12.15
>
> **Societal features which influence the incidence of malingering**
>
> - Cultural and legislative framework that recognises the existence of relevant debilities
> - Chances of malingering increased for those debilities which are simply social constructions, those with quantitative rather than qualitative symptomatology, and those with uncertain uncontrollability
> - Authorised gatekeepers must find it easier to allow false claims than deny real ones
> - Should be minimum post-decision checking and no sanctions for recoveries
> - Acceptability of such conduct by subcultures will encourage false claims and foster the belief that elites and those in authority are feathering their own nests inappropriately.

> ### Box 12.16
>
> **Challenges in detecting dissimulation of pain**
>
> - Understanding patient objectives in seeking health-care consultation
> - Frequent absence of physical pathology that could explain complaints and symptoms
> - Misguided concerns about functional/psychological overlays
> - Validity of self-report as an index of subjective states
> - Distinction between pain experience and pain expression
> - Necessity of establishing conscious intent to dissemble.
>
> From Craig & Badali (2004)

features which influence the incidence of malingering. These are shown in Box 12.15.

He concludes 'since all these conditions can be found in contemporary Britain it is not surprising that malingering in PSA and PER is widespread' (p. 132). Deception and malingering, however, does not appear to be confined to injured or sick people. Wynia (2003) investigates US physicians' deception of insurers to help their patients; a theme developed further by Locascio (2003) in his analysis of malingering among medical providers of disability-related programmes.

Deception

The nature of deception

According to Craig & Badali (2004), in varying degrees, all contacts between people include at least some appraisal of the other person's competence, sincerity and credibility, and

> *Deception is a generic term describing a broad range of social actions ranging from culture specific conformity and impression management to lying and exploitative dishonesty. The former can be positively sanctioned and maintain positive social interactions, whereas the latter can lead to criminal charges and almost invariably are regarded as morally reprehensible (p. 377).*

They are evident early in childhood (Talwar & Lee 2002) and occur throughout the animal kingdom (Byrne & Stokes 2003). Craig & Badali (2004) have identified a number of challenges in detecting dissimulation of pain. They are shown in Box 12.16.

The disjunction between pathology and pain poses a particularly difficult problem. Thus it has been estimated that up to 85% of individuals who report low-back pain have no discernible pathology (AMA 2000). In commenting on clinicians who find themselves faced with a patient reporting pain for which they cannot identify sufficient physical pathology to provide an explanation, they may seek refuge in pseudopsychological formulations and thus 'avoid the social consequences of charging patient with deception or malingering, but do signal that practitioners are suspicious and are prepared to attribute the source of the complaints to selfish motives' (Craig & Badali 2004, p. 379). Accusations of deception or malingering are, of course, serious matters.

Malingering

The nature of malingering

Malingering has been defined as 'the willful, deliberate and fraudulent feigning or exaggerating of the symptoms of illness or injury, done for the purpose of a consciously desired end' (Dorland 1974). Wessley (2003) traces modern concepts of malingering to the development of social insurance legislation as a counter to socialism in Germany where 'between 1880 and 1900 German neurologists were apparently classifying about one third of cases of so-called functional nervous diseases as due to malingering' (p. 33). The subsequent beginnings of the welfare state in Britain and development of the physician as a medical gatekeeper sanctioning entry to benefits can thus be seen as a part of a 'moral crusade'. Wessley continues:

> It was the physician's duty to stem the flood of idleness and deceit unleashed by the new legislation. The detection of malingering was thus a semi-class war, with the workman assumed to be trying to outwit the physician to gain money, and the physician standing to uphold the rights and resources of the state against this deception (p. 34).

Malingering does not have a clear place within the psychiatric pantheon, for although it is included among a number of conditions that might be 'a focus of clinical attention' it is not classified as a mental disorder in either the DSM-IV (DSM-IV-TR 2000) or in the ICD-10 (ICD 1992).

Mendelson & Mendelson (2004) draw attention to an interesting survey of orthopaedic surgeons and neurosurgeons by Leavitt & Sweet (1986) who found that although 60% of the respondents considered that malingering was relatively infrequent and occurred in less than 5% of patients, 10% of the respondents considered that malingering occurred in more than 25% of cases and one surgeon estimated the frequency of malingering as 75%. Perhaps, in the attribution of malingering, we learn more about the assessor than the patient.

Having viewed a range of methods for the evaluation of malingered pain (including questionnaires, clinical examination, facial expression, mechanical testing, differential spinal blocks, thermography and amytal/pentothal administration) Mendelson & Mendelson (2004) conclude:

> Malingering defined as the simulation of disease is not a medical or psychiatric diagnosis but a legal finding that must be based on the facts presented to the appropriate tribunal, jury or judge (p. 430).

Approaches to the detection of malingering are reviewed earlier in this chapter.

Exaggeration

The nature of exaggeration

In chronic pain assessment, consideration of 'malingering' should be concerned primarily not with the

Box 12.17

Assumed equivalences in the judgement of 'mismatch'

- Accident and injury
- Injury and damage 'physical signs'
- Signs and symptoms
- Symptoms and limitations (disability)
- Disability and work compromise.

detection of fraud as such, or with the identification of primary diagnosable psychiatric disorder, but with an appraisal of the extent to which there is evidence of *exaggeration* in the presentation of symptoms. There are difficulties both in the identification and in the interpretation of exaggeration.

Difficulties in the identification of exaggeration in the context of chronic pain

There are three general difficulties for the medicolegal assessors in the assessment of exaggeration.

1 There are wide variations in symptoms, disability and work compromise which cannot be accurately predicted from injury or supposed damage.

2 Disability and work compromise are multiply determined.

3 Psychosocial factors are far more important than physical factors in the development of chronic disability.

A competent assessment of all these facets would seem to be beyond the competence of most medicolegal assessors, but the law requires a medical opinion nonetheless. It may be helpful therefore to see exaggeration from a slightly different perspective in terms of firstly the problem of 'mismatch'. Legally the term 'exaggeration' doesn't imply *intent* as such; but some sort of mismatch is implied. Attribution of mismatch, however, implies an underlying set of fundamental equivalences, as shown in Box 12.17.

Clinical research, in contrast, has demonstrated a wide range of variation amongst these facets of illness and dysfunction. Indeed, arguably, one of the most important factors in the move from the pathology-based medical model to the biopsychosocial model of illness was recognition of the poor correlation between

Box 12.18

General approach to the evaluation of exaggeration

- Identification
- Consideration of description and validity
- Postulated mechanisms
- Clinical interpretation and explanation
- Implications for forensic judgement.

symptoms, signs and the development of pain-associated disability (Waddell 1998).

General approach to the evaluation of exaggeration

The general approach to evaluation of exaggeration is summarised in Box 12.18.

Identification

The manner and context in which evidence of exaggeration has been obtained should be carefully considered in terms of alternative explanations.

Consideration of description and validity

The actual assessment should be based on careful measurement, wherever possible relying on validated tools with an acceptable scientific pedigree and acceptable in legal contexts. Suspected inaccuracy in measurement should be highlighted and described in simple terms.

Consideration of mechanisms

In a medicolegal assessment, the assessor should determine whether the 'over-reaction' is mediated by distress, is based on misunderstandings about pain, hurt and harming or has become part of a 'learned behaviour pattern'. (In arriving at such an assessment the assessor may be guided by standardised psychometric assessment in addition to clinical history and symptom presentation.)

Clinical interpretation and explanation

Reference should be made to the expert's familiarity with the clinical condition, drawing attention to the specific features of the claimant's history which are typical or untypical of patients with the condition, and of those involved in litigation.

Box 12.19

Key questions in interpretation of exaggeration

- Evidence of inconsistency suggestive of exaggeration?
- Type of misrepresentation:
  - Amplification or minimisation?
- Intentionality:
  - Deliberate or unconscious?
  - If deliberate, what is the intent?
- Purpose:
  - Is it with the intent to convince or to deceive?

Implications for forensic judgement

The evidence should be presented without prejudice in an endeavour to assist the court in arriving at a view about the exaggeration.

Difficulties in the interpretation of exaggeration

A particularly difficult feature of clinical assessment is the ascription of motive to the claimant. It is trivially true that all claimants in prosecuting a claim have an interest in outcome, whether financial or in terms of redress for a perceived injustice. In a minority of cases, the prime mover behind litigation appears to be a third party, such as a relative or representative. If there appears to be evidence of exaggeration, however defined, the first question is whether or not the exaggeration is intended or deliberated. It is not possible at this juncture to enter into extended debate about conscious or unconscious processes, but it would certainly seem to be the case that a proportion of claimants are unaware that they have been inconsistent in their self-report, and that deliberate exaggeration may be offered as an explanation for this inconsistency.

Viewed simplistically, mismatch might be taken de facto as evidence of exaggeration. There are, however, a number of important issues in the interpretation which need to be addressed. They are shown in Box 12.19.

Evidence of inconsistency suggestive of exaggeration

Without convincing evidence of some sort in inconsistency in clinical presentation, in stated or observed pain-associated limitations or in extent of work capability, the question of exaggeration may not be raised. It is important at the outset, however, to be clear about the basis of the alleged (or identified) exaggeration before further clarification is sought.

Type of misrepresentation

There are a number of ways in which the term exaggeration is used. Although usually used to describe *amplification* of symptoms, or pain-associated incapacities, it may also be used in the sense of *minimisation* of previous health problems, thereby potentially enhancing the specific impact of the accident in question.

Intentionality

If it seems that there is a case to answer in terms of identifiable exaggeration (however defined), the question of *intent* arises. Is the exaggeration deliberate (i.e. with conscious intent) or unconscious? This may be a critical issue as far as the court is concerned and perhaps therefore merits some further reflection.

Deliberate exaggeration

What do we make of deliberate exaggeration? Is it simply a clinical correlate of malingering? Claimants may exaggerate for different reasons. Taking a robust view, all such deliberate exaggeration might be viewed as deceit. A distinction can, however, be made between 'exaggeration with the intent to convince' and 'exaggeration with the intent to deceive'. In what circumstances might the former arise? As for example when the claimant is convinced that they are not being believed, whether as a consequence of the reaction of family, of workmates, of health-care personnel or of previous medicolegal assessors. In extreme cases, they may discover they have been the subject of videotape surveillance. *If* they perceive themselves as having a genuinely disabling chronic condition, they may believe they have to exaggerate to convince the assessor of their genuineness.

It could be argued of course that deliberate exaggeration, of whatever nature, is deceitful and casts trenchant doubt on the entire claim. On the other hand, it is easy to understand how in the morass of medicolegal assessment a claimant can become confused and make errors of judgement. Should deliberate exaggeration be established, however, it is a matter for the court rather than the expert witness to take a view on it.

Unconscious exaggeration

It may be difficult to explain inconsistency in terms of genuine variation in clinical symptomatology. Clinically,

chronic pain patients frequently present as distressed, disaffected or confused, and may appear to exaggerate. They may be bemused also not only about the persistence of their pain, but also about the medicolegal process itself.

Perhaps 'unconscious exaggeration' is a contradiction in terms and the term 'over-reaction' would be preferable (although use of this term also carries a danger of ascribing motive rather than just describing mismatch or inconsistency).

Purpose of misrepresentation

If it appears that deliberate exaggeration has occurred it is relevant to ask a further question. Is it exaggeration with the intent to *convince* or exaggeration with the intent to *deceive?*

Exaggeration with the intent to convince

Thus, a strong history of iatrogenic confusion/distress and previous insinuations of faking or malingering are likely to strengthen the conviction of the claimant that they need to convince the expert witness of the genuineness of their symptoms. Specific investigation of the psychological impact of both their previous treatment, and of the impact of the medicolegal process may be illuminating in this regard.

Exaggeration with the intent to deceive

This is a serious state of affairs and must have positive evidence to support it, rather than be assumed because of the lack of alternative evidence. Such a formulation may lead to a finding by the court of fraud or malingering. If the expert witness can find no explanation for the exaggeration, he/she should say so.

Deception, malingering and exaggeration: some concluding reflections

In order to seek redress for injury, suffering and pain-related compromise, a claimant has to establish that a tort (negligent act) has occurred and the resulting symptoms or incapacities are a consequence of it. The burden of proof is on the claimant, and in the case of chronic pain problems the claimant's account is a core part of the evidence. The defendant equally has the right to defend the claim and the detection of malingering is an important facet of defence. To the extent that the claimant is reliant on self-report, the veracity of the claimant may become a central part of the case.

It has been argued in this chapter that in cases of personal injury, while completely fabricated or feigned symptoms (true malingering) is probably relatively rare, apparent inconsistencies in symptom presentation are commonplace. The proper role of the expert witness is to assist the court in the identification and description of the evidence germaine to their specific professional expertise. Adjudication per se properly is a matter for the court.

It has also been argued that inconsistencies per se therefore are not inherently suspicious but have to be understood as a consequence of inevitable imprecision in the attempted mapping of work compromise on to pain-associated limitations, on to symptoms, on to physical impairment and on injury sustained in the accident in question. Some suggestions have been made about how the expert witness might approach the identification and assessment of these factors.

Conclusion

There is now considerable consensus that chronic pain and pain-associated incapacity need to be understood within a biopsychosocial perspective. In this chapter particular attention has been directed at the influence and impact of economic factors, of which the medicolegal context has been identified as particularly complex.

Disentangling of the complexity of psychological and social forces on the individual with incapacitating pain can be a daunting task, since the individuals themselves may not be fully aware of the influences that have shaped their beliefs, emotions and behaviour. In terms of pain management, however, economic factors must be addressed as potential obstacles to recovery. Individuals may need to make some difficult choices as far as their futures are concerned. It must be recognised that failure to assess and understand the powerful influence of economic factors affecting symptom presentation and recovery will lead to ineffective or inappropriate treatment, thus contributing to the distress and chronic incapacity which pain management is designed to ameliorate.

Key points

- Chronic pain, pain-associated incapacity and work disability represent a massive cost to society in terms of costs of health care, benefits and lost productivity
- There are a number of factors which influence the economic impact on the individual of inability to work
- Adverse economic factors can influence not only an individual's health and well-being but also their acceptance of and response to treatment
- Chronic pain patients may seek redress following painful injury
- Without a 'no-fault' compensation system, the claimant will have to adduce evidence of injury
- Both the nature of the injury and its credibility may be challenged
- As a consequence, involvement in litigation may be extremely stressful in its own right
- Assessment of the psychological component in chronic pain following personal injury is a complex task, very different in nature from a routine clinical assessment
- Economic factors can have an impact on the perception of pain, adjustment to it and response to treatment
- With chronic pain patients, such factors need to be carefully evaluated before clinical decisions are made
- It cannot be assumed that such factors influence all patients equally and patients should be assessed on an individual basis.

References

AMA 2000 Guides to the evaluation of permanent impairment, 5th edn. American Medical Association, Chicago, IL

Arbisi P A, Butcher J N 2004 Psychometric perspectives on detection of malingering and pain: use of the Minnesota Multiphasic Personality Inventory – 2. Clinical Journal of Pain 20:383–391

Aylward M 2003 Origins, practice and limitations of disability assessment medicine. In: Halligan P, Bass C, Oakely D (eds) Malingering and illness deception. Oxford University Press, Oxford, ch 22, pp 287–300

Aylward M 2004 Personal communication

Backcare 2005 http://www.backpain.org/pdfs/backfacts-UK-2005.pdf

Belsey J 2002 Primary care workload in the management of chronic pain: a retrospective study using a GP database to identify resource implications for UK primary care. Journal of Medical Economics 5:39–52

Ben-Shaker G, Furedy J J 1990 Theories and applications in the detection of deception. Springer-Verlag, New York

Bogduk N 2004 Diagnostic blocks: a truth serum for malingering. Clinical Journal of Pain 20:409–414

Byrne R W, Stokes S 2003 Can monkeys malinger? In: Halligan P, Bass C, Oakely D (eds) Malingering and illness deception. Oxford University Press, Oxford, ch 4, pp 54–67

Chatterji M, Tilley C J 2002 Sickness, absenteeism, presenteeism and sick pay. Oxford Economic Papers 54:669–687

Collie J 1913 Malingering and feigned sickness. Edward Arnold, London

Craig K D, Badali M A 2004 Introduction to the special series on pain deception and malingering. Clinical Journal of Pain 20:377–382

De Paulo B M, Lindsay J J, Malone B E et al 2003 Clues to deception. Psychology Bulletin 129:74–118

Dorland 1974 Dorland's illustrated medical dictionary, 25th edn. W B Saunders, Philadelphia, PA

DSM-IV 1994 Diagnostic and statistical manual of mental disorders, 4th edn. American Psychiatric Association, Washington, DC

DSM-IV-TR 2000 Diagnostic and statistical manual of mental disorders, 4th edn. American Psychiatric Association, Washington, DC

DWP 2005 Department for Work and Pensions. http://www.dwp.gov.uk/asd/asd1/ib_sda/ib_sda_feb05_rounded.xls

Employers' Health Coalition 2000 Healthy people/ Productivity Survey 1999 (restricted access)

Faust D 1995 The detection of deception. In: Weintraub M I (ed) Neurologic clinics, malingering and conversion reactions. W B Saunders, Philadelphia, pp 255–265

Fishbain D A Cutler R B, Rosomoff H L et al 2004 Is there a relationship between nonorganic physical findings (Waddell signs) and secondary gain/malingering? Clinical Journal of Pain 20:399–408

Frederick R I 2003 Neuropsychological tests and techniques that detect malingering. In: Halligan P, Bass C, Oakely D (eds) Malingering and illness deception. Oxford University Press, Oxford, ch 25, pp 323–335

Greene R L 1997 Assessment of malingering and defensiveness by multiscale personality inventories. In: Rogers R (ed) Clinical assessment of malingering and deception, 2nd edn. The Guilford Press, New York, ch 9, pp 169–207

Halligan P W, Bass C, Oakley D A 2003 Willful deception as illness behaviour In: Halligan P W, Bass C, Oakley D A (eds) Malingering and illness deception. Oxford University Press, Oxford, ch 1, pp 3–28

Helmes E, Reddon J R 1993 A perspective on developments in assessing psychopathology: a critical review of the MMPI, MMPI-2. Psychology Bulletin 113:453–471

Iacano W G, Patrick C J 1997 Polygraphy and integrity testing. In: Rogers R (ed) Clinical assessment of malingering and deception, 2nd edn. The Guilford Press, New York, ch 13, pp 252–281

ICD-10 1992 The ICD-10 Classification of mental and behavioural disorders. Clinical descriptions and diagnostic guidelines. Geneva, World Health Organisation

Keller L S, Butcher J N 1991 Assessment of chronic pain patients with the MMPI-2. MMPI-2 monographs. University of Minnesota Press, Minneapolis, MN

Kennedy F 1946 The mind of the injured worker: its effects on disability periods. Compensation Medicine 1:19–21

Kitchen 2004 Investigating benefit fraud and deception in the United Kingdom. In: Halligan P, Bass C, Oakely D (eds) Malingering and illness deception. Oxford University Press, Oxford, ch 24, pp 313–322

Leavitt F, Sweet J J 1986 Characteristics and frequency of malingering among patients with low back pain. Pain 25:357–364

Locascio J 2003 Malingering, insurance medicine and the medicalisation of fraud. In: Halligan P W, Bass C, Oakley D A (eds) Malingering and illness deception. Oxford University Press, Oxford, ch 23, pp 301–310

Main C J 1999 Medicolegal aspects of pain: the nature of psychological opinion in cases of personal injury. In: Gatchel R J, Turk D C (eds) Psychosocial aspects of pain. Guilford Press, New York, ch 9, pp 132–147

Main C J 2003 The nature of chronic pain: a clinical and legal challenge. In: Halligan P, Bass C, Oakely D (eds) Malingering and illness deception. Oxford University Press, Oxford, ch 13, pp 171–183

Main C J, Spanswick C C 1995 'Functional overlay' and illness behaviour in chronic pain: distress or malingering? Conceptual difficulties in medico-legal assessment of personal injury claims. Journal of Psychosomatic Research 39:737–753

Main C J, Waddell G 1998 Behavioural responses to examination: a re-appraisal of the interpretation of 'non-organic signs'. Spine 23:2367–2371

Main C J, Wood P L R, Hollis S, Spanswick, C C, Waddell C 1992 The distress assessment method: a simple patient classification to identify distress and evaluate risk of poor outcome. Spine 17: 42–50

Mandiakis N, Gray A 2000 The economic burden of back pain in the UK. Pain 84:95–103

Mendelson G 1988 Psychiatric aspects of personal injury claims. Thomas, Springfield, IL

Mendelson G 2003 Outcome-related compensation. In: Halligan P, Bass C, Oakely D (eds) Malingering and illness deception. Oxford University Press, Oxford, ch 17, pp 220–231

Mendelson G, Mendelson D 2004 Malingering pain in the medicolegal context. Clinical Journal of Pain 20:423–432

Miller H 1961 Accident neurosis. British Medical Journal I: 919–925

Phillips C P, Main C J Aylward M et al 2006 Putting the pain in policy making. (submitted)

Robinson M E, Dannecker E A 2004 Critical issues in the use of muscle testing for the determination of sincerity of effort. Clinical Journal of Pain 20:392–398

Robinson W P 2003 The contemporary cultural context for deception and malingering in Britain. In: Halligan P W, Bass C, Oakley D A (eds) Malingering and illness deception. Oxford, Oxford University Press, ch 10, pp 132–143

Shapiro A P, Teasell R W 1998 Misdiagnosis of chronic pain as hysteria and malingering. Current Review of Pain 2:9–28

Spence S, Farrow T, Leung D et al 2003 Lying as an executive function. In: Halligan P W, Bass C, Oakley D A (eds) Malingering and illness deception. Oxford University Press, Oxford, ch 20, pp 256–266

Sullivan M 2004 Exaggerated pain behavior: By what standard? Clinical Journal of Pain 20:433–439

Talwar V, Lee K 2002 Emergence of white-lie telling in children between 3 and 7 years of age. Merrill Palmer Quarterly 48:160–181

Vrij A, Mann S 2003 Deceptive responses and detecting deceit. In: Halligan P W, Bass C, Oakley D A (eds) Malingering and illness deception. Oxford University Press, Oxford, pp 348–362

Waddell G 1998 The back pain revolution. Churchill Livingstone, New York

Waddell G 2004 The back pain revolution, 2nd edn. Churchill Livingstone, New York

Waddell G, McCulloch J A, Kummel E et al 1980 Non-organic signs in low-back pain. Spine 5:117–125

Wessley S 2003 Malingering; historical perspectives. In: Halligan P W, Bass C, Oakley D A (eds) Malingering and illness deception. Oxford University Press, Oxford, ch 2, pp 31–41

Wynia M K 2003 When the quantity of mercy is strained: US physicians' deception of insurers for patients. In: Halligan P W, Bass C, Oakley D A (eds) Malingering and illness deception. Oxford University Press, Oxford, ch 15, pp 197–206

Chapter Thirteen

13

Psychological perspectives on work

Historical perspective

Early attempts in scientific management focused primarily on work efficiency and the division of labour. Essentially, work was simplified and standardised, leading to the design of repetitive and monotonous jobs within which skill variety was a minimum and workers had no control over the work processes. As the workforce became more educated, however, individuals aspired to better working conditions and job design theorists began to incorporate human performance factors, including individual needs. Herzberg (1974), in developing *job enrichment theory*, distinguished 'intrinsic' factors relating to the work conditions (such as degree of control, relationships and skill development) from 'extrinsic' factors (such as financial rewards or benefits and the physical environment).

Hackman & Oldham (1976) similarly, in their *job characteristics theory*, advocated the view that specific characteristics of the job (such as skill variety, task significance and autonomy) in combination with individual characteristics (such as growth need strength) would determine personal and work outcomes. Finally, Davis (1980), in his development of *sociotechnical systems theory*, recommended a 'flattened' management structure that would promote participation, interaction between and across groups of workers, enriched jobs, and, most important, meeting individual needs. According to Carayon & Lim (1999), this theory offers the foundation for current understandings of the relationship between social and technical factors. Thus although certain 'objective' work characteristics can be distinguished from 'perceived' work characteristics, different work organisations will produce very different psychosocial work factors, and so these factors need to be understood within specific contexts.

Stress and work

The nature of work stress

The nature of work stress has been a major focus of research. It has been implicated as a cause of sickness absence, and, by implication, as a potential obstacle to return to work, particularly important in the context of recovery from injury (whether considered in terms of work rehabilitation or work retention).

Smith & Carayon-Sainfort (1989) in the *balance theory of job design*, identified five elements of the work system which interacted to produce a 'stress load' (Box 13.1). According to this theory, psychosocial factors are multiple and diverse.

The principal psychosocial work factors and their facets suggested by Carayon & Lim (1999) are shown in Box 13.2. They stress that such factors need to be understood in the context of societal changes in the economic, social, technological, legal and physical environments.

Specific models of work stress (adapted from Cox 1993)

Cox (1993) identifies three different, but overlapping approaches to the definition and study of stress. His three major models are shown in Box 13.3.

According to the 'engineering' model, stress is conceptualised as an aversive or noxious characteristic of the work environment and is construed essentially as an environmental *cause* of ill-health. The model has been criticised on the grounds of oversimplicity, since specific stimuli such as noise may be stressful or beneficial depending on a number of other factors.

Box 13.1

Elements of the work system producing 'stress load'

1 The individual
2 Tasks
3 Technology and tools
4 Environment
5 Organisational factors.

Box 13.2

Selected psychosocial work factors and their facets

1 Job demands
- Quantitative workload
- Variance in workload
- Work pressure
- Cognitive demands.

2 Job content
- Repetitiveness
- Challenge
- Utilisation and development of skills.

3 Job control
- Task/instrumental control
- Decision/organisational control
- Control over the physical environment
- Resource control
- Control over workplace: machine-pacing.

4 Social interactions
- Social support from supervisor and colleagues
- Supervisor complaint, praise, monitoring
- Dealing with (difficult) clients/customers.

5 Role factors
- Role ambiguity
- Role conflict.

6 Job future and career issues
- Job future ambiguity
- Fear of job loss.

7 Technology issues
- Computer-related problems
- Electronic performance monitoring.

8 Organisational and management issues
- Participation
- Management style.

Carayon & Lim (1999, Table 15.2, p. 278)

Box 13.3

Major models of stress

- The 'engineering' model
- The 'physiological' model
- The 'psychological' model.

In the 'physiological' model, stress is defined in terms of the physiological *response* to a threatening or dangerous environment. This model has been criticised because of differences in physiological responses to the same stressor, and difficulties in identifying unambiguously responses which are specifically stress responses (rather than orienting responses for example).

Both models have been criticised for ignoring individual differences in the cognitive and perceptual processing of information, and ignoring the interactions between the individual and his/her environment and organisational *contexts* of work stress.

Finally, in a third model, the 'psychological' model, stress is conceptualised in terms of the *dynamic interaction* between the person and their work environment. Lack of fit, whether defined objectively or subjectively (in terms of the individual's perceptions) has been recognised as a potential stress (French et al 1974).

In such 'transactional' models, stress involves elements of both cognition (such as appraisal) and emotion. The appraisal process may be thought of in five stages, beginning with no more than a hazy recognition of the existence of a problem, and leading via an *ongoing* process of interaction between coping strategies, reappraisal and redefinition of the problem.

According to Cox (1993):

> The experience of stress is therefore defined, first, by the realisation that they are having difficulties in coping with demands and threats to their well being and, second, that coping is important and the difficulty in coping depresses or worries them (p. 17).

Coping with occupational stress

Stress affects people differently. Whether or not they become ill appears to depend to a considerable extent on what they think about the stressor and how they cope with it. Researchers have studied individual differences both in the way stressors are perceived and also the extent to which these appraisals might moderate the relationship between stress and health (Payne 1988). A number of characteristics of the psychological processes mentioned in the literature are shown in Box 13.4 for illustrative purposes. They are addressed in much more detail elsewhere (Griffiths 1998).

As can be seen, a wide range of work organisational characteristics have been associated with stress and ill-health and musculoskeletal disorders, but they are confounded with physical work load (Bongers et al 1993, Vingård & Nachemson 1999, Davis & Heaney 2000); most studies to date have been unable to quantify either their individual importance or specific interactions. Nevertheless, the available evidence provides most support for influence of the factors shown in Box 13.5 (Bongers et al 1993, Vingård & Nachemson 1999), and it seems that workers' reactions to psychosocial

Box 13.4

Psychological features associated with poor health and well-being

- Working under time pressures
- Having too much or too little to do
- Monotonous tasks and too little variety
- Long working hours
- Poor communication systems
- Organisational change
- Lack of understanding of organisational structure or goals
- Lack of participation in decision making
- Lack of control (e.g. over work methods, pace or work environment)
- Inadequate and unsupportive supervision
- Poor relationship with co-workers
- Bullying, harassment and violence
- Isolated or solitary work
- Job insecurity
- Career stagnation
- Lack of recognition and feedback
- Unfair or unclear performance evaluation
- Being overskilled or underskilled for the job
- Unclear or conflicting roles
- Continuously dealing with other people's problems
- Conflicting demands of work and home.

From Griffiths (1998, pp. 217–218)

Box 13.5

Work organisational factors most clearly associated with occupational stress/musculoskeletal disorders

- High demand and low control
- Time pressure/monotonous work
- Lack of job satisfaction
- Unsupportive management style
- Low social support from colleagues
- High perceived workload.

aspects of work may be more important than the actual aspects themselves (Davis & Heaney 2000), with stress acting as an intermediary (Bongers et al 1993).

Common sense would suggest that with such a wide variety of working circumstances and individual differences in the perception of work, that it would be inappropriate to try to develop a concept that encompassed all such factors within a single model. From a more general viewpoint, it would appear that negative appraisals associated with ineffective coping strategies appear to be lead to frustration, even anger, and to significant work stress, deterioration in health and absence from work. In the context of musculoskeletal injury, however, there appears to have been specific research neither into the appraisal of stress at work nor into strategies specifically for coping with stress at work.

Conclusion: what lessons can be learned from the occupational stress literature?

The occupational stress literature has been important in the identification of adverse features of the working environment. Many different organisational characteristics have been associated with ill-health, sickness absence or impaired productivity. Certain characteristics of the working environment appear to constitute risk factors in their own right, but it seems that *perceptual* factors may be even more important than objective characteristics. Most jobs have irritating, difficult or stressing features which can be thought of as risk factors for sickness or ill-health. Individuals, however, vary in their reaction to difficult circumstances or adversities, and the extent to which a specific individual copes with such risk factors will influence job satisfaction, morale and psychological well-being. The principal lessons from the occupational stress literature are shown in Box 13.6.

In recovery from musculoskeletal injury, an adverse view of work may become an additional obstacle to return to work.

Traditional perspectives on musculoskeletal symptoms and injury

Traditionally, occupational prevention and rehabilitation has focused primarily on biomechanics, ergonomics and the reduction of risk. Identification of psychological features of work, and in particular the relationship between work stress and ill-health, does not appear

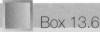

Box 13.6

Lessons from the occupational stress literature

- Aspects of work can have an adverse psychological impact in terms of stress
- Work stress can adversely affect health and lead to sickness absence
- A number of the key influences on health have been identified
- Coping styles and strategies may mediate or moderate the relationship between work stress, ill-health and work absence
- Perception of work may be more important than actual working conditions or characteristics
- There has, however, been no systematic research into the relationship between occupational stress, musculoskeletal symptomatology and recovery from injury.

to have had a significant influence on the management of musculoskeletal symptoms or in the management of injury.

Biomechanical and ergonomic perspectives

Burton (1997) has highlighted an apparent contradiction in the way in which occupational injury is viewed and managed:

On the one hand, ergonomists and biomechanists strive to reduce physical stress in the work place with the intent of lowering the risk of musculoskeletal problems, while clinical scientists and psychologists are suggesting not only that psychological factors are important, but that rehabilitation of the back-injured worker should involve physical challenges to the musculoskeletal system (p. 2575).

This dilemma illustrates not only a management problem, as Burton asserts, but also illustrates a fundamental conflict in models of injury. At the heart of the debate lies the nature of mechanisms of chronicity.

The basic 'injury/damage' model is based on the commonly held view that physically demanding work is detrimental to the back in the sense that it can cause injury through sudden or cumulative trauma, and the injury in turn leads to pain and disability. Much clinical and non-clinical scientific research has been directed at the nature of injury and the possible underlying mechanisms. There are have been many variants on the basic themes, but in the field of occupational injury, the primary focus has been on biomechanical analysis of the physical stresses sustained during various movements or postures under various conditions of load. It might appear that there ought to be a direct relationship between the physical demands of work and the occurrence of injury, but in fact there are significant inconsistencies in the scientific literature (Burton & Main 2000a).

Certainly there is evidence of increased risk of work-related disorders affecting the back, neck and upper limbs with certain types of work, but not all workers become injured, and certainly not all become significantly disabled. Marras et al (1993) found that risk of musculoskeletal symptoms could be predicted from a combination of five trunk motion and workplace risk factors, but since not all jobs with high injury rates require the same physical abilities (Halpern 1992), the relationship between these risk factors and actual injury is not straightforward.

There is, however, evidence that many workers *perceive* their musculoskeletal symptoms to be work-related. In one UK Survey (Jones et al 1998) of individuals reporting musculoskeletal symptoms, nearly 80% identified a work task, or set of tasks, as leading to their complaint. The evidence seems to show that the back can certainly be injured in various ways (whether at work or leisure), but the 'injury model' is not able to explain the wide variation in resultant disability.

The primary focus of the biomechanical and ergonomic perspective has been on prevention. There have been energetic attempts to improve the working environment, with ergonomic redesign, to reduce the risk of injury. Most ergonomic interventions focus on strategies to reduce spinal loading, but the only intervention which has been formally evaluated has been worker training in manual handling techniques. Occupational guidelines for manual handling designed to constrain task performance to within safety limits of lifting and handling, have been produced. It appears that while lifting techniques can be improved, it has not been possible to demonstrate a corresponding reduction of injury rates (Smedley & Coggan 1994). The explanation for the lack of success in preventing injury is perhaps not all that surprising. According to Burton (1997), although epidemiological studies can link the occurrence of initial back pain with certain physical stressors (such as spinal loading and physical usage), there is little evidence that the symptoms are due to irreversible damage to spinal structures. Furthermore, there is increasing evidence

that recurrence and disability are mediated by psycho-social phenomena such as the perception of comfort and the ability to cope (Hadler 1997).

In a recent review of the available evidence, Burton et al (1998) concluded:

The possible role of ergonomics for reducing recurrence rates seems at best equivocal, but there is no convincing evidence that continuation of work is detrimental in respect of disability. It is likely that much back pain is only work-related in as much that people of working age get painful backs. It is becoming clear that reducing spinal loads or awkward postures is likely to have only a small impact on the overall pattern of back pain. Non-biomechanical approaches (organisational and social) seemingly are more effective in maintaining ability to work (p. 1134).

Risks of work-related illness and injury

Identification and management of risk factors for work-related disability will be addressed specifically in Chs 14 and 15, but a brief review of the development of modern approaches is relevant at this juncture. Much of the emphasis on primary prevention of injury has relied on epidemiological studies which have addressed principally anthropomorphic and physical risks factors, with a heavy biomechanical and ergonomic emphasis. This specific focus on primary prevention has perhaps hindered proper analysis of the mechanisms of recovery from injury, many of which seem to be psychosocial rather than biomechanical or ergonomic. Recognition, particularly in North America, of the increasing costs of long-term disability led to investigations into its predictors and a number of researchers examined a wide range of presenting characteristics in an effort to find predictors of chronicity.

In a prescient review of risk factors in industrial low-back pain, Bigos et al (1990) implicated four major types of risk factors in industrial low-back pain (Box 13.7). In their view, methodological problems significantly compromised accurate evaluation of these factors, but recognition of the importance of addressing individual and workplace factors on the one hand, and both physical and psychological factors on the other, is consistent with the 'systems approach' we recognise later in this book.

Similarly, and contemporaneously, Cats-Baril & Frymoyer (1991), in a study of employees with between 2 and 6 weeks' work compromise, identified four main risk factors for long-term disability (Box 13.8). Job

Box 13.7

Four major risk factors in industrial low-back pain

- Individual factors (mainly demographic and anthropomorphic)
- Physical findings (mainly radiographic)
- Workplace factors (including various work characteristics)
- Psychological factors (determined from psychological tests or evidence of substance abuse).

Box 13.9

Specific psychological factors predicting return to work

- Lower pain severity
- Pain drawing scores
- Higher treatment satisfaction
- Higher cooperativeness during treatment
- Lower levels of hypochondriasis
- Distrust/stubbornness
- Depression
- Pre-morbid pessimism.

Box 13.8

Four major risk factors for long-term disability

- Job characteristics
- Aspects of job satisfaction
- Clinical history
- Educational level.

characteristics considered important were: work status at time of the survey, past work history and type of occupation. The important elements of job satisfaction comprised pre-retirement policies and benefits, perception about whether the injury was compensable, who was at fault and whether a lawyer had been contacted.

However, the utility of their predictive model was criticised on methodological grounds specifically because of their failure to control for duration of disability, and because of the likely influence of psychological factors in terms of expectation (Lehmann et al 1993):

> *The population of patients who have already incurred two weeks of off-work time secondary to low back trouble probably are anticipating long-term disability, and, perhaps more importantly, so are their health care providers, employers, and insurers. These expectations may trigger illness behaviours that help establish long-term disability* (p. 1110).

The criticism, although appropriate, seems a little harsh. Research design in such studies is significantly problematic, and it is only recently that research guidelines have been systematised (Linton et al 2005).

Psychological features of work

Specific psychological features have been investigated in more detail in a number of other studies in the 1990s. Carosella et al (1994) found that patients with low return-to-work expectations and heightened perceived disability, pain and somatic focus, had problems complying with an intensive work rehabilitation programme. Haazen et al (1994) have shown that change in distorted pain cognitions, worker's compensation status and use of medication were the most important predictors in behavioural rehabilitation of low-back pain (they were, however, pessimistic about the overall level of prediction achieved). The above studies, although tantalising, do not identify the putative psychological factors with sufficient degree of accuracy to evaluate their specific importance.

Feuerstein et al (1994) categorised variables predicting return to work by 1 year into five categories: medical history, demographics, physical findings, pain and psychological indices.

The specific psychological factors identified by them in different studies are shown in Box 13.9.

In addition to these clinical psychological variables, Feuerstein & Huang (1998) grouped the factors associated with delayed recovery into medical, ergonomic and psychosocial (although they did not subclassify the latter specifically into clinical and occupational perceptions). Feuerstein & Zastowny (1999) did, however, recognise that in occupational rehabilitation the psychological problems specifically associated with job stress and work re-entry should be specific targets for psychological intervention (in addition to the usual clinical targets).

Finally, in two controlled studies, a large difference in prevalence of musculoskeletal disorders in Dutch and Belgian nurses was explained not by workload, or attribution of work as a cause, but by attitudes to work and depressive symptoms (Burton et al 1997). In another study, Burton et al (1996), in a comparison of musculoskeletal complaints among police in Northern Ireland and in Manchester (UK), found that the proportion of officers with persistent (chronic) back complaints did not depend on length of exposure to physical stressors, but to psychosocial factors such as distress and blaming work.

According to an influential review by Bongers et al (1993):

> Monotonous work, high perceived work load, and time pressure are related to musculoskeletal symptoms. The data also suggest that low control on the job and lack of support by colleagues are positively associated with musculoskeletal disease. Perceived stress may be an intermediary in the process (p. 297).

It would seem that there is now overwhelming evidence that psychosocial factors influence musculoskeletal symptomatology and effect on work. Studies have been carried out in a wide range of settings, with varying degrees of precision and differences in measurement tools. The studies have offered evidence in the form of statistical associations between a range of psychosocial variables, work performance and illness characteristics. In an attempt to integrate some of these findings, consideration will now be given specifically to the psychological effects of work absence and on recovery from injury.

The psychological effects of work absence

Stress, especially if prolonged, is likely to lead to ill-health or sickness absence. Absence from work, however, is in itself a risk factor for further absence and delayed recovery. Extended absence from work can have a marked effect on the perception of the work environment. Interpersonal relationships at work for example may be an important determinant of successful return to work. Good relationships with colleagues, a sense of being valued, and worry about letting one's colleagues down, may act as important incentives to return to work after injury; while an unpleasant or difficult interpersonal environment may represent a significant obstacle to return to work. The specific effect of these absences as a result of physical injury can have an even more marked effect since the individual may

be anxious about coping not only with the stressful work environment but also with the physical demands of work. Appraisal of such factors, combined with a loss of self-confidence and anxiety about not being able to perform satisfactorily on return to work may also represent a specific hindrance.

A clinical perspective on chronic incapacity and recovery from injury

Recent clinical studies into the outcome of treatment for low-back pain have, however, offered a more specific evaluation of the role of different sorts of psychological variables in the prediction of chronic incapacity (as determined by self-reported disability) than is currently available in most occupational studies. The findings of such studies for the understanding of the nature and development of chronic incapacity may have relevance also to secondary prevention in occupational settings. Examples of these studies will now be reviewed.

In a study of attitudes, beliefs and absenteeism among workers in a biscuit factory, Symonds et al (1996) showed that workers who had taken in excess of 1 week's absence due to low-back trouble had significantly more negative attitudes and beliefs (when compared with workers who had taken shorter absences, or with those who reported no history of back trouble). Beliefs about the inevitability of back pain, fears of hurting or harming and perceived disability were significantly associated with absenteeism. In an associated study (Symonds et al 1995), introduction of a psychosocial pamphlet, designed to correct mistaken beliefs about back pain (e.g. confusing hurting with harming) and reduce avoidance behaviour, successfully reduced extended sickness absence resulting from low-back trouble.

It is clear from these studies that there is a fair degree of consensus about the sort of factors which appear to affect recovery from incapacity in occupational settings, but there does not seem to be a conceptual framework within which to encompass the diverse and specific research findings.

Occupational factors and recovery from injury: a conceptual framework

Recognition of the considerable costs of work-related incapacity has spurred considerable effort directed at the identification of risk factors associated with chronic incapacity. Although many of the studies have been able to quantify the relative risk of a range of factors in association with poor outcome, frequently they have had to rely upon the information which has been available and have not included standardised or validated assessment tools. Studies have frequently offered little more than a series of estimates of the specific importance of each of the variables with little attempt to examine their influence on each other or locate their findings within an overall theoretical framework. While undoubtedly it is important to identify characteristics associated with chronic incapacity, not all such risk factors are targets for intervention, and the risk ratios in many of the epidemiological studies are too low to inform clinical or management decision making in the individual case.

In the context of pain management, the focus needs to be on the identification more specifically on *obstacles to recovery*. Despite the acknowledged methodological weaknesses in many of the studies, the general picture is clear. Certain working conditions and adverse work characteristics place an individual at increased risk of ill-health and associated absence from work. These occupational features, in the context of individual vulnerabilities or additional external stressors, may lead to impaired performance and work absence. In the context of injury, they may delay recovery and return to work. It is within this framework that the importance of clinical and occupational features now will be considered. Initiatives in the field of non-specific low-back pain will be used to illustrate this new perspective.

Flags and obstacles to recovery from an occupational perspective

The development, description and use of red, orange and yellow flags has already been presented in previous chapters. It is important to recognise that the yellow flags (Kendall et al 1997) were developed not only from a clinical perspective but also from an occupational perspective and consisted of both psychological and socio-occupational risk factors. This is also evident in the behaviour management guidelines reproduced in Box 13.10.

Further conceptual development

In tackling obstacles to recovery, whether from the perspective of actual clinical management or occupational rehabilitation, it seems necessary, however, to distinguish concerns that the individual has about their personal well-being from specific concerns about work. It was decided therefore to subdivide the yellow flags into

> **Box 13.10**
>
> **Behaviour management guidelines**
>
> 1 Provide a *positive* expectation that the individual will return to work
> 2 Be directive in scheduling regular reviews of progress
> 3 Keep the individual active and at work
> 4 Acknowledge difficulties of daily living
> 5 Help maintain positive cooperation
> 6 Communicate that having more time off work reduces the likelihood of successful return
> 7 Beware of expectations of 'total cure' or expectation of simple 'techno-fixes'
> 8 Promote self-management and self-responsibility
> 9 Be prepared to say 'I don't know'
> 10 Avoid confusing the report of symptoms with the presence of emotional distress
> 11 Discourage working at home
> 12 Encourage people to recognise that pain can be controlled
> 13 If barriers are too complex, arrange multidisciplinary referral.

clinical yellow flags and occupationally focused blue flags (Main & Burton 1998, Burton & Main 2000b).

The occupational component of the original New Zealand yellow flags focused on the perception of work, but in terms of obstacles to recovery, it is necessary to make a distinction also between two types of occupational risk factors. They can be thought of as factors concerning the *perception* of work (blue flags) and objective work characteristics (black flags). This distinction is similar to the distinction between *intrinsic* and *extrinsic* factors by Herzberg (1974), and with differentiation between Type-I (worker-centred) and Type-II (workplace or system-centred factors) (Sullivan et al 2005) but with a focus on obstacles to recovery, i.e. potential targets for a some sort of biopsychosocial intervention. These perspectives are explored in depth in Chapters 14 and 15.

Blue flags

The blue flags have their origin in the stress literature reviewed above. They are *perceptions* of work which are generally associated with higher rates of symptoms, ill-health and work loss which in the context of injury may delay recovery, or constitute a major obstacle to it. They

Box 13.11

Possible reasons for failure of work retention programmes

- In general, we have failed to distinguish adequately between risks for chronicity, modifiable risk factors and obstacles to recovery
- More specifically, we have failed to understand that sustained work retention or rehabilitation of the individual may require addressing both clinical and occupational obstacles to recovery
- Finally, even the most sharply focused intervention designed to remove the relevant yellow and blue flags may fail as a consequence of insuperable obstacles in the form of black flags.

are characterised by features such as high demand/low control, unhelpful management style, poor social support from colleagues, perceived time pressure and lack of job satisfaction. Individual workers may differ in their perception of the same working environment.

A large number of factors in the literature could be termed blue flags, and a definitive typology has not as yet been developed. The most useful grouping to date seems to be that of Carayon & Lim (1999) outlined above in Box 13.2. The first five factors: job content (perception of), perceived job demand, job control, job role (particularly clarity and conflict) and social interactions (with supervisor and workmate) could reasonably be described as types of blue flag. (Further work on classification of both the blue and black flags currently is underway.)

Bigos et al (1990) opined that perception may be more important than the objective characteristics since:

Once an individual is off work, perception about symptoms, about the safety of return to work, and about impact of return to work on one's personal life can affect recovery even in the most well-meaning worker (p. 184).

This was confirmed in a recent evaluation of the HSE 'stress tool' in the UK, when individual's *perceptions* of work (i.e. blue flags) were more powerfully associated than objective work characteristics with both sickness absence and self-rated performance (Main et al 2005).

Black flags

Black flags are *not* a matter of perception, and affect all workers equally. They include both nationally established

policy concerning conditions of employment and sickness policy and working conditions specific to a particular organisation. They are described in detail in Chapter. 15.

The need for an integrated approach to obstacles to recovery

There are in our view several major reasons that we have been so unsuccessful in work retention and in rehabilitation following musculoskeletal dysfunction. Some of the principal reasons are outlined in Box 13.11.

Conclusions and preliminary recommendations

The incorporation of the principles of pain management into work retention and work rehabilitation are discussed fully in Chapters 14 and 15, but it is important at this juncture to recognise the need for an integrated conceptual framework linking assessment and management. During the last two decades, the powerful influence of psychosocial factors has been demonstrated. Early studies into the psychological components have been followed by investigations into the influences of economic and occupational factors on the perception of pain and development of disability. Disentangling of the complexity of psychological and social forces on the individual with incapacitating pain is frequently a daunting task, since the individual themselves may not be fully aware of the influences which have shaped their beliefs, emotions and behaviour. In terms of pain management, however, occupational factors must be considered not only as potential obstacles to recovery, but also as potential targets for intervention and opportunities for change.

Failure to assess and understand the powerful influence of occupational factors affecting symptom presentation and recovery will lead to ineffective or inappropriate treatment, thus contributing to distress and chronic incapacity which pain management is designed to ameliorate.

We believe that our previous recommendations (Burton & Main 2000b) for the assessment and management of occupationally related musculoskeletal disorders still have merit in terms of specifics; they are reproduced in Box 13.12.

However, in Chapters 14 and 15 we have attempted to update the findings from more recent studies into the identification and management of pain-related work disability, developing a sharper focus on different types of intervention, at both an individual and organisational level.

Box 13.12

Recommendations for assessment and management of occupationally related musculoskeletal disorders

- Recognise that the workers' perception of their work is fundamental to understanding recovery from injury
- Understand the inherent risks in certain occupational environments for producing extended sickness absence and delayed recovery after injury
- Facilitate a system for early reporting of musculoskeletal symptoms to appropriately trained personnel
- Identify mistaken beliefs about the nature of pain, hurting/harming and unnecessary fears of prolonged injury, and recognise other psychological characteristics of the individual (yellow flags)
- Identify aspects of work perceived to be problematic by the injured worker (blue flags)
- Distinguish yellow flags and blue flags from lack of motivation to work
- Provide a psychosocial preventative approach to the individual, promoting self-help, establishing confidence and reducing unnecessary apprehension
- Facilitate return to work as soon as possible; restricted duties (if required) should be brief and time-limited. Maintain management of the worker within the occupational environment so far as is possible.

From Burton & Main (2000b)

References

Bigos S J, Battie M C, Nordin M et al 1990 Industrial low back pain. In: Weinstein J, Wiesel S (eds) The lumbar spine. W B Saunders, Philadelphia, pp 846–859

Bongers P M, de Winter C R, Kompier M A J et al 1993 Psychosocial factors at work and musculoskeletal disease. Scandinavian Journal of Work and Environmental Health 19:297–312

Burton A K 1997 Back injury and work loss: biomechanical and psychosocial influences. Spine 22:2575–2580

Burton A K, Main C J 2000a Relevance of biomechanics in occupational musculoskeletal disorders. In: Mayer T G, Gatchel R J, Polatin P B (eds) Occupational musculoskeletal disorders. Lippincott Williams and Wilkins, Philadelphia, ch 10, pp 157–166

Burton A K, Main C J 2000b Obstacles to recovery from work-related musculoskeletal disorders. In: Karwowski W (ed) International encyclopaedia of ergonomics and human factors. Taylor and Francis, London, pp 1542–1544

Burton A K, Tillotson K M, Symonds T L et al 1996 Occupational risk factors for first onset of low back trouble: a study of serving police officers. Spine 21:2612–2620

Burton A K, Symonds T L, Zinzen E et al 1997 Is ergonomic intervention alone sufficient to limit musculoskeletal problems in nurses? Occupational Medicine 47:25–32

Burton A K, Battie M C, Main C J 1998 The relative importance of biomechanical and psychosocial factors in low back injuries. In: Karwowski W, Marras W S (eds) The occupational ergonomics handbook. CRC Press, Boca Raton, FL, ch 61, pp 1127–1138

Carayon P, Lim S-Y 1999 Psychosocial work factors. In: Karwowski W, Marras W (eds) The occupational ergonomics handbook. CRC Press, Boca Raton, FL, ch 15, pp 275–283

Carosella A M, Lackner J M, Feuerstein M 1994 Factors associated with early discharge from a multidisciplinary work rehabilitation program for chronic low back pain. Pain 57:69–76

Cats-Baril W L, Frymoyer J W 1991 Identifying patients at risk of becoming disabled because of low-back pain: The Vermont Rehabilitation Engineering Center predictive model. Spine1 6:605–607

Cox T 1993 Stress research and stress management: putting theory to work. HSE Books, Sudbury, Suffolk

Davis K G, Heaney C A 2000 The relationship between psychosocial work characteristics and low back pain: underlying methodological issues. Clinical Biomechanics 15:389–406

Davis L E 1980 Individuals and the organisation. California Management Review 22:5–14

Feuerstein M, Huang G D 1998 Preventing disability in patients with occupational musculoskeletal disorders. American Pain Society Bulletin 8:9–11

Feuerstein M, Zastowny T R 1999 Occupational rehabilitation: multidisciplinary management of work-related musculoskeletal pain and disability. In: Gatchel R, Turk D C (eds) Psychological approaches to pain management: a practitioner's handbook. Guilford Press, New York, pp 458–485

Feuerstein M, Menz L, Zastowny T R et al 1994 Chronic back pain and work disability: vocational outcomes following multidisciplinary rehabilitation. Journal of Occupational Rehabilitation 4:229–251

French J P R, Rogers W, Cobb S 1974 A model of person-environment fit. In: Coehlo G W, Hamburg D A, Adams J E (eds) Coping and adaptation. Basic Books, New York

Griffiths A 1998 The psychosocial work environment. In: McCaig R, Harrington M (eds) The changing nature of occupational health. HSE Books, Sudbury Suffolk, ch 11, pp 213–232

Haazen I W C J, Vlaeyen J W S, Kole-Snidjers A M K et al 1994 Behavioral rehabilitation of chronic low back pain: searching for the predictors of treatment outcome. Journal of Rehabilitation Science 7:34–43

Hackman J R, Oldham G R 1976 Motivation through the design of work: test of a theory. Organisational Behaviour and Human Performance 16:250–279

Hadler N M 1997 Back pain in the workplace. What you lift or how you lift matters far less than whether you lift or when. Spine 22:935–940

Halpern M 1992 Prevention of low back pain: basic ergonomics in the workplace and clinic. In: Nordin M, Vischer T L (eds) Common low back pain: prevention of chronicity. Bailliere Tindall, London, pp 705–730

Herzberg E 1974 The wise old turk. Harvard Business Review Sep/Oct:70–80

Jones J R, Hodgson J T, Clegg T et al 1998 Self-report of work-related illness in 1995. HSE Books, Sudbury, Suffolk

Kendall N A S, Linton S J, Main C J 1997 Guide to assessing psychosocial yellow flags in acute low back pain: risk factors for long term disability and work loss. Accident Rehabilitation and Compensation Insurance Corporation of New Zealand and the National Health Committee, Wellington, NZ

Lehmann T R, Spratt K F, Lehmann K K 1993 Predicting long term disability in low back injured workers presenting to a spine consultant. Spine 18:1103–1112

Linton S J, Gross D, Schultz I Z et al 2005 Prognosis and the identification of workers risking disability: research issues and directions for future research. Journal of Occupational Rehabilitation 15:457–474

Main C J, Burton A K 1998 Pain mechanisms. In: McCaig R, Harrington M (eds) The changing nature of occupational health. HSE Books, Sudbury Suffolk, ch 12, pp 233–254

Main C J Glozier N, Wright I A 2005 Validation of the HSE Stress Tool: an investigation within four organisations by the Corporate Health and Performance Group (CHAP). Occupational Medicine 55:208–214

Marras W S, Lavender S A, Leurgans S et al 1993 The role of dynamic three-dimensional trunk motion in occupationally related low back disorders: the effects of workplace factors, trunk position and trunk motion characteristics on injury. Spine 18:617–628

Payne R 1988 Individual differences in the study of occupational stress. In: Cooper C L, Payne R (eds) Causes, coping and consequences of stress at work. Wiley and Sons, Chichester

Smedley J, Coggan D 1994 Will the manual handling regulations reduce the incidence of back disorders? Occupational Medicine 44:63–65

Smith M J, Carayon-Sainfort P 1989 A balance theory of job design for stress reduction. International Journal of Industrial Ergonomics 4:67–79

Sullivan M J L, Feuerstein M, Gatchel R J et al 2005 Integrating psychosocial and behavioral interventions to achieve optimal rehabilitation outcomes. Journal of Occupational Rehabilitation 15:475–489

Symonds T L, Burton A K, Tillotson K M et al 1995 Absence resulting from low back pain can be reduced by psycho-social intervention at the workplace. Spine 20:2738–2745

Symonds T L, Burton A K, Tillotson K M et al 1996 Do attitudes and beliefs influence work loss due to low back trouble? Occupational Medicine 22:2612–2620

Vingård E, Nachemson A 1999 Work related influences on neck and low back pain. In: Nachemson A, Jonsson E (eds) Swedish SBU report. Evidence based treatment for back pain. Swedish Council on Technology Assessment in Health Care (SBU), Stockholm (English trans: Lippincott, Philadelphia)

Chapter Fourteen

14

Pain and work: individually focused interventions

Introduction

The case for tackling pain-associated work limitations in terms of costs to the individual and society has already been made. A review of clinically focused interventions has already been offered in Chapters 10 and 11. It is relevant at this juncture to make three general observations.

Firstly, the focus of this chapter will be on Type I (worker-focused) interventions (Sullivan et al 2005a), having the individual worker as the prime focus of intervention. In the next chapter we shall adopt a more organisational perspective considering primarily the Type II (system- or organisation-focused) interventions. However, since organisational changes should of course impact on the individual the distinction may seem somewhat arbitrary, but the nature of the interventions is rather different.

Secondly, adopting the 'flag' terminology, although a major focus of this chapter will be on blue flags (i.e. perceptions of work) as potentially modifiable risk factors for sickness absence or prolonged disability, since by definition black flags have been defined as 'system' obstacles to return to work (RTW) or optimal function, it will be argued in the next chapter that, taking a 'systems approach', black flags may in fact become opportunities for change and thereby could be said to fall within the general framework of work retention or work rehabilitation.

Thirdly, some clarification of our use of the term 'work rehabilitation' is appropriate. For convenience, we include rehabilitation into work of those already off sick as well as efforts to prevent work absence in the first place, considering initiatives often subsumed under the category of 'prevention of work disability', but we also make mention of the problem of 'presenteeism', both in terms of condition-specific underperformance at work, and also more generally in terms of influences on suboptimal performance, but this will be discussed more specifically in Ch. 16. In this regard we are adopting a broader definition of 'rehabilitation' than Waddell & Watson (2004).

The nature of clinical and occupational rehabilitation

Research studies have demonstrated that disability is multifactorial and that chronic disability needs to be understood within a biopsychosocial framework. In occupational settings, interventions have been based primarily on biomedical or ergonomic principles, but investigations into predictors of outcome have shown that the specific influence of psychosocial factors may be more important than has been previously recognised. Furthermore, clinical studies into the psychosocial mechanisms associated with the development of chronic incapacity (or failure to recover after musculoskeletal injury) appear to indicate a real opportunity for the design of interventions targeted specifically at prevention. Rehabilitation per se is usually considered to fall within the remit of the health services, but in occupational settings there would appear to be considerable potential benefit in adopting a biopsychosocial perspective towards both work rehabilitation and work retention. Waddell & Watson (2004) offer a synthesis of the main principles of rehabilitation, in which occupational components are clearly in evidence (Box 14.1).

Inconsistency in terms of definition and boundary is confusing, and such clarification is helpful, but in attempting to provide an overreaching framework, there is a danger of underestimating the importance of variation in focus, objectives and outcomes which appears to characterise the literature. The primary outcome measures of existing interventions are usually: work retention (or prevention of work disability), reduction in sickness absence days/costs and RTW rates. However, because of this variety of methods and concepts in such interventions, and a lack of defined successful outcomes, there are few substantial conclusions of what works, on whom and when (Krause et al 1998).

Clinical interventions and RTW

Clinical interventions (Chs 9, 10 and 11) can help reduce pain, reduce distress, enhance pain coping strategies and increase function. For some patients/employees, an individualised pain management intervention

Box 14.1

Principles of rehabilitation

Key principles
- Good clinical management is fundamental
- The primary goal for patients and health care is pain relief, but
- For patients who do not recover quickly, health care alone is not enough.

The three components of rehabilitation
- Reactivation and progressive increase in activity levels
- Address dysfunctional beliefs and behaviour
- An occupational component or setting.

In addition
- Patient, health professional(s), and employer must communicate and work together to common agreed goals
- Identify and address obstacles to return to work
- The main goal is job retention and (early) return to work.

Delivery
- Timing
- Setting
- Organisational/policy framework
- Culture of rehabilitation and return to work.

Outcome
- The measure of successful rehabilitation is sustained return to regular work.

Waddell & Watson (2004, p. 396, Box 18.2)

from a health-care professional may be all that is needed to enable the symptomatic worker to remain at work or enable the individual to return to work. Many of the early pain management programmes were funded in order to get people back to work, since the costs of work disability were so high, a modest success rate in terms of overall outcomes from such programmes was nonetheless cost-effective and seen therefore as a satisfactory return on investment (ROI). Such funding arrangements, however, are vulnerable to changes in market forces, such as the costs of health care and the availability for work. The focus and content of such programmes usually is on function rather than work per se. As will be discussed below, it seems that multidisciplinary programmes that include psychosocial pain management interventions are more effective in reducing work disability than programmes that do not include psychosocial interventions but there is little evidence of clinical programmes dealing specifically with occupational obstacles to recovery.

There are many ways of clustering interventions. In this chapter, for convenience, more clinically focused approaches such as exercise, physical therapy and pain management will precede consideration approaches such as back schools, functional restoration programmes and work modification, and will conclude with examples of some recent RTW initiatives in the UK. Finally, more recent approaches to secondary prevention of work disability, including the specific targeting of risk factors, will be addressed.

Exercise and physical therapy

Individual physical therapy is often offered following injury in an effort to assist return to work. Many physiotherapeutic modalities are fairly passive in nature and little is required of the patient, but recommendation of specific exercises and attempts at reactivation offer an approach to rehabilitation that involves *active* participation. 'Prescription' of exercise and activity is sometimes used in conjunction with specific physical therapy (such as manipulation and mobilisation).

Cherkin et al (1998) compared physical therapy, chiropractic manipulation and the use of an educational booklet for the treatment of patients with low-back pain, and found no significant differences amongst the groups in the numbers of days of reduced activity, in missed work or in recurrences of back pain. Additionally, in a review of four types of intervention including back and aerobic exercises, Lahad et al (1994) concluded that there was limited evidence to recommend exercise to prevent low-back pain in asymptomatic individuals. However, evidence exists suggesting that, when combined with other approaches, exercise may be very beneficial. For example, Lindstrom et al (1992) found that a graded activity programme coupled with a behavioural approach encouraging patients to return to work through operant techniques returned patients to work 5.1 weeks earlier on average than the patients in the control groups.

A clear and direct focus on activity clearly has intuitive appeal. Outcome, however, is frequently evaluated in terms of some sort of functional criterion such as attainment of an acceptable level of functioning. In occupational settings, 'acceptability' may be defined in terms of how well an individual performs a set of tasks. Indeed rehabilitation may have been tailored to the individual in this respect. If recovery of function were determined solely by functional attainment, then results of such specifically focused rehabilitation might be more impressive. As mentioned in previous chapters, however, back injury claims and RTW are influenced by

Box 14.2

Efficacy of exercise programmes

- Rehabilitation can reduce pain and increase activity levels, regardless of the type of exercise used to engage the patient in the rehabilitation process
- Specific physical exercises can produce specific physical and psychological effects
- Improvements in specific physical performance measures do not predict improvement in disability and return to work
- Programmes involving intense physical exercise are no more effective than those that involve moderate exercise
- Exercise programmes that also address psychosocial issues are likely to be more effective.

Adapted from Waddell (2004, p. 380)

psychosocial as well as biomechanical factors directed primarily at work content. Thus, aiming to increase function to perform a specific task at work as the sole criterion of success may not be adequately addressing the entirety of the problem.

A summary of the efficacy of exercise programmes is presented in Box 14.2.

Pain management programmes and RTW

As highlighted in previous chapters, multidisciplinary pain management programmes (PMPs) compare favourably with other approaches in the clinical rehabilitation of the chronic pain patient. PMPs were described in detail in Chapter 11, but for convenience their defining characteristics are reproduced in Box 14.3.

It may be of course that work-related goals are identified as targets for treatment, and general recovery of confidence in the management of pain may be important in tackling problems of work, but there is often no *explicit work focus* in such programmes. This may explain why although research reviews have found superiority for cognitive–behavioural programmes over other forms of treatment on clinical measures such as pain, pain coping strategies and pain behaviour, there is no clear evidence of significant effect on RTW (Morley et al 1999, Peat et al 2001, Van Tulder & Koes 2002). Thus it would seem that for chronic pain patients even comprehensive interdisciplinary pain management does not guarantee successful occupational outcomes.

There is, however, some encouragement for earlier intervention (or secondary prevention) in terms of occupational outcomes. Linton & Andersson (2000) developed a brief pain management programme, focused primarily on developing and practising coping skills, comprising six weekly 2-hour sessions. The content of the programme is shown in Table 14.1. Although there is some occupational focus in sessions 2 and 3, there is no specific reactivation or exercise component and such and no specific work interventions. The programme reduced the risk of long-term sickness absence ninefold in the following six months. In a population cohort of people with recurrent low-back pain, the programme produced a greater reduction in sickness over the following 6 months, in comparison with a control group (Linton & Ryberg 2001).

Finally, Marhold et al (2001) reduced future sick leave in patients with short-term absence, but not with long-term absence.

Occupational health services

In the UK, variants of occupational health provision have been available for more than a century, and it might be assumed that the development of occupational health services would offer an opportunity not only for

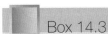

Box 14.3

Defining characteristics of PMPs

- Behavioural rather than a disease perspective
- Focus on pain management rather than cure
- Blend of ingredients
- Interdisciplinary skill-mix
- Incorporation of group therapy
- Emphasis on active rather than passive approaches to treatment
- Promulgation of self-help and patient responsibility
- Behavioural rather than a disease perspective.

Table 14.1 Linton's cognitive–behavioural programme		
Session	**Focus**	**Skills**
1	Causes of pain and prevention of chronic problems	Problem solving Applied relaxation Learning about pain
2	Managing your pain	Activities; maintaining daily routines Activity scheduling Relaxation training
3	Promoting good health; controlling stress at home and at work	Warning signals Cognitive appraisal Beliefs
4	Adapting for leisure and work	Communication skills Assertiveness Risk situations Applying relaxation
5	Controlling flare-ups	Plan for coping with flare-ups Coping skills review Applied relaxation
6	Maintaining and improving results	Risk analysis Plan for adherence

From Waddell (2004, Table 18.6, p. 382), with permission of Elsevier Ltd.

earlier intervention, but for a clearer 'occupational' component in the intervention. In practice, however, occupational health provision is extremely patchy, appears to be under recurrent financial pressure and appears to have an established role only with large employers. Even then, occupational health provision often seems to represent little more than clinical provision in an occupational setting and in the context of pain management is little different in content from what might be expected in a clinical setting. Indeed many occupational services are now 'outsourced' to independent health-care providers who offer a variety of health-care products and programmes for specific clinical conditions. (These issues are discussed further in Ch. 15.)

Interventions with a clear occupational focus

It must be admitted that a precise delineation between programmes with and without a specific work focus is somewhat hazardous since programmes are often not described in sufficient detail to identify the specific occupational component. Typical clinical interventions have already been described in the previous section. For convenience, the rest of the interventions will be subsumed under back schools (and other primarily educational approaches), functional restoration programmes (FRP), modified work (although the latter is also addressed in the next chapter) and recent RTW initiatives in the UK:

Back schools combine back pain education and strengthening exercises, and are a popular intervention technique. Back pain education can include topics related to back care: the structure and function of the spine, safe lifting, ergonomics, pain control and relaxation techniques (Brown et al 1992).

Functional restoration is based on quantitative measurement of physical and functional capacity, with a psychosocial assessment of barriers to recovery. It purports to offer a medically directed, interdisciplinary team in an individualised, intensive treatment programme to achieve specific socio-economic valued outcomes, namely RTW and work retention. Advocates of this approach state that it permits motivated, disabled individuals to reach their highest possible functional level (Garcy et al 1996).

Modified work recognises the individual's perceptions of function and limitation, and reorganises job duties accordingly. Types of modified work include: light duty, graded work exposure, work trial, supported employment and sheltered employment. This approach conveys a sense of understanding the psychosocial aspects of work and disability for work, as well as the physical and financial aspects (Yamamoto 1997), but also it may be a component of a phased RTW strategy required by the individual's employer (discussed further in Ch. 15).

RTW initiatives. Over the last decade in the UK, there has been a plethora of new initiatives for the management of back pain, instigated by a variety of agencies, but particularly at the instigation of the Department for Work and Pensions or DWP (and its predecessors).

Many rehabilitation programmes aiming to prevent low-back pain and unnecessary work disability employ variants of these methods, which although different in specific configuration nonetheless contain the essence of these approaches. Although their importance in overcoming this problem is not denied, evidence of such rehabilitation programmes to date shows limited success.

Back schools

Back schools and educational types of intervention are widely utilised in low-back pain rehabilitation, and are relatively easy to carry out in a workplace or clinical setting. However, demonstration of successful outcome may depend on what specific outcome is measured (i.e. RTW, work retention or a reduction of injury reporting). A study by Daltroy et al (1997) showed that over 5.5 years an educational programme designed to prevent low-back injury did not reduce the median cost per injury, the time off from work per injury, the rate of related musculoskeletal injuries or the rate of repeated injury after return to work; only the subject's knowledge of safe behaviour was increased by the training.

In a meta-analysis of the efficacy of back school programmes, Di Fabio (1995) concluded that back schools were most efficacious when coupled with a comprehensive rehabilitation programme. Efficacy was supported for the treatment of pain and physical impairments and for education/compliance outcomes, but work, vocational and disability outcomes were not improved significantly by either the comprehensive or the primary prevention back school programmes.

Back schools and educational programmes, in aiming to teach safe behaviour and knowledge of the mechanics of the back, contain the essentials of primary prevention. Primary prevention aims to prevent injury or reinjury, and implies that back pain can be avoided, which may not be true. An episode of low-back pain may be inevitable and is in itself fairly inconsequential; the problem lies with such episodes leading to low-back pain disability. As Hadler (1999) states, 'a year without at least one episode of backache is unusual for most people. Coping successfully is healthfulness' (p. 259). This suggests that, in order to address the factors that may lead to disability, recovery from musculoskeletal injury needs to be understood in the context of such individuals, their lifestyle and their beliefs.

Functional restoration

Mayer et al (1985) first advocated functional restoration, a derivative of a sports medicine approach (Mayer & Gatchel 1988) and in their approach to rehabilitation, focused on maximising functional ability. The objectives of their functional restoration programme were 'the restoration of joint mobility, muscular strength, endurance and conditioning, as well as cardiovascular fitness leading to restoration of the ability to perform specific functional tasks such as lifting, bending, twisting, and tolerance of prolonged static positioning'. They claimed not only that quantitative functional capacity measures could provide 'objective evidence' of patient abilities but, since consistency in data required maximal effort, could also thereby give a measure of 'effort'. Although primarily used for chronic rather than acute or subacute groups of patients, the approach deserves comment in the context of considering different approaches to occupational rehabilitation.

Mayer et al (1985) and Hazard et al (1989), in claiming respectively an 85% and 81% success rate in returning patients to work, have attracted methodological criticisms in their lack of proper control groups, and failure to include dropouts in the treatment groups (resulting in an overestimation of their success rates). A review of major studies of functional restoration was undertaken by Waddell (1998), who concluded, 'Functional restoration for chronic low back pain looks promising, but there is a lack of good evidence that it does actually return patients to work' (p. 363).

Functional restoration can be criticised also on conceptual grounds. Although it has the appeal of being an optimal, tailored intervention, which is designed to measure the individual's ability and capacities, an 'objective' intervention such as this does not incorporate explicitly the many important subjective factors involved in response to rehabilitation. Functional restoration makes the further claim that its focus on objectivity permits an appraisal of effort and motivation to recover. The approach has attracted interest by assessors attempting to identify malingerers. (In fact all that the 'objective' evaluation offers is a description of performance, which is determined by a wide range of subjective factors such as, for example, fears that activity may be harmful. The inferential leap therefore appears to be unwarranted.)

In conclusion, while the idea of a truly objective measurement that identifies clear deficits has obvious appeal, the apparent objectivity is illusory; what is obtained is a measure of *performance*, which is itself subject to a variety of influences. The worker's *perception* appears to be more influential than the actual work characteristics. In fact this was recognised in an early study by Magora (1973) who was one of the first to note that workers' perceptions about the nature of their jobs were critical factors in whether they recalled or reported back pain, and it seems that functional restoration or work hardening programmes yield better RTW outcomes when they include a cognitive–behavioural component (Schonstein et al 2004).

Nonetheless, in an update of the earlier review, Waddell & Watson (2004) concluded 'It is probably the best and most powerful *physical* approach ever devised for the rehabilitation of back pain. Yet, on critical examination, the evidence is that it does not achieve the goal of getting patients back to work' (p. 393).

Modified work

A more recent approach, which takes into account the importance of context as well as content of the job, has been the modification of the actual work. Although modified work is regarded by some as a breakthrough in the job rehabilitation process, little is known about the structure, effectiveness, and efficiency of such programmes.

In a systematic review of modified work and RTW literature, Krause et al (1998) concluded that modified work programmes facilitate return to work for both temporarily and permanently disabled workers. These authors also found that injured workers who are offered modified work then return to work about twice as often as those who are not; similarly, modified work programmes cut the number of lost work days in half. A possible reason for this reported success is that the approach aims at not only reducing workers' compensation costs, but also the financial, psychological and physical strain placed on workers when a disabling injury occurs.

Modified work also aims to facilitate an early return to work, with the opinion that intervening quickly will reduce the negative, potentially disabling effects of taking time away from normal lifestyle activities such as work. The idea of intervening quickly was studied by Hazard et al (1997) who stated that a quick identification of the small number of back-injured workers who become disabled would facilitate more efficient targeting. Other supporters of the early intervention are Yassi et al (1995), Sinclair et al (1997), Ryan et al (1995) and Galvin (1999) who all maintain that early assessment and timely rehabilitation would prevent further disability, restore optimal work capacity and reduce dependency on compensation benefits. Von Korff et al (1993) believe a critical period lies between 4 and 12 weeks after onset for an intervention to be successful, and Nachemson (1983) supports this by stating that adverse biological and psychosocial consequences compound the pain, and therefore should be addressed as soon as possible.

RTW initiatives

During the last decade, in the UK, there has been a particular focus on the management of low-back pain. Waddell (2004) provides an interesting summary of the major initiatives concerned (Table 14.2).

Since then there have been a number of further initiatives yielding major reports, including the Wales Health-Work Report (Main et al 2004), Screening of DWP for long-term incapacity (Waddell et al 2003), the IUA/ABI Working Party Report on Psychology, Personal Injury and Rehabilitation (IUA 2004), Obstacles to recovery from musculoskeletal disorders in industry (Burton et al 2005), work, health and wellbeing (Waddell & Burton 2006), and a report on case management (Hanson et al 2006), all of which address facets of the health–work interface.

It is clearly impossible within the constraints of this chapter to give details of all these reports. However, mention will be made of two specific initiatives from which some lessons perhaps can be learned.

The UK Back in Work initiative funded 18 small pilot studies to tackle back pain in the workplace. These pilots were widely varied in focus, content and manner of delivery, but Brown (2002) concluded that although there were some interesting new collaborations, there were no really innovative approaches, and despite satisfaction expressed by the health-care professionals and workers, the employers' reactions were more mixed and 'there is no evidence that any of the pilot schemes had any real impact on back pain, sickness absence, or long-term incapacity' (cited by Waddell 2004 p. 389).

However, another small study permits a degree of optimism. Watson et al (2004) designed an occupationally focused rehabilitation programme for unemployed benefit recipients with low-back pain as the stated reason for unemployment. The programme included clinical pain management, with a strong reactivation focus,

specific attention directed at both yellow and blue flags, establishment of job-seeking skills and assistance from a job placement adviser. The 84 participants had been symptomatic on average for 7 years, and out of work for an average of 38 months. Despite their apparent poor prognosis, 97% of those who started completed the programme, and at 6 months approximately 40% were employed, with a further 26% engaged in purposeful activity (job training, education or undertaking voluntary work). Further evaluations of this approach currently are under way.

Targeting risk factors for work disability

It is difficult to draw clear or confident conclusions from such a heterogeneous group of studies, with such varying contents in terms of interventions and with such disparate outcomes, particularly as far as work is concerned. Considered overall, however, it would seem therefore that clinical interventions for chronic pain patients may be necessary, but are unlikely to be sufficiently powerful to achieve sustained RTW for the majority of chronic pain sufferers. Once employees have been off work for a significant length of time, the obstacles to sustained RTW appear to increase in number and complexity. There are, however, some reasons for optimism. We know that PMPs can diminish certain of the clinical concomitants of chronic pain, the Watson et al (2004) study offers some optimism that a 'systems approach' may be successful, even in patients with long-established back disability, in returning them to employment, and the early intervention studies of Linton and his colleagues hold out promise in terms of early intervention (and secondary prevention).

Research highlighting the important role of psychosocial factors in pain and disability has prompted the development of intervention approaches designed to target psychosocial risk factors associated with musculoskeletal conditions. The following section, relying principally on our recent review (Sullivan et al 2005a) describes different psychosocial intervention programmes that have either been specifically designed to facilitate RTW, or have implications for RTW programmes. The primary focus is on secondary prevention.

The term cognitive–behavioural does not refer to a specific intervention, but rather to a range of intervention strategies (as outlined in Chs 9 and 10). The principal applications of such interventions are listed in Box 14.4. Interventions have included population health interventions (Buchbinder et al 2001), primary-care

Table 14.2 UK initiatives on clinical management and health services for back pain

Date	Source	Product	Reference
May 1994	Clinical Standards Advisory Group (CSAG)	Report on NHS services for LBP. Appendix: Management guidelines for LBP	CSAG (1994)
Jan 1996	Health Care Evaluation Unit	*Low Back Pain: An Evaluation of Therapeutic Interventions*	Evans & Richards (1996)
Sept 1996	Royal College of General Practitioners (RCGP: multidisciplinary)	Clinical guidelines for the management of acute LBP	
Sept 1996	The Stationery Office	*The Back Book* (a booklet for patients)	Roland et al (1996)
Feb 1999	Royal College of General Practitioners (multidisciplinary)	*Clinical Guidelines for the Management of Acute LBP*, 2nd edn	RCGP (1999) www.rcgp.org.uk
1999–2001	Joint Dept of Health (DoH)/Health and Safety Executive (HSE)	Back in Work pilot initiatives	DoH/HSE (2001)
Mar 2000	Faculty of Occupational Medicine	*Occupational Health Guidelines for the Management of Low Back Pain*	Carter & Birrell (2000), www.facoccmed.ac.uk
August 2000	Institute for Musculoskeletal Research and Clinical Implementation	Audit toolkit for acute back pain	Breen et al (2000) www.imrci.ac.uk
Oct 2000	HSE	European Week for Health and Safety at Work: Turn your back on musculoskeletal disorders *Back in work: managing back pain in the workplace:* a leaflet for employers and workers	HSE (2000): www.hse.gov.uk
	HSE/Health Education Board of Scotland	Launch of Working Backs Scotland campaign	www. working backsscotland.com
2002	National Institute for Clinical Excellence	Piloting guide on referral practice, based on RCGP guidelines	www.nice.org.uk
2002	RCGP Scottish Programme of Improving Clinical Effectiveness in primary care	GP quality improvement programme. Desk-top memo, recording, and audit system	www.ceppc.org/spicc
2002	NHS Modernisation Agency	National Back Pain Collaborative	www.modern.nhs.uk/ orthopaedics
2003	Dept for Work and Pensions (formerly Dept of Social Security)	Job retention and rehabilitation pilot schemes	

NHS, National Health Services; LBP; Low-back pain. From Waddell (2004, Table 19.5, p. 415), with permission of Elsevier Ltd.

Box 14.4

Principal applications of psychosocial risk factor targeting

- Population health interventions
- Primary care interventions
- Clinic-based cognitive–behavioural interventions
- Community-based cognitive–behavioural interventions.

interventions (Von Korff et al 1998), clinic-based cognitive–behavioural interventions (Linton et al 2006), and community-based cognitive–behavioural interventions (Sullivan & Stanish 2003, Sullivan et al 2005b).

Buchbinder et al (2001) developed an innovative programme based on a public information advertising campaign, which illustrated how attitudes and beliefs associated with work disability might be targeted on a broad scale, even before work injury occurs. For two and half years the Australian campaign, targeting the state of Victoria, was associated with a significant shift in societal attitudes toward injury and disability, and led to a decline in the number of compensation claims for back pain.

Most secondary prevention programmes have been implemented within the health-care system. There has been considerable emphasis placed on the role of the primary-care physician in the provision of what has been termed medical reassurance. Medical reassurance refers to communication from health-care providers aimed at correcting erroneous beliefs, reducing fear associated with pain symptoms, and encouraging return to an active lifestyle in spite of the persistence of pain symptoms. Current medical practice guidelines recommend providing patients with reassurance and clear advice about the importance of continuing their daily activities (Koes et al 2001). (The nature of reassurance in the context of GP interventions is discussed further in Ch. 9.)

However, reassurance has also been directed specifically at the reduction of work disability, and investigations support the effectiveness of reassurance and recommendations for self-management as a means of reducing the duration of work disability (Indahl et al 1998, Linton et al 1993).

Advice to stay active and information aimed at reducing fear can lead to significant reductions in sick days and higher RTW rates (Indahl et al 1998, Hagen et al 2003, Malmivaara et al 1995) but not all studies have supported the efficacy of brief medical reassurance/activity advice interventions. In one study, occupational physicians were provided with guidelines for early medical reassurance, but results 1 year later showed no

significant benefit when compared to a group receiving usual primary care (Verbeek et al 2002). Von Korff et al (2005) screened back pain patients for functional difficulties approximately 2 months after their initial visit. Those with significant functional problems were randomised to an activation–reassurance group or to a control group. Although the activation–reassurance group was more active and reported fewer functional limitations, there were no differences between the groups at the follow-up on disability compensation benefits.

As aforementioned, reviews of the literature indicate that multidisciplinary programmes that include psychosocial pain management interventions are more effective in reducing work disability than programmes that do not include psychosocial interventions (Crook et al 2005, Guzman et al 2004). Also, functional restoration or work hardening programmes yield better RTW outcomes when they include a cognitive–behavioural component (Schonstein et al 2004). These reviews support the utility of cognitive–behavioural approaches in the secondary prevention of work disability, but the unique contribution of cognitive–behavioural interventions is difficult to determine within the context of a multidisciplinary programme.

There have been efforts to develop cognitive–behavioural interventions that target psychosocial factors that are more directly linked to work disability. For example, van den Hout et al (2003) studied the effects of teaching problem-solving skills to back pain patients off work for less than 6 months. Patients were randomised to a group receiving graded activity training and education or to a group receiving graded activity and problem solving. Those receiving problem-solving skills training had better RTW outcomes. Marhold et al (2001) examined the effects of teaching specific RTW skills. Patients off work for an average of 3 months were randomised to a treatment-as-usual control group or a cognitive–behavioural group that included specific RTW skills training. Results demonstrated that participants who received RTW skills training had significantly less absenteeism at 1-year follow-up than did the treatment-as-usual control group.

An extensive discussion of screening was offered in Chapter 5, but further mention of it in the context of work disability is relevant at this juncture. Gatchel et al (2003) developed a statistical algorithm for differentiating acute low-back pain patients who were designated as either high or low risk for developing chronic disability. In one study, high-risk acute patients were randomly assigned to one of two groups: an early functional restoration group with a cognitive–behavioural approach or a treatment-as-usual group. Results showed that, relative to the treatment-as-usual group, the functional restoration group displayed significantly fewer indices of chronic pain disability on a wide range of work, health-care utilisation, medication use and self-reported pain variables.

Linton & Andersson (2000) also used a risk screening procedure to select patients for a secondary prevention intervention. They compared the effects of a 6-week cognitive–behavioural group intervention to two information-provision comparison groups for individuals who were identified as higher risk, based on their scores on the Örebro Screening Questionnaire for Pain (Boersma & Linton 2003). All groups showed comparable improvements in pain severity, mood and activity level. However, follow-up analyses showed that the cognitive–behavioural intervention led to a significantly lower probability of being on long-term sick leave compared to the two information groups.

More recently, Linton et al (2006) showed that participation in a cognitive–behavioural intervention was associated with greater reduction in work disability than guideline-based treatment-as-usual. Participants with short-term back pain in a primary-care setting who had higher-risk profiles on a screening instrument were selected for inclusion in the clinical trial. Participants were randomly assigned to one of three intervention conditions: (1) a standardised, guideline-based, treatment-as-usual condition, (2) a 6-week cognitive–behavioural group condition, or (3) the combination of a 6-week cognitive–behavioural group and physical therapy condition. The two groups receiving cognitive–behavioural interventions had fewer days off work for back pain during the 12-month follow-up than did the guideline-based treatment-as-usual group.

Other investigations have pointed to the potential benefit of matching intervention approaches to specific psychosocial risk profiles. In a programme of intervention developed by Vlaeyen et al (2002), individuals with high levels of pain-related fears are gradually exposed to activities that have been avoided with an approach similar to that which would be used for the treatment of phobic conditions, and a clinical trial has shown that this type of intervention can be effective in reducing levels of fear, pain and pain-related disability (George et al 2003).

Community-based intervention programmes, such as the Pain-Disability Prevention (PDP) Program, have also been developed to specifically target certain psychosocial risk factors (Sullivan & Stanish 2003). The intervention is currently provided by a network of trained psychologists widely distributed in various regions of four Canadian provinces. By adding a psychosocial component to usual care (medical care and physiotherapy), the objective is to create virtual multidisciplinary teams at the community-based level. Individuals are selected for treatment if they obtain elevated scores (above the 50th percentile) on risk factors addressed by the intervention programme (pain catastrophising, fear of movement/reinjury, perceived disability and depression). The PDP Program is a standardised 10-week intervention that uses structured activity-scheduling strategies and graded activity involvement to target risk factors such as fear of movements/reinjury and perceived disability. Thought-monitoring and cognitive-restructuring strategies are used to target catastrophic thinking and depression. A preliminary study yielded encouraging results with 60% of PDP-treated clients returning to work, compared to an 18% base rate of return. A recent study showed that, in a sample of 215 injured workers who completed the PDP Program, treatment-related reductions in pain catastrophising significantly predicted RTW (Sullivan et al 2005b).

Given the limited number of psychologists available to provide cognitive–behavioural interventions, translation to community practice is challenging. A key step forward has been described in a programme developed for front-line rehabilitation professionals such as physiotherapists and occupational therapists (Sullivan et al 2006). The Progressive Goal Attainment Program (PGAP) is also a standardised community-based intervention that aims to reduce risk factors for prolonged work disability such as pain catastrophising, fear of movement and reinjury and perceived disability. As with the PDP Program, individuals are selected for the intervention based on elevated scores on measures of psychosocial risk factors targeted by the intervention. The rationale behind the development of the programme was that increasing front-line rehabilitation professionals' ability to detect and intervene on psychosocial risk factors would facilitate early implementation of risk-factor-targeted interventions. In a recent clinical trial with a sample of individuals who had been work disabled due to whiplash symptoms, 75% of individuals in the PGAP group returned to work compared to 50% who followed usual treatment (Sullivan et al 2006).

Finally, it should be noted that superior RTW outcomes were achieved without demonstrating a greater magnitude of pain reduction. For example, in the Linton et al (2006) study, there were no significant differences in pain reduction among treatment conditions. Nevertheless, the groups receiving the cognitive–behavioural interventions were able to be more active, and had fewer days of work absence despite the fact that their reported pain levels were similar to the comparison group. Similarly, Sullivan et al (2005b) reported that pain reduction was not associated with a higher probability of RTW when reductions in other psychosocial risk factors were statistically controlled.

Taken together, these findings suggest that treatment-related reduction in psychosocial risk factors are important determinants of RTW, independent of reductions in pain, and the approach would seem to merit further investigation.

Conclusions

Conclusions and general recommendations are summarised in the key points; they are discussed below.

Importance of distinguishing worker-related (Type I) from workplace/system related (Type II) factors. There is a wide variety of initiatives which might sit under the umbrella of work rehabilitation and this makes the evaluation of initiatives designed to reduce work disability extremely difficult. It would seem helpful, however, to attempt to make a clear distinction in the first instance between worker-related (Type I) and workplace/system factors (Type II).

Central role of yellow and blue flags in work disability. In addressing the assessment and management of Type I factors in particular, the further differentiation into yellow and blue flags would seem to offer further strategic help in terms of a plan for intervention.

Need for a specific occupational focus within a pain management approach. For chronic pain patients, cognitive–behavioural approaches to treatment, at their most developed in interdisciplinary PMPs, can produce positive outcomes for clinical parameters, but in tackling work disability need an additional specific occupational focus which is not routinely available in traditional clinical PMPs.

Encouraging evidence for occupationally focused cognitive–behavioural approaches in secondary prevention. A number of recent studies have produced encouraging evidence of the efficacy of secondary prevention using a CBT approach in the reduction of future sick leave (work disability).

No clear evidence for back schools and/or FRPs in reducing work disability. There is no evidence that back schools reduce future work disability and the early promising results for FRPs do not seem to have been sustained.

Work modification may be useful as part of an overall strategy for reducing work disability. While work modification may be viewed as an organisational rather than a worker-related intervention, the provision of appropriate modified work may lessen the impact of perceived obstacles to return to work.

Strong interest in the UK in development of new RTW strategies, within an overall 'systems approach'. In the management of musculoskeletal disorders, and low-back pain in particular, in the UK there have been a large number of governmental initiatives designed to facilitate return to work and decrease the general burden to society of work disability. Unfortunately there have been significant problems in the practical implementation of some of these seemingly well-intentioned initiatives and some of the newer initiatives await evaluation. It would seem, however, that the need to adopt a biopsychosocial approach to the prevention and management of pain-associated work disability is now accepted.

Specific targeting of psychosocial risk factors for work disability represents an encouraging development. There is now some encouraging evidence from prospective studies that a pro-active approach to the early identification and targeting of psychosocial risk factors can reduce work disability, and currently a number of initiatives under way in a variety of settings should enable further appraisal of such initiatives. Although Shaw et al (2006) consider that not all benefits of RTW interventions are easily explicable by risk-factor reduction, 'assigning early intervention strategies based on risk factor assessment remains a promising, yet untested approach' (p. 601).

Despite significant technical and methodological problems in linking screening, targeting and interventions, this approach would seem to merit further attention. There remain significant technical problems in the development and establishment of accurate screening procedures enabling targeted interventions directed specifically at modifiable risk factors. However, the development and validation of new assessment tools, and the delivery of more sharply focused interventions, should enable the design of research trials of sufficient rigour to gather the evidence of what works for whom, when, how and where, and thus reduce the impact of work disability.

Key points

- **Importance of distinguishing worker-related (Type I) from workplace-system-related (Type II) factors**
- **Central role of yellow and blue flags in work disability**
- **Need for a specific occupational focus within a pain management approach**
- **Encouraging evidence for occupationally focused cognitive–behavioural approaches in secondary prevention**

(Continued)

- **No clear evidence for back schools and/or FRPs in reducing work disability**
- **Work modification may be useful as part of an overall strategy for reducing work disability**
- **Strong interest in the UK in development of new RTW strategies, within an overall 'systems approach'**

- **Specific targeting of psychosocial risk factors for work disability represents an encouraging development**
- **Despite significant technical and methodological problems in linking screening, targeting and interventions, this approach would seem to merit further attention.**

References

Boersma K, Linton S J 2003 Early identification of patients at risk of developing a persistent back problem: the predictive validity of the Örebro musculoskeletal pain questionnaire. Clinical Journal of Pain:19:80–86

Brown D 2002 Initiative evaluation report: back in work. HSE Contract Research Report 441. HSE Books, London

Brown K C, Sirles A T, Hilyer J C et al 1992 Cost-effectiveness of a back school intervention for municipal employees. Spine 17:1224–1228

Buchbinder R, Jolley D, Wyatt M 2001 Effects of a media campaign on back pain beliefs and its potential influence on management of low back pain in general practice. Spine 26:2535–2542

Burton A K, Bartys S, Wright I A et al 2005 Obstacles to recovery from musculoskeletal disorders in industry. HSE Research Report RR323. HSE Books, HMSO Norwich

Cherkin D C, Deyo R A, Battie M et al 1998 A comparison of physical therapy, chiropractic manipulation, and provision of an educational booklet for the treatment of patients with low back pain. New England Journal of Medicine 339:1021–1029

Crook J, Milner R, Schultz I Z et al 2005 Determinants of occupational disability following a low back injury: a critical review of the literature. In: Schultz I Z, Gatchel R J (eds) Handbook of complex occupational disability claims: early risk identification, intervention and prevention. Springer, New York, pp 169–189

Daltroy L H, Iversen M D, Larson M G et al 1997 A controlled trial of an educational program to prevent low back injuries. New England Journal Medicine 337:322–328

Di Fabio R P 1995 Efficacy of comprehensive rehabilitation programs and back school for patients with low back pain: a meta-analysis. Physical Therapy 75(10):865–878

Galvin D E 1999 Employer-based disability management and rehabilitation programs. Annual Review of Rehabilitation 5:215

Garcy P, Mayer T, Gatchel R J 1996 Recurrent or new injury outcomes after return to work in chronic disabling spinal disorders: tertiary prevention efficacy of functional restoration treatment. Spine 21:952–959

Gatchel R J, Polatin P B, Noe C E et al 2003 Treatment- and cost-effectiveness of early intervention for acute low back pain patients: a one-year prospective study. Journal of Occupational Rehabilitation 13:1–9

George S Z, Fritz J M, Bialosky J E et al 2003 The effect of a fear-avoidance-based physical therapy intervention for acute low back pain: results of a randomized control trial. Spine 28:2551–2560

Guzman J, Esmail R, Karjalainen K et al 2004 Multidisciplinary bio-psycho-social rehabilitation for chronic low-back pain. The Cochrane Database of Systematic Reviews, The Cochrane Library

Hadler N M 1999 Occupational musculoskeletal disorders, 2nd edn. Lippincott Williams & Wilkins, Philadelphia, PA

Hagen E M, Grasdal A, Eriksen H R 2003 Does early intervention with a light mobilization program reduce long-term sick leave for low back pain: a 3-year follow-up study. Spine 28:2309–2316

Hanson M A, Burton A K, Kendall N A S et al 2006 The costs and benefits of active case management and rehabilitation for musculoskeletal disorders. HSE Books, London

Hazard R G, Fenwick J W, Kalisch S M et al 1989 Functional restoration with behavioural support: a one-year prospective study of patients with chronic low-back pain. Spine 14:157–161

Hazard R G, Haugh L D, Reid S et al 1997 Early physician notification of patient disability risk and clinical guidelines after low back injury. Spine 22:2951–2958

Indahl A, Haldorsen E H, Holm S et al 1998 Five-year follow-up study of a controlled clinical trial using light mobilization and an informative approach to low back pain. Spine 23:2625–2630

IUA 2004 IUA/ABI working party report: psychology, personal injury and rehabilitation. International Underwriting Association of London

Koes B W, van Tulder M W, Ostelo R et al 2001 Clinical guidelines for the management of low back pain in primary care: an international comparison. Spine 26:2504–2513

Krause N, Dasinger L K, Neuhauser F 1998 Modified work and return to work: a review of the literature. Journal of Occupational Rehabilitation 8:113–139

Lahad A, Malter A, Berg A O et al 1994 The effectiveness of four interventions for the prevention of low back pain. Journal of the American Medical Association 272:1286–1291

Lindstrom I, Ohlund C, Eek C et al 1992 The effect of graded activity on patients with subacute low back pain: a randomized prospective clinical study with an operant-conditioning behavioural approach. Physical Therapy 72:279–290

Linton S J, Andersson T 2000 Can chronic disability be prevented? A randomised trial of a cognitive-behavioural intervention and two forms of information in patients with spinal pain. Spine 25:2825–2831

Linton S J, Ryberg M 2001 A cognitive-behavioural group intervention as prevention for persistent neck and back pain in a non-patient population: a randomised controlled trial. Pain 90:83–90

Linton S J, Hellsing A L, Andersson D 1993 A controlled study of the effects of an early intervention on acute mus-culoskeletal pain problems. Pain 54:353–359

Linton S J, Boersma K, Jansson M et al 2006 The effects of cognitive-behavioral and physical therapy preventive interventions on pain related sick leave: a randomized controlled trial. Clinical Journal of Pain, in press

Magora A 1973 Investigation of the relation between low back pain and occupation. V: psychological aspects. Scandinavian Journal of Rehabilitation Medicine 5:191–196

Main C J, Phillips C J, Thomas A P, Farrell A 2004 The Wales health work report. Welsh Assembly Government (and Dept for Work & Pensions UK)

Malmivaara A, Hakkinen U, Aro T et al 1995 The treatment of acute low back pain – bed rest, exercises, or ordinary activity? New England Journal of Medicine 332:351–355

Marhold C, Linton S J, Mellin L 2001 A cognitive-behavioural return-to-work programme: effects on pain patients with a history of long-term versus short-term sick leave. Pain 91:155–163

Mayer T, Gatchel R 1988 Functional restoration for spinal disorders: the sports medicine approach. Lea & Febiger, Philadelphia, PA

Mayer T G, Gatchel R J, Kishino N et al 1985 Objective assessment of spine function following industrial injury. Spine 10:482–494

Morley S, Eccleston C, Williams A 1999 Systematic review and meta-analysis of randomised controlled trials of cognitive-behavioural therapy and behaviour therapy for chronic pain in adults, excluding headache. Pain 80:1–13

Nachemson A 1983 Work for all: for those with low back pain as well. Clinical Orthopaedics and Related Research 179:77–85

Peat G M, Moores L, Goldingay S et al 2001 Pain manage-ment program follow-ups. A national survey of current practice in the United Kingdom. Journal of Pain and Symptom Management 21:218–226

Ryan W E, Krishna M K, Swanson C E 1995 A prospective study evaluating early rehabilitation in preventing back pain chronicity in mine workers. Spine 20:489–491

Schonstein E, Kenny D T, Keating J et al 2004 Work con-ditioning, work hardening and functional restoration for workers with back and neck pain. The Cochrane Database of Systematic Reviews, The Cochrane Library

Shaw W S, Linton S J, Pransky P 2006 Reducing sickness absence from work due to low back pain: how well do intervention strategies match modifiable risk factors? Journal of Occupational Rehabilitation 16:591–605

Sinclair S J, Hogg-Johnson S, Mondloch M V et al 1997 The effectiveness of an early active intervention program for workers with soft-tissue injuries: the early claimant cohort study. Spine 22:2919–2931

Sullivan M J L, Stanish W D 2003 Psychologically based occupational rehabilitation: The Pain-Disability Prevention Program. Clinical Journal of Pain 19:97–104

Sullivan M J L, Feuerstein M, Gatchel R J et al 2005a Integrating psychosocial and behavioral interventions to achieve optimal rehabilitation outcomes. Journal of Occupational Rehabilitation 15:475–489

Sullivan M J L, Ward L C, Tripp D et al 2005b Secondary prevention of work disability: community-based psycho-social intervention for musculoskeletal disorders. Journal of Occupational Rehabilitation 15:377–392

Sullivan M J L, Adams H, Rhodenizer T et al 2006 A psycho-social risk factor targeted intervention for the prevention of chronic pain and disability following whiplash injury. Physical Therapy 86:8–18

van den Hout J H, Vlaeyen J W, Heuts P H et al 2003 Secondary prevention of work-related disability in non-specific low back pain: does problem-solving therapy help? A randomized clinical trial. Clinical Journal of Pain 19:87–96

Van Tulder M, Koes B W 2002 Low back pain and sciatica: chronic. Clinical Evidence 8:1171–1187 (available online at www.clinicalevidence.com)

Verbeek J H, van der Weide W E, van Dijk F J 2002 Early occupational health management of patients with back pain: a randomized controlled trial. Spine:27:1844–1851

Vlaeyen J W, De Jong J R, Onghena P et al 2002 Can pain-related fear be reduced? The application of cognitive-behavioral exposure in vivo. Pain Research and Management 7:144–153

Von Korff M, Deyo R A, Cherkin D et al 1993 Back pain in primary care: outcomes at one year. Spine 18(7):855–862

Von Korff M, Moore J E, Lorig K et al 1998 A randomized trial of a lay person-led self-management group intervention for back pain patients in primary care. Spine 23:2608–2615

Von Korff M, Balderson B H, Saunders K et al 2005 A trial of an activating intervention for chronic back pain in primary care and physical therapy settings. Pain 113:323–330

Waddell G 1998 The back pain revolution. 1st edn. Churchill Livingstone, Edinburgh

Waddell G 2004 The back pain revolution. 2nd edn. Churchill Livingstone, Edinburgh

Waddell G, Burton A K 2006 Is work good for your health and well-being? The Stationary Office, London

Waddell G, Watson P J 2004 Rehabilitation. In: Waddell, G (ed) The back pain revolution, 2nd edn. Churchill Livingstone, Edinburgh, ch 18, pp 371–399

Waddell G, Burton A K, Main C J 2003 Screening of DWP clients for risk of long-term incapacity: a conceptual and scientific review. Royal Society of Medicine Monograph. Royal Society of Medicine Press, London

Watson P, Booker C K, Moores L et al 2004 Returning the chronically unemployed with low back pain to employment. European Journal of Pain 8(4):359–369

Yamamoto S 1997 Guidelines on worksite prevention of low back pain. Labour Standards Bureau notification no 57. Industrial Health 35:143–172

Yassi A, Tate R, Cooper J E et al 1995 Early intervention for back injuries in nurses at a large Canadian tertiary care hospital: an evaluation of the effectiveness and cost benefits of a two-year pilot project. Occupational Medicine 45:209–214

Chapter Fifteen

Pain and work: organisational perspectives

With Kay Greasley

CHAPTER CONTENTS

Introduction

The major emphasis of this chapter is also on the health–work interface, with particular emphasis on pain and its impact, but we shift focus to the organisational perspective. We shall comment on organisation structures and processes, but our primary focus will be on interventions designed to target organisational risk factors with a view to achieving optimal organisational outcomes, in terms of work rehabilitation and work retention. While the clinical status of the employee on return to work (RTW) after injury or illness might be assumed to be the most important factor influencing RTW, the actual timing of RTW is likely to be influenced also by the economic implications of working, or not, for the employee and the organisational factors enabling or preventing RTW. Of equal importance is the employee's decision about whether to return to work. A number of the key influences on work retention and rehabilitation are shown in Box 15.1. The organisational factors in particular will be explored further in this chapter.

In fact, decisions about whether or not to return to work after injury can be complex, with major differences between employees having a similar clinical condition in terms of their decision and the influences on it. Traditionally, much of the focus of work rehabilitation has been on clinical status, in terms of residual physical restrictions or restricted capacity to work, and potential risks to the employers of further injury, but the primary focus of this chapter is to consider organisational factors which may prevent or hinder successful RTW. To assist appraisal of the relevant issues a degree of further conceptual clarification is offered.

Attempts to depict the employee–organisation interface

There have been many attempts to construct models or conceptual frameworks linking employee characteristics with organisational structures and processes, and indeed the linking of the Type I–Type II distinction (Sullivan et al 2005a) between individually focused and organisationally focused interventions with the flags is one of the most recent attempts to do this. It is, however, relevant to pass comment on a number of other models.

Box 15.1

General influences on return to work after injury/illness

- Clinical status
- Employee decision:
  - economic factors
  - other personal factors.
- Organisational factors:
  - employer's contractual obligations
  - system of sick certification
  - system for human resource and occupational health monitoring
  - requirement for fitness to RTW certification.

Rochester model of work disability

The influential Rochester model of work disability (Feuerstein 1991) is shown in Figure 15.1. The Rochester model was one of the earliest models explicitly implicating medical status, physical capabilities, specific psychological factors and aspects of work (work demands) in a model of work disability. Although conceptual rather than statistically derived, it offered an important alternative to impairment models, which seemed to pay little regard to occupational factors, or to the prevailing disability models with their emphasis almost entirely on ergonomic or biomechanical factors.

Sherbrooke model

An increasing number of factors have been implicated in work disability. The complexity of the situation is reflected in the Sherbrooke model (Loisel et al 2001a, Loisel & Durand 2005, Loisel et al 2005). In the latest adaptation (Fig. 15.2), the influences of a variety of legislative and funding factors, specific organisation or workplace factors, aspects of health-care provision and personal factors are depicted.

This conceptualisation inspired the implementation of a randomised clinical trial (Loisel et al 1997) on subacute work-related back pain comparing a clinical intervention, an occupational intervention, a combined intervention and a (usual care) control group. Only

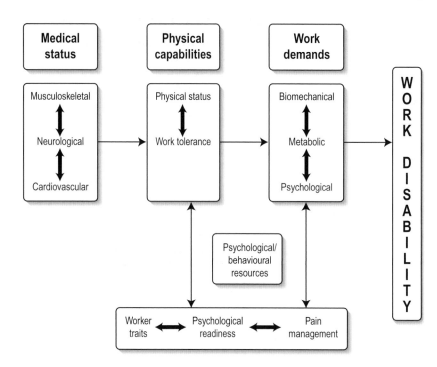

Figure 15.1 • The Rochester model of work disability (Feuerstein 1991).

the combined approach was superior to the usual care approach in terms of faster RTW.

Finally, by way of introduction, Truchon et al (2006) in a prospective longitudinal study of workers on sick leave due to back pain used staged structural equation modelling to try to disentangle some of the determinants of disability. Some of their major findings are shown in Box 15.2. Following extensive statistical analysis, both cross-sectionally and longitudinally, inter alia they concluded:

> *Two factors are particularly useful in predicting chronic disability. These were distress and fear of work ... the most innovative outcome of this analysis was the capacity of work support to predict fear of work ... These findings suggest that workplace characteristics merit equal consideration to improve our understanding of chronic disability (p. 66).*

Black flags: economic and organisational obstacles to RTW

The nature of black flags

In previous chapters a distinction has been made between primary clinical flags (red, orange and yellow) and occupational flags (blue). From a work retention or work rehabilitation perspective, however, a further distinction has been made between two different types of occupational risk factors: those concerning the perception of work (blue flags) and organisational obstacles to recovery, comprising objective work characteristics and conditions of employment (black flags) (Main & Burton 2000).

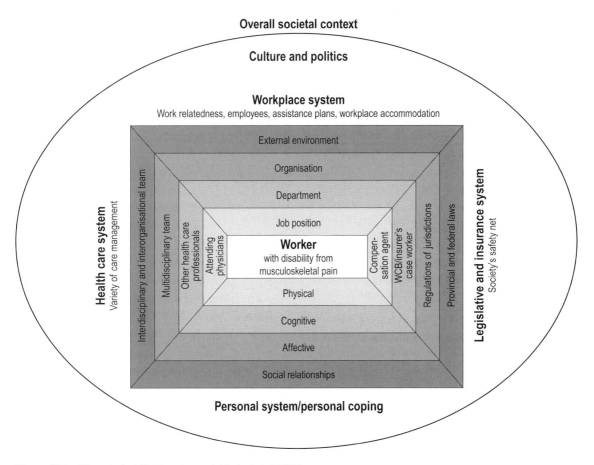

Figure 15.2 • The adapted Sherbrooke model (Loisel et al 2005).

Box 15.2

The determinants of chronic disability

- Environmental demands (stressors over the previous six months) and the fear of movement (cognitive appraisal of threat) generated psychological distress (anxiety, depression, anger and catastrophising), predicting 24% of the variance
- This distress, combined with fear of movement had a direct effect on the use of coping strategies that centred on avoidance of physical activities, explaining 42% of the variance
- Avoidance and distress directly influenced functional status (disability)
- The factors in combination accounted for 54% of the variance in outcome (functional status)
- Emotional distress and fear of work were consistent predictors of functional status, work status (returned vs absent) and number of days of sickness absence at 6-month follow-up
- Fear of work in turn was predicted by emotional distress, fear of movement and perceived absence of work support (in terms of adequate polices and practices)
- The biological variables showed 'enormous variance' but significant correlations were found between biological response (cortisol levels) and psychosocial variables, giving some support for disturbance to the stress response system as a possible precursor of disability.

Truchon et al (2006)

Box 15.3

Black flags I: job context and working conditions

National
- Rates of pay
- Nationally negotiated entitlements:
  - sick certification
  - benefit system
  - wage reimbursement rate.

Local
- Sickness policy:
  - entitlements to sick leave
  - role of occupational health in 'signing off' and 'signing on' requirement for full fitness
  - possibility of sheltered work
  - possibility of restricted duties.
- Management style:
  - supervisor/line manager support
  - response to pain-associated limitations
  - facilitation of RTW.
- Social climate:
  - co-worker support
  - attitudes to pain (illness), absence and work restrictions.
- Trades union support/involvement
- Organisational size and structure.

Box 15.4

Black flags II: content-specific aspects of work

- Ergonomic:
  - job heaviness
  - lifting frequency
  - postures
  - sitting/standing postural requirements.
- Temporal characteristics:
  - number of working hours
  - shift pattern.

Black flags are *not* a matter of perception, and affect all workers equally. They include both nationally established policy concerning conditions of employment and sickness policy and working conditions specific to a particular organisation.

There are also content-specific aspects of work, which characterise certain types of jobs, and which are associated with higher rates of illness, injury or work loss. These features of work, following injury, may require a higher level of working capability to maintain successful work retention. After certain types of injury, such jobs may be specifically contra-indicated and therefore constitute an absolute obstacle to RTW.

For convenience these are differentiated into black flags associated with job context and general working conditions (Box 15.3) and black flags associated with content-specific aspects of work (Box 15.4).

There are two important caveats concerning blue and black flags.

Blue–black flag overlap

Firstly, it is important to understand the overlap between blue and black flags. Certain characteristics of work are in general associated with absence and suboptimal performance, and as such can reasonably be viewed as black flags. However, there may be considerable variation among employees about how such characteristics are viewed, and to that extent they may function as blue flags. The distinction may be important when consideration is given to solutions. Thus changes to management style focused on changing the behaviour of a supervisor properly is an organisational intervention (a Sullivan Type II intervention), while changing an employee's perception of or attitude to his/her supervisor would require a blue flag intervention focused on the individual (a Sullivan Type I intervention).

From obstacles to opportunities

Black flags, although potential obstacles to recovery may become opportunities for change. At the core of the 'flag' construct is a conceptual shift from risks (many of which may be immutable) to *obstacles to recovery*, which may be individual clinical factors, perceptions of work or organisation, and which may in turn require a range of solutions from individual clinical interventions and work reintegration strategies to fundamental redesign of the individual/organisation interface. Unnecessary low-back pain disability is unhelpful to both employer and worker.

(It should be noticed in this context, however, that the term *obstacles to recovery* does not necessary imply a complete resolution of symptoms and should be understood as shorthand for *obstacles to recovery/optimal function* or viewed from a slightly different perspective as *obstacles to engagement in the recovery process*.)

Prior to consideration of possible solutions the relationship between organisational processes and work absence will be examined.

Organisational structures and processes

A number of the key occupational influences on work retention and rehabilitation are shown in Box 15.5.

Organisational structures

Function of human resources

Large organisations need a system for monitoring performance and employee management. Frequently this will fall to a department of human resources (HR). The function of HR departments, however, can vary between organisations and the traditional HR functions

Box 15.5

Key organisational influences on work retention and rehabilitation

- Function of human resources:
  - organisational performance evaluation
  - absence monitoring
  - organisational 'temperature checks'
  - individual performance evaluation
  - attendance management
  - channels of communication.
- With workforce
- With individual employees
- Access to occupational health:
  - in house
  - externally resourced.
- Specific organisational procedures and practices:
  - legal obligations as an employer
  - health and safety
  - conditions of employment
  - sick leave
  - RTW polices and procedures.

are sometimes blended into departments of organisational development (OD). For the purpose of this chapter the term HR will be preferred.

Historically HR departments have derived from personnel departments, which seemed to have a stronger focus on care of the employee rather than the modern HR department, which may have a range of functions, both at an organisational and at an individual employee level. At an organisational level HR may be required to conduct organisational performance evaluation, including absence monitoring and organisation-wide 'temperature checks' on the health of the workforce. This may include specific surveys of factors such as job stress, job satisfaction, work–life balance, and health. They may also have a responsibility for individual performance evaluation and attendance management, including what are sometimes euphemistically termed 'counselling' sessions with employees who have reported sick more than a certain number of times during a specified period. Potentially, therefore, HR departments have key channels of communication with all aspects of the organisation from the workforce as a whole to individual employees and in the context of RTW may have to liaise not only with the employee but also with the employee's line manager and with occupational health.

Access to occupational health

The availability and content of occupational health is widely variable across organisations. Larger organisations may have 'in house' provision of a range of occupational services including specialised physical therapy or counselling in addition to a general 'GP function'. Increasingly, however, such services are being outsourced to independent health-care providers who offer a range of health products targeted at specific health conditions and sometimes including as part of the package a system of risk assessment derived from questionnaires completed by employees. Often these are completed on a confidential basis, leading to risk profiling from which employees can elect to sign up for a range of employee assistance products (such as stress reduction, smoking cessation and exercise programmes).

At a simple level, therefore, occupational health may offer a fast track to the sort of individual clinical services available in the health-care system, but it would also seem to have potential as a vehicle for prevention at an organisational level not so much in terms of primary prevention but in terms of secondary prevention, i.e. in offering programmes to assist in the management of symptoms for those still at work, thereby reducing the impact of symptoms on performance and reducing sickness absence.

Traditionally occupational health has been derived from a sickness and disability perspective although at the time of writing there appears to be a growing interest in the UK not only in illness management, but also on enhancement of well-being (Waddell & Burton 2006). Unfortunately there is as yet little controlled research on the comparative worth of such interventions, whether initially or in combination.

Specific organisational policies and practices

There is a range of specific legal obligations which fall upon any organisation in its role as an employer. These vary from country to country (Waddell et al 2002), as does the extent to which they are monitored by inspectorates such as the Health and Safety Executive (HSE) in the UK. During the twentieth century the primary focus of legislation was on safety and, as a derivative, on the provision of a safe and non-toxic work environment with a clear focus on the prevention of accidents. Identification of potential physical risk factors has led to the development of strategies designed to minimise exposure to risks of injury. In the musculoskeletal context such initiatives have led to the development of general guidelines for lifting and handling and specific

task and job design. Clearly jobs may differ greatly in terms of physical demand but the particular focus in terms of musculoskeletal injury has been on ergonomic design in relationship to the physical demands of work. There has until recently been very little focus on psychosocial risk factors.

In addition to externally imposed legal requirements, each organisation is characterised by a set of specific organisational procedures and practices, crystallised in conditions of employment including policies and procedures for sickness management, which may have a direct bearing on the transition from sickness absence back into work. Employees in most Western countries have a degree of financial protection in the form of insurance cover or access to sickness benefits which may ease the financial burden of absence from work. However, the degree of protection in terms of wage replacement and the time over which this extends is widely variable but it is important to consider as a major potential influence on RTW.

The impact on work retention and RTW

Traditionally the clinical condition of the employee in terms of fitness to work has been seen in terms of clinical management of the condition and clearance for RTW following a risk appraisal by the employer. Clinical treatment has tended to focus on specific physical or psychological symptoms without specific regard to perceptions of work or organisational obstacles to satisfactory and sustained RTW. It has become increasingly clear, however, that a wide range of psychosocial factors can have a powerful influence on health for those at work and on RTW for those who are off sick (Truchon et al 2006, Waddell et al 2003, Linton et al 2005).

A number of general influences on RTW were shown in Box 15.1 where it can be seen not only that there are more than clinical factors which may be operating but also that there are a number of 'key players' who may become involved in permitting or sanctioning RTW, whether fully or with work restrictions.

(It will be argued later that optimal management of the health–work interface requires a 'systems approach' in which a range of stakeholders may need to become involved.)

Defining workplace interventions

There are numerous definitions of workplace interventions. Shaw et al (2002) make a helpful link between risk factor domains, focus on secondary prevention and

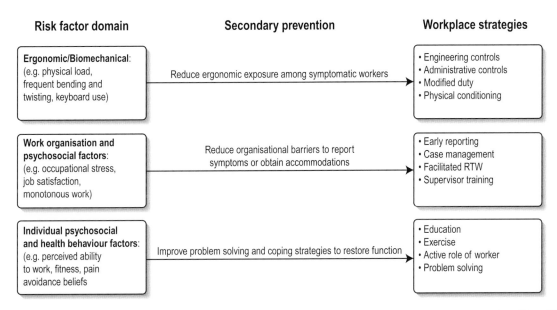

Risk factor domain	Secondary prevention	Workplace strategies
Ergonomic/Biomechanical: (e.g. physical load, frequent bending and twisting, keyboard use)	Reduce ergonomic exposure among symptomatic workers →	• Engineering controls • Administrative controls • Modified duty • Physical conditioning
Work organisation and psychosocial factors: (e.g. occupational stress, job satisfaction, monotonous work)	Reduce organisational barriers to report symptoms or obtain accommodations →	• Early reporting • Case management • Facilitated RTW • Supervisor training
Individual psychosocial and health behaviour factors: (e.g. perceived ability to work, fitness, pain avoidance beliefs	Improve problem solving and coping strategies to restore function →	• Education • Exercise • Active role of worker • Problem solving

Figure 15.3 • Conceptual framework for the secondary prevention of musculoskeletal disorders in the workplace (From Shaw et al 2002), with permission from Elsevier Ltd.

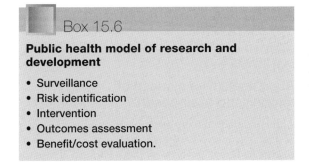

Box 15.6

Public health model of research and development

- Surveillance
- Risk identification
- Intervention
- Outcomes assessment
- Benefit/cost evaluation.

specific workplace strategies. Their conceptual model is shown in Figure. 15.3. The interaction between flags can be seen. Thus the reduction of ergonomic exposure would be an example of a black flag intervention (and Type II in Sullivan et al's classification); the reduction of organisational barriers as described are blue–black flag interventions (and Type II), while improving problem solving and coping strategies to restore function are addressing mainly yellow and blue flags (and Type I).

Shaw et al (2002) further distinguish primary and secondary prevention initiatives into a public health model of research and development, the stages of which are shown in Box 15.6. This would seem to be a helpful conceptual framework for considering the focus and purpose of appraisals and interventions.

Franche et al (2005b) recommend a further general distinction between work environment modification (such as changes in rotation and workstation reorganisation) and graduated RTW (e.g. modified hours, duties or both). Later in this chapter the evidence for impact of various interventions will be reviewed, but as a precursor, the nature of organisations will be considered from a number of more general perspectives.

Organisation management and work absence

In the rest of this chapter we consider absence in the workplace from a variety of perspectives. We review the nature of organisational management of absence, and in particular how supervisors, policies and RTW programmes impact on absence and presenteeism. We explore health management policies and their relationship with workplace absence, specifically highlighting the role of employers and modified work within such policies. We then examine potential barriers to health management and absence policy, incorporating the experience of the employee and the importance of dynamic relationships. Finally we offer a number of recommendations for health and absence management within an organisational context.

The importance of absence from the workplace

The costs of absence

Absence has been described as the largest single source of lost productivity in business and industry (Harvey & Nicholson 1993) with 90% of businesses citing absence as a significant cost (Chartered Institute of Personnel Development, CIPD 2005a). It is argued that this is a problem for all organisations and is particularly problematic for public sector organisations (Johnson et al 2003, McHugh 2001). The cost of this absence to the UK economy is estimated to be £13 billion (IDS 1998). Research instigated by the Confederation of British Industry (CBI) estimated that in 1998, 200 million days were lost through absence. This equates to an average employee having 8.5 days absent from work per year. More recent figures indicate a reduction in the number of days employees are absent from work to 7.2 per annum (IDS 2004). However, a CIPD survey (2005b) estimates that 8.4 days is the average number of days absent.

The absence figures according to the CIPD (2005c) vary considerably according to industry sector, with public sector levels of absence standing at 10.3 days in comparison to 6.8 days in the private sector, and this gap is widening. Thus while there is some variance in absentee level, there is agreement that it is a significant cost to British industry with the average cost of absence as £601 per employee, per annum. This figure rises to £645 for public sector organisations (CIPD 2005c).

Short-term vs long-term absence

Absence can be classified into two main categories: short term and long term. A recent CIPD survey found that of all absence 60% is attributed to absence of 5 days or less, just under a fifth is for between 5 days and 4 weeks with a similar proportion for 4 weeks or more (CIPD 2005c).

Major causes of absence in manual and non-manual workers

The major cause of short-term absence is linked to minor illness for both manual and non-manual employees. Back pain and musculoskeletal injuries were found to be subsequent causes of short-term absence for manual workers. Causes of long-term absence (4 weeks or more) are related to stress and mental health for non-manual employees; however, musculoskeletal injuries and back pain remain a predominant cause of long-term absence for manual workers (CIPD 2005a).

Direct and indirect costs

Precise responsibilities of employers vary across countries and jurisdictions, but it is important to realise that there are direct and indirect costs associated with absence which are met by the employing organisations (Berger et al 2001). The direct costs result from the direct payment of sick pay to the employee, particularly as the employer may need to bring in alternative staff to provide cover for absent personnel, in essence, paying twice (Dunn & Wilkinson 2002). This has led many employers to review and revise their absence control policies in an attempt to reduce these costs (Edwards & Whitson 1993). The drivers of these efforts have arisen due to three interrelated factors, the need to cut costs, especially when operating in a highly competitive market, the avoidance of disruption that is caused when staff are absent and the change in statutory sick pay (IRS 1994), which now means that the employer makes a more substantial contribution to this direct cost (Cunningham & James 2000). Despite the apparent need to manage the costs of absence a recent survey by the CIPD found that less than half of the employers monitor the cost of absence (CIPD 2005a).

Absenteeism as a cause of 'organisational ill-health'?

Although much of the literature focuses on the costs of absent employees, high absenteeism may be indicative of a deeper problem of organisational ill-health. Saratoga (1998) highlights how high absence levels are a clear indicator of organisational misbehaviour, indicating disaffection with the organisation. Individual and organisational health are interdependent, and an unhealthy organisation is ill-equipped to face organisational challenges (McHugh 2001, Cooper 1994, Ho 1997).

Factors associated with absenteeism

There are a variety of opinions as to the specific causes of absenteeism, but there would appear to be a general consensus that organisation and managerial practice is a strong determinant of absence, whether by actually inducing illness or injury or by contributing to low levels of employee motivation and employee attitude.

An adequate understanding of this complex matrix thus appears to require an understanding both of the general organisational features (black flags) and the individual work perceptions (blue flags). Many studies investigating health indicators will include a mixture of the two. As examples, some of the more common diagnoses have been linked to increased pressure of work, stress and organisational change (Seccombe 1995), especially when the change process has been badly managed (Bennett 2002). Employee commitment to the organisation has been found to be positively correlated with lower rates of absenteeism (Dalton & Mesch 1990), commitment can be negatively linked to absenteeism and labour turnover (Cotton & Tuttle 1986), and concepts such as 'discretionary effort' are now appearing. Lack of trust and respect between management and staff has been identified as a contributor to absenteeism while, conversely, relationships that are good may foster a higher level of attendance (Bennett 2002). The author argues that additional job demands and a more pressing environment result in an increased level of employee stress which contributes both directly and indirectly to high levels of absenteeism. Other organisational influences on employee absence which have been identified include: task and work context organisation, management hierarchy, levels of employee responsibility, autonomy, job satisfaction and the structure of the organisation (Dalton & Mesch 1990, Rentsch & Steel 1998, Cotton & Tuttle 1985). Organisational cultural norms also seem to be highly influential on the level of absenteeism, and individuals seem to learn what are viewed as 'acceptable' levels of absence from their peers and management (Gellatly & Luchak 1998). Thus organisational climate may have a powerful influence on the levels of absenteeism.

Attitudes towards absenteeism

While an extensive body of research exists on the causes and management of absence, the prime interest from an HR perspective is its management (i.e. attendance management), but it seems there is a tendency to avoid examination of genuine injury and illness (Cunningham & James 2000), such as cancer and trauma, i.e. tangible and unambiguous health problems in which the effect on work is uncontroversial.

Perceptions of legitimacy: the influence of visibility and timing

The type of illness or injury seems to have an influence on attitudes towards absenteeism. Perceptions

---

> ### Box 15.7
>
> **Principal categories of absence**
>
> - Actual injury or illness, which may be partly attributable to how the organisation is managed
> - Absent, without any physical ailment
> - Absence attributable to low job satisfaction (or similar issues).

of whether a complaint is genuine are often based on visibility and time (Taylor et al 2003). For example, accidents that occur in the workplace with immediate consequences are seen as a legitimate cause of absence. In contrast, health complaints such as stress or repetitive strain injury, which may not emerge for some time and are difficult to identify, are less likely to be seen as legitimate. There is of course an obvious advantage to employers in holding the view that absences are voluntary, for to concede that many absences are legitimate is to admit, at least in part, that the cause lies in the working environment (Taylor et al 2003) and that the employer has a degree of responsibility. Such issues may become sharply focused in the context of compensation for work injury (Ch. 12).

Perceived responsibilities for the management of short-term and long-term absence

The management of long-term conditions is considered to be the responsibility of occupational health, and the focus of attendance management therefore tends to be on short-term absences often predicated on the assumption that workers are away from the workforce for other reasons than ill-health and the management of absence that stems from 'genuine illness and injury' is not properly addressed.

It is important, however, to explore the arrangements that organisations have in place to facilitate all workers on the road back into work (Cunningham & James 2000). Bennett (2002) identifies three principal categories of absence, shown in Box 15.7, illustrating commonly held views on absence. Two out of three reasons are partly or wholly attributable to the organisation, a finding supported by McHugh (2001) who considered that the root cause of illness may be partly attributable to the way organisations are managed.

These interesting issues would seem to be badly in need of some sharply focused research.

Managing organisational absence

Addressing absence: towards solutions

Recognition of the interdependence of individual and organisational well-being and the importance of inter-related organisational factors (McHugh 2001) necessitates a more person-centred approach. As previously indicated, these factors may include: the structure of the organisation, management hierarchy, the way in which tasks or the work context are organised, levels of employee responsibility, morale, motivation and job satisfaction. All of these factors have been shown to impact on employee absence (Dalton & Mesch 1990, Rentsch & Steel 1998). Similarly, Belbo & Ortlieb (2006) found that home life and the working environment impacted on absence with autonomy, strain and the social environment in the workplace playing key roles on absence levels. Furthermore, the level of employee commitment has been positively related to lower levels of absence (Bennett 2002). Hence any approach that will successfully address absence will require a multifaceted approach. There are, however, a number of specific factors which seem to merit priority for attention.

Facilitating communication among interested parties (i.e. the key 'stakeholders')

Miscommunications are ineffective and costly and can delay return to optimal function. Information is often communicated and shared on a piecemeal or ad hoc basis, developed in response to a particular legal or management requirement, and without attention to either the accuracy or effectiveness of the communication. Communication is important both within the workplace, particularly in the context of provision of modified or restricted work as part of the reintegration process, but also between the workplace and the treating clinicians. Although occupational health would seem to be ideally placed to serve as an appropriate conduit, many organisations outsource occupational health and so this is not always a practical proposition. (As will be discussed below, the role of the patient/worker's line manager or supervisor therefore is extremely important.)

The social climate at work: the importance of relationships

The relationships between individuals within the organisational context play a crucial role in the RTW process and the relationship specifically between the employee and their immediate colleagues has been identified as highly influential on this process. Baril et al (2003) found that when the returning worker was given a modified work task this could cause resentment from other colleagues, especially if this task is seen as being reserved for senior staff. This situation, however, could be avoided if co-workers were given the opportunity to provide input into how tasks would be modified and distributed. A more positive relationship can also be fostered by sharing information about the changes in tasks performed and the health problem of the returning employee. Without sufficient or correct information, misunderstandings with fellow workers can occur and this can have negative consequences as the emotional atmosphere at the workplace has considerable influence on sickness absence (Nordqvist et al 2003).

The key role of the supervisor on employee absence

It has long been recognised that the supervisor plays a crucial role in the implementation of absence policies (Torrington & Hall 1995, Storey 1992). He/she is often in a unique position in being both the link between upper management and the worker but also in being the link between the health-care provider and the worker.

Thus employers often rely on supervisors to support the RTW process of absent employees and often the supervisor or department managers would be required to make first contact with the absent employee to enquire about their reasons for absence. Further, the supervisor is most likely to be responsible for conducting the RTW interview (Cunningham & James 2000). In line with this crucial role it is recommended that supervisors receive training so that they have a full understanding of the policies and are able to manage poor attendees (Havergal 1996, CIPD 2005a).

Where the supervisor actively accepts the responsibility for their role in the absence management policy, absence levels are reported to be lower or improving (Bennett 2002). However, it is not always clear who is responsible for the implementation of policy and often supervisors feel that while they have some awareness of the policy the main responsibility rests with the HR department. At the same time a significant proportion of HR practitioners felt that supervisors are not implementing the absence policy and felt that it was failing because of the reluctance to accept responsibility. Dunn & Wilkinson (2002, p. 233) highlighted how the management of absence was akin to 'pass the baton' as managers attempt to involve HR and vice versa, and in contrast to the findings of Bennett (2002) have not found evidence to suggest that devolving this responsibility to line managers would be successful. This lack of clear distinction in responsibility can result in a case of 'muddling through' (Dunn & Wilkinson 2002, p. 241). Franche et al (2005a) recommend some key aspects of the role of the supervisor. They are shown in Box 15.8.

The relationship between the employee and their supervisor is also recognised as key in the implementation of health and absence management policies. The employees' colleagues are also important in creating a positive emotional atmosphere (Nordqvist et al 2003). For example, employee perceptions of the RTW interview are very much dependent upon the relationship they have with their supervisor. If it is good the interview was seen positively, whereas if it is negative the employees viewed it as an unnecessary control mechanism (Bennett 2002). The importance of the supervisor is underlined by Shaw et al (2003) who found that the supervisory relationship may be as important as physical work accommodation to facilitate RTW after an injury.

When supervisors are involved in the planning and implementation of RTW programmes they experience fewer role conflicts (Baril et al 2003). The attitude of the supervisors towards RTW programmes is also influenced by the overall managerial and workplace attitude towards injured workers. If senior management value and understand the reasons for an RTW programme it is more likely that the programme will succeed. Thus, any policy needs the interrelated support of the employee, supervisor and management. When all stakeholders coordinate their efforts this can have a significant impact on the success of the RTW programme (Friesen et al 2001), but to achieve this goal there needs to be a climate of trust and respect, within which positive relationships and good communication can thrive (Baril et al 2003).

As health management and absence policies require the interaction of many different parties, Cunningham & James (2000) have recommended a case study approach so that the dynamic interplay between the organisation and the various individuals can be understood. The complexity and interrelatedness of these issues is reiterated by Friesen et al (2001) who state:

> RTW is influenced by multiple factors and systems. No system is isolated; an action on the part of one person, or a policy developed within one system, has an impact which often influences the responses of people within another system (p. 19).

Hence it is necessary to look at the individuals within their organisational context. This point is particularly pertinent as the attitudes of one group may contrast sharply with that of other stakeholders. In one study HR managers attributed resistance to modified work to a lack of worker motivation, while workers referenced organisational factors and elements of workplace culture (Baril et al 2003). Therefore it is essential to incorporate the views of all key stakeholders.

Impact of policies on organisational absence

A number of reflections on the impact of policies on organisational absence are shown in Box 15.9.

Box 15.8

Key features of the role of the supervisor

- Must have a vested interest in improving RTW outcomes
- Disability management practices should feature in the performance evaluation of the supervisor
- They must be supported by senior management in their efforts to promote well-being and safety, even when this adversely affects production schedules
- They need some first-aid skills to be able to gauge the seriousness of the worker's health complaints and recommend/support appropriate workplace accommodations.

Box 15.9

Key issues in successful policy implementation

- Need for systematic approach to data collection
- Influence of stringently controlled absence management
- Differences between management of long-term and short-term sickness absences
- Enthusiasm for 'robust' attendance management policies and procedures
- Risks of an 'over-robust' approach.

Need for systematic approach to data collection

It has been argued that monitoring and control procedures help to decrease the level of sickness absence (Seccombe 1995). Thus a more systematic approach to the collection of absence data is associated with lower levels of employee absence (Bennett 2002). The CIPD argue that managing absence effectively is achieved through accurate and reliable measurement, and monitoring is the only way an organisation can understand if it has a problem with absenteeism (CIPD 2005a). According to Dunn & Wilkinson (2002) an absence policy that is established by a legitimate source authority and implemented with clear and enforced legal sanctions should improve employee attendance. The clarity of the attendance management policies in place is reiterated by a CIPD report with states that policies must be clear and supportive of the organisations objectives and culture (CIPD 2005a).

Influence of stringently controlled absence management

In essence it may be perceived that stringent and controlled absence management policies are associated with lower levels of absence. However, the claim that absence control policies reduce absenteeism has been disputed (Cunningham & James 2000) as little evidence has been produced that more rigorous absence control procedures actually reduce the overall levels of absence (Wooden 1988, Edwards & Whitson 1993).

Differences between management of long-term and short-term sickness absences

The issue has already been addressed in general terms, but it bears restatement in terms of its specific impact. According to the CIPD (2005c) 60% of absences are short term in nature, but according to Clarke et al (1995), since the majority of days lost is through long spells of employee absence from the workplace, the focus of management policy on short-term absence is misdirected. Absence control policies may also, ironically, encourage absence. For example, if the policy is triggered after 10 days then it may encourage employees to take up to 9 days (Dunn & Wilkinson 2002).

Enthusiasm for 'robust' attendance management policies and procedures

HR managers may attribute low absence to a lack of tolerance within the organisation, reflective of the strict absence management policies in place. They may believe that the main reason for absence is the fact that employees do not lose out financially (Bennett 2002), based on the suppositions that employees are only interested in the financial outcome and that employees considering absence from work for illegitimate reasons will attend if it impacts on their salary. According to HR practitioners around 14% of all absences are taken for illegitimate reasons (CIPD 2005c). Low absence rates were viewed as a consequence of their rigorous management and the fact that employees knew they could not 'get away' with absence, rather than any motivation from the employee to attend (Bennett 2002).

Risks of an 'over-robust' approach

The success of absence control policies has been linked to how organisations can deter rather than encourage absenteeism. However, the policy should 'not include punishing an employee for being absent or direct discipline of any kind; rather, the reductions in absenteeism may merely reflect the existence of some reasonable policy which does not encourage employee absenteeism' (Dalton & Todor 1993, p. 207). It is therefore important that the policy should not be seen as draconian and unfair to the genuinely sick as this results in low employee morale (Taylor et al 2003). Furthermore, it can result in employees being pressured into returning to work before they are ready, in order to avoid disciplinary action. Paradoxically this can serve to raise absence as they return to work before they are fully fit and so may relapse and any contagious diseases may be spread amongst the workforce (Taylor et al 2003).

Absenteeism, presenteeism and suboptimal performance

Costs of absenteeism

Ill-health is not only a buren to individuals and society but also to employers. The costs of work absence or absenteeism have long been recognised. It has been suggested that the principal causes of absenteeism can be classified into five main categories: personal illness, family issues, personal needs, entitlement mentality and reported stress (Woo et al 1999, Atchiler & Motta 1994). Health promotion programmes have been advocated as a way of addressing absenteeism (Aldana & Pronk 2001).

The additional challenge of 'presenteeism' or suboptimal performance

In the UK, the annual cost of absenteeism has been estimated at over 1% of the GDP (Chatterji & Tilley 2002) but it is known that health risk factors and disease also adversely affect worker productivity (Burton et al 1999); it has been estimated that 3–11 hours per week in terms of productivity is lost to employers. Perhaps unsurprisingly, mental illness such as depression has a powerful influence on absenteeism, but job performance is also affected. It has been shown that depressed workers are seven times more likely to have poor job performance than non-depressed workers. The authors concluded 'because of presenteeism, previous reports of absenteeism may represent only a fraction of the cost of depression in the workplace' (Druss et al 2001, p. 733). Specific studies have examined the influence of physical disease on absenteeism. In another study sponsored by the Employers' Health Coalition of Tampa, Florida, based on a 1999 analysis of 17 diseases, researchers found that lost productivity due to presenteeism was on average 7.5 times greater than productivity due to absenteeism. For some conditions – notably allergies, arthritis, heart disease, migraine and neck/back/spine pain – the ratio was 15 to 1, 20 to 1 or even approaching 30 to 1 (Employers' Health Coalition 2000).

The idea of staff staying at work when they should be off sick, that is, 'presenteeism' remains a relatively unexplored area (Grinyer & Singleton 2000). McKevitt et al (1997) considers that the reasons for this lack of research relate to an assumption that presenteeism does not present an economic or managerial problem. However, Grinyer & Singleton (2000) argue that attendance management policies in place may encourage presenteeism and paradoxically result in higher levels of absence. They argue that there may be a number of reasons for this, summarised in Box 15.10.

Similarly Hansson et al (2006) found that employees are reluctant to take sick leave and thus may remain in the workplace when ill. Hansson et al (2006), like Grinyer & Singleton (2000), link the causes of presenteeism to absence management policies in place, for the employee will attend the workplace even if ill so as to avoid RTW interviews and trigger points. Employees consider that these features are punitive and disciplinary in nature, and therefore something to avoid. Furthermore, they find that if they are absent this damages relationships with colleagues, especially if working in a small team, and may also limit their opportunities for promotion (Grinyer & Singleton 2000). If as suggested, presenteeism, encouraged by absence management policies, ultimately results in higher levels of absence then clearly these policies are costly and not effective.

Finally, Chatterji & Tilley (2002) argue from an economic perspective that the costs associated with presenteeism mean that it is not always advantageous to reduce absence levels, and indeed the authors argue that some absence may be necessary in order to reduce the hidden costs of presenteeism.

The role of health management policies and RTW programmes

A number of important influences on RTW programmes are shown in Box 15.11.

The importance of agreement regarding goals

Health management policies in the workplace may be defined as an approach to workplace health which

Box 15.10

Costs of presenteeism

- Unwell employees coming into work could spread contagious illness
- Attendance management policies that have 'trigger points' may result in employees extending a period of absence rather than having further episodes of absence
- Continuing in the workplace when unfit to do so may then delay recovery or even exacerbate ill-health
- Being in work while ill may increase stress, particularly if annual leave is taken to avoid the associated penalties of absence.

Adapted from Grinyer & Singleton (2000)

Box 15.11

Influences on RTW programmes

- Unwell employees coming into work could spread contagious illness
- The importance of agreement regarding goals
- Impact of return to work programmes on absenteeism
- The role of employers
- Modified work
- Paths back into sustained employment
- Organisational difficulties in optimising health management.

can include health promotion, disease prevention, safety management and organisational development (Chu & Dwyer 2002). Employers have been found to be accepting a greater responsibility in this area with a move towards employer-based programmes for the rehabilitation of employees (Shrey 1996). Despite this shift there is limited literature on why and how workplace RTW programmes are effective (Baril et al 2003). Furthermore, there is little understanding of the beliefs and attitudes of those involved in the RTW programme. As Young et al (2005) have pointed out, the perception of what is a good RTW outcome depends upon the stakeholder interests and this needs to be recognised if a full understanding of RTW interventions is to be realised. RTW interventions thus need to be seen as a worthwhile process for all parties.

Impact of RTW programmes on absenteeism

RTW programmes represent the arrangements that organisations adopt to facilitate the return to work of ill and injured workers (Cunningham & James 2000). Hence the assumption of RTW policies is that employees are genuinely ill or injured and therefore need support to aid their re-entry into the workplace. The presence of RTW policies has been linked with favourable trends in absence (although not overall absence levels, Cunningham & James 2000). Additionally, RTW interventions have been found to reduce disability duration and the associated costs; however, outcomes related to quality of life remain unclear (Franche et al 2005b).

In comparison with interventions targeting Type I psychosocial risk factors (worker-related), few studies have addressed the impact of interventions targeting Type II (workplace- or system-related) risk factors and specific trials are needed (Sullivan et al 2005a). Nonetheless, a pro-active stance towards health management is supported by the CIPD who argue that effective management of health and welfare results in competitive benefits for the organisation (CIPD 2005d). Furthermore, organisations with RTW programmes have lowered injury costs and are related to satisfaction among both workers and managers (Friesen et al 2001). Despite this claim the number of organisations that implement a successful RTW programme is low, nor is it known why or how RTW programmes are effective (ibid). Similarly the CIPD found that while occupational health professionals are seen as the most effective method of managing long-term absence, only 62% use them (CIPD 2006), offering this service mostly through outsourcing methods (CIPD 2005d). Establishing a

clearer understanding of RTW policies is necessary if we are to understand what makes them effective and how they relate to absenteeism levels.

The role of employers

Recent literature has emphasised the importance of an employer-established RTW programme as a key factor that influences the return to work of employees who are absent due to back diagnoses (Nordqvist et al 2003). The authors describe how the respondents in their study raised this issue even though the researcher did not directly introduce it, thus indicating the importance of the employer. Recommendations for RTW programmes based on this study include contacting the absent employee, providing information and feedback from the supervisor to other workers and establishing routines which should be clear to all members of the workplace. Their essential argument rests on the premise that the RTW programme needs to be simple and unambiguous. Other work has emphasised the importance of a pro-active policy and an interdisciplinary, almost holistic approach to the management of health in the workplace (Chu & Dwyer 2002).

The environment that the organisation creates is crucial to the development of health management policies. Thus the culture and policies need to facilitate employee participation, professional growth and teamwork (Chu & Dwyer 2002). Furthermore, the creation of a positive emotional atmosphere should be sought and this, it is argued, can be provided by the employees' supervisor (Nordqvist et al 2003).

Modified work

Employers can also support their health management policy through the introduction of modified work for employees. By adjusting the work demands placed on an employee on their return to work, it is possible to change the working environment in order to suit the employees' needs. A number of studies have demonstrated that modifying work for injured and disabled workers shows that levels of absenteeism are reduced (Krause et al 1998, Nordqvist et al 2003). It is argued that employees who are offered modified tasks return to work twice as often as those who are not (Krause et al 1998, Crook & Moldofsky 1995). Indeed if done quickly, lost time from work may be reduced by 30% (Sinclair et al 1998).

Despite the clear indications as to the success of modified work on absenteeism the application of such

Box 15.12

Conclusions regarding modified work

- There is some evidence that modifying work for injured and disabled workers reduces absenteeism
- The application of such initiatives is not widespread, may be fairly nominal or instigated for too short a time period
- Despite this lack of implementation, ergonomic modifications remain the most common form of work modification
- The least common form of work modification relates to work organisation and sickness absence policies, even though these issues may be the most crucial.

initiatives is not widespread (Strunin & Boden 2000). Where modified work is offered, employees may feel that such adjustments, for example, light work, are in name only or that they are offered for too short a time period. On a similar theme it was found that during a participatory ergonomics programme only half of the suggested solutions were implemented (Loisel et al 2001a). Hence the evidence suggests that implementation of modified work in terms of ergonomics and task organisation while having a significant presence is not as common as might be anticipated. Despite this lack of implementation, ergonomic modifications remain the most common form of work modification. The least common form of work modification relates to work organisation and sickness absence policies, even though it is argued that these issues are the most crucial influences on employee absence (Taylor et al 2003). A number of the key issues regarding modified work are shown in Box 15.12.

Paths back into sustained employment

The employee experience of returning to work after a period of absence can vary considerably. Strunin & Boden (2000) identified three main paths that employees may encounter when re-entering employment. The first and most common route is described as 'welcome back' whereby the employer wants the worker to return and provides an environment that responds to the needs of the individual. The second path, 'business as usual', occurs when the employer recognises the worker's condition but neither assists or hinders the RTW

process. The third and final path, 'you're out', is where the employer either refuses to rehire the worker or their employment is terminated soon after the return, as the employer finds fault with the performance of the employee. Hence according to these authors the employer plays the crucial role in how RTW is experienced by the employee. When the employee perceives that the RTW process is driven by management attempts at cost control there is a distinct lack of motivation to participate in any RTW paths implemented by management (Baril et al 2003).

Organisational difficulties in optimising health management

Managers often feel that they are unable to implement particular health management policies, as they believe it will leave their organisation uncompetitive. Notably they are reluctant to amend targets and breaks due to perceived constraints of competitive pressures (Taylor et al 2003). Similarly Baril et al (2003) found that while modified work would be accommodated initially, an increase in production demands would result in an abandonment of such modifications so that production targets could be met. This conflict was felt greatly by supervisors who would try to meet the demands of production targets and accommodate the employees' needs. Thus the supervisor can act as a barrier to or enabler of necessary accommodations and they may be reluctant to help if it hinders their work (Shaw et al 2003). However, unless management are prepared to tackle these work organisational issues, the problems of occupational ill-health cannot be resolved (Taylor et al 2003). Hence there is a call for a much greater focus on the workplace *context* in which RTW interventions take place (Pransky et al 2004, Loisel et al 2005). This focus should include an identification and understanding of the organisational barriers that may compromise the successful implementation of new practical strategies (Loisel et al 2001a).

Targeting workplace or system-related psychosocial risk factors

Workplace or system-related psychosocial risk factors

Qualitative and quantitative surveys have begun to address more systematically the psychosocial dimensions of the work environment as potential risk factors for prolonged work disability. For example, job stress and co-worker support have been shown to be related to the duration of work disability (Elfering et al 2002). Hoogendoorn et al (2002) reported that the lack of social support at work and work dissatisfaction were predictors of prolonged work disability. Pransky et al (2001) reported that employer attitudes toward work disability might also impact RTW outcomes. Van Duijin et al (2004) reported the results of a survey of occupational health physicians and human resources managers showing that lack of co-worker support for modified work re-entry programmes was perceived as a major obstacle to successful RTW. Based on a review of the literature, Teasell & Bombardier (2001) reported that lack of availability of modified work and lack of autonomy in the workplace were predictors of prolonged work disability.

Interventions targeting psychosocial risk factors for work disability

Only recently have intervention programmes targeting psychosocial risk factors been implemented with the goal of preventing prolonged work disability. For example, the Sherbrooke model for back pain management was developed as an integrated approach, directed at both the worker and the workplace. It is composed of three integrated components: an occupational intervention, a clinical intervention and early rehabilitation (Loisel et al 1997). A clinical trial demonstrated better RTW outcomes and lower overall costs for patients in the Sherbrooke model intervention compared to usual care (Loisel & Durand 2005).

There is some emerging evidence that RTW rates can be improved by intervening on risk factors such as supervisor attitudes and co-worker support (Shaw & Feuerstein 2004). Similarly, ergonomic and modified RTW programmes such as those described in the Sherbrooke model might improve RTW rates, at least in part, through the reduction of psychosocial risk factors such as pain-related fears and perceived disability. Pransky et al (2001) reported the results of a pilot study suggesting promising RTW outcomes for a support and guidance intervention aimed at increasing employers' involvement in facilitating the RTW process.

In a recent study, occupational health nurses and case managers from the workers' compensation system were trained to provide early intervention to back injured workers at elevated risk for disability (Schultz & Crook 2004). The intervention involved an individual session of motivational interviewing and RTW planning with the worker. The intervention also included phone communication with the worker's family physician, work-place visit, focused case management and follow-up with the worker and employer after the return to work. The preliminary outcomes have been positive with respect to duration of disability, compared to conventional treatment.

Recommendations for action

Need for better measurement

To date, however, research on the role of worker attitudes, motivation and feelings of shame has been limited to surveys of employers' or stakeholders' views of RTW obstacles. More research is needed with respect to the operational definition and assessment of these variables in order to elucidate further how these variables might impact on work disability.

Factors such as social support in the workplace, job satisfaction, job stress and work autonomy have been shown to be associated with RTW outcomes, and this research has been important in highlighting how social or interpersonal dimensions of the work environment might influence RTW outcomes, but the role of these factors in the RTW process needs to be investigated more systematically. There is a need for more precise operational definitions of relational, attitudinal and support variables in the workplace, and more research is also needed in the development of methods of assessing these.

Developing a focus on RTW skills

An emerging trend in the secondary prevention of work disability is the development of interventions that specifically address RTW skills. Greater attention is also being given to dose- and time-dependent factors that might influence RTW outcomes. The evidence suggests that cognitive–behavioural interventions have a more pronounced impact on RTW outcomes the earlier they are implemented following the onset of work disability (Marhold et al 2001). A time-dependent dose–response relation may exist where brief interventions (e.g. medical reassurance) may yield improved outcomes in the very early stages (e.g. acute stage) of work disability, but interventions of longer duration addressing multiple dimensions of pain and disability may be required for individuals who have been absent from work for longer periods of time (Linton 2002, Haldorsen et al 2002).

Matching to risk profiles

There has been more consideration of the potential benefits of matching interventions to specific risk profiles. There are indications that the selection of candidates for treatment on the basis of 'at risk' profiles might be a rational and perhaps more cost-effective approach to the use of limited secondary prevention treatment resources (Sullivan & Stanish 2003, Linton & Andersson 2000). More research is needed to evaluate whether matching interventions to risk profiles yields better outcomes than traditional approaches that do not consider psychosocial risk profiles.

Does reduction in risk factors increase probability of RTW?

An assumption that has guided the development of risk-factor-targeted interventions for the prevention of work disability is that reductions in risk factors will be associated with a higher probability of returning to work. To date, there have been few investigations designed to verify the tenability of this assumption. Although research has pointed to psychosocial risk factors predictive of work disability, little is known about the relation between risk-factor reduction and RTW outcomes. More research is required to investigate the nature and degree of risk-factor reduction required to improve RTW outcomes.

Available research suggests that interventions provided by case managers or occupational health nurses might be an effective means of managing or preventing the development of workplace- or system-related psychosocial risk factors (Pransky et al 2001, Schultz & Crook 2004). This is clearly an area that will require more research attention in the future.

Need for a multifaceted approach

The need for multipronged integrated approaches for secondary prevention of work disability is being echoed in recent theorising on the determinants of successful RTW (Feuerstein 1991, Loisel & Durand 2005). Franche & Krause (2005) have put forward a conceptual framework to account for the variety of dynamic social, psychological and economic factors that influence disability and RTW. There seems to be an emerging consensus that the most significant gains in secondary prevention will likely emerge from intervention programmes that simultaneously target both individual and organisational psychosocial risk factors (Sullivan et al 2005a).

It is expected that future developments in the secondary prevention of work disability will ultimately reduce the proportion of individuals who continue along a chronic trajectory. It is important to acknowledge, however, that in spite of improved treatment outcomes, a certain number of individuals will not respond favourably to intervention. As such, there will be a continued need for multidisciplinary tertiary prevention programmes.

In the future it is recommended that employers take a lead role in the management of workplace health by becoming change agents and visionary leaders in this area (Chu & Dwyer 2002). When instigating changes and developing health management and absence initiatives, employers must recognise the interrelatedness of organisational and individual factors which contribute to its success or failure. Any improvements should consider the issue holistically:

> *Improvements should be seen as mutually supportive, rather than as a cafeteria menu from which the least contentious, individual items are selected (p. 454).*

Hence it is not sufficient for management to select solutions which just suit their own needs, any changes need to support the health management and absence policy in its entirety. Further recommendations include participation and empowerment of the worker, which is vital to the well-being of the worker on their return to work. Similarly, it is important that all stakeholders (i.e. not just management) are involved in the planning and implementation of any initiative (Friesen et al 2001). Information sharing is also recognised as crucial in this process (Pransky et al 2004, Freisen et al 2001, Nordqvist et al 2003). Through effective information exchange (a two-way process) relationship building is enabled and this may be especially important in reaching a consensus on any RTW programme (Pransky et al 2004). Furthermore, Amick et al (2000) reported that a more open and receptive communication demonstrated by employers was linked with superior disability management outcomes. The important role of communication reflects earlier statements of the need to keep co-workers informed of the returning employee's condition and modified work task (Nordqvist et al 2003). Therefore communication throughout the organisation appears to be a crucial component of any health management and absence policy.

It is evident that RTW activities, health management and absence policies are important areas of research as these issues have many implications for both the individual and the organisation. Cunningham & James

(2000) support this view and recommend that research should focus on a number of issues, including exploration of variations of presence, content and operation of policies between organisations, the nature and extent of sickness absence and the extent to which their impact is affected by the structure and climate of manager–worker relations. Further research in this area needs to examine the perceptions of individual stakeholders, particularly on the perspectives of the employers and employees (Feuerstein 2003), the dynamic relationships within the organisation and the organisational climate if a coherent account of health management and absence policies is to be established.

Conclusions

Interaction between flags

For convenience, in terms of conceptualisation, and in consideration of types of intervention, a fairly sharp distinction has been made between the more clinically focused flags (red, orange and yellow) and the more occupationally focused flags (blue and black). Design of work retention and work rehabilitation, however, is about individual workers, or groups of individual workers, who may be 'surrounded' by flags of different colours. Management of the flags, whether as specific targets for intervention in their own right, or as risk factors for suboptimal performance or absence will often involve a series of stakeholders, and require a 'systems approach' (as was conceptualised in the development of the yellow flags and demonstrated by Loisel et al (1997) who, in their randomised controlled trial, demonstrated the need to tackle both the clinical and occupational components of work disability).

A developmental model of work disability

Young et al (2005) offer an illuminating approach to work disability (or, in other parlance, rehabilitation of the injured worker), inspired by the WHO's classification of functioning, disability and health. As a precursor they offer clarification of their use of key terms which is reproduced for illustrative purposes in Box 15.13 as a helpful way to understand the RTW process.

They then consider RTW in terms of four phases: Off work; Re-entry, Maintenance and Advancement, which they use primarily as a research framework for linking key RTW actions with associated outcomes. They are reproduced in Table 15.1.

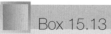

Box 15.13

Suggestions for clarification of key terms (from Young et al 2005)

Work disability

The result of a condition that causes a worker to miss at least one day of work and includes time off work as well as any ongoing work limitations.

Return-to-work (RTW)

When RTW is used without a qualifier (stakeholder, process, outcome, goal, etc.) it refers to RTW as a phenomenon encompassing both the process and associated outcomes.

RTW stakeholder

A person, organisation or agency that stands to gain or lose based on the results of the RTW process. The primary stakeholders are workers, employers, health-care providers, payers and society.

Return-to-work goal

A mutually acceptable RTW target; usually a safe, sustainable and timely RTW with the previous employer at preinjury levels of productivity and wages. In other cases, an alternative RTW goal may be set; RTW goals are not assumed to be static (and the RTW process may include goal review and change based on information that becomes available).

Return-to-work process

Refers to the process workers go through in order to reach, or attempt to reach, their final RTW goal. It encompasses a series of events, transitions and phases and includes interactions with other individuals and the environment. The process begins at the onset of work disability and concludes when a satisfactory long-term outcome has been achieved.

Return-to-work outcome

Describes a measurable characteristic of the worker's RTW status or experience. Outcomes can occur through the process and include such variables as employment status, productivity, job satisfaction, promotion and satisfaction with disability management activities.

As Sullivan et al (2005a) point out,

at the present time, little is known about the manner in which Type I (worker-related) and Type II (workplace or system-related) psychosocial risk factors summate or interact to influence the duration of work disability (p. 483).

Table 15.1 Key RTW and associated outcomes

Phase	Key RTW actions	Associated Outcomes
1. Off Work	Determine abilities	Able vs unable to work
	Determine work intentions	Intend to resume working vs not
	Determine employment goal	Goal formulated (inc. hours, duties, remuneration, productivity & advancement opportunities)
	Formulate plan for achieving goal	Plan formulated
	Perform behaviours required to achieve goal	Behaviours performed
	Identify suitable work option	Suitable option identified
	Determine readiness for work re-entry	Assessed as ready for work re-entry
	Secure suitable position	Suitable position secured
2. Re-entry	Return to work-place	Achieved vs not
	Determine job suitability	Job suitable (i.e. good use of skills, safe, acceptable remunerations) vs not
	If job unsuitable, determine if this can be changed	Job has potential to be suitable vs not
	If unsuitable job can be changed, determine a plan for doing so	Formulate plan for change vs not
	If unsuitable job cannot be changed, seek alternative	Alternative identified
	Reassess work abilities	Abilities reassessed
	Determine if work abilities can be improved	Potential for improvement vs not
	Reassess employment goal	Appropriate vs not
	If goal not appropriate, reformulate goal	Goal reformulated (inc. hours, duties, remuneration, productivity & advancement opportunities vs not)
	Determine progress towards achieving goal	Progressing satisfactorily vs not
	Determine when goal status has been initiated	Goal status achieved vs not
3. Maintenance	Demonstrate consistent performance	Goal status maintained vs not
	Reassess employment goal	Advancement desired vs advancement not desired vs decide to withdraw from the labour force
4. Advancement	Maintain employment gains	Goal status maintained vs not
	Formulate plan for advancement	Plan formulated vs not
	Perform activities required to advance	Performing advancement seeking vs not
	Find suitable advancement opportunity	Suitable opportunity identified vs not
	Achieve advancement	Advancement achieved vs not

From Young et al (2005, Fig. 2, p.564).

Nonetheless, although further research into the determinants of work absence is clearly needed, we have identified a number of the important individual and organisational factors associated with outcome. However, we now need to move beyond attempted identification of individual predictors to hypothesis-driven investigations, using appropriate metrics within a conceptual framework which includes the key elements, players and processes necessary to focus interventions on modifiable targets and, wherever possible, attempting to turn apparent obstacles into opportunities for change.

Key points

- In considering pain-related work compromise, it is important to appraise the nature and implementation of organisational policies and practice concerning ill-health and sickness absence
- Distinguishing national policies and legislation regarding employment from local organisation-specific agreements and practices may offer opportunities for improving sickness management
- Employers' attendance management policies may be a major obstacle to work retention and return to work
- However, what may appear to be significant obstacles to successful and sustained RTW (black flags) may present opportunities for organisation interventions
- Detailed analysis of the human resource/occupational health interface is a prerequisite for developing a successful work retention or RTW strategy

(Continued)

- Prolonged absence is multiply determined, and its costs are often identified, but the costs of short-term absence and health-related work compromise in those still at work may represent an important 'hidden' cost and, as such, merit specific consideration
- An overall strategy, incorporating health-related work compromise, not only for those with prolonged absence but also for those with short-term absences and those still at work, but struggling, is required
- In reshaping and designing policy to optimise work retention and facilitate successful RTW, clear and effective communication among all key stakeholders is required
- For those with recurrent or prolonged absences, adoption of a 'case-management' framework may be helpful
- The social climate at work, particularly with reference to ill-health, needs to be considered at the level both of management and of working colleagues
- Key players include the employee, occupational health, and human resources, but the role of the line manager or supervisor is critical, and merits special attention.

References

Aldana S G, Pronk N P 2001 Health promotion programs, modifiable health risks and employee absenteeism. Journal of Occupational and Environmental Medicine 43:36–46

Amick, III B, Habeck R, Hunt A et al 2000 Measuring the impact of organizational behaviors on work disability prevention and management. Journal of Occupational Rehabilitation 10(20):21–38

Atchiler L, Motta R 1994 Effects of aerobic and non-aerobic exercise on anxiety, absenteeism and job satisfaction. Journal of Clinical Psychology 50:829–840

Baril R, Clare J, Friesen M et al, the Work Ready Group 2003 Management of return-to-work programs for workers with musculoskeletal disorders: a qualitative study in three Canadian Provinces. Social Science and Medicine 57:2101–2114

Belbo M, Ortlieb R 2006 The impact of working conditions and household context on employee absenteeism. 24th International Labour Process Conference, University of London, 10–12 April

Bennett H 2002 Employee commitment: the key to absence management in local government? Leadership and Organizational Development Journal 23(8):430–441

Berger M L, Murray J F, Xu J et al 2001 Alternative valuations of work loss and productivity. Journal of Occupational and Environmental Medicine 43:18–24

Bloch F S, Prins R 2001 Who returns to work and why. Transaction Publishers, New Brunswick

Burton W N, Conti D J, Chen C Y et al 1999 The role of health risk factors and disease on worker productivity. Journal of Occupational and Environmental Medicine 41:863–877

Chatterji M, Tilley C J 2002 Sickness, absenteeism, presentee-ism, and sick pay. Oxford Economic Papers 54:669–687

Chu C, Dwyer S 2002 Employer role in integrative workplace health management: a new model in progress. Disease Management and Health Outcomes 10(3):175–186

CIPD 2005a Absence management. www.cipd.co.uk

CIPD 2005b Sickness continues to hit public sector employers harder than private services sector. Press Office. www.cipd.co.uk

CIPD 2005c Annual survey report. Absence management: a survey of policy and practice. www.cipd.co.uk/onlineinfodocuments/surveys

CIPD 2005d Occupational health and organisational effectiveness. www.cipd.co.uk

CIPD 2006 A barometer of HR trends and prospects. Overview of CIPD surveys. www.cipd.co.uk

Clarke S, Elliot R, Osman J 1995 Occupation and sickness absence. Occupational Health: Decennial Supplement, HMSO, London

Cooper C 1994 The costs of healthy work organisation. In: Cooper C, Williams S, Creating healthy work organisations. John Wiley, Chichester

Cotton J L, Tuttle J M 1986 Employee turnover: a meta-analysis and review with implications for research. Academy of Management Review 11:55–70

Crook J, Moldofsky H 1995 Prognostic indicators of disability after a work-related musculosketal injury. Journal of Musculoskeletal Pain 3(2):155–159

Cunningham I, James P 2000 Absence and return to work: towards a research agenda. Personnel Review 29(1):33–47

Dalton D, Mesch D 1990 The impact of flexible scheduling on employee attendance and turnover. Administrative Science Quarterly 35(20):370–388

Dalton D R, Todor W D 1993 Turnover, transfer, absenteeism: an interdependent perspective. Journal of Management 19:193–219

Druss B G, Schlesinger M, Allen H M (Jr) 2001 Depressive symptoms, satisfaction with health care and 2-year work outcomes in an employed population. American Journal of Psychiatry 158:731–734

Dunn C, Wilkinson A 2002 Wish you were here: managing absence. Personnel Review 31(2):228–246

Edwards P, Whitson C 1993 Attending to work: the management of attendance and shop floor order, Blackwell, Oxford

Elfering A, Semmer N K, Schade V et al 2002 Supportive colleague, unsupportive supervisor: the role of provider-specific constellations of social support at work in the development of low back pain. Journal of Occupational Health Psychology 7:130–140

Employers' Health Coalition 2000 Healthy people/productivity community survey 1999. Restricted access

Feuerstein M 1991 Multidisciplinary approach to the prevention, evaluation and management of work disability. Journal of Occupational Rehabilitation 11:5–12

Feuerstein M 2003 Editorial. In their own words: qualitative studies of employers and workers. Journal of Occupational Rehabilitation 13:127

Franche R L, Krause N 2005 Readiness for return to work following injury or illness: conceptualizing the interpersonal impact of health care, workplace and insurance factors. In: Schultz I Z, Gatchel R J (eds) Handbook of complex occupational disability claims: early risk identification, intervention and prevention. Springer, New York, ch 4 pp 67–91

Franche R L, Baril R, Shaw W et al 2005a Workplace-base return-to-work interventions: optimizing the role of

stakeholders in implementation and research. Journal of Occupational Rehabilitation 15:525–542

Franche R L, Cullen K, Clarke J et al, the Institute for Work & Health (IWH) 2005b Workplace-based RTW Intervention Literature Review Research Team. Workplace-based return-to-work interventions: a systematic review of the quantitative literature. Journal of Occupational Rehabilitation 15:607–631

Friesen M N, Yassi A, Cooper J 2001 Return-to-work: the importance if human interactions and organizational structures. Work 17:11–22

Gellatly I R, Luchak A A 1998 Personal and organisational determinants of perceived absence norms. Human Relations 51(8):1085–1103

Grinyer A, Singleton V 2000 Sickness absence as risk-taking behaviour: a study of organisational and cultural factors in the public sector. Health, Risk and Society 2(1):7–21

Haldorsen E M, Grasdal A L, Skouen J S et al 2002 Is there a right treatment for a particular patient group? Comparison of ordinary treatment, light multidisciplinary treatment, and extensive multidisciplinary treatment for long-term sick-listed employees with musculoskeletal pain. Pain 95:49–63

Hansson M, Bostrom C, Harms-Ringdahl K 2006 Sickness absence and sickness attendance: what people with neck or back pain think. Social Science and Medicine 62:2183–2195

Harvey J, Nicholson N 1993 Incentives and penalties as a means of influencing attendance: a study in the UK public sector. International Journal of Human Resource Management 4(4):641–855

Havergal M 1996 Lies, damned lies and absence statistics. Health Manpower Management 22(1):30–31

Ho J T 1997 Corporate Wellness programmes in Singapore: effects on stress, satisfaction and absenteeism. Journal of Managerial Psychology 12(3):177–180

Hoogendoorn W E, Bongers P M, de Vet H C et al 2002 High physical work load and low job satisfaction increase the risk of sickness absence due to low back pain: results of a prospective cohort study. Occupational and Environmental Medicine 59:323–328

IDS 1998 Managing absence. Incomes Data Services, London

IDS 2004 Incomes Data Services report on the CBI survey in IDS HR Studies 782 – September 2004 that reviews sickness and absence surveys by CIPD, CBI. www.incomes-data.co.uk

IRS (Industrial Relations Services) 1994 Sick pay trends, absence control developments and the impact of SSP changes. IRS Employment Trends 569:8–16

Johnson C J, Croghan E, Crawford J 2003 The problem and management of sickness absence in the NHS: considerations for nurse managers. Journal of Nursing Management 11:336–342

Krause N, Dasinger L K, Neuhauser F 1998 Modified work and return to work: a review of the literature. Journal of Occupational Rehabilitation 8(2):113–139

Linton S J 2002 New avenues for the prevention of chronic musculoskeletal pain and disability pain research and clinical management, vol 12. Elsevier, Amsterdam

Linton S J, Andersson T 2000 Can chronic disability be prevented? A randomized trial of a cognitive-behavioural intervention and two forms of information for patients with spinal pain. Spine 25:2825–2831

Linton S J, Gross D, Schultz I Z et al 2005 Prognosis and the identification of workers risking disability: research issues and directions for future research. Journal of Occupational Rehabilitation 15:457–474

Loisel P, Durand M J 2005 Working with the employer: the Sherbrooke model. In: Schultz I Z, Gatchel R J (eds) Handbook of complex occupational disability claims: early risk identification, intervention and prevention. Springer, New York, ch 26, pp 479–488

Loisel P, Abenhaim L, Durand P et al 1997 A population-based randomised clinical trial on back pain management. Spine 22:2911–2918

Loisel P, Durand M J, Berthelette D et al 2001a Disability prevention: new paradigm for the management of occupational back pain. Disease Management Health Outcomes 9:351–360

Loisel P, Gosselin L, Durand P et al 2001b Implementation of participatory ergonomics program in the rehabilitation of workers suffering from subacute back pain. Applied Ergonomics 32:53–60

Loisel P, Buchbinder R, Hazard R et al 2005 Prevention of work disability due to musculoskeletal disorders: the challenge of implementing evidence. Journal of Occupational Rehabilitation 15:507–524

McHugh M 2001 Employee absence: an impediment to organisational health in local government. The International Journal of Public Sector Management 14(1):43–58

McKevitt C, Morgan M, Dundas D et al 1997 Sickness absence and 'working through' illness: a comparison of two professional groups. Journal of Public Health Medicine 19:295–300

Main C J, Burton A K 2000 Economic and occupational influences on pain and disability. In: Main C J, Spanswick C C (eds) Pain management: an interdisciplinary approach. Churchill Livingstone, Edinburgh, ch 4, pp 63–87

Marhold C, Linton S J, Melin L 2001 A cognitive-behavioral return-to-work program: effects on pain patients with a history of long-term versus short-term sick leave. Pain 91:155–163

Nordqvist C, Holmqvist C, Alexanderson K 2003 Views of laypersons on the role employers play in return to work when sick-listed. Journal of Occupational Rehabilitation 13(1):11–20

Overmeer T, Linton S J, Boersma K 2004 Do physiotherapists recognise established risk factors? Swedish physiotherapists evaluation in comparison to guidelines. Physiotherapy 90:35–41

Pransky G, Shaw W S, McLellan R K 2001 Employer attitudes, training, and return to work outcomes: a pilot study. Assistant Technologist 13:131–138

Pransky G S, Shaw W S, Franche R L et al 2004 Disability prevention and communication among workers, physicians, employers and insurers – current models and opportunities for improvement. Disability and Rehabilitation 26(11):625–634

Pransky G, Gatchel R, Linton S J et al 2005 Improving return to work research. Journal of Occupational Rehabilitation 15(4):525–542

Rentsch J R, Steel R P 1998 Testing the durability of job characteristics as predictors of absenteeism over a six year period. Personnel Psychology 51(1):165–191

Rowlinson K, Berthoud R 1998 Disability benefits and employment. DSS Research Report No 54. London, HMSO

Saratoga 1998 The European/United Kingdom human asset effectiveness report, 5th edn. Saratoga, Oxford

Schultz I, Crook J 2004 Application of a risk-for-disability questionnaire in the identification of subacute low back injured workers who require early intervention. Journal of Pain 4(suppl 1):8

Seccombe I 1995 Sickness absence and health at work in the NHS. Health Manpower Management 21(5):6–11

Shaw W S, Feuerstein M 2004 Generating workplace accommodations: lessons learned from the integrated case management study. Journal of Occupational Rehabilitation 14:207–216

Shaw W S, Feuerstein M, Huang G D 2002 Secondary prevention and the workplace. In: Linton S J (ed) New avenues for the prevention of chronic musculoskeletal pain and disability. Pain Research and Clinical Management, vol 12. Elsevier Ltd, Amsterdam, pp 215–235

Shaw W S, Robertson M M, Pransky G et al 2003 Employee perspectives on the role of supervisors to prevent workplace disability after injuries. Journal of Occupational Rehabilitation 13(3):129–142

Shrey D E 1996 Disability management in industry. Disability and Rehabilitation 18(8):408–414

Sinclair F J, Hogg-Johnson S, Shannon H et al 1998 Preventing disability from work-related low-back pain. New evidence gives new hope – if we can just get all the players onside. Canadian Medical Association Journal 158:12

Storey J 1992 Developments in the management of human resources. Basil Blackwell, Oxford

Strunin L, Boden L I 2000 Paths of re-entry: employment experiences of injured workers. American Journal of Industrial Medicine 38:373–384

Sullivan M J L, Stanish W D 2003 Psychologically based occupational rehabilitation: the pain-disability prevention program. Clinical Journal of Pain 19:97–104

Sullivan M J L, Feuerstein M, Gatchel R J et al 2005a Integrating psychosocial and behavioral interventions to achieve optimal rehabilitation outcomes. Journal of Occupational Rehabilitation 15:475–489

Sullivan M J L, Ward L C, Tripp D et al 2005b Secondary prevention of work disability: community-based psycho-social intervention for musculoskeletal disorders. Journal of Occupational Rehabilitation 15:77–392

Taylor P, Baldry C, Bain B et al 2003 'A unique working environment': health, sickness and absence management in UK call centres. Work, Employment and Society 17(3):435–458

Teasell R W, Bombardier C 2001 Employment-related factors in chronic pain and chronic pain disability. Clinical Journal of Pain 17:S39–S45

Torrington D, Hall L 1995 Personnel management, 3rd edn. Prentice-Hall, London

Truchon M, Fillion L, Cote P et al 2006 Déterminantes de l'incapacité chronique: étude prospective longitudinale de travailleurs en arrêt de travail en raison d'une lombagie. (Determinants of chronic disability: a prospective longitu-dinal study of workers on sick leave due to low back pain.) Report to ISST

van Duijn M, Miedema H, Elders L et al 2004 Barriers for early return-to-work of workers with musculoskeletal disorders according to occupational health physicians and human resources managers. Journal of Occupational Rehabilitation 14:31–41

Waddell G, Burton A K 2006 Is work good for your health and well-being? The Stationary Office, London

Waddell G, Aylward M, Sawney P 2002 Back pain, incap-acity for work and social security benefits: an international literature review and analysis. Royal Society of Medicine Press, London

Waddell G, Burton A K, Main C J 2003 Screening to identify people at risk of long-term incapacity for work: a concep-tual and scientific review. Royal Society of Medicine Press, London

Woo M, Yap A K, Oh T G et al 1999 The relationship between reported stress and absenteeism. Singapore Medical Journal 40:1–12

Wooden M 1988 Management of labour absence: an inventory of strategies and measures. National Institute of Labour Studies, Flinders University of South Australia, Working Paper 97

Young A E, Wasiak R, Roessler R T et al 2005 Return-to-work outcomes following work disability: stakeholder motiv-ations, interests and concerns. Journal of Occupational Rehabilitation 15(4):543–556

Section **Six**

Conclusions

In Chapter 16 we consider possible future developments of relevance to pain management, such as use of functional magnetic resonance imaging (fMRI), evolutionary perspectives and phenomenology and their potential for shedding further light on the pain experience. We consider that reappraisal of the nature of chronicity and the determinants of consulting may prove helpful. We recommend reappraisal of the role of psychological assessment in particular, with the design of new targeted interventions in the context of a clearer understanding of the importance of *context* as well as content in the delivery of pain management, and a broadening of perspective to include consideration of well-being as well as sickness, and performance as well as absence. In extending the reach of pain management, we consider the use of new vehicles for service delivery, and identify the importance of fully addressing issues of diversity, within an evidence-based culture and research framework.

Chapter **Sixteen**

Conclusions

CHAPTER CONTENTS

New models of pain and disability: opportunities for pain management

With the rapid development of sophisticated tools such as functional magnetic resonance imaging (fMRI) we are being offered new insights into the structure and function of the nervous system, the brain and pain processing. It can be expected that this new knowledge will in turn lead to new understanding of fundamental pain mechanisms. In parallel with investigation of the anatomical and physiological substrates of nociception and pain perception, adoption of an evolutionary perspective offers an understanding of pain as part of an adaptive biological response to the human environment (Williams 2002). Studies of consciousness within a constructivist framework shed further light on the pain experience (Chapman et al 1999). This 'internal representation of reality' allows us into the world of phenomenology, beginning with the primacy of the pain experience and offering an interface for the biological and psychological components of pain. When we deconstruct the experience of pain into its cognitive and emotional components, we begin to understand the suffering of the pain patient. Consideration of the patient's view of him/herself in terms of their schema about pain and illness can help us understand the differences between their 'enmeshed' image of themselves (Pincus & Morley 2001) as pain patients, as contrasted with their 'prepain' self, with others and with their own futures. Thus considering patients in terms of their 'possible selves' (Morley et al 2005) allows us to investigate the processes of psychological adjustment and consideration of pain management strategies, whether in terms of reactivation and re-engagement or in terms of acceptance (McCracken & Eccleston 2003, McCracken et al 2004). The full emotional impact of suffering is still insufficiently understood (Wall 1999), although there have been importance advances in the role of fear (Vlaeyen et al 1995, Vlaeyen & Linton 2000). Pain, however, also has its behavioural component and an adequate understanding of pain behaviour cannot be understood without appreciation of its social context. This of course was well understood by luminaries such as Fordyce (1976), the full force of whose insights has underpinned modern pain management, and Turk et al (1983) who were amongst the first to realise the importance of addressing both the cognitive and behavioural aspects of chronic pain and who inspired the recent development of the biopsychomotor model of pain (Sullivan 2007) with a focus on secondary prevention (Linton et al 1989, Linton & van Tulder 2000) and the targeting of risk factors for chronicity (Sullivan et al 2005). This broadening of perspectives not only allows us a wider range of possible therapeutic approaches for the individual in pain, but also to the adoption of 'system approaches' focusing on the social context of the pain patient, in terms of participation in society and work.

New understandings of chronicity

A second theme which has emerged during the gestation of this textbook has been the difficulties in moving from a static to a dynamic view of pain and the development of chronicity. We have long understood that there are differences between acute pain and chronic pain. Although in the early days of the single-handed anaesthetist-led pain relief clinics, the difference seems to have been used primarily in terms of treatment failure or the simple passage of time, rather than appreciation of the psychological and physiological changes that have become apparent with investigation of psychological mechanisms, the postulation of the 'neuromatrix' (Melzack 1999) and identification of neuroplasticity (Woolf & Salter 2000).

Traditionally, the concept of tissue-healing time, derived from an understanding of inflammatory processes, led to a view that most pain 'should get better' by around 6 weeks. This in combination with a number of studies looking at recovery rates after injury (Crook & Moldovsky 1994) may have contributed inadvertently to an underestimation of the extent of individual differences and helped establish an oversimplistic view of the extent and nature of chronicity. There has often been

an assumption that cessation of consultation and resolution of symptoms were the same but we now know they are not. Many people report ongoing symptoms of pain and disability but they do not consult and may not even be absent from work. Why this is so has received little attention, as research has been so preoccupied with those who adopt a sick role, but it may be useful and informative to investigate positive coping to help inform future management.

Clinical research trials clearly need inclusion and exclusion criteria for patients entering the study. In terms of prognosis and outcome it is clearly important to attempt to study a homogeneous group of patients and criteria based on length of present episode are frequently employed. Indeed the early studies demonstrating differences between acute and chronic patients could not have been undertaken without some sort of 'classification rules'. However, given the proportion of patients who recover fairly quickly, decisions about inclusion or exclusion are influenced not so much by a clear understanding of the process of chronicity, but by expediency and cost. In a cost-constrained health-care system, it would seem wasteful to allocate resources to the investigation or treatment of patients with acute pain problems who are going to get better in any event. In terms of prevention of prolonged pain or continued disability, however, having perhaps excluded the majority who recover quickly, there would appear to be a window of opportunity (between perhaps 3 and 12 weeks), where identification of prognostic predictors and attempts at secondary prevention would seem to be worthwhile. That said, there is a danger of underestimating the importance of individual differences within such a window. We know that the strength of predictors varies with the passage of time (Waddell et al 2003) and that in a significant proportion of back patients, the pattern is recurrent rather than chronic. We need to gain a clearer understanding of the *process* of chronicity itself and may need less simplistic classifications in our research. Recent attempts at classification based on presence of prognostic factors for chronicity (Von Korff & Miglioretti 2006, Dunn et al 2007) may prove helpful. We also require much more sharply focused studies of change in the individual, and response to targeted interventions, assisted by more powerful and imaginative research designs such as single-case methodology (Morley & Vlaeyen 2005), with specific targeting perhaps of modifiable risk factors for chronicity. Failure to grasp the challenge of addressing such individual differences may result in failure to advance beyond the present models in increasing our success rate in prevention and in leaving individuals vulnerable to well-intentioned, but misdirected initiatives such as *Back Pain in the Workplace* (Fordyce 1995).

Determinants of consulting

We still do not have a clear understanding of the determinants of consulting in the individual case. The reasons for consulting are not always self-evident, and not always clear, even in the mind of the patient.

In developing teaching about, and training in, early intervention, it has become our practice to structure our assessment such that it *begins* with an explicit focus on determining the patient/worker's reason for consultation; whether it has been self-initiated, instigated by a family member or other clinician, or mandated as a requirement for sick certification or entry into a work rehabilitation programme. There remains a fertile area of research in determining why a person identifies a symptom as significant and the factors motivating subsequent consultation. In this book we have already looked at the potential for public health initiatives in the modification of beliefs about back pain with the potential for an impact upon consultation and work absence. Other researchers have identified people with unhelpful beliefs about pain in a working population with specific interventions to correct these and so prevent work absence. Once again, imaginative interventions introduced early seem to be key. Waiting until the 'person' becomes a 'patient' could mean we lose the initiative in the prevention of chronicity.

Role of psychological assessment

We have focused much on this topic earlier in the book, because of the increasing recognition of the powerful influence of psychological factors in prognosis. Firstly, we should like to offer an initial observation. There are different types of psychological assessment, and we have tried to make a clear distinction between the psychological aspects of pain, disability and work (yellow and blue flags), the assessment of which should be within the competence of all health-care and rehabilitation personnel, and the assessment of significant psychological factors (orange flags) requiring careful appraisal by a suitably qualified mental health professional as a precursor of reconsideration of 'routine' pain management. Secondly, specifically in terms of pain management, we should like to offer two specific recommendations. We need to change our focus of psychological assessment from depicting the psychological backdrop to purposive assessment of targets for interventions. In tertiary-care programmes for patients with significant pain and high levels of disability, the potential targets for intervention may be clearly evident. In considering secondary prevention potential targets may be much less evident and necessitate a focus on modifiable risk factors for prolonged pain or disability. We acknowledge that many health-care professionals are uncomfortable taking on these additional skills. We do not expect them to become psychologists; that is inappropriate and is not required. But they must become proficient in identifying and managing simple problems which will lead to suboptimal outcome regardless of how technically proficient they are within their own discipline (e.g. medicine, manual therapy).

New types of interventions

While it is always important to develop new interventions and types of interventions, it would seem that we now have quite a large armamentarium on which to draw. It is to be expected that there will be further developments in, and refinements of, specific psychological techniques such as mindfulness, meditation, cognitive restructuring and acceptance therapy. It seems, however, that the challenge at this time is not so much devising radically new approaches to intervention, but in customising more effectively the techniques already at our disposal and gaining a clearer understanding of contextual influences on acceptance of, and response to, treatment. The emphasis should be not so much on new techniques but on better selection and moving these interventions appropriately upstream, nearer to the start of the episode of pain.

Clearer understanding of potential for pain management in different settings

In developing the new edition of this textbook we have been struck by the potential for the extension of modern pain management into other parts of the health-care system and occupational environment. As a first step in the 'roll-out' of pain management, we have focused in particular on primary-care, secondary-/tertiary-care and occupational settings. We recognise that this distinction is not only somewhat imprecise, and health-care system dependent, but, at least for now, we feel that such differentiation may be helpful. It is clear that there are related but distinct challenges for pain management in each of these settings.

Primary care

In primary care, effort needs to be focused on optimal early management, possibly incorporating systems of screening and targeting, but perhaps assisted by media campaigns and development of optimal self-care advice, using information technology to deliver 'best advice' focused not only on symptom management, but also on the promulgation of well-being in its various guises. It has to be accepted that pain is a part of life, but unnecessary suffering and significant compromise to participation and work is not. Given the propensity of our citizens to 'catastrophise' and health-care professions to 'overmedicalise' pain, we must direct our efforts to optimise secondary prevention. Musculoskeletal pain is a common event for most people, incapacity in varying degrees is likely in a few, disability to the point of social exclusion should be unacceptable and can be avoided.

Secondary/tertiary care

In secondary/tertiary care, although tertiary pain clinics and rehabilitation programmes may be viewed as the seedbed of modern pain management, much remains to be done. It would seem fair to say that there has been a significant improvement in the management of chronic 'benign' pain within chronic pain programmes. It is undoubtedly true that the economic impact of musculoskeletal disability has been an important driver in this process. However, we need to recognise that chronic pain is a component of a wide range of conditions, but through the vagaries of referral systems and the politics of health care, the management of chronic pain in patients with comorbid conditions frequently seems to be suboptimal. Thus for example, patients with chronic non-specific musculoskeletal conditions seem to be better served in terms of access to modern pain management, than do for example patients with visceral pain, renal pain, gynaecological pain, genito-urological pain or headache. Similarly, although cardiac patients, neurological/neurosurgical patients and cancer patients seem to have access to a broader spectrum of treatment and pain management than some of the aforementioned groups, specialised pain management seldom seems to have prominence in their profile of care. It sometimes seems that pain management is the last resort of those with benign or non-specific pain and that in patients with 'identifiable' conditions medical management remains the focus. These somewhat random reflections are offered merely as illustrations of the underprovision in our view of optimal pain management in secondary-/tertiary-care settings. The reasons for this state of affairs are undoubtedly complex, as are any solutions. Recognition of pain *in its own right*, as has happened in some jurisdictions, might be a first step in redirecting resources to the improvement of the management of pain in secondary-/tertiary-care settings.

In the previous edition of this book we focused mainly on those people who had come to the end of medical investigations and interventions. Many institutions still require that patients are not seeking other interventions as a prerequisite to inclusion in a pain management programme. We need to become more imaginative in how we can combine medical investigations with pain management techniques. This will require close and honest cooperation between the members of the team and the agreement with the patient of the aims of treatment and the expected outcomes. Although much progress has been made in the areas of rheumatoid disease there remains much more work to be done on how to successfully marry the two.

Occupational settings

Perhaps the most noticeable difference between the first edition of the textbook and this new edition has been the increased focus on the pain/work interface. We have attempted firstly to distinguish clinical from occupational perspectives, not only in terms of their nature, but in terms of their implications for action. This was crystallised specifically into our subdivision of the original yellow flags for chronicity (Kendall et al 1997) into clinical yellow flags and occupational blue and black flags (Main & Burton 2000). We have stressed the importance of distinguishing *perceptions* of work from *objective* work characteristic, which in terms of potential obstacles to recovery/optimal function map onto the blue and black flags respectively. Finally, in terms of moving from obstacles to recovery to opportunities for intervention, we have distinguished Type I (worker-centred) interventions from Type II (workplace or system) interventions (Sullivan et al 2005).

There are, however, some additional emerging perspectives which merit mention.

From absenteeism to presenteeism

It is known that health risk factors and disease not only lead to sickness absence but also adversely affect worker productivity (Burton et al 1999). Hansson et al (2006) found that employees are reluctant to take sick leave and thus may remain in the workplace when ill. 'Presenteeism', or suboptimal performance through ill-health is a burden not only to individuals and society but also to employers. In another recent study, Main et al (2005) found that negative impact of symptoms had an even greater influence on performance than absence and that perceptions of work (blue flags) had a more powerful influence than objective work characteristics. Thus pain management for symptomatic workers, possibly in conjunction with the management of other symptoms, would seem to merit consideration in the context of the minimisation of work compromise and future work absence.

From sickness management to well-being

As was previously discussed (particularly in Ch. 15), symptoms of ill-health (including pain) are usually addressed primarily from a 'sickness management' perspective. Studies of organisational stress had identified aspects of the working environment and aspects of work which are associated with ill-health. Factors have ranged from temperature and lighting to the social environment at work. Legislation has been introduced to establish minimum standards in terms of temperature, light and air quality, such that organisations can be held to account in the event of failure of meeting the requisite standards. Yet it has been known for many years that the social climate at work can also have a powerful influence of performance and well-being. Managers are now trained in the identification and prevention of bullying and harassment. It has always been understood that some jobs by their very nature can be unpleasant, monotonous and inherently unsatisfying. In such situations, improvements in the working environment can act as a 'buffer' against the tedium and unpleasantness of work. It the UK, in particular, there has been a tendency to overemphasise the negative aspects of work. Indeed it has been assumed that work, in terms of health primarily is a hazard. Recently, however, there has been an increasing recognition that work can have many positive features over and above the obvious financial rewards.

In 2005, the UK government published a *Health, Work and Well-being* strategy (HM Government 2005) in which there was an explicit recognition of the need for a shift in focus from sickness to well-being. In a later, but associated evidence-based review, Waddell & Burton (2006) concluded:

> *There is a strong evidence base that work is generally good for physical and mental health and wellbeing. Worklessness is associated with poorer physical and mental health and wellbeing. Work can be therapeutic and can reverse the adverse health effects of unemployment (p. ix).*

While it is clear that there are many different ways in different individuals in which objective work characteristics and perceptions of work may influence both ill-health and well-being, there are important implications for pain management. Given that a significant proportion of the population have recurrent pain problems at best, and persistent pain-associated limitations at worst, enhancement of pain *tolerance* may be the best we can achieve. Strategies for the enhancement of well-being therefore may be viewed as a facet of pain management. This area, however, has not as yet been set in a research framework.

New vehicles for service delivery

There is now a much wider range of methods by which the pain patient can become informed about his/her condition, and there seems to be an increasing appetite among the general public for information about all sorts of pain conditions. Distance-learning courses have for several decades been an important facet of higher education, and are likely to continue to be so, but most pain patients want much more direct and personally relevant information about their condition. Popular magazines, of course, have been around for decades, and frequently contain articles and comment on aspects of pain, but patients now have in addition the world-wide web.

World-wide web

With the increasing sophistication in information technology, and marketplace competition, it has become clear that speed of access to information is an important parameter. Ease of access also is continually improving, so that information can be downloaded onto highly portable devices such as mobile phones while people are on the move. Typing simple terms such as 'pain' into web-based search engines yields a vast number of websites ranging from simple and sensible educational material to potentially harmful, bizarre and illegal sources of information. There is a multitude of chat-rooms and blogs within which surfers can compare their experiences of pain, its impact and its treatment. Unfortunately such material is unregulated and not therefore subject to quality control. This problem has been addressed to an extent by the provision of evidence-based guidelines and media campaigns developed on the basis of professional consensus. Competent and helpful advice has also been developed by patient-led organisations, which have the additional advantage of offering a degree of psychological support by those who have become burdened by their pain. Self-management has always been a core component of modern pain management. Researchers are now beginning to explore the use of the web as a vehicle for service delivery. Unfortunately by its very nature this is an exceedingly difficult area to research, but there would certainly appear to be opportunities to explore this approach for the increasing group of patients who are comfortable with, and experienced in, use of the web.

Multiskilled professionals

In the first section of this chapter, we attempted to portray the way in which our increased understanding of the nature of pain has led to a much wider range of possibilities for pain management. This clearly has implications in terms of required skills and competencies needed by health-care and occupational professionals. It is frequently observed that basic professional training seldom is sufficient to equip individuals to deliver pain management. It is assumed that each profession has ownership of a set of core professional skills, required in terms of their accreditation, and offering protection to the general public in terms of legally sanctioned practice. Pain management, however, is a relatively new discipline, and indeed within some health-care jurisdictions, is not yet accepted as a discipline in its own right. There are of course commonalities, in terms of required competencies, such as assessment skills, communication skills and provision of simple advice and reassurance, across professional groups, but many pain professionals have expressed the view that the importance of these common skills may not have been recognised specifically as part of their training. (Some of the difficulties in incorporating these common principles into clinical management in primary care were illustrated in Ch. 9.)

The history of medicine has been characterised by increasing specialisation, and although it is tempting to suggest that an obvious solution to the underemphasis of general skills, in contrast to core professional skills, is the establishment of a new type of health-care professional, such a suggestion is probably unrealistic and not particularly helpful. A preferred solution would be to develop a broadening of perspective to incorporate illness and not just disease, thus moving towards a genuine biopsychosocial framework within which each profession's core professional skills can be located. There has been a move towards more 'patient-centred' training amongst professional groups. In terms of pain management, this is a shift which is to be welcomed, with the proviso that we must retain the important 'bio' part of the biopsychosocial framework and avoid the danger of 'over-psychologising' pain.

Case management

In insurance-funded jurisdictions, such as the workmen's compensation boards in Canada, health maintenance organisations (HMOs) in the USA, and private health care in the UK, the funding of elements of health care have always required authorisation prior to health-care spending and provision. For many specific, acute health-care problems the system, if bureaucratic, seems to work reasonably well. Cover for chronic, and less clearly defined health conditions has always been much more problematic. Multidisciplinary treatment programmes represent a still greater challenge in terms of funding. Concern about costs has led to increasing requirement for the specification of elements of treatment packages and parts of the body being treated. Thus there may be cover for a range of ICD-10-defined physical or psychiatric conditions, and for pain modality treatments, but not for the type of patient-centred approach to pain management we have been advocating. Unfortunately if the costs of rehabilitation and secondary prevention cannot be sanctioned, society will end up with an increasing burden of preventable ill-health, increasing work disability and higher social support and benefit costs. Clearly it is for each society to take a view on the obligations and entitlements it requires of, or offers to its citizens, but it could plausibly be argued that in the scenario outlined, there are actually no winners, and the burden of pain has simply been shifted, rather than removed.

In earlier chapters we have highlighted the disjunction between clinical and occupational management, and it would certainly seem that at this time, particularly in the UK, this is a problem which has not yet been solved. Hanson et al (2006), however, have investigated the costs and benefits of active case management and rehabilitation for musculoskeletal disorders (MSDs). Their stated aim was to collate the evidence on the costs and benefits associated with active case management and rehabilitation programmes for those with MSDs; to identify potential motivators for, and obstacles to, the adoption of these programmes; and from this to develop a model programme based on the evidence and assess its acceptability to stakeholders. They defined case management as a goal-oriented approach to keeping employees at work and facilitating an early return to work. They state that:

> *There is good scientific evidence that case management methods are cost-effective through reducing time off work and lost productivity, and reducing healthcare costs. There is even stronger evidence that best-practice rehabilitation approaches have the very important potential to*

Box 16.1

The key components of successful and cost-effective case management

- Individual worker has their own case manager
- Case manager facilitates safe and sustainable return to work by recognising and addressing personal and occupational obstacles to secure safe and sustainable return to work
- Case manager interfaces with health-care services, but is not also the provider of health care
- Best clinical practice guidelines are available and followed
- Case manager monitors all aspects of treatment – appropriateness, timeliness, adherence, outcome and cost
- Case manager makes treatment funding decisions
- Duration management techniques are available (using normative data on likely absence durations for conditions, the case manager can identify when a case has exceeded a typical absence period, and this triggers a review of the case)
- Case manager liaises directly with employer about return to work
- Case manager negotiates transitional work arrangements
- Early intervention focus.

Box 16.2

Myths commonly held in relation to MSD absence

- The employee must be 100% fit before they return to work
- Concern about a risk of reinjury through work activities
- It's not the employer's problem
- Workers *must* be given light duties on return to work
- A GP sick note means the worker cannot work
- People with pain want to stay off as long as possible
- The employer shouldn't contact people who are off sick.

early, and the organisation staying in touch with the individual during absence.

Clearly a case management approach is relevant potentially to other sorts of sickness absence and work retention, but is offered at this juncture as a type of vehicle which seems to enable the blending of both clinical and occupational perspectives for pain management. As described it is applicable particularly to organisational settings, but it would seem that there are lessons which may be useful also for more clinical settings in recognition of the need for a properly managed process with clear objectives, and careful monitoring based on efficient and effective communication and use of resources.

Research agenda

Given the breadth of modern pain management as outlined above, the challenges clearly are considerable. It has been argued, however, that development of a new focus for pain management represents considerable opportunities, and in the era of evidence-based medicine, research is of paramount importance. While there always has to be a place for research into fundamental pain mechanisms, and outcome of treatment, a major thrust of this textbook has been to make the case for secondary prevention in clinical and occupational settings. It has been argued that a specific focus on modifiable risk factors, in the context of obstacles to recovery may enhance the relevance and effectiveness of pain management.

In the context of clinical pain management, we have still a lot to learn in terms of patient selection, tailoring

significantly reduce the burden of long-term sickness absence due to MSDs (p. vii).

They undertook a literature review, and developed a consultation process with organisations, including a survey, focus group discussions, and a further survey of those of working age with MSDs in terms of obstacles to remaining in or returning to work. In the second phase, they developed and validated a management model. The key components of successful and cost-effective case management they identified are shown in Box 16.1.

The report also identified the characteristics of effective case managers, in which the role of communication was highlighted. The report includes an interesting discussion of both blue and black flags. Having identified a number of commonly held myths in relation to absence with MSDs (Box 16.2), they concluded that the key components of successful programmes have been identified, and include providing early access to appropriate advice, remaining at work or returning of treatment and optimising outcome. There may be a limit to what we can learn from studies of groups of patients. Individual differences in responsiveness of apparently similar patients to similar treatment remain a clinical and research challenge. Vlaeyen & Morley (2005) have advocated the use of more imaginative research designs to investigate treatment in the individual case.

Again, since we are never likely either to prevent or cure all pain, an increased understanding of prognostic factors for prolonged pain and disability needs to become a major focus for research. Participants at the Liberty Mutual Conference on Work Disability in 2005 agreed a set of recommendations for the improvement in prognosis research (Linton et al 2005). They are shown in Table 16.1.

There needs to be an ongoing interactive process between clinical practice and research, such that clinical practice sets the questions, which are then evaluated and refined by research, thereby improving clinical understandings and outcomes, thereby setting further research questions.

Policy/political agenda

Some further reflections on economic influences

This textbook has not primarily been focused on issues of policy and economics, but, as has been stated in Chapter 12, economic factors can have a powerful influence on pain and response to treatment. In the UK, they come into sharp focus in the medicolegal arena in which clinical treatment and rehabilitation can become compromised by the fact of involvement in litigation, and settlement of compensation can be significantly delayed by difficulties in obtaining early effective treatment. The reasons for this state of affairs lie partly in the lack of a no-fault compensation system, but also in the underlying concepts of physical impairment derived from neurorehabilitation, and the Cartesian disjunction between physical and mental disorders. Increasing costs of compensation, delay in case closure, and recognition of the

Table 16.1 Hopkinton recommendations for prognosis research

Issue	Definition
Sampling	Strictly outline inclusion/exclusion criteria
	State enrolment time point clearly
	For many questions, clear, early enrolment is necessary ($<$3 weeks following onset)
	Representative sampling techniques (random selection or consecutive cases)
Design	Prospective, inception cohorts required or RCTs
Prognostic indicators	Strictly define constructs of measure
	Selection should flow from conceptual framework, recognising the multifactorial nature of the problem
	Use standardised, psychometrically sound instruments
Analysis	Multivariable techniques to adjust for all potential confounders
	Avoid overfitting the data (too many covariates for sample size)
	Prospective validation in homogenous cohorts required
Follow-up	Strictly define outcome(s) of interest
	Adequate duration of follow-up (years)
	Strive for $>$80% follow-up rate
	Patterns of attrition should be investigated to determine if they are random or systematic
	Blinded outcome measurement with standardised, psychometrically sound instruments
Conceptual framework	Strictly define the construct of the problem being studied
	Account for the recurrent and multifactorial nature of back pain disability
	Overarching theory requires identifying specific hypothesised relationships between variables
	Broaden the view to include factors outside of the usual professional/discipline boundaries

Linton et al (2005, Table 1, p. 460).

importance of psychosocial factors led the International Underwriting Association of London and the Association of British Insurers to reappraise the litigation process itself and to establish a joint working party on *Psychology, Personal Injury and Rehabilitation*. In their report (IUA 2004), they accepted the role of psychological factors, articulated the limitations of the physical model of injury, and identified the inadequacies of the medical 'stepped care' approach and, in legal/insurance practice, in the ways cases were managed. Inter alia, they considered that 'monitoring and, where necessary, responding to psychological and social factors can produce faster and better recovery' (p. 10), recognised a shortfall in appropriated qualified clinical experts, and stated the need for improvement in the medico-legal assessment of psychological and social risk factors in assessment of prognosis. They concluded:

> The ideal aim would be to create a fully co-ordinated effective, timely and appropriately funded response to any case of personal injury. This would include mechanisms that take proper account of psychological and social factors at each turn (p. 11).

If indeed this aspiration is realised, it may be that the mutually unhelpful interface between clinical management and the litigation process can be dismantled. However, despite the clear advantages of the funding of earlier more appropriate clinical interventions by insurance companies, it is difficult to be optimistic regarding the future of the adversarial 'tort' system of compensation, which will always, to a greater or lesser extent, remain a burden for the chronic pain patient involved in litigation.

Extending the reach of pain management

Health-care systems arguably are designed by the policy makers on the basis of the information available about the general population, on the instructions of politicians at the behest of their constituents. Inevitably, and perhaps appropriately, consideration is given in the first instance to the needs of the majority. It is easy to make assumptions of commonalities in perceptions of symptoms, illness health-care usage and work, and underestimate the needs of minorities. The principles of equity of entitlement and access to health care, social support and work are now enshrined in European legislation. In the development of a generic approach to pain management, it seems that failure to take into account special

circumstances of various sorts has meant that the nature of health-care provision, and of pain management in particular, as it has developed is not of equal help to all pain patients. Specifically, implications of gender, age, disability, special needs and ethnicity all need to be taken into account. Only a brief reflection on each is possible at this juncture.

Gender

There are both sex and gender differences in perception of pain, health-care usage and response to treatment (Ch. 3). While it is to be hoped that at least some of the more blatant gender inequalities have been addressed with legislation, it is necessary where possible to design pain evaluations and interventions to facilitate the maximum degree of self-disclosure and enablement of participation in treatment.

Age

Assessment of pain problems, and in particular of the psychosocial context, is particularly difficult in children and adolescents. There are difficulties not only in factoring in the influence of the development process, but in the nature of the pain management intervention and in the extent to which it is appropriate to focus self-help as a key component of the process. The development of specific expertise with this population in impressive units such as the National Hospital for Rheumatic Diseases in Bath, UK, may serve as a spur to the development of further programmes.

Similarly, the needs of older people have not been taken into account sufficiently in the way health care has developed. There are important issues of comorbidity, access to treatment, and engagement in treatment, all of which need to be considered (Crome et al 2007), and it may be that the potential specifically of a cognitive–behavioural approach to pain management, with involvement of carers has been underestimated (Main et al 2007). In addition to this the research in the area of the management of pain in the elderly remains poor; most research uses a cut-off age of no higher than 70. As the number of older people increases in society and the number of active people in this age group increases, the expectations of this group with regards to health care and the demands on the service are likely to change. At present we believe pain management as a service in most countries is ill-equipped to deal with this.

Disability rights

There are complex issues concerning whether or not it is helpful to consider pain as a form of disability. All people with disabilities are of course entitled to equal access to and provision of treatment, and every effort should be made to accommodate special difficulties in both pain assessment and in pain management. Whether pain per se should be considered a disability in its own right requires careful consideration. If a person is disadvantaged in terms of participation or suffering, perhaps special allowance should be made for this. On the other hand, some pain patients do not wish to be viewed or treated as different from anyone else. Indeed a specific ethos underpinning much of pain management is to try to enable the person to recover as much normal function as possible, thereby attempting to minimise their actual or perceived identity as a pain patient.

Special needs

There are pain patients with specific cognitive problems, both inherited and acquired, which may significantly limit both their clinical evaluation and their participation in treatment. It may simply not be possible to involve them in a group programme or an approach to pain management requiring detailed cognitive appraisal. In such circumstances every effort should be made to identify the behavioural concomitants of pain and pain-associated suffering. Much more research is needed into the development of effective pain management for this population.

Implications for ethnic diversity

Modern pain management has developed particularly in English-speaking countries, or the more affluent European countries which can or choose to afford a high quantity and quality of health-care provision. Pain management programmes in such countries will tend to be developed in the language of that country embracing the philosophical approaches of, mainly, the West. There are differences not only in language but in perceptions of disease and expectations of health care. There is also evidence of poorer health-care access in minority groups (Ch. 4). However, progressively more basic pain assessment tools are now being translated into different languages and it is to be hoped that a broader range of ethnically and culturally tailored pain management programmes will be developed. However, much further research is needed into how to customise such programmes to achieve optimal pain management.

Expert patient groups

The idea of training patients to be expert advisors in the management of common illnesses developed in the

1990s. The aim was to inform the patient about their condition and develop disease-specific as well as general self-management skills (Lorig et al 1999). The programmes are relatively short and are delivered to a predetermined format. The majority of time is spent on general coping and health management skills. This initially demonstrated good effect in studies conducted in the USA. However, the earlier studies were often conducted with people who responded to advertisements to participate and so might be seen as a self-selecting group.

More recent data appears to demonstrate that such programmes have a limited acceptability in the patient population, and extending the programmes into primary care and offering them to a wider range of patients leads to reduced efficacy (Solomon et al 2000, Buszewicz et al 2006). Systematic reviews presented evidence that the programmes are more effective where patients have a 'specific' disease (e.g. asthma and diabetes) than on those who have more generalised or non-specific disease (e.g. osteoarthritis) or pain (Warsi et al 2004). Health-care funders obviously have an interest in these programmes as they are normally led by informed volunteers at a low cost. In the UK, the Government is committed to the development of these programmes and has recently formed a not-for-profit company to provide these services more widely. It is not clear where these programmes fit with reference to the interventions described in this book. They are certainly not a substitute for pain management programmes for patients with a high degree of psychological distress. However, it is likely that this initiative will expand, in the UK at least. Further research is required to identify the characteristics of the patients who benefit from such programmes and how pain management and expert patient programmes can cooperate to best effect.

Recommendations: where now for pain management?

It is difficult in a textbook of this length and breadth to draw it to a close, but considered overall, there seems to be a number of recommendations and shifts in emphasis from the first edition.

Firstly, we have suggested a significant broadening in approach for pain management. In attempting to blend the worlds of pain management and work disability, we might be accused by some of 'carpet-bagging' or overextending the proper reach of pain management; this has not been our intention. We do not see management as being owned exclusively by clinical pain specialists.

Secondly, in recommending a broadening of focus from traditional targets of pain management to the identification of modifiable risk factors as potential targets for intervention, we unashamedly have tried to move pain management upstream. We have suggested that it needs to extend beyond specialist pain clinics to secondary clinics/primary care, and across to occupational settings. In advocating such developments, we are mindful of the need for sensitivity to context, and of applications that reflect this.

Thirdly, in advocating the flag terminology, at least for now, and in requesting a specific focus on obstacles to recovery, we have attempted not only to differentiate between clinical and occupational factors, but we have placed a huge and acknowledged emphasis on the patient or worker's perception of his/her pain and its effects. As such, we are open to the charge of over-emphasising psychosocial factors, but as things stand, on the current evidence base, we believe that our view is justified. Nonetheless we have also identified the need for system-based solutions.

Fourthly, in recommending a systems approach and distinguishing between worker-centred and workplace- or system-centred interventions, we have tried to find a way of turning obstacles to recovery into possibilities for intervention. While we believe it is helpful to an extent in considering the needs of the individual, to distinguish individual-centred and system-centred interventions, to make a significant impact on pain-associated limitations, a combined approach involving interorganisational working (Loisel et al 2005) may be required.

Challenges

There remain many challenges for pain management. Many of these have already been discussed, but we should like to conclude with three specific observations.

Firstly, we believe that the importance of the appropriate use of language in communicating about pain has been significantly underestimated, in clinical settings (both with patients and between colleagues), within the workplace, between clinical and occupational agencies, and in the media. We are hampered by Cartesian terminology and the 'mind–body' split. We still tend to view chronic pain with inherent suspicion and mistrust the chronic pain patient. In our view incompetent, insensitive and even malicious use of language underpin much of the iatrogenic confusion and distress which can develop in patients/workers with chronic pain. We believe specific research in this field might prove illuminating.

Secondly, we believe we should embark on a redefinition of professional roles and responsibilities in the field of pain management. Much of our education and training, as currently delivered, does not seem to be based sufficiently on a biopsychosocial framework, and in our view it is time for reconsideration of the professional expertise we require to deliver modern pain management.

Thirdly, we view the development of pain management as an evolutionary and ongoing process which needs to be able to adapt to new developments in knowledge and understanding. Although we have advocated a significant enlarging of the traditional canvas for pain management, we still believe it should rest on foundations of concerted effort on the part of health-care and occupational professionals to deliver the best possible help for pain sufferers. For most pain sufferers, however, optimal pain management cannot be achieved without active engagement on their part in the process. While some of pain management is, and should be, set in the context of delivery of an optimal degree of pain relief, we believe that in many circumstances, particularly in the context of secondary prevention, a more appropriate role for the health-care or occupational professional is as a coach, attempting to maximise the patient/worker's capacity for self-help, both in maximising function, but also in enhancing well-being.

Postscript: some thanks and an apology

We should like to conclude by acknowledging the considerable debt to our many professional colleagues and the wide community of researchers whose ideas have inspired us to produce this new edition. We have unashamedly relied upon a wide range of scientific articles and reports in order to shape our view of the status and practice of modern pain management. In this process we will undoubtedly have underrepresented or misrepresented the views of some of our colleagues. We have not done so intentionally, and apologise unreservedly for occasions where we have done so. Our biases and prejudices we are sure are clearly evident and we have to take responsibility for them. We hope nonetheless that the textbook will be of some help not only to those interested in finding out what pain management is about, and where it came from, but also to those finding themselves in a position to help those struggling with pain. If this book has made a small contribution to that endeavour, it will have been worthwhile.

References

Burton W N, Conti D J, Chen C Y et al 1999 The role of health risk factors and disease on worker productivity. Journal of Occupational and Environmental Medicine 41:863–877

Buszewicz M, Rait G, Griffin M et al 2006 Self management of arthritis in primary care: randomised controlled trial. British Medical Journal 333:879

Chapman C R, Nakamura Y, Flores L Y 1999 Chronic pain and consciousness: a constructivist perspective. In: Gatchel R J, Turk D C (eds) Psychosocial perspectives in pain. The Guilford Press, New York, ch 3, pp 35–55

Crome P, Main C J, Lally F (eds) 2007 Pain in older people. Oxford, Oxford University Press

Crook J, Moldovsky H 1994 The probability of recovery and return to work from work disability as a function of time. Quality of Life Research 3:Suppl 1

Dunn K M, Croft P R, Main C J et al 2007 A prognostic approach to defining chronic pain: replication in a UK primary care low back pain population. Accepted for publication in *Spine*.

Fordyce W E 1976 Behavioral methods for chronic pain and illness. C V Mosby, St Louis, MS

Fordyce W E (ed) 1995 Back pain in the workplace. IASP Press, Seattle

Hanson M A, Burton A K, Kendall N A S et al 2006 The costs and benefits of active case management and rehabilitation for musculoskeletal disorders. HSE Research Report 493. Sudbury, HSE Books

Hansson M, Bostrom C, Harms-Ringdahl K 2006 Sickness absence and sickness attendance: what people with neck or back pain think. Social Science and Medicine 62:2183–2195

HM Government 2005 Health, work and well-being – caring for our future. Dept for Work and Pensions, London (www.dwp.gov.uk/publications/dwp/2005/health_and_ wellbing.pdf)

IUA 2004 Psychology, personal injury and rehabilitation: Report of the IUA/ABI Working Party. International Underwriting Association of London, London

Kendall N A S, Linton S J, Main C J 1997 Guide to assessing psychosocial yellow flags in acute low back pain: risk factors for long term disability and work loss. Accident Rehabilitation and Compensation Insurance Corporation of New Zealand and the National Health Committee, Wellington NZ

Linton S J, van Tulder M W 2000 Preventative interventions for back pain and neck pain. In: Nachemson A, Jonsson E (eds) Neck pain and back pain: the scientific evidence of causes, diagnoses and treatment. Lippincott, Williams and Wilkins, Philadelphia, ch 6, pp 127–147

Linton S J, Bradley L A, Jensen I et al 1989 The secondary prevention of low back pain: a controlled study with follow-up. Pain 36:197–207

Linton S J, Gross D, Schultz I Z et al W 2005 Prognosis and the identification of workers risking disability: research issues and directions for future research. Journal of Occupational Rehabilitation 15:457–474

Loisel P, Durand M-J, Baril R et al 2005 Interorganisational collaboration in occupational rehabilitation: perceptions of an interdisciplinary rehabilitation team. Journal of Occupational Rehabilitation 15:581–590

Lorig K, Sobel D S, Stewart A L et al 1999 Evidence suggesting that a chronic disease self-management program can improve health status while reducing hospitalization. A randomized trial. Medical Care 37:5–14

McCracken L M, Eccleston C 2003 Coping or acceptance: what to do about chronic pain? Pain 105:197–204

McCracken L M, Carson J W, Eccleston C et al 2004 Acceptance and change in the context of chronic change. Pain 107:4–7

Main C J, Burton A K 2000 Economic and occupational influences on pain and disability. In: Main C J, Spanswick C C (eds) Pain management: an interdisciplinary approach. Churchill Livingstone, Edinburgh, ch 4, pp 63–87

Main C J, Glozier N, Wright I A 2005 Validation of the HSE stress tool: an investigation within four organisations by the Corporate Health and Performance Group (CHAP). Occupational Medicine 55:208–214

Main C J, Waters S J, Keefe F J 2007 Cognitive behaviour therapy. In: Crome P, Main C J, Lally F (eds) Pain in older people. Oxford, Oxford University Press, pp 109–119

Melzack R 1999 Pain and stress: a new perspective. In: Gatchel R J, Turk D C (eds) Psychosocial perspectives in pain. The Guilford Press, New York, ch 6, pp 89–106

Morley S, Vlaeyen S W J 2005 Epilogue to special series. Clinical Journal of Pain 21:69–72

Morley S, Davies C, Barton S 2005 Possible selves in chronic pain: self-pain enmeshment, adjustment and acceptance. Pain 115:84–94

Pincus T, Morley S 2001 Cognitive processing bias in chronic pain: a review and integration. Psychology Bulletin 127:599–617

Solomon D, Warsi A, Brown-Stevenson T et al 2000 Does self-management education benefit all populations with arthritis? A randomised controlled trial in a primary care physician network. Journal of Rheumatology 29(2):362–368

Sullivan M J L 2007 Toward a biopsychomotor conceptualisation of pain. Clinical Journal of Pain (in press)

Sullivan M J, Feuerstein M, Gatchel R et al 2005 Integrating psychosocial and behavioral interventions to achieve optimal rehabilitation outcomes. Journal of Occupational Rehabilitation 15:475–489

Turk D C, Meichenbaum D H, Genest M 1983 Pain and behavioral medicine: a cognitive-behavioral perspective. Guilford Press, New York

Vlaeyen J W, Linton S J 2000 Fear-avoidance and its consequences in chronic musculoskeletal pain: a state of the art. Pain 85:317–332

Vlaeyen J W, Morley S 2005 Cognitive-behavioural treatments for chronic pain. What works for whom? Clinical Journal of Pain 21:1–8

Vlaeyen J, Kole-Snijders A M J, Boeren R G B et al 1995 Fear of movement/(re)injury in chronic low back pain and its relation to behavioral performance. Pain 62:363–372

Von Korff M, Miglioretti D L 2006 A prospective approach to defining chronic pain. In: Flor H, Kalso E, Dostrovsky J O (eds) Proceedings of the 11th World Congress on Pain. IASP Press, Seattle, ch 66, pp 761–769

Waddell G, Burton A K 2006 Is work good for your health and well-being? London, TSO

Waddell G, Burton A K, Main C J 2003 Screening of DWP clients for risk of long-term incapacity: a conceptual and scientific review. Royal Society of Medicine Monograph. Royal Society of Medicine Press, London

Wall P D 1999 Pain: the science of suffering. Weidenfield and Nicholson, London

Warsi A, Wang P, LaValley M et al 2004 Self-management education programs in chronic disease: a systematic review and methodological critique of the literature. Archives of Internal Medicine 164:1641–1649

Williams A C de C 2002 Facial expression of pain: an evolutionary account. Behavioral and Brain Sciences 25:439–455

Woolf C, Salter M W 2000 Neuronal plasticity: increasing the gain in pain. Science 288:1765–1768

Index